Iron Metabolism in Health and Disease

Edited by

Jeremy H. Brock PhD
University Department of Immunology, Western Infirmary, Glasgow, Scotland

June W. Halliday AM, BSc, PhD
Chairperson, Liver Unit, Queensland Institute of Medical Research, The Bancroft Center, Brisbane, Australia and Professor, Department of Medicine, University of Queensland

Martin J. Pippard BSc, MB, ChB, MRCPath, FRCP
Professor of Haematology, Ninewells Hospital & Medical School, University of Dundee, Dundee, Scotland

Lawrie W. Powell AC, MD, PhD, FRCP(Lond), FRACP
Professor of Medicine, The University of Queensland, and Director, Queensland Institute of Medical Research, The Bancroft Center, Brisbane, Australia

W.B. Saunders Company Ltd
London Philadelphia Toronto Sydney Tokyo

This book is printed on acid-free paper

W. B. Saunders   24–28 Oval Road
Company Ltd   London, NW1 7DX

                     The Curtis Center
                     Independence Square West
                     Philadelphia, PA 19106-3399, USA

                     55 Horner Avenue
                     Toronto, Ontario, M8Z 4X6, Canada

                     Harcourt Brace & Company (Australia) Pty Ltd
                     30–52 Smidmore Street
                     Marrickville
                     NSW 2204, Australia

                     Harcourt Brace Japan Inc.
                     Ichibancho Central Building, 22-1 Ichibancho
                     Chiyoda-ku, Tokyo 102, Japan

©1994 W. B. Saunders Company Ltd

A CIP record for this book is available from the British Library

ISBN 0-7020-1732-9

Typeset by Dobbie Typesetting Limited, Tavistock, Devon
Printed in Great Britain by Hartnolls Limited, Bodmin, Cornwall

Contents

Foreword

Meetings on clinical aspects of iron metabolism were held in Aix-en-Provence in 1963 and in Arosa in 1969. However, the first conference at which fundamental aspects were addressed was organized by Philip Aisen, Pauline Harrison and Ernest Huehns and was held in London in the summer of 1973. Its title, *The First International Conference on the Proteins of Iron Storage and Transport*, indicated its special focus but at subsequent meetings the interests have widened and the conferences have provided workers from differing scientific backgrounds with unique opportunities to exchange ideas and broaden their personal perspectives. The international character of the 11 conferences that have thus far been held is reflected by the venues – the United Kingdom (twice), the United States (twice), Canada, Belgium, France, Israel, Switzerland, Japan and Australia.

It is against this background that the current book must be seen. Virtually all the contributors have been actively involved in the regular conferences on iron and have thus had the opportunity to see their own work in a much wider context. The resultant sense of 'holism' is a major feature of *Iron Metabolism in Health and Disease*. The reader gets the feeling that the authors of each of the chapters have prepared them with a sense of how they will relate to what comes before and after. As a result, there is a strong thread of continuity throughout, with no sharp divide between basic aspects and the more applied. The overall cohesion of this multi-authored book is further reinforced by careful editing and by extensive cross-referencing. The second impression is an equally vivid one. Each of the chapters is written by experts who have contributed significantly to the fields about which they are writing. The result is a book which is not only 'state of the art' but which is also stamped with authority.

The stage is set by a chapter which shows that the proteins of iron metabolism are joined to each other genetically, structurally and functionally by strong evolutionary ties. The introduction is followed by a detailed consideration of the major pathway of internal iron exchange, the red cell cycle. This leads on to a consideration of the role of transferrin and its receptor in the transport and cellular uptake of iron, and of the role of ferritin as a storage protein. Particularly exciting are new insights relating to homeostatic control of the proteins involved in cellular iron metabolism. In this novel mechanism a common *cis*-acting RNA element (IRE) and a common *trans*-acting protein (IRE-BP) modulate at least two genes. Iron deprivation reduces translation of the mRNA encoding ferritin and at the same time protects the mRNA encoding the transferrin receptor from degradation. This coordinated mechanism seems to be fundamental to cellular iron homeostasis.

The first chapters set the stage for the more clinically orientated ones that follow. Various aspects of haem and non-haem iron absorption are reviewed, with special emphasis on the effects of dietary composition on iron nutrition. The two major disorders of iron balance, iron deficiency and iron overload, are then considered.

Quantitative aspects of iron deficiency have now been defined with some precision and screening measures are being progressively refined. In this latter context, the level of the serum transferrin receptor appears particularly promising as a measure of tissue iron deficiency. Of great potential importance, too, is a growing body of evidence that iron deficiency causes nervous system dysfunction in young children. Primary and secondary iron overload are extensively reviewed. HLA-linked haemochromatosis is the focus of particular interest, since elucidation of the genetic defect promises to provide wider insights into normal iron transport mechanisms. While tantalizingly close, the 'holy grail' remains elusive. The pathological sequelae of parenchymal iron overload have been the subject of intensive investigation and the mechanisms involved in iron toxicity, including lipid peroxidation and free radical-mediated injury, are described in a separate chapter. This is followed by a review of the role of iron in infection, immunity, inflammation and neoplasia. Although the pathophysiology of these relationships has been investigated in a variety of experimental settings it is still not clear as to whether changes in iron status actually predispose to infections, inflammatory or neoplastic disease. While desferrioxamine has been used for over 30 years in the therapy of the iron overload complicating thalassaemic syndromes, the search for new chelators continues to excite major interest. The topic of chelation is reviewed not only in the context of iron overload but in relation to the prevention of hydroxyl radical formation in a variety of clinical settings, including port-ischaemic reperfusion injury, organ transplantation and drug toxicity. Exciting evidence that chelators may have a role in inhibiting tumour growth and the growth of malarial parasites is also reviewed. The book concludes with a chapter documenting the changes that occur in measurements of iron status at different ages in the two sexes and with a critical review of the individual measurements and their clinical interpretation.

To have synthesized the wealth of information on iron metabolism that has accumulated in the last few years into a coherent whole is a signal achievement, especially when it is presented in such a logical and readable manner. Equally important is the clear definition of gaps in our current understanding. Many of these will, I am sure, be filled by the time the second edition appears.

T. H. Bothwell

Preface

The exponential growth in knowledge of human iron metabolism over the past decade has been breath-taking. This has resulted in large part from the unprecedented advances in molecular and cell biology and particularly recombinant DNA technology which are now beginning to reveal the mysteries of cellular metabolism, its genetic regulation and the aberrations which result in human disease. At the same time, the importance of iron metabolism has been extended beyond the traditional areas of erythropoiesis and nutrition, so that it is now recognized as a key element in fields such as oncology, pathology and infectious disease.

To collate this staggering accumulation of information has proved a somewhat daunting prospect which the present editors have accepted in the belief that, given the time that has elapsed since the classic works of Bothwell and colleagues (1979) and Jacobs and Worwood (1980), there is a pressing need for a comprehensive review of the present state of knowledge of mammalian iron metabolism. While this has been no easy task, it has been a stimulating one which has been aided enormously by the excellent response of the contributors, all of whom are actively involved in basic or clinical research into human iron metabolism.

Our aim has been to review the many recent advances in knowledge of normal and aberrant human iron metabolism and particularly to attempt to satisfy the needs of basic scientists on the one hand and practising clinicians on the other. Thus we hope that these chapters will provide a useful update and reference source for those at the laboratory bench as well as those in the clinic.

We are indebted to Dr Susan King especially for helping to initiate the project, Mr Sean Duggan and his colleagues at W. B. Saunders for their patience and enthusiasm and for their assistance in expediting the final product once the manuscripts were to hand.

J. H. Brock
J. W. Halliday
M. J. Pippard
L. W. Powell

Contributors

Professor **Philip Aisen** MD
Professor of Physiology and
  Biophysics and Professor of Medicine
Albert Einstein College of Medicine,
Bronx, NY 10461, USA

Professor **Bruce R. Bacon** MD
Professor of Internal Medicine and
  Director, Division of Gastro-
  enterology and Hepatology
St Louis University Medical Center
St Louis, MO 63110, USA

Dr **Erica Baker** BSc(Hons), PhD
Senior Research Fellow of the
  National Health and Medical
  Research Council
Department of Physiology
The University of Western Australia
Nedlands
Perth WA 6009
Australia

Professor **Roy D. Baynes** MB, BCh,
  FCP, MMed, PhD, FACP
Professor of Medicine
Department of Medicine
Division of Hematology
The University of Kansas Medical
  Center
3901 Rainbow Boulevard
Kansas City, Kansas 66160, USA

Professor **Gary M. Brittenham** MD
Professor of Medicine
Case Western Reserve University
  School of Medicine
Metro Health Medical Center
2500 Metro Health Drive, R369
Cleveland, OH 44109-1998, USA

Dr **Robert S. Britton** PhD
Department of Internal Medicine
Division of Gastroenterology and
  Hepatology
St Louis University Medical Center
3635 Vista Avenue
St Louis, MO 63110, USA

Dr **Jeremy H. Brock** PhD
University Department of Immunology
Western Infirmary
Glasgow G11 6NT, Scotland, UK

Professor **June W. Halliday** AM, BSc,
  PhD
Chairperson – Liver Unit
Queensland Institute of Medical Research
The Bancroft Center
PO Royal Brisbane Hospital
Brisbane 4029 QLD, Australia
and Professor, Department of Medicine
University of Queensland
Brisbane, Australia

Dr **J. Harford** PhD
Director of Biochemistry and Cell Biology
RiboGene, Inc.
21375 Cabot Boulevard
Hayward
CA 94545, USA

Professor **Chaim Hershko** MD
Professor and Head
Department of Medicine
Shaare Zedek Medical Center and
Department of Human Nutrition and
  Metabolism
Hebrew University Hadassah Medical
  School
PO Box 3235, Jerusalem 91031, Israel

Dr Elizabeth Jazwinska PhD
Queensland Institute of Medical
   Research
Liver Unit
The Bancroft Center
300 Herson Road
Brisbane 4029 QLD
Australia

Dr Richard D. Klausner MD
Cell Biology and Metabolism Branch
National Institute of Child Health
   and Development
National Institutes of Health
Bethesda
MD 20892
USA

Professor Evan H. Morgan PhD, DSc
Department of Physiology
The University of Western Australia
Nedlands
Perth WA 6009
Australia

Professor Martin J. Pippard BSc,
   MB, ChB, FRCP, MRCPath
Professor of Haematology and Honorary
   Consultant Haematologist
Ninewells Hospital and Medical School
University of Dundee
Dundee DD1 9SY
Scotland
UK

Professor Lawrie W. Powell AC,
   MD, FRCP(Lond), FRACP
Professor of Medicine
The University of Queensland and
   Director
Queensland Institute of Medical
   Research
The Bancroft Center
300 Herson Road
Brisbane 4029 QLD
Australia

Dr G. A. Ramm BSc(Hons), PhD
Department of Internal Medicine
Division of Gastroenterology and
   Hepatology
St Louis University Medical Center
PO Box 15250, St Louis,
MO 63110-0250, USA

Dr Tracey B. Rouault MD
Head, Unit on Iron Metabolism
Cell Biology and Metabolism Branch
National Institute of Child Health and
   Development
National Institutes of Health
Bethesda, MD 20892, USA

Professor Barry Skikne MBBCH,
   FCP, FACP
Professor of Medicine
Department of Medicine
Division of Haematology
University of Kansas Medical Center
3901 Rainbow Boulevard, Kansas City
KS 66160, USA

Professor Anthony S. Tavill MD,
   FRCP
Professor of Internal Medicine
Case Western Reserve University and
   Director
The Maurice and Sadie Friedman Center
   for Digestive and Liver Disorders
Mount Sinai Medical Center
One Mount Sinai Drive
Cleveland, Ohio 44106, USA

Dr Mark Worwood BSc, PhD, FRCPath
Reader in Haematology
University of Wales College of Medicine
Heath Park, Cardiff CF4 4XN, UK

Dr Ray Yip MD, MPH
Chief, Maternal and Child Nutrition
   Section
Division of Nutrition
Department of Health and Human
   Services
Centers for Disease Control
Atlanta, GA 30333, USA

1. Iron Metabolism: An Evolutionary Perspective

P. AISEN

Departments of Physiology and Biophysics, and Medicine, Albert Einstein College of Medicine, 1300 Morris Park Avenue, Bronx, New York 10461, USA

'Signatures of all things I am here to read.'
S. Dedalus

1. INTRODUCTION: THE USES OF IRON IN BIOLOGY

The versatility of uses Nature has found for iron originates in the simple aqueous chemistry of this essential transition metal. Of the diverse chemical reactions of iron in solution the most important is the facile and reversible one-electron oxidation–reduction reaction that takes iron between its two common oxidation states, the ferrous and the ferric. This is the reaction exploited by most iron-dependent enzymes involved in electron transport or oxygen carriage, and responsible for the threat to

Table 1.1 Major events in the evolution of iron metabolism

Event	Date
The Big Bang: Time begins	15–18 billion years ago
Formation of the earth and solar system	4.5–5 billion years ago
Prokaryotic life begins	3.5 billion years ago
Photosynthesis by cyanobacteria: bacterioferritin	3 billion years ago
Oxygen-rich atmosphere: aerobic iron metabolism	2 billion years ago
Appearance of eukaryotic cells	850 million years ago
Multicellular organisms: ancestral transferrin gene	650 million years ago
Eukaryotic ferritins	
Transferrin gene duplication and fusion: appearance of two-sited transferrin	350–500 million years ago
Speciation of transferrins: ovotransferrin	180 million years ago
Speciation of transferrins: lactoferrin and serum transferrin	5 million years ago

life posed by excess iron in acute and chronic iron overload. Recent studies suggest that this reaction may underlie the origin of life as well. Major events in the evolution of iron metabolism are summarized in Table 1.1.

1.1. Iron in the Prebiotic Earth

Some 4.5 billion years ago, when the earth had just condensed and cooled to a globe approximating the one we know today, the atmosphere was free of molecular dioxygen in substantial concentration. It was more likely neutral, consisting largely of nitrogen and carbon dioxide, or perhaps slightly reducing due to the presence of small amounts of hydrogen (Cairns-Smith, 1978). Iron, the fourth most abundant element of the earth's crust and the second most prevalent metal (aluminium is the first), probably existed in the ferrous state at a concentration in sea water estimated to be 10^{-4} M (Mauzerall, 1992). The problem faced by life in its early struggles was how to convert carbon dioxide to organic form and nitrogen to ammonia. An intriguing and plausible suggestion is that iron assumed a dominant role in this process (Borowska and Mauzerall, 1988).

Using UV radiant energy to drive the reaction, slightly alkaline solutions of ferrous iron can evolve molecular hydrogen (Schrauzer and Guth, 1976), apparently by transfer of electrons from Fe(II) to water of hydration in a pH dependent fashion, yielding Fe(III) and H_2 (Borowska and Mauzerall, 1988). Similar photoreduction of water (or, equivalently, photo-oxidation of aquated ferrous ion) has been proposed to account for the formation of ferric hydroxide in geological 'banded iron formations', principal repositories of the world's iron (Cairns-Smith, 1978). Thus, ferrous iron may have been a rich source of electrons for geological formations as well as for atmospheric and aqueous reactions. The question then arises whether inorganic (or preorganic) Fe(II) can also use radiant energy to reduce carbon dioxide of the primitive atmosphere.

Photochemically-driven reduction of nitrogen, using ferrous iron in sea water as a catalyst in a crude mimicking of nitrogenase, may have provided ammonia for the molecules of life (Mauzerall, 1992). Early exploratory studies suggested that solar UV light can promote the reduction of carbon dioxide in aqueous solution to formaldehyde, formate, methane and methanol in the presence of suitable transition metal ion catalysts, most importantly ferrous iron (Borowska and Mauzerall, 1988). These species can then serve as precursors for the synthesis of sugars, amino acids and nucleic acids. Although the efficiency of the iron(II)-catalysed reaction has recently been called into question (Mauzerall, 1991), a role for iron in the photochemical generation of hydrogen which could then contribute to formation of reduced carbon compounds by lightning still seems possible. The chemistry underlying the beginnings of life is very much in dispute – after all, the necessary experiments are difficult to reproduce, and appropriate controls have never been performed. Nevertheless, the possibility that iron was involved in the initiation of life remains intriguing and appealing, particularly since life, once established, inescapably depends upon iron (Neilands, 1972).

1.2. Iron and Early Life

No other element exhibits the adaptability of iron in the electron transport reactions central to life. The redox potentials of iron in its biological complexes range from -750 mV in enterochelin, the iron transporter (siderophore) of *E. coli* (Cooper *et al.*, 1978), to $+350$ mV for the high potential iron sulfur protein of *Chromatia* (Dus *et al.*, 1967), to $+770$ mV for simple aquated iron ions. Thus, iron can function as the strongest of reducing agents or the most powerful of oxidants in a biological milieu. Since the exploitation of chemical free energy by living systems usually depends on redox reactions, the versatility of iron complexes finds application in energy transduction and biosynthesis in organisms at all levels of sophistication. The redox responsiveness of iron also underlies its role in switching metabolic pathways of facultative anaerobes like *E. coli* when they experience a change in atmosphere (Spiro and Guest, 1991). Iron serves as a redox sensor in the regulatory pathways of enzymes expressed in response to alterations in ambient oxygen tension. In like fashion, iron functions in higher organisms as a redox sensor governing the activity of the purple acid phosphatases with binuclear iron centres (Doi *et al.*, 1988). Even as the simple aquated ion, iron can carry out reactions for which specialized enzymes have evolved, although at greatly reduced rates compared with those provided by such enzymes. For example, catalase and peroxidase activity has been observed with inorganic iron, while the reactions of Fe(II) with oxygen are primitive models of cytochrome oxidase function (Granick, 1953; Cotton and Wilkinson, 1988). Photoreduction of nitrogen in the presence of Fe(II) has also been observed (Schrauzer and Guth, 1976), a reaction anticipatory of nitrogenase without which the evolution of life would have come to a stop. A reasonable sequence for the evolution of iron-dependent enzymes has been proposed (Kamaluddin *et al.*, 1986). Initial dependence on free Fe(II) to catalyse simple reactions borrowed from the prebiotic globe is followed by use of Fe(II)-cyanide complexes for more sophisticated chemistry. Mixed-ligand cyanide–amino acid complexes of Fe(II) then evolve to macro-molecular complexes of iron, and the enzymes we know today. Even template-directed polynucleotide synthesis may have begun on the surfaces of ferric hydroxide gels (Schwartz and Orgel, 1985). It is easy to see why Nature has turned to iron to catalyse or regulate reactions without which life, in the simplest or most complex organisms, cannot proceed.

Once having bounded themselves from the non-living world by lipid membranes, ancient cells faced the new problem of guarding themselves from iron overload in an oxygen-free milieu where ferrous iron abounded. Studies with cells from contemporary higher organisms show that Fe(II) by itself penetrates cell membranes to enter cellular metabolic and synthetic pathways (Egyed, 1988; Morgan, 1988). In part the problem of avoiding iron excess must have been mitigated by a high concentration of H_2S in the primitive pools where life is thought to have started. The solubility product of ferrous sulfide is about $10^{-18} M^2$ (Smith and Martell, 1976), so that the solubility of Fe(II) in neutral aqueous solution saturated with H_2S is only $10^{-13} M$ (Smith and Emery, 1982). Thus, sulfide may have served the same protective function and posed the same problems for the iron-dependent protocell as hydroxyl ion does for the cells we know today.

Reactions of Fe(II) could also have provided metabolic energy for the earliest life on earth. The dependence today of *Thiobacillus ferrooxidans* on the energy provided by oxidation of ferrous iron for its metabolic needs may have originated in pathways developed by much more ancient organisms (Lane *et al.*, 1992). Abundance of FeS in muds and soils of the prebiotic era is compatible with another reaction that might be sunlight-driven to yield metabolic energy (Williams, 1990):

$$H_2O + 2FeS + CO \rightarrow 2FeO + \rangle CHOH + 2S.$$

Although, as indicated above, the efficiency of such reactions is uncertain, the possibility persists that primitive cells may have captured and exploited colloidal iron sulfides for biological catalysis. Williams (1990) offers the provocative suggestion that the surfaces of mineralized iron sulfides could have catalysed reactions like those now seen in proteins with iron-sulfur clusters – the dehydrogenases and dehydratases, for examples. No great imagination is required for the conceptual leap from catalysis by inorganic ferrous sulfide to catalysis by iron-sulfur enzymes, species long antedating the coming of dioxygen to biology. The universe of bio-inorganic chemistry borrowed much from the simpler world of inorganic chemistry.

Because life on earth began in an anaerobic milieu, insights into the regulation of iron metabolism by the earliest life forms, including the presumptive 'universal ancestor' of life (Woese *et al.*, 1990), might be gleaned from inquiries into iron transport and storage in anaerobic bacteria. Remarkably little attention has been directed at these intriguing problems, however. Anaerobic cultures of *E. coli*, often assumed to satisfy their requirements for iron by uptake of ferrous iron, are competent to sequester iron from siderophores such as enterobactin and ferrichrome, despite the specificity of these agents for ferric iron (Lodge and Emery, 1984). The anaerobic uptake of iron borne by siderophores appears to involve the same energy-dependent mechanisms operating under the same genetic regulation as iron uptake by aerobic cultures. Whether obligate anaerobes make use of siderophores, specific for either Fe(II) or Fe(III), to harvest iron, or simply depend on the membrane-traversing facility of aquated Fe(II), has not been determined.

The dissimilatory sulfate-reducing organism *Desulfovibrio gigas*, an obligate anaerobe, has a high requirement and correspondingly avid appetite for iron. Although the uptake pathway is not known, an interesting observation has been reported about the fate of iron once it has been acquired by the organism. A highly insoluble black protein, bearing about 6% iron and accounting for 90% of the organism's content of iron, has been isolated from *D. gigas* (Smith and Emery, 1982). This iron-bearing protein is thought to reside in an electron-dense layer between the outer and cytoplasmic membranes of *D. gigas*. Because of its insolubility, detailed molecular characterization of the protein was not possible. In its crude, presumably native, state, the protein resisted loss of iron to dilute acid, to Fe(II) chelators such as bathophenanthroline, ferrozine and dipyridyl, and to the siderophore Ferrichrome A. When solubilized by SDS, however, the protein readily relinquished its iron to dialysis against Tris buffer, pH 7.6. Removal of iron appeared to be reversible, since a black, insoluble preparation, representing about 90% of the solubilized protein, could be recovered by further dialysis against finely powdered ferrous sulfide in 3% β-mercaptoethanol. The solubilized protein showed one major 14 kDa band on SDS-polyacrylamide gel electrophoresis, suggesting a multimeric structure in the native protein. An appealing but highly speculative hypothesis is that the protein is a ferrous analogue of ferritin, with a protein shell surrounding a core of ferrous sulfide.

A protein with the salient characteristics of a true ferritin has recently been isolated from the obligate anaerobe *Bacteroides fragilis* (Rocha *et al.*, 1992). The molecule is composed of 24 subunits, each of molecular mass 16.7 kDa. A 30-residue N-terminal sequence of each subunit shows 43% homology with the corresponding sequence of human H-chains, and somewhat lesser homology with bacterial ferritins. The protein incorporated iron from an inorganic source to a limited extent – only three atoms per molecule – during growth of its host organism; its ultimate capacity for iron storage was not evaluated. Presumably, the anaerobic ferritin functions not only to store iron, but to shield *B. fragilis*, an organism devoid of such protective enzymes as catalase and superoxide dismutase, from noxious iron-catalysed reactions which may ensue with even brief exposure to oxygen.

1.3. Possible Remnants of Anaerobic Ancestry in Contemporary Aerobic Life

1.3.1. *Magnetotactic Bacteria*

Many organisms, from bacteria through honey bees to homing pigeons, make use of the earth's magnetic field in seeking environments most supportive of their particular physiological needs. For most of these organisms, the magnetic sensor is magnetite, a mixed oxide of Fe(II) and Fe(III) with the overall composition Fe_3O_4. Magnetite is best viewed as a composite crystalline structure ('inverse spinel') of FeO and Fe_2O_3. Half of the ferric ions are distributed in an octahedral lattice, with the other half arranged in tetrahedral interstices together with the Fe(II) ions (Cotton and Wilkinson, 1988). The electron spins of Fe(II) and Fe(III) are coupled to each other in opposing (antiferromagnetic) fashion, but because their magnetic moments are unequal residual magnetism persists at ordinary temperatures. Thus, a particle of magnetite will orientate itself in an external field, and so inform its host organism of the field. At sufficiently high temperature, well beyond the physiological range, thermal energy may overcome the antiferromagnetic coupling, and magnetite will lose its magnetism.

In the magnetotactic bacteria, the magnetite exists in lipid-enveloped structures known as magnetosomes (Blakemore and Blakemore, 1991). These structures are ordered in strings within the bacterial cell, an arrangement which enhances their magnetic interaction with the earth's field. The bacteria are ancient organisms, their fossils having been identified in 2-billion-year-old Precambrian rocks (Blakemore and Blakemore, 1991; Vali and Kirschvink, 1991). Related contemporary organisms may be microaerophilic or anaerobic (Bazylinski, 1991), suggesting that the earlier species also required an anaerobic environment.

Membrane-bounded ferrimagnetic structures similar to magnetite, but consisting of mixed sulfides of iron with the overall formula Fe_3S_4 ('greigite'), have recently been identified in a magnetotactic bacterium common in brackish, sulfide-rich water and sediment (Mann et $al.$, 1990). These magnetic particles probably result from reduction of sulfate, possibly using hydrogen as reductant; their host cells (thought but not yet shown to be obligatory anaerobes) may therefore represent the most ancient of magnetotactic organisms. What possible advantage can magnetotaxis be to a bacterium struggling for survival in a hostile environment?

Organisms collected in the magnetic southern hemisphere are south-seeking, while those from the northern hemisphere are north-seeking. In each case, the earth's field is used as a directional indicator, a kind of magnetic plumb-line (Lins de Barros et $al.$, 1990) pointing the bacteria to deeper, oxygen-poor regions of the waters and muds in which they seek survival. Magnetotaxis may therefore have originated in organisms dependent on electron transfer to sulfur for energy transduction. Nothing is known of when these organisms first appeared in geological time, but they are probably ancient species. It has even been suggested that the lipid bilayer of the magnetosome of magnetotactic bacteria represents an evolutionary step toward genesis of true prokaryotic cells (Vali and Kirschvink, 1991). Exploitation of magnetism for direction-finding persists in much more recent and more developed species, such as the homing pigeon and honey bee.

1.4. A Novel Function of Magnetite in Contemporary Organisms

Magnetite is distinguished not only for its magnetic properties, but for its hardness and durability. These latter characteristics are exploited by the chiton, a barnacle-like organism, and the limpet in the fabrication of their teeth or radulae (Webb et $al.$, 1989). These radulae are rasping structures for securing nutrients from or attachments to the rocks upon which they live (van der Wal, 1991). The magnetite is thought to be formed by reduction of Fe_2O_3 (as ferrihydrite in the chiton and goethite in the limpet), in a reaction sequence somewhat similar to that taken by microbes in their synthesis of magnetite. Whether the genetic information for such synthesis persisted from earlier times, or was rediscovered by the marine molluscs, is not yet known.

1.5. Photosynthesis and its Implications for Iron Metabolism

By far the most important event in the evolutionary history of iron metabolism occurred more than three billion years ago when ancestors of the cyanobacteria (blue-green algae) learned to attach phytol side chains to modified porphyrin rings that trapped Mg^{2+} to generate the light-capturing chlorophyll molecule (Loomis, 1988). Solar energy could then be put to biological use in photosynthesis, liberating dioxygen to the atmosphere and making possible aerobic existence. Over the next billion years, as the cyanobacteria held sway, atmospheric concentration of dioxygen increased, and abundant and soluble ferrous iron was converted to the ferric form. By two billion years ago, the atmosphere had become oxygen-rich (Futuyma, 1986) and eukaryotic cells made their appearance. To survive, organisms had to evolve new kinds of molecules to harvest and maintain iron in soluble, non-toxic and bioavailable form. Iron metabolism as we know it today was the inevitable consequence of life with oxygen.

Perhaps the most dramatic indication of the importance of iron-binding molecules in the preservation of species is presented by the organisms responsible for their evolution – the cyanobacteria. In their fight for life, success may be determined by the ability to secure iron in the face of high demand for limited reserves of the metal (Murphy *et al.*, 1976). Organisms that synthesize hydroxamate chelators of iron, making the metal available to themselves but not to competing cells, endure while less resourceful types succumb. The prevalence of a species in the aquatic ecosystem may reflect, in a large part, its ability to capture iron from a hostile environment.

1.6. Adaptive Responses in Higher Organisms

The interdependence of oxygen management and iron metabolism in oxygen-dependent species is ineluctable. As solitary cells organized into colonies and then into complex organisms, iron proteins evolved for the transport of oxygen in circulatory systems, for the facilitated diffusion of oxygen in cells demanding great fluxes of oxygen, for energy transduction by oxidative phosphorylation, and for non-redox group transfer reactions as in the iron-dependent hydratases–dehydratases and phosphatases. Specialized proteins of iron metabolism, the ferritins and transferrins, were evolved to manage the storage and transport of iron when ferric iron is the thermodynamically stable form of the metal. Even the evolution of proton-pumping compartments of cells or organs, including the stomach, has been put to use in liberating and solubilizing iron for physiological needs. The ingenious inventions of Nature (Granick, 1953) are amply applied in regulation of iron metabolism.

2. PROTEINS OF IRON METABOLISM: THE TRANSFERRINS

2.1. Toward a Definition of the Transferrins

The transferrins have been traditionally characterized as a class of two-sited iron-binding proteins found in the extracellular fluids and specialized intracellular structures of organisms in the phylum Chordata. Although once adequate, the emphasis of modern molecular biology on the unity of life compels a definition of transferrins that is less restrictive and more precise.

The unique feature of iron binding by transferrins is that it depends upon concomitant binding of a suitable anion, ordinarily (but not necessarily) carbonate. Cooperativity between anion and metal ion is almost absolute: neither is strongly bound without the other, but together they bind tightly (Aisen et al., 1967; Harris and Aisen, 1989). This interdependent 1:1 binding may be taken as a single defining characteristic of the transferrins: proteins exhibiting it are proper transferrins. Iron-binding proteins which do not depend on anion-binding may be iron transporters or even evolutionary precursors of the transferrins but are not full-fledged members of the transferrin class of iron-binding proteins.

Transferrins are customarily divided into three broad categories, depending upon their origin. Serum transferrins (sometimes called serotransferrins) are found in blood and extracellular fluids; lactoferrins or lactotransferrins are so named because of their presence in milk, but are also found in a variety of secreted fluids and in the specific granules of neutrophils; ovotransferrins are present in egg whites. Chick ovotransferrin and serum transferrin are encoded by the same gene, but lactoferrin is the product of a gene distinct from that specifying transferrin, although both are found on human chromosome 3 (Miller et al., 1983; Teng et al., 1987). For this reason, and to avoid confusion, the term lactoferrin may be preferable to lactotransferrin. True milk transferrin appears identical to serum transferrin, from which it may be derived (Baker et al., 1968). Mammary epithelial cells also appear to secrete transferrin (Lee et al., 1984), presumably as the product of the same gene expressed in liver.

Recently, a new class of transferrin, melanotransferrin, has been identified in the membranes of malignant melanoma cells (Brown et al., 1982; Plowman et al., 1983). The amino acid sequence of melanotransferrin is about 40% homologous with other members of the transferrin family (Rose et al., 1986), but melanotransferrin has a functional metal-binding site only in its N-terminal half (Baker et al., 1992).

Crystallographic studies have shown that transferrins are bilobal proteins (Fig.1.1: Bailey et al., 1988; Anderson et al., 1987, 1989) consisting of approximately 680 amino acids, there being about 40% amino acid sequence homology between the lobes (Mazurier et al., 1983; Metz-Boutigue et al., 1984). Homology between corresponding halves of transferrins from different species generally exceeds homology between N- and C-lobes of the same transferrin (Williams, 1982). Each lobe is further organized into two dissimilar sub-domains of about 160 amino acids, separated by a cleft that contains the metal-binding site.

With the exception of the protein from trout (Stratil et al., 1983), transferrins are glycoproteins. In all species so far studied, glycosylation sites are invariably at asparaginyl residues. Human transferrin bears two carbohydrate chains, accounting for about 6% of the mass of the protein, both attached to the C-terminal lobe at residues N414 and N611 (Metz-Boutigue et al., 1984). No specific function of the carbohydrate is known, although partial loss of terminal sialic residues are a distinctive finding in alcoholism (Stibler, 1991; Mihas and Tavassoli, 1992).

2.2. Characteristics of Metal Binding by Transferrins

In addition to the interdependence of anion and metal binding functions, members of the transferrin class share a number of other characteristics (Harris and Aisen, 1989;

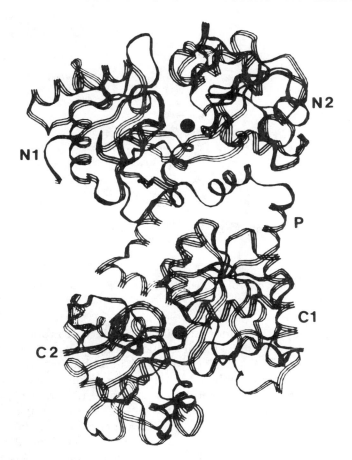

Fig. 1.1 Ribbon diagram showing the characteristic folding of transferrins into two lobes (N-lobe above, C-lobe below), and four domains (N1, N2, C1 and C2). Iron atoms are shown as filled circles. The inter-lobe connecting peptide (P) is helical in lactoferrin (shown here), but irregular in transferrin. From Baker and Lindley (1992) with permission.

Aisen, 1989). Detailed crystallographic structures are available only for human lactoferrin (Anderson *et al.*, 1987, 1989, 1990) and rabbit serum transferrin (Bailey *et al.*, 1988), but the similarities of these suggest that the ligand structure of the binding sites is common to all mature transferrins. Briefly, each site offers one aspartyl (D60 referenced to the N-terminal lobe of human lactoferrin) carboxylate donor oxygen, the phenolate oxygens of two tyrosines (Y92 and Y192) in *cis* relationship to each other, and one histidyl (H253) nitrogen to its bound metal (Fig. 1.2). Charge transfer from tyrosyl oxygen donors to bound Fe(III) is responsible for the characteristic salmon-pink colour of iron-laden transferrin; the iron-free apoprotein is perfectly colourless. The protein provides four of the six ligand atoms required to coordinate iron; the remaining two are satisfied by oxygens of the carbonate co-anion (Anderson *et al.*, 1989). This carbonate, in bidentate ligation to iron, is further fixed to the protein by hydrogen bonding to peptidyl nitrogen atoms of a helix protruding into the cleft bearing the binding site. Electrostatic linkage to arginine, originally thought to be the anchoring group for the anion, is supplemented

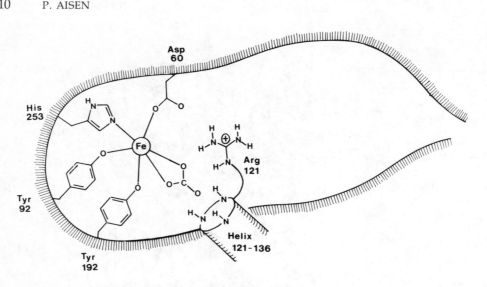

Fig. 1.2 The metal-binding site of human lactoferrin. Reprinted, with permission, from Anderson *et al.* (1989).

by hydrogen bonding to the N-terminus of helix 5, which protrudes into the binding cleft, and to the hydroxyl group of a threonine (Shongwe *et al.*, 1992). This network of hydrogen bonding is a distinctive feature of anion binding to the transferrins. Of chemical interest, but probably not of physiological importance, is the ability of other bifunctional anions to substitute for carbonate (Aisen *et al.*, 1967). To be acceptable to transferrin, the anions must possess a carboxyl group and a Lewis base function separated by no more than 7Å (Schlabach and Bates, 1975). Spectroscopic studies indicate that the Lewis base coordinates to the bound metal ion (Schneider *et al.*, 1984). Carbonate is bound more strongly than other anions (Aisen *et al.*, 1967), and its presence usually precludes involvement of any other anion unless such anion is present in great excess (Shongwe *et al.*, 1992).

Why Nature should have evolved the complexity of a ternary structure of iron, protein and anion for the control of iron transport (and such other functions as the transferrins may carry out) is not clear. Without the co-anion, the ligands provided by the protein are insufficient to guard iron from hydrolysis; with the anion, binding is sufficiently stable to resist removal by all but the strongest chelators. Since the first pK of carbonic acid, about 6.1, is within a range accessible to cells, one conjecture is that the arrangement provided by Nature makes possible reversible binding. By protonating the bound carbonate, the cell might facilitate disruption of the anion-metal or anion-protein bond of transferrin, thus freeing iron for its needs while leaving the protein intact (Aisen and Leibman, 1973). Recent EXAFS (Garratt *et al.*, 1991) and crystallographic (Smith *et al.*, 1991) studies of anion binding in copper complexes of chicken ovotransferrin and human lactoferrin, showing considerable flexibility in the coordination of the anion, appear consistent with this view.

Binding and release of iron by transferrin are accompanied by a remarkable conformational change in the protein. In the absence of metal, the two domains of the binding cleft swing apart on their hinge to assume an 'open' configuration (Fig. 1.3). Occupation of the binding site by metal takes the protein to a 'closed' state

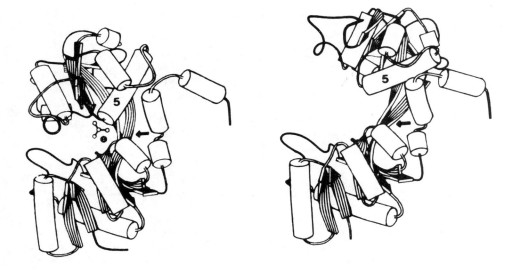

Fig. 1.3 Schematic diagram showing folding of (a) closed, and (b) open forms of a transferrin lobe, taken from the conformational change seen for the N-lobe of human lactoferrin. Helices are shown as cylinders, β-sheets as arrows. The arrows indicate the appproximate position of the hinge in the two 'backbone' strands. From Baker and Lindley (1992) with permission.

as the domains pivot to enclose the bound metal (Anderson *et al.*, 1990; Baker and Lindley, 1992). Crystallographic studies have nicely demonstrated this for the N-lobe of lactoferrin, but the C-lobe retains its closed configuration in the lactoferrin crystal even when unoccupied (Anderson *et al.*, 1990). However, low-angle X-ray scattering studies clearly show that both lobes of lactoferrin and transferrin in solution can assume open or closed states depending on their occupancy by metal (J. G. Grossman *et al.*, 1992). The grasping jaw effect may be exploited by the transferrin receptor in facilitating release of iron within the acidified endosome (Bali *et al.*, 1991).

General agreement prevails about differences in the metal-binding properties of the two sites. The N-terminal site is much more acid-labile (Princiotto and Zapolski, 1975; Lestas, 1976; Aisen *et al.*, 1978; Evans and Williams, 1978), differs in kinetic properties and exhibits distinctive spectroscopic features compared with its partner site in the C-terminal lobe (Zak and Aisen, 1985). Release of iron from each site also responds differently to binding of transferrin to the transferrin receptor (Bali and Aisen, 1991, 1992). Whether these differences are mapped into the functional domain is still controversial, however. Some workers have reported equal iron-donating ability or equal occupancy of the sites in the human circulation (Beguin *et al.*, 1988), but others have found unequal cellular uptake of iron from the sites or unequal occupancy in the circulation (Williams and Moreton, 1980; van Eijk and van Noort, 1986; Zak and Aisen, 1986). Quite possibly, the discord results from use of differing methodologies for distinguishing the four possible species of transferrin – apotransferrin, monoferric transferrin loaded at the C-terminal site, monoferric transferrin loaded at the N-terminal site and diferric transferrin. Both isoelectric focusing and urea gel electrophoresis have been used toward this end. One suggestion is that isoelectric focusing, because of the low isoelectric point of iron-bearing transferrin (pH 5.0–5.4) and the iron-chelating properties of the supporting

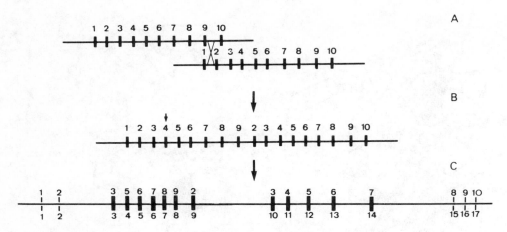

Fig. 1.4 Proposed scheme for the origin of present-day transferrin genes. The primordial single-sited ancestral gene is postulated to have had ten exons, including exon 1 coding for the signal peptide. Duplication and intragenic crossing-over (A) led to a double gene in which a 3'-terminal exon and the following leader exon had been lost (B). During subsequent evolution, exon 4 in the 5' end of the gene was lost, and intron lengths were modified. In the representation of the human transferrin gene (C), upper numbers correspond to exon numbers in (A) and (B), and lower numbers to exons of the modern gene. For details, see Park *et al.* (1985), from which this scheme is reprinted with permission.

ampholytes used, promotes depletion or scrambling of iron from transferrin (Zak and Aisen, 1986; D'Alessandro *et al.*, 1988; Oratore *et al.*, 1989). Even with studies restricted to urea-gel electrophoresis, however, discord persists (Vogel *et al.*, 1989), so the question of functional differences remains unsettled and vexed.

The iron-binding sites of transferrin can accommodate many metal ions other than ferric iron (Morgan, 1981), although iron is bound more strongly and will displace other metals if present in competitive concentrations. Whether or not binding of other metals has any physiological significance is uncertain, although there is evidence that plasma manganese (Scheuhammer and Cherian, 1985), aluminium (Fatema *et al.*, 1991) and chromium (Hopkins and Schwarz, 1964) are at least partly bound to transferrin.

Like the protein it encodes, the human transferrin gene is arranged in two parts, corresponding to the two lobes of the protein molecule (Park *et al.*, 1985). The intron–exon organization is identical in both parts, with introns interrupting the coding sequences to create homologous patterns of coding sequences in each. Thus, two-sited transferrins must have evolved by duplication and fusion of an ancestral gene specifying a single-sited protein (Greene and Feeney, 1968; MacGillivray *et al.*, 1983). Very likely, this event took place early in vertebrate evolution, even before the appearance of chordates.

A plausible model for the origin of the present-day gene entails unequal crossing-over by recombination between ten coding sequences of the putative original gene, leading to tandem duplication in an 18-exon intermediate gene (Park *et al.*, 1985; Schaeffer *et al.*, 1987). Subsequent loss of one exon in the 5' region produced 17 exons separated by 16 introns in the transferrin gene of today (Fig. 1.4). The evolutionary significance of this series of events is not certain. Possibly, the ancestral gene coded for a fixed, membrane-bound protein of size too small to escape filtration by the glomerular kidney (Williams *et al.*, 1982). When this putative transferrin ancestor was selected to transport iron in the circulation, its doubling in size assured that it would resist loss in a filtration kidney. Other evolutionary advantages may also obtain. At the least, a two-sited protein can carry twice as much iron as its single-sited precursor. The Fletcher–Huehns conjecture that a two-sited transferrin allows fine tuning of cellular iron uptake (Fletcher and Huehns, 1968), although controversial, still has its appeal.

2.3. A Brief Overview of Transferrin–Cell Interactions

Most cells depend on receptor-mediated uptake of iron from circulating transferrin to obtain the element for synthesis of iron enzymes or for storage in ferritin. Details of the transferrin-to-cell limb of the metabolic iron cycle have been extensively studied in the past decade (Dautry-Varsat *et al.*, 1983; Klausner *et al.*, 1983) and the way in which this mechanism operates in different cells and tissues is discussed in detail in Chapter 3. The initial event is the recognition and binding of transferrin bearing one or two ferric ions by the cell surface transferrin receptor, a disulfide-linked homodimer of 90 kDa carbohydrate subunits (Hu and Aisen, 1978; Seligman *et al.*, 1979; Enns and Sussman, 1981; Jing and Trowbridge, 1987). Formation of the complex of transferrin and its receptor triggers internalization of the complex into a clathrin-coated vesicle (Harding *et al.*, 1983) which matures into a proton-pumping endosome (Yamashiro *et al.*, 1983). As the endosome reaches a pH near 5.5, iron is released from transferrin, and makes its way by an unknown route across the endosomal membrane for disposition by the cell. Meanwhile, the acidified compartment bearing iron-depleted transferrin still joined to its receptor, returns to the cell surface. There, again encountering a pH of 7.4, apotransferrin is released from the receptor to the circulation for a new cycle of iron transport. Particularly noteworthy features of the transferrin-to-cell interaction include:

1. Transferrin is accompanied by its receptor throughout its journey in the cell.
2. At extracellular pH, the receptor binds iron-transferrin much more tightly than iron-free transferrin (Young *et al.*, 1984). Thus, the cell-surface receptor can selectively seize iron-loaded transferrin even in the face of competition by a great excess of apotransferrin. At the pH of the acidified endosome, apotransferrin is more tightly bound by receptor than iron-laden transferrin (Ecarot-Charrier *et al.*, 1980), ensuring that the complex of receptor and its ligand will persist.
3. The entire cycle is completed in most cells within 2–3 min.

Recent studies suggest a new role for the receptor in modulating iron release from transferrin (Bali *et al.*, 1991; Bali and Aisen, 1991). At the pH of the cell surface, where release is to be avoided so that iron-catalysed oxidation of membrane lipids does not occur, the receptor impedes release of iron from transferrin. At endosomal pH, in contrast, the receptor facilitates release, thereby accounting in large part for release rates observed within cells. Binding of transferrin to its receptor modulates release from each site, and from diferric and monoferric transferrins, distinctively. Whether these effects offer an advantage to cells is yet to be determined.

2.4. Evolutionary History of the Transferrins

The earth is estimated to be 4–4.5 billion years old, with another billion years required for the common ancestor of life to gain its first hold on the planet. After an indeterminate time, probably 500 000 000–1 000 000 000 years, differentiation of the common ancestor into the diverse species of biology began as the lineage of eubacteria (including the photosynthesizing cyanobacteria) separated from the archaea (archaebacteria) (Woese *et al.*, 1990). About 850 000 000 years ago the eukaryotes made their first appearance (Noguchi, 1978), branching off the primary stem of archaea. Fossil records suggest that complex multicellular animals first appeared about 640 million years ago (Futuyma, 1986). Divergence between insects and vertebrates occurred some 250 million years later, with mammals making their entry about 250–300 million years ago. The point of interest is the debut of transferrin on the evolutionary scene.

The oldest existing species in which transferrin-like molecules have been found are the tobacco hornworm (*Manduca sexta*) (Bartfeld and Law, 1990), the tarantula *Dugesiella hentzi* (Lee *et al.*, 1978) and the Dungeness crab *Cancer register* (Huebers *et al.*, 1982). A single-chain glycoprotein of $M_r = 77 000$ and capable of binding one ferric ion has been isolated from the haemolymph of the hornworm, a true insect. Although its iron-binding properties were not studied in detail, the amino acid sequence deduced from its cDNA showed 26–28% identity with known sequences of vertebrate transferrins. Like the vertebrate proteins, the putative insect transferrin shows internal homology between N- and C-terminal halves, although the extent of homology, 19%, is considerably less than that observed in vertebrate transferrins (33–46%). Particularly striking are the similarities in cysteine arrangements of insect and vertebrate proteins: 23 of 24 cysteine residues are conserved among the hornworm protein, hen ovotransferrin, human serum transferrin and human lactoferrin. Of considerable interest, therefore, would be detailed studies of the iron-binding site.

All insects lack myoglobin, and most lack haemoglobin as well (Locke and Nichol, 1992). Demands for iron are correspondingly restricted to the synthesis of iron-dependent enzymes of general cellular metabolism. Nevertheless, insects express ferritin for storage of iron (Huebers *et al.*, 1988), and possibly for iron transport as well. The transferrin-like protein in the haemolymph of *Manduca* is probably used to carry iron from gut to cells, which incorporate haemolymph by pinocytosis. If this is the sole mechanism for cellular uptake of transferrin and its iron, transferrin receptors in the insect world would seem to be unnecessary. Experimental study of this intriguing question has apparently not been undertaken.

The putative crab transferrin is a single-chain polypeptide of molecular weight near 150 000 that can accept two iron atoms per molecule (Huebers *et al.*, 1982). Binding of iron results in formation of a visible absorption band like that of the transferrins. The crab protein apparently meets the proposed chemical criterion for classification as a transferrin, since bicarbonate facilitates formation of a coloured complex with iron. Whether carbonate actually binds to the protein in 1:1 stoichiometry with iron has not been investigated. *Magister* transferrin is an effective donor of iron to rat reticulocytes (Huebers *et al.*, 1982). Rat transferrin successfully competes with the arthropod protein in providing iron to reticulocytes, an observation which points to participation of the rat transferrin receptor in the process of iron uptake from the crab protein. This is surprising, since the more recently evolved ovotransferrin is virtually ineffective in binding to rabbit reticulocytes or providing iron to the cells (Zapolski and Princiotto, 1976).

Perhaps the most intensively scrutinized of the putative prevertebrate transferrins is that from the ascidian sea squirt, *Pyura stolonifera* (Martin *et al.*, 1984), and its close relative, *Pyura haustor* (Bowman *et al.*, 1988). These aquatic creatures are prochordates, having notochords only during larval development. A single-sited single-chain iron-binding protein of molecular weight near 41 000 was isolated by labelling *Pyura* blood with ^{59}Fe, and using the label to sort the iron-binding fraction by gel filtration chromatography and preparative electrophoresis (Martin *et al.*, 1984). Titration with ferrous ammonium sulfate established the stoichiometry of binding, and demonstrated the development of an absorption band at 450 nm upon iron binding. This peak is reasonably close to the peak absorption at 465–470 nm associated with true vertebrate transferrins. Association of iron binding with (bi)carbonate binding was shown using [^{14}C]-bicarbonate; when iron was removed from the protein with deferroxamine, the ^{14}C label was also lost. In final corroboration of the placement of the *Pyura* protein among the transferrins was the demonstration that it could serve as an iron source for iron-deficient rat reticulocytes in a process that is apparently receptor-mediated. Although rates of iron uptake by the cells from the protein were not reported, uptake saturated at a protein concentration of about 4.5×10^{-6} M, and was competitively inhibited by human diferric transferrin. This is a particularly noteworthy observation, since half-ovotransferrin fragments fail to bind to their respective receptor unless present in combination (Brown-Mason and Woodworth, 1984).

These remarkable findings prompted further study of *Pyura* iron-binding protein using the technology of molecular biology (Bowman *et al.*, 1988). Genomic DNA from the ascidian *Pyura haustor* was digested with restriction endonucleases. Hybridization of the resulting fragments, separated by electrophoresis, to a human transferrin cDNA probe was observed even under highly stringent conditions. Thus, the transferrin gene sequence may have been largely conserved during the 400–500 million years separating prochordates and human beings, although the *Pyura* sequence seems to be significantly smaller than its human counterpart. Interestingly, the regulatory sequence and factors which specify tissue-specific expression of the transferrin gene (Mendelzon *et al.*, 1991) may also have been conserved during evolution since the human cDNA probe, used to identify transferrin mRNA transcripts, hybridized selectively to digestive cells of *Pyura*. These cells are believed to be the anlage of vertebrate liver, the principal site of transferrin synthesis in vertebrates.

Taken together, these structural, functional and genetic studies are compelling evidence that the *Pyura* protein is, or is closely related to, the putative transferrin precursor gene specifying a single-sited molecule. The primitive excretory apparatus of *Pyura* does not depend on filtration (Martin *et al.*, 1984), so that this organism can retain a half-sized transferrin that would be eliminated by more advanced species. The ability of the *Pyura* and crab proteins to donate iron to mammalian reticulocytes has been interpreted as suggesting that the transferrin receptor may be of origin as ancient as transferrin (Martin *et al.*, 1984). Since functional transferrin receptors have not yet been identified in prevertebrate species, an alternative possibility is that the receptor evolved only after transferrins were firmly established, and was tailored to accommodate the iron-binding protein.

In the vertebrate world circulating two-sited transferrins identical in important respects to human transferrin have been found in hagfish (Aisen *et al.*, 1972) and lamprey (D. Macey and P. Aisen, unpublished observations), species identified in fossil remains from at least 300 million years ago (Bardack, 1991). The evolutionary emergence of vertebrates must therefore have been accompanied or preceded by emergence of the two-sited transferrin we know today. Presumably, the appearance of the filtration kidney demanded the gene duplication and fusion event for survival of the organism dependent upon iron.

Also noteworthy is the fact that genes for transferrin (Yang *et al.*, 1984), lactoferrin (Teng *et al.*, 1987; McCombs *et al.*, 1988), melanotransferrin (Plowman *et al.*, 1983) and the transferrin receptor (Miller *et al.*, 1983; Rabin *et al.*, 1985) are all found on human chromosome 3. Given the structural similarity of the proteins, the likelihood is that genes for lactoferrin and transferrin differentiated from a common precursor relatively late in evolution, hence their presence on the same chromosome. Whether the location of the transferrin receptor gene on that chromosome is more than coincidence is a matter for speculation. Sequence homologies in 18-nucleotide regions of transferrin cDNA and the complement (antisense) of receptor cDNA have been recognized. This may be too faint an event to make much of, but the temptation to do so can be irresistible (Bowman *et al.*, 1988).

2.5. Regulation of Transferrin Expression

Two features of the regulation of transferrin expression are noteworthy: its tissue specificity and its responsiveness to iron deficiency. In mammals, the hepatocyte is by far the major site of transferrin synthesis and the source of plasma transferrin, although many other cells are capable of transferrin synthesis (Morgan, 1981; Idzerda *et al.*, 1986; Lum *et al.*, 1986). Cells separated from the circulation by organ-specific barriers, such as brain oligodendrocytes and astrocytes (Espinosa de los Monteros *et al.*, 1990) and testis (Griswold *et al.*, 1988), also secrete transferrin. Expression of transferrin by liver cells is transcriptionally regulated and responsive to iron status. Deficiency of the element results in a two- to four-fold increase in the rate of synthesis and a 2.4-fold increase in the level of transferrin mRNA (McKnight *et al.*, 1980; Idzerda *et al.*, 1986), mostly associated with polysomes (McKnight *et al.*, 1980), although very recently evidence for translational regulation of transferrin through an iron-responsive element in the mRNA has been reported (Cox and Adrian, 1993). The clinical corollary is that iron deficiency is often associated with a modest increase in plasma transferrin, while iron overload is accompanied by a decrease in plasma transferrin. In the oviduct, however, expression is insensitive to iron status but stimulated by oestrogen and progesterone with a two- to three-fold increase in the rate of mRNA transcription (McKnight and Palmiter, 1979). By contrast, transferrin synthesis in the lactating mammary glands of some species can exceed that in the liver, leading to a higher concentration of the protein in milk than in plasma (Jordan *et al.*, 1967). Like ferritin synthesis (Tsuji *et al.*, 1991), transferrin expression can be affected by cytokines. Transferrin synthesis in mouse macrophages is up-regulated by γ-interferon but indifferent to iron; human macrophages do not express transferrin at all (Djeha *et al.*, 1992). Since only one functioning transferrin gene is known to exist (Bowman *et al.*,

1988), regulation of transferrin gene expression must have evolved differently in different cells.

Considerable progress has been made in elucidating the mechanism of tissue-specific expression of the transferrin gene. When a 659-bp fragment (-620 to 39) of the human transferrin gene was cloned into a plasmid upstream of its CAT (chloramphenicol acetyltransferase) gene, and the vector then used to transfect human cell lines, expression of CAT was observed only in hepatoma-derived cells and not in HeLa cells (Brunel *et al.*, 1988). Thus, the tissue-specific regulatory sequences must be located in the cloned fragment.

Promoter, enhancer and negative *cis*-acting elements were then localized to discrete sequences of the 5'-flanking region (Ochoa *et al.*, 1989; Schaeffer *et al.*, 1989). Deletion analysis showed that different subsets of promoter sequences are activated by at least three trans-acting nuclear factors (Ochoa *et al.*, 1989), of which two (Tf-LF1 and C/EBP) are responsible and sufficient for conferring liver-specific transcriptional activity through interaction with two proximal promoter elements (Schaeffer *et al.*, 1989; Mendelzon *et al.*, 1991). Liver nuclear factors binding to a 10-base motif in enhancer elements have also been isolated (Mendelzon *et al.*, 1991; Petropoulos *et al.*, 1991). Sertoli cells, obliged to synthesize transferrin because of the impenetrability of the blood–testis barrier (Griswold *et al.*, 1988), express their own distinctive nuclear regulatory factors. These bind to a TATA box or to their own promoter regions of the transferrin gene (Guillou *et al.*, 1991). Whether all of these regulatory factors are members of a common family of evolutionarily related proteins is yet to be determined.

3. PROTEINS OF IRON METABOLISM: THE FERRITINS

3.1. Introduction and Overview

Nowhere is the impact of an aerobic atmosphere on iron metabolism more clearly revealed, and rarely is structure more closely tailored to function, than in the hierarchy of ferritins. These proteins are essential in iron-dependent organisms ranging from bacteria to man (Harrison *et al.*, 1987; Theil, 1987). The ferritin molecule of all species so far studied is a hollow protein shell comprised of 24 subunits (Fig. 1.5), surrounding a core of polynuclear iron oxide deposited as ferrihydrite (FeOOH) and holding as much as 4000–4500 iron atoms. Most mammalian subunits are of two types, designated H (for heavy or heart) and L (for light or liver) respectively. Each of these subunits is specified by its own gene, and each gene is situated on a different chromosome. A cDNA for a third type of subunit with intermediate mobility on SDS gels, and therefore designated M, has been identified in immature erythrocytes of the bullfrog tadpole (Dickey *et al.*, 1987). Because ferritins from the bullfrog and the parasitic worm *Schistosoma mansoni* (Dietzel *et al.*, 1992) resemble H-chains more closely than they do L-chains, it has been suggested that the H-subunit may have been the evolutionary forerunner of ferritin subunits (Harrison *et al.*, 1991). Atypical ferritins (Linder *et al.*, 1989) and ferritin subunits (Moroz *et al.*, 1989) have also been reported.

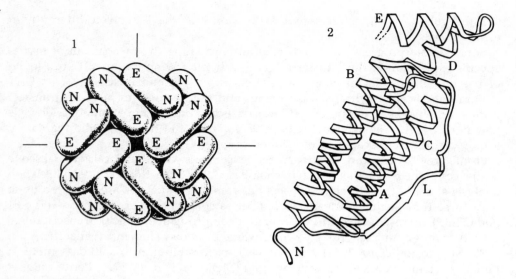

Fig. 1.5 Structure of ferritin. In (1), a schematic representation of the complete 24-subunit molecule is shown, viewed down a molecular four-fold axis illustrating 4 3 2 symmetry. In (2), a ribbon diagram of the α-carbon backbone of a ferritin subunit is shown. The main body of the subunit is a bundle of four long helices (A, B, C and D) with a short helix (E) lying at an acute angle to the bundle axis. The N-terminus of the molecule (N) lies at the opposite end from the helix E, and in (1) the orientation of the subunits in the complete molecule is indicated by the positions of N and E. The loop L joins helices B and C together. From Ford *et al.* (1984) with permission.

The subunit composition of ferritins varies with the tissues and species from which they are isolated; horse spleen ferritin, the subject of most laboratory studies, is about 85–90% L-subunit. Different proportions of H- and L-subunits in a ferritin molecule give rise to isoferritins with characteristic isoelectric points, and therefore separable by isoelectric focusing (Arosio *et al.*, 1978). Administration of iron results in a preferential synthesis of L-subunits and therefore of L-rich isoferritins (Bomford *et al.*, 1981). Studies with recombinant proteins, however, indicate that the H-subunit, because of a 'ferroxidase' site not found in its L-counterpart, is particularly active in taking up ferrous iron in the early stages of core formation (Wade *et al.*, 1991). Nevertheless, isoferritins with a high proportion of H-subunits are found in tissues, such as heart (Powell *et al.*, 1975) and blood cells (Jones *et al.*, 1983), which are not primarily involved in iron storage. As discussed in Chapter 4, H-rich ferritins may be primarily involved in iron detoxification, while L-rich ferritins are mainly involved in long-term iron storage.

The ferroxidase site functions in true catalytic manner, accepting ferrous iron, promoting its oxidation by molecular dioxygen, and releasing the resulting ferric iron for deposition in the core. Site-selective mutagenesis studies incriminate two glutamate (Glu27, Glu62) and one histidine (His65) in ferroxidase function of the human H-chain (Lawson *et al.*, 1989). These three residues, along with a water molecule, comprise a tetrahedral binding site for iron in a site surrounded by four helical bundles of the same subunit (Fig. 1.6). Two additional residues (Glu 107 and Gln 141) make hydrogen bonds to the coordinated water, and so may have a role in

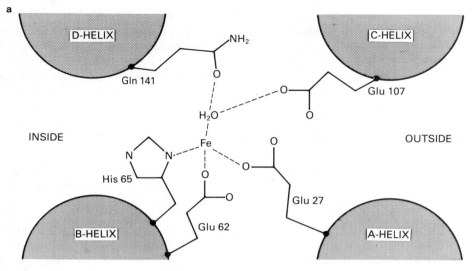

Fig. 1.6 Ferroxidase site of human ferritin H-subunit. Reprinted, with permission, from Harrison *et al.* (1991).

metal binding at this site (Harrison *et al.*, 1991; Lawson *et al.* 1991), particularly since these five residues are conserved in rat, chicken and human H-chains. The ferroxidase centre is embedded in a four-helix bundle of the H-subunit, rather than on the outside of the molecule as once believed. Access of iron to and from the site may be through narrow channels through the bundle, facilitated by thermal fluctuations in channel size, 'pushed' by incoming Fe(II) seeking oxidation on its way to core formation or 'pulled' by a concentration gradient to the core. How electrons are transferred from ferrous iron to dioxygen – whether via direct binding of oxygen to metal or by conduction through the protein to remotely bound oxygen – is still essentially unknown.

Ferric iron in its complex with dihydrolipoate also has access to the interior of an empty or nearly empty ferritin molecule, although to a limited extent (Bonomi and Pagani, 1991). In general, however, substantial loading of ferritin with iron *in vitro* demands presentation of the metal in its ferrous form.

Horse spleen ferritin is pierced by eight hydrophilic channels along the molecule's three-fold axes of symmetry, and six hydrophobic channels related to its three four-fold axes. The hydrophilic channels are lined with glutamate and aspartate residues at their outside and inside termini, respectively, and with serines, histidines and cysteines along their courses. Hydrophobic channels are largely walled by leucines. Earlier suggestions that the channels serve as principal conduits for iron entry into ferritin now seem unlikely since such entry is remarkably insensitive to site directed mutations of channel walls (Wade *et al.*, 1991). Uptake, oxidation and stable deposition of iron in the ferritin core is an organized process competing with oxidation, hydrolysis and precipitation in bulk solution. Only when the kinetics of all processes entailed in stable core formation is favourable to core formation will iron deposition in ferritin prevail.

Little is known of the mechanisms brought to bear within cells to release iron from ferritin. Superoxide radical generated by physiological (or pathophysiological) enzyme systems, such as xanthine–xanthine oxidase, has been proposed (Reif, 1992) and questioned (Bolann and Ulvik, 1990) as an intracellular means for freeing iron from the ferritin core. Although release may be accomplished *in vitro* by incubating iron-laden ferritin with reducing agents (Jones *et al.*, 1978), including reducing free radicals (Reif *et al.*, 1988), such release has usually been driven by the presence of potent Fe(II) chelating agents. Without such agents being present, the ferritin molecule accommodates reduced iron in its core quite comfortably (Watt *et al.*, 1985; Rohrer *et al.*, 1987). Perhaps, therefore, the cell must resort to degradation of ferritin to capture its iron, a process that may also give rise to haemosiderin formation (see Chapter 4). In all, however, the ferritin molecule is well structured for its buffering role in iron metabolism, accepting and detoxifying iron in times of surfeit, holding it in conditions of sufficiency, and making it available when iron deficiency threatens.

3.2. Evolution of the Ferritins: Conservative or Convergent?

In general, ferritins of all species share the broad characteristics of iron uptake, nucleation and core formation. However, structural, and even functional, features may vary with origin. Probably the most ancient of known ferritins is that isolated from the cyanobacterium *Synechocystis* (Laulhère *et al.*, 1992). On native gradient-gel electrophoresis this protein has a molecular mass near 400 kDa, and on SDS gel electrophoresis consists entirely of 19 kDa subunits. The likelihood, then, is that the *Synechocystis* ferritin molecule is assembled of 24 subunits, similar to its counterparts from more advanced species. As isolated, the protein carries an average of 2300 iron atoms per molecule. Like other bacterial ferritins, the cyanobacterial ferritin contains haem (0.25 groups/subunit), a moiety absent in vertebrate ferritins, and higher concentrations of phosphate (1500 groups/molecule) than are found in most eukaryotic ferritins. The presence of haem suggests that the protein may function, or have evolved from a protein that functions, in electron transport. Indeed, bacterioferritin from *E. coli* has been identified with cytochrome b_1 from that species (Smith *et al.*, 1988b). Whether electron transfer by the haem groups is exploited in the uptake of iron by bacterioferritin is an intriguing but unanswered question. When exposed to labelled iron, *Synechocystis* cells rapidly accumulate the element in their ferritin, but they do not react to iron stress by altering their total concentration of the protein. Such apparent failure to regulate ferritin synthesis in response to iron status distinguishes this prokaryote from more advanced cells, and casts doubt on the role of its ferritin in long-term iron storage.

Ferritins from more recently evolved bacterial species, *Azotobacter vinelandii* and *E. coli*, have been studied in even greater depth. Like the cyanobacterium ferritin, both of these are haem proteins classifiable as b-type cytochromes (Stiefel and Watt, 1979; Yariv, 1983). The haem content of bacterioferritins may vary with species; the protein from *Pseudomonas aeruginosa* has been found to bear one haem per subunit (Kadir and Moore, 1990), while other bacterioferritins may possess one b-type haem for every two protein subunits (Andrews *et al.*, 1991b). Low resolution crystallographic data are consistent with an overall structure of the *E. coli* protein very similar to that of horse spleen ferritin (Smith *et al.*, 1988a). Haem may influence the reduction potential of iron in bacterial ferritin, – 420 mV and invariant between pH 6 and pH 8 for *A. vinelandii* ferritin (Watt *et al.*, 1986), compared with – 190 mV (pH 7) to $-416\,mV$ (pH 9) for iron in horse spleen ferritin (Watt *et al.*, 1985; Chasteen *et al.*, 1991). It is not evident that this effect has any physiological significance, particularly since the mechanism of iron release from ferritin *in vivo* is not known. The relatively large number of haem groups per molecule may indicate an electron storage, as well as iron storage, role for the bacterioferritins.

Bacterioferritin cores are also richer in phosphate than those from their vertebral counterparts, containing from 1.5–2 phosphate groups per iron (Laulhère *et al.*, 1992). Phosphate accelerates the autoxidation of ferrous iron by horse spleen ferritin and the formation of EPR-silent clusters of Fe(III), particularly in the early stages of core formation (Cheng and Chasteen, 1991). Whether this effect offers an advantage to bacteria that is no longer needed by more complex organisms is not known. Core formation in bacterioferritin is similar to that in horse spleen ferritin in its inhibition by zinc ions (Mann *et al.*, 1987).

In general, the cores of bacterial ferritins closely resemble those of vertebrate ferritins. On Mössbauer spectroscopy, the 'blocking temperature', a measure of the transition rate between magnetically ordered and averaged structures, is appreciably lower (20–22 K) for *A. vinelandii* ferritin (Watt *et al.*, 1986) than for horse spleen ferritin (38 K). This is consistent with a smaller average volume for the core of the bacterioferritin, as evidenced by electron microscopic measurements (Mann *et al.*, 1987).

All of the known bacterial ferritins are related by sequence identities or similarities. The first 54 N-terminal amino acids of the *Synechocystis* ferritin subunit are 50% identical and 73% similar to the corresponding residues of *E. coli* ferritin, and 40% identical and 60% similar to ferritin from *Nitrobacter winogradskyi* (Laulhère *et al.*, 1992). Even greater homologies are found when *Azotobacter vinelandii* ferritin is taken as the reference structure (Andrews *et al.*, 1991a; Harrison *et al.*, 1991). Immunological cross-reactivity is also displayed by bacterioferritins from *E. coli*, *A. vinelandii* and *Pseudomonas aeruginosa* (Andrews *et al.*, 1991a), further establishing the close structural relationships among these ferritins from bacteria.

Similarities among ferritins cross kingdom boundaries. Amino acid residues comprising the putative ferroxidase centre of vertebrate H-chain ferritins are conserved or conservatively substituted in the helix bundle centres of bacterioferritins from *A. vinelandii*, *E. coli* and *N. winogradskii* (Andrews *et al.*, 1991b). Recently a gene specifying a polypeptide of 165 amino acids with 25% overall sequence identity to human H-chain ferritin, and 50% identity in the 20 N-terminal amino acids, has been cloned from *E. coli* (Izuhara *et al.*, 1991). Although it has not yet been shown that the polypeptide gene product is capable of assembly into a functional ferritin, its size and sequence suggest that this is likely to be the case.

Plant ferritins from soybean and pea seed also bear close structural similarities to each other, with 89% conservation of amino acids between the two proteins when about half of the total amino acid sequences are compared (Ragland *et al.*, 1990). The ferritin subunits show substantial homologies in amino acid residues when sequences are aligned with those from vertebrates. Of particular interest, residues from subunit interfaces thought to be involved in iron binding are especially well conserved.

A major difference between plant and animal ferritins is their cellular locations. Animal ferritins are free in the cytoplasm, but plant ferritins are contained within membrane-bound plastids. Available evidence, including the demonstration of a transit peptide that is ultimately cleaved from the ferritin subunit (Ragland *et al.*, 1990), indicates that the ferritin is specified by the plant cell genome, rather than the prokaryotic genome of the plastid (Laulhère *et al.*, 1992). The plastid is generally believed to be the evolutionary result of a photosynthesizing cyanobacterium invading the primitive plant cell band to set up mutually beneficial residence there. Why then did the bacterioferritin disappear from the prokaryotic chloroplast, only to be replaced by the eukaryotic ferritin of the plant cell (Laulhère *et al.*, 1992)?

One possibility is that expression of the prokaryotic ferritin gene is insensitive to iron levels, while the plant gene responds to iron by regulating expression at the level of transcription (Lescure *et al.*, 1991; Laulhère *et al.*, 1992). Since plastid function is accompanied by oxygen evolution, the organelle must be protected against iron-catalysed reactions generating noxious oxygen species. To accomplish this, an iron-sensing ferritin-synthesizing apparatus is provided by the host plant cell, thereby ensuring that potentially toxic iron will be safely sequestered in the storage protein.

The central question is whether the ferritins we know today represent a convergence of once diverse structures to a molecule uniquely fitted to its iron storage function, or conservation and modification of an ancestral protein that evolution could not substantially improve. Overall similarities in morphology, homologies in amino acid sequence and virtual equivalence in iron storage argue compellingly for conservative evolution from a common progenitor. Divergences, as they arose, may have been mutational events generating new molecules tailored to meet specialized needs of organisms.

The evolutionary relationships between bacterioferritins and vertebrate ferritins have recently been considered in depth (M. J. Grossman *et al.*, 1992). Sequence identity between bacterioferritin from *A. vinelandii* and eukaryotic ferritins ranged from 24% with rat H-subunit ferritin to 29% with rat L-subunit. To exclude the possibility that these identities merely reflect similarities in amino acid composition, rather than true sequence homologies, the bacterioferritin sequence was randomized by computer, and the randomized sequence again compared with sequences of eukaryotic ferritins. Sequence identities then vanished. A computer-generated global alignment of the bacterioferritin sequence with eukaryotic ferritin sequences was undertaken, ignoring all available structural information. Of 58 residues conserved in all the eukaryotic ferritins, 19 were found in *A. vinelandii* bacterioferritin (assuming a glutamate/aspartate equivalence). Furthermore, three of the five helices and the long loop joining helix B to helix C achieve consensus alignment without the need for insertions or deletions. Finally, four of the five key residues implicated in ferroxidase activity are conserved in the prokaryotic ferritin and the fifth is flanked by hydrophilic residues which serve a hydrogen-bonding function. The evidence supporting an evolutionary relationship between bacterioferritins and eukaryotic ferritins is therefore compelling.

4. REPRISE

Another unifying theme binds proteins of iron metabolism together in an evolutionary sense. As described in detail in Chapter 5, the transferrin receptor (Müllner and Kühn, 1988; Müllner *et al.*, 1989; Kühn, 1991), animal ferritins

(Rouault *et al.*, 1988) and aminolevulinic acid synthase (Cox *et al.*, 1991) are all regulated by short palindromic *cis*-acting sequences in untranslated regions of their respective mRNAs. Because of their effects on mRNA function, these looped sequences have come to be known as Iron Regulatory Elements or IREs. The IRE, in turn, responds to the presence of a *trans*-acting cytoplasmic IRE-binding protein (Kaptain *et al.*, 1991), which may be the primary sensor of iron status in the cell. IRE-binding proteins were sought for and found in human, mouse, chicken, frog, fish and fruit fly and annelid worm tissues (Rothenberger *et al.*, 1990). All of these proteins, which are now thought to be identical with cytoplasmic aconitase (Chapter 5) were found to have the same molecular weight and IRE-binding activity, and so may be linked in evolution as are the transferrins and ferritins.

Genetically, structurally and functionally, then, proteins of iron metabolism are joined by strong evolutionary ties to each other. The first synthesis of ferritin in an iron-dependent cyanobacterium must have been compelled by its photosynthetic activity, an event long antedating appearance of eukaryotes and multicellular organisms. When organisms shielded themselves from the nutrients (and hazards) of their environment by an integument, a circulatory system and the transferrins became necessary. Parsimony of natural processes then led to the conservation of ferritins and transferrins during evolution, simply because they did their jobs so effectively. Proteins of iron metabolism we know today were commissioned when life turned to light from the sun to sustain itself.

ACKNOWLEDGEMENT

Preparation of this manuscript was supported in part by Grant DK-15056 from the National Institutes of Health, US Public Health Service.

REFERENCES

Aisen, P. (1989) Physical biochemistry of the transferrins: Update, 1984–1988. In: *Iron Carriers and Iron Proteins* (eds T. M. Loehr, H. B. Gray and H. B. P. Lever), VCH Publishers, Weinheim.

Aisen, P. and Leibman, A. (1973) The role of the anion-binding site of transferrin in its interaction with the reticulocyte. *Biochim. Biophys. Acta* **304**, 797–804.

Aisen, P. *et al.* (1967) Bicarbonate and the binding of iron to transferrin. *J. Biol. Chem.* **242**, 2484–2490.

Aisen, P., Leibman, A. and Sia, C.-L. (1972) Molecular weight and subunit structure of hagfish transferrin. *Biochemistry* **11**, 3461–3464.

Aisen, P., Leibman, A. and Zweier, J. (1978) Stoichiometric and site characteristics of the binding of iron to human transferrin. *J. Biol. Chem.* **253**, 1930–1937.

Anderson, B. F., Baker, H. M., Dodson, E. J. *et al.* (1987) Structure of human lactoferrin at 3.2-Å resolution. *Proc. Natl. Acad. Sci. USA* **84**, 1769–1773.

Anderson, B. F., Baker, H. M., Norris, G. E., Rice, D. W. and Baker, E. N. (1989) Structure of human lactoferrin: Crystallographic structure analysis and refinement at 2.8 Å resolution. *J. Mol. Biol.* **209**, 711–734.

Anderson, B. F., Baker, H. M., Norris, G. E., Rumball, S. V. and Baker, E. N. (1990) Apolactoferrin structure demonstrates ligand-induced conformational change in transferrins. *Nature* **344**, 784–787.

Andrews, S. C., Findlay, J. B. C., Guest, J. R., Harrison, P. M., Keen, J. N. and Smith, J. M. A. (1991a) Physical, chemical and immunological properties of the bacterioferritins of *Escherichia coli, Pseudomonas aeruginosa* and *Azotobacter vinelandii*. *Biochim. Biophys. Acta* **1078**, 111–116.

Andrews, S. C., Smith, J. M. A., Yewdall, S. J., Guest, J. R. and Harrison, P. M. (1991b) Bacterioferritins and ferritins are distantly related in evolution: Conservation of ferroxidase-centre residues. *FEBS Lett.* **293**, 164–168.

Arosio, P., Adelman, T. G. and Drysdale, J. W. (1978) On ferritin heterogeneity: Further evidence for heteropolymers. *J. Biol. Chem.* **253**, 4451–4458.

Bailey, S., Evans, R. W., Garratt, R. C. *et al.* (1988) Molecular structure of serum transferrin at 3.3-Å resolution. *Biochemistry* **27**, 5804–5812.

Baker, E, Shaw, D. C. and Morgan, E. H. (1968) Isolation and characterization of rabbit serum and milk transferrins. Evidence for difference in sialic acid content only. *Biochemistry* **7**, 1371–1378.

Baker, E. N. and Lindley, P. F. (1992) New perspectives on the structure and function of transferrins. *J. Inorg. Biochem.* **47**, 147–160.

Baker, E. N., Baker, H. M., Smith, C. A. *et al.* (1992) Human melanotransferrin (p97) has only one functional iron-binding site. *FEBS Lett.* **298**, 215–218.

Bali, P. K. and Aisen, P. (1991) Receptor-modulated iron release from transferrin: Differential effects on N- and C-terminal sites. *Biochemistry* **30**, 9947–9952.

Bali, P. K. and Aisen, P. (1992) Receptor-induced switch in site-site cooperativity during iron release by transferrin. *Biochemistry* **31**, 3963–3967.

Bali, P. K., Zak, O. and Aisen, P. (1991) A new role for the transferrin receptor in the release of iron from transferrin. *Biochemistry* **30**, 324–328.

Bardack, D. (1991) First fossil hagfish (Myxinoidea): A record from the Pennsylvanian of Illinois. *Science* **254**, 701–703.

Bartfeld, N. S. and Law, J. H. (1990) Isolation and molecular cloning of transferrin from the tobacco hornworm, *Manduca sexta*. Sequence similarity to the vertebrate transferrins. *J. Biol. Chem.* **265**, 21684–21691.

Bazylinski, D. A. (1991) Anaerobic production of single-domain magnetite by the marine magnetotactic bacterium, strain MV-1. In: *Iron Biominerals* (eds R. B. Frankel and N. A. Blakemore), Plenum Press, New York, pp. 69–77.

Beguin, Y., Huebers, H. and Finch, C. A. (1988) Random distribution of iron among the two binding sites of transferrin in patients with various hematologic disorders. *Clin. Chim. Acta* **173**, 299–304.

Blakemore, R. P. and Blakemore, N. A. (1991) Magnetotactic magnetogens. In: *Iron Biominerals* (eds R. B. Frankel and R. P. Blakemore), Plenum Press, New York, pp. 51–67.

Bolann, B. J. and Ulvik, R. J. (1990) On the limited ability of superoxide to release iron from ferritin. *Eur. J. Biochem.* **103**, 899–904.

Bomford, A. B., Conlon-Hollingshead, C. and Munro, H. N. (1981) Adaptive responses of rat tissue ferritins to iron administration. *J. Biol. Chem.* **256**, 948–955.

Bonomi, F. and Pagani, S. (1991) Uptake of iron by apoferritin from a ferric dihydrolipoate complex. *Eur. J. Biochem.* **199**, 181–186.

Borowska, Z. and Mauzerall, D. (1988) Photoreduction of carbon dioxide by aqueous ferrous ion: An alternative to the strongly reducing atmosphere for the chemical origin of life. *Proc. Natl. Acad. Sci. USA* **85**, 6577–6580.

Bowman, B. H., Yang, F. and Adrian, G. S. (1988) Transferrin: evolution and genetic regulation of expression. *Adv. Genetics* **25**, 1–38.

Brown, J. P., Hewick, R. M., Hellstrom, I., Hellstrom, K. E., Doolittle, R. F. and Dreyer, W. J. (1982) Human melanoma-associated antigen p97 is structurally and functionally related to transferrin. *Nature* **296**, 171–173.

Brown-Mason, A. and Woodworth, R. C. (1984) Physiological levels of binding and iron donation by complementary half-molecules of ovotransferrin to transferrin receptors of chick reticulocytes. *J. Biol. Chem.* **259**, 1866–1873.

Brunel, F., Ochoa, A., Schaeffer, E. *et al.* (1988) Interactions of DNA-binding proteins with the 5' region of the human transferrin gene. *J. Biol. Chem.* **263**, 10180–10185.

Cairns-Smith, A. G. (1978) Precambrian solution photochemistry, inverse segregation, and banded iron formations. *Nature* **276**, 807–808.

Chasteen, N. D., Ritchie, I. M. and Webb, J. (1991) Stepped potential microcoulometry of ferritin. *Anal. Biochem.* **195**, 296–302.

Cheng, Y. G. and Chasteen, N. D. (1991) Role of phosphate in initial iron deposition in apoferritin. *Biochemistry* **30**, 2947–2953.

Cooper, S. R., McArdle, J. V. and Raymond, K. N. (1978) Siderophore electrochemistry: relation to intracellular iron release mechanism. *Proc. Natl. Acad. Sci. USA* **75**, 3551–3554.

Cotton, F. A. and Wilkinson, G. (1988) *Advanced Inorganic Chemistry*, 5th edn, John Wiley & Sons, New York, pp. 709–725.

Cox, L. A. and Adrian, G. S. (1993) Posttranscriptional regulation of chimeric human transferrin genes by iron. *Biochemistry* **32**, 4738–4745.

Cox, T. C., Bawden, M. J., Martin, A. and May, B. K. (1991) Human erythroid 5-aminolevulinate synthase: Promoter analysis and identification of an iron-responsive element in the mRNA. *EMBO J.* **10**, 1891–1902.

D'Alessandro, A. M., D'Andrea, G. and Oratore, A. (1988) Different patterns of human serum transferrin on isoelectric focusing using synthetic carrier ampholytes or immobilized pH gradients. *Electrophoresis* **9**, 80–83.

Dautry-Varsat, A., Ciechanover, A. and Lodish, H. F. (1983) pH and the recycling of transferrin during receptor-mediated endocytosis. *Proc. Natl. Acad. Sci. USA* **80**, 2258–2262.

Dickey, L. F., Sreedharan, S., Theil, E. C., Didsbury, J. R., Wang, Y.-H. and Kaufman, R. E. (1987) Differences in the regulation of messenger RNA for housekeeping and specialized-cell ferritin. A comparison of three distinct ferritin complementary DNAs, the corresponding subunits, and identification of the first processed pseudogene in amphibia. *J. Biol. Chem.* **262**, 7901–7907.

Dietzel, J., Hirzmann, J., Preis, D., Symmons, P. and Kunz, W. (1992) Ferritins of *Schistosoma mansoni*: Sequence comparison and expression in female and male worms. *Mol. Biochem. Parasitol.* **50**, 245–254.

Djeha, A., Pérez-Arellano, J. L., Hayes, S. L. and Brock, J. H. (1992) Transferrin synthesis by macrophages: up-regulation by gamma-interferon and effect on lymphocyte proliferation. *FEMS Microbiol. Immunol.* **5**, 279–282.

Doi, K., Antanaitis, B. C. and Aisen, P. (1988) The binuclear iron center of uteroferrin and the purple acid phosphatases. *Struct. Bond.* **70**, 1–26.

Dus, K., de Klerk, H., Sletten, K. and Bartsch, R. G. (1967) Chemical characterization of high potential iron proteins from *Chromatium* and *Rhodopseudomonas gelatinosa*. *Biochim. Biophys. Acta* **140**, 291–311.

Ecarot-Charrier, B., Grey, V. L., Wilcynska, A. and Schulman, H. M. (1980) Reticulocyte membrane transferrin receptors. *Can. J. Biochem.* **58**, 418–426.

Egyed, A. (1988) Carrier mediated iron transport through erythroid cell membrane. *Br. J. Haematol.* **68**, 483–486.

Enns, C. A. and Sussman, H. H. (1981) Physical characterization of the transferrin receptor in human placentae. *J. Biol. Chem.* **256**, 9820–9823.

Espinosa de los Monteros, A., Kumar, S., Scully, S., Cole, R. and de Vellis, J. (1990) Transferrin gene expression and secretion by rat brain cells in vitro. *J. Neurosci. Res.* **25**, 576–580.

Evans, R. W. and Williams, J. (1978) Studies of the binding of different iron donors to human serum transferrin and isolation of iron-binding fragments from the N- and C-terminal regions of the protein. *Biochem. J.* **173**, 543–552.

Fatema, S. J. A., Kadir, F. H. A. and Moore, G. R. (1991) Aluminium transport in blood serum. Binding of aluminium by human transferrin in the presence of human albumin and citrate. *Biochem. J.* **280**, 527–532.

Fletcher, J. and Huehns, E. R. (1968) Function of transferrin. *Nature* **218**, 1211–1214.

Ford, G. C., Harrison, P. M., Rice, D. W. *et al.* (1984) Ferritin: design of an iron-storage molecule. *Phil. Trans. R. Soc. Lond. B* **304**, 551–565.

Futuyma, D. J. (1986) *Evolutionary Biology*, 2nd edn, Sinauer Associates, Inc., Sunderland, Massachusetts.

Garratt, R. C., Evans, R. W., Hasnain, S. S., Lindley, P. F. and Sarra, R. (1991) X.a.f.s. studies of chicken dicupric ovotransferrin. *Biochem. J.* **280**, 151–155.

Granick, S. (1953) Inventions in iron metabolism. *American Naturalist* **87**, 65–75.

Greene, F. C. and Feeney, R. E. (1968) Physical evidence for transferrins as single polypeptide chains. *Biochemistry* **7**, 1366–1371.

Griswold, M. D., Hugly, S., Morales, C. and Sylvester, S. (1988) Evidence for *in vivo* transferrin synthesis and the relationship between transferrin mRNA levels and germ cells in the testis. *Ann. NY Acad. Sci.* **513**, 302–303.

Grossman, M. J., Hinton, S. M., Minak-Bernaro, V., Slaughter, C. and Stiefel, E. I. (1992) Unification of the ferritin family of proteins. *Proc. Natl. Acad. Sci. USA* **89**, 2419–2423.

Grossman, J. G., Neu, M., Pantos, E. *et al.* (1992) X-ray solution scattering reveals conformational changes upon iron uptake in lactoferrin, serum and ovo-transferrins. *J. Mol. Biol.* **225**, 811–819.

Guillou, F., Zakin, M. M., Part, D., Boissier, F. and Schaeffer, E. (1991) Sertoli cell-specific expression of the human transferrin gene. Comparison with the liver-specific expression. *J. Biol. Chem.* **266**, 9876–9884.

Harding, C., Heuser, J. and Stahl, P. (1983) Receptor-mediated endocytosis of transferrin and recycling of the transferrin receptor in rat reticulocytes. *J. Cell Biol.* **97**, 329–339.

Harris, D. C. and Aisen, P. (1989) Physical biochemistry of the transferrins. In: *Iron Carriers and Iron Proteins* (eds T. M. Loehr, H. B. Gray and A. B. P. Lever), VCH Publishers, Weinheim, pp. 239–351.

Harrison, P. M., Andrews, S. C., Ford, G. C., Smith, J. M. A., Treffry, A. and White, J. L. (1987) Ferritin and bacterioferritin: iron sequestering molecules from microbes to man. In: *Iron Transport in Microbes, Plants and Animals* (eds G. Winkelmann, D. van der Helm and J. B. Neilands), VCH, Weinheim, pp. 445–475.

Harrison, P. M., Andrews, S. C., Artymiuk, P. J. *et al.* (1991) Probing structure–function relations in ferritin and bacterioferritin. *Adv. Inorg. Chem.* **36**, 449–486.

Hopkins, L. L. and Schwarz, K. (1964) Chromium(III) binding to serum proteins specifically siderophilin. *Biochim. Biophys. Acta* **90**, 484–491.

Hu, H.-Y. Y. and Aisen, P. (1978) Molecular characteristics of the transferrin–receptor complex of the rabbit reticulocyte. *J. Supramol. Struct.* **8**, 349–360.

Huebers, H. A., Huebers, E., Finch, C. A. and Martin, A. W. (1982) Characterization of an invertebrate transferrin from the crab *Cancer register*. *J. Comp. Physiol.* **148**, 101–109.

Huebers, H. A., Huebers, E., Finch, C. A. *et al.* (1988) Iron binding proteins and their roles in the tobacco hornworm, *Manducca sexta*. *Comp. Physiol. B* **158**, 291–300.

Idzerda, R. L., Huebers, H., Finch, C. A. and McKnight, G. S. (1986) Rat transferrin gene expression: tissue-specific regulation by iron deficiency. *Proc. Natl. Acad. Sci. USA* **83**, 3723–3727.

Izuhara, M., Takamune, K. and Takata, R. (1991) Cloning and sequencing of an *Escherichia coli* K12 gene which encodes a polypeptide having similarity to the human ferritin H subunit. *Mol. Gen. Genet.* **225**, 510–513.

Jing, S. and Trowbridge, I. S. (1987) Identification of the intermolecular disulfide bonds of the human transferrin receptor and its lipid-attachment site. *EMBO J.* **6**, 327–331.

Jones, B. M., Worwood, M. and Jacobs, A. (1983) Isoferritins in normal leucocytes. *Br. J. Haematol.* **55**, 73–81.

Jones, T., Spencer, R. and Walsh, C. (1978) Mechanism and kinetics of iron release from ferritin by dihydroflavins and dihydroflavin analogues. *Biochem. J.* **17**, 4011–4017.

Jordan, S. M., Kaldor, I. and Morgan, E. H. (1967) Milk and serum iron and iron-binding capacity in the rabbit. *Nature* **215**, 76–77.

Kadir, F. H. A. and Moore, G. R. (1990) Bacterial ferritin contains 24 haem groups. *FEBS Lett.* **271**, 141–143.

Kamaluddin, M. S., Singh, M. and Deopujari, S. W. (1986) Chemical evolution of iron containing enzymes: mixed ligand complexes of iron as intermediary steps. *Origins of Life* **17**, 59–68.

Kaptain, S., Downey, W. E., Tang, C. *et al.* (1991) A regulated RNA binding protein also possesses aconitase activity. *Proc. Natl. Acad. Sci. USA* **88**, 10109–10113.

Klausner, R. D., Ashwell, J. V., VanRenswoude, J. B., Harford, J. and Bridges, K. (1983) Binding of apotransferrin to K562 cells: explanation of the transferrin cycle. *Proc. Natl. Acad. Sci. USA* **80**, 2263–2266.

Kühn, L. C. (1991) Annotation. mRNA–Protein interactions regulate critical pathways in cellular iron metabolism. *Br. J. Haematol.* **79**, 1–5.

Lane, D. J., Harrison, A. P., Jr, Stahl, D. *et al.* (1992) Evolutionary relationships among sulfur- and iron-oxidizing eubacteria. *J. Bacteriol.* **174**, 269–278.

Laulhère, J.-P., Labouré, A.-M., Van Wuytswinkel, O., Gagnon, J. and Briat, J.-F. (1992) Purification, characterization and function of bacterioferritin from the cyanobacterium *Synechocystis* P.C.C. 6803. *Biochem. J.* **281**, 785–793.

Lawson, D. M., Treffry, A., Artymiuk, P. J. *et al.* (1989) Identification of the ferroxidase centre in ferritin. *FEBS Lett.* **254**, 207–210.

Lawson, D. M., Artymiuk, P. J., Yewdall, S. J. *et al.* (1991) Solving the structure of human H ferritin by genetically engineering intermolecular crystal contacts. *Nature* **349**, 541–544.

Lee, M. Y., Huebers, H., Martin, A. W. and Finch, C. A. (1978) Iron metabolism in a spider, *Dugesiella hentzi*. *J. Comp. Physiol.* **127**, 349–354.

Lee, Y.-H., Parry, G. and Bissell, M. J. (1984) Modulation of secreted proteins of mouse mammary epithelial cells by the collagenous substrata. *J. Cell Biol.* **98**, 146–155.

Lescure, A.-M., Proudhon, D., Pesey, H., Ragland, M., Theil, E. C. and Briat, J.-F. (1991) Ferritin gene transcription is regulated by iron in soybean cell cultures. *Proc. Natl. Acad. Sci. USA* **88**, 8222–8226.

Lestas, A. N. (1976) The effect of pH upon human transferrin: selective labelling of the two iron-binding sites. *Br. J. Haematol.* **32**, 341–350.

Linder, M. C., Goode, C. A., Gonzalez, R., Gottschling, C., Gray, J. and Nagel, G. M. (1989) Heart tissue contains small and large aggregates of ferritin subunits. *Arch. Biochem. Biophys.* **273**, 34–41.

Lins de Barros, H. G. P., Esquivel, D. M. S. and Farina, M. (1990) Magnetotaxis. *Sci. Progress* **74**, 347–359.

Locke, M. and Nichol, H. (1992) Iron economy in insects: transport, metabolism, and storage. *Ann. Rev. Entomol.* **37**, 195–215.

Lodge, J. S. and Emery, T. (1984) Anaerobic iron uptake by *Escherichia coli*. *J. Bacteriol.* **160**, 801–804.

Loomis, W. F. (1988) *Four Billion Years. An Essay on the Evolution of Genes and Organisms*, Sinauer Associates, Inc., Sunderland, Mass.

Lum, J. B., Infante, A. J., Makker, D. M., Yang, F. and Bowman, B. H. (1986) Transferrin synthesis by inducer T lymphocytes. *J. Clin. Invest.* **77**, 841–849.

MacGillivray, R. T. A., Mendez, E., Shewale, J. G., Sinha, S. K., Lineback-Zins, J. and Brew, K. (1983) The primary structure of human serum transferrin. The structures of seven cyanogen bromide fragments and the assembly of the complete structure. *J. Biol. Chem.* **258**, 3543–3553.

Mann, S., Williams, J. M., Treffrey, A. and Harrison, P. M. (1987) Reconstituted and native iron-cores of bacterioferritin and ferritin. *J. Mol. Biol.* **198**, 405–416.

Mann, S., Sparks, N. H. C., Frankel, R. B., Bazylinski, D. A. and Jannasch, H. W. (1990) Biomineralization of ferrimagnetic greigite (Fe_3S_4) and iron pyrite (FeS_2) in a magnetotactic bacterium. *Nature* **343**, 258–261.

Martin, A. W., Huebers, E., Huebers, H., Webb, J. and Finch, C. A. (1984) A mono-sited transferrin from a representative deuterostome: the ascidian *Pyura stolonifera* (Subphylum urochordata). *Blood* **64**, 1047–1052.

Mauzerall, D. (1991) Retraction. *Proc. Natl. Acad. Sci. USA* **88**, 4564.

Mauzerall, D. C. (1992) The photochemical origins of life and photoreaction of ferrous ion in the archaean oceans. *Origins of Life* **20**, 293–302.

Mazurier, J., Boutigue-Metz, M. H., Jolles, J., Spik, G., Montreuil, J. and Jolles, P. (1983) Human lactotransferrin: molecular, functional and evolutionary comparisons with human serum transferrin and hen ovotransferrin. *Experientia* **39**, 135–141.

McCombs, J. L., Teng, C. T., Pentecost, B. T., Magnuson, V. L., Moore, C. M. and McGill, J. R. (1988) Chromosomal localization of human lactotransferrin gene (LTF) by in situ hybridization. *Cytogenet. Cell Genet.* **47**, 16–17.

McKnight, G. S. and Palmiter, R. D. (1979) Transcriptional regulation of the ovalbumin and conalbumin genes by steroid hormones in chick oviduct. *J. Biol. Chem.* **254**, 9050–9058.

McKnight, G. S., Lee, D. C., Hemmaplardh, D., Finch, C. A. and Palmiter, R. D. (1980) Transferrin gene expression. Effects of nutritional iron deficiency. *J. Biol. Chem.* **255**, 144–147.

Mendelzon, D., Boissier, F. and Zakin, M. M. (1991) The binding site for the liver-specific transcription factor Tf-LF1 and the TATA box of the human transferrin gene promoter are the only elements necessary to direct liver-specific transcription *in vitro*. *Nucleic Acids Res.* **18**, 5717–5721.

Metz-Boutigue, M.-H., Jolles, J., Mazurier, J. *et al.* (1984) Human lactotransferrin: amino acid sequence and structural comparisons with other transferrins. *Eur. J. Biochem.* **145**, 659–676.

Mihas, A. A. and Tavassoli, M. (1992) Laboratory markers of ethanol intake and abuse: A critical appraisal. *Am. J. Med. Sci.* **303**, 415–428.

Miller, Y. E., Jones, C., Scoggin, C., Morse, H. and Seligman, P. (1983) Chromosome 3q(22-ter) encodes the human transferrin receptor. *Am. J. Hum. Genet.* **35**, 573–583.

Morgan, E. H. (1981) Transferrin, biochemistry, physiology and clinical significance. *Mol. Aspects Med.* **4**, 3–123.

Morgan, E. H. (1988) Membrane transport of non-transferrin-bound iron by reticulocytes. *Biochim. Biophys. Acta* **943**, 428–439.

Moroz, C., Shterman, N., Kupfer, B. and Ginzburg, I. (1989) T-cell mitogenesis stimulates the synthesis of a mRNA species coding for a 43-kDa peptide reactive with CM-H-9, a monoclonal antibody specific for placental ferritin. *Proc. Natl. Acad. Sci. USA* **86**, 3282–3285.

Müllner, E. W. and Kühn, L. C. (1988) A stem-loop in the 3′ untranslated region mediates iron-dependent regulation of transferrin receptor mRNA stability in the cytoplasm. *Cell* **53**, 815–825.

Müllner, E. W., Neupert, B. and Kühn, L. C. (1989) A specific mRNA binding factor regulates the iron-dependent stability of cytoplasmic transferrin receptor mRNA. *Cell* **58**, 373–382.

Murphy, T. P., Lean, D. R. S. and Nalewajko, C. (1976) Blue-green algae: their excretion of iron-selective chelators enables them to dominate other algae. *Science* **192**, 900–902.

Neilands, J. B. (1972) Evolution of biological iron binding centers. *Struct. Bond.* **11**, 145–170.

Noguchi, T. (1978) A hybrid clock for molecular evolution and an evolutionary clock. In: *Evolution of Protein Molecules* (eds H. Matsubara and T. Yamanaka), Japan Scientific Societies Press, Tokyo, pp. 61–75.

Ochoa, A., Brunel, F., Mendelzon, D., Cohen, G. N. and Zakin, M. M. (1989) Different liver nuclear proteins bind to similar DNA sequences in the 5′ flanking regions of three hepatic genes. *Nucleic Acids Res.* **17**, 119–133.

Oratore, A., D'Alessandro, A. M. and D'Andrea, G. (1989) Effect of synthetic carrier ampholytes on saturation of human serum transferrin. *Biochem. J.* **259**, 909–912.

Park, I., Schaeffer, E., Sidoli, A., Baralle, F. E., Cohen, G. N. and Zakin, M. M. (1985) Organization of the human transferrin gene: Direct evidence that it originated by gene duplication. *Proc. Natl. Acad. Sci. USA* **82**, 3149–3153.

Petropoulos, I., Augé-Gouillou, C. and Zakin, M. M. (1991) Characterization of the active part of the human transferrin gene enhancer and purification of two liver nuclear factors interacting with the TGTTTGC motif present in this region. *J. Biol. Chem.* **266**, 24220–24225.

Plowman, G. D., Brown, J. P., Enns, C. A. *et al.* (1983) Assignment of the gene for human melanoma-associated antigen p97 to chromosome 3. *Nature* **303**, 70–72.

Powell, L. W., Alpert, E., Isselbacher, K. J. and Drysdale, J. W. (1975) Human isoferritins: organ specific iron and apoferritin distribution. *Br. J. Haematol.* **30**, 47–55.

Princiotto, J. V. and Zapolski, E. J. (1975) Difference between the two iron binding sites of transferrin. *Nature* **255**, 87–88.

Rabin, M., McClelland, A., Kühn, L. C. and Ruddle, F. H. (1985) Regional localization of the human transferrin receptor gene to 3q26.2-qter. *Am. J. Hum. Genet.* **37**, 1112–1116.

Ragland, M., Briat, J.-F., Gagnon, J., Laulhère, J.-P., Massenet, O. and Theil, E. C. (1990) Evidence for conservation of ferritin sequences among plants and animals and for a transit peptide in soybean. *J. Biol. Chem.* **265**, 18339–18344.

Reif, D. W. (1992) Ferritin as a source of iron for oxidative damage. *Free Radic. Biol. Med.* **12**, 417–427.

Reif, D. W., Schubert, J. and Aust, S. D. (1988) Iron release from ferritin and lipid peroxidation by radiolytically generated reducing radicals. *Arch. Biochem. Biophys.* **264**, 238–243.

Rocha, E. R., Andrews, S. C., Keen, J. N. and Brock, J. H. (1992) Isolation of a ferritin from *Bacteroides fragilis*. *FEMS Microbiol. Lett.* **95**, 207–212.

Rohrer, J. S., Joo, M.-S., Dartyge, E., Sayers, D. E., Fontaine, A. and Theil, E. C. (1987) Stabilization of iron in a ferrous form by ferritin. *J. Biol. Chem.* **262**, 13385–13387.

Rose, T. M., Plowman, G. D., Teplow, D. B., Dreyer, W. J., Hellstrom, K. E. and Brown, J. P. (1986) Primary structure of the human melanoma-associated antigen p97 (melano-transferrin) deduced from the mRNA sequence. *Proc. Natl. Acad. Sci. USA* **83**, 1261–1265.

Rothenberger, S., Müllner, E. W. and Kühn, L. C. (1990) The mRNA-binding protein which controls ferritin and transferrin receptor expression is conserved during evolution. *Nucleic Acids Res.* **18**, 1175–1179.

Rouault, T. A., Hentze, M. W., Caughman, S. W., Harford, J. B. and Klausner, R. D. (1988) Binding of a cytosolic protein to the iron-responsive element of human ferritin messenger RNA. *Science* **241**, 1207–1210.

Schaeffer, E., Lucero, M. A., Jeltsch, J.-M. *et al.* (1987) Complete structure of the human transferrin gene. Comparison with analogous chicken gene and human pseudogene. *Gene* **56**, 109–116.

Schaeffer, E., Boissier, F., Py, M.-C., Cohen, G. N. and Zakin, M. M. (1989) Cell type-specific expression of the human transferrin gene. Role of promoter, negative and enhancer elements. *J. Biol. Chem.* **264**, 7153–7160.

Scheuhammer, A. M. and Cherian, M. G. (1985) Binding of manganese in human and rat plasma. *Biochim. Biophys. Acta* **840**, 163–169.

Schlabach, M. R. and Bates, G. W. (1975) The synergistic binding of anions and Fe^{3+} by transferrin. *J. Biol. Chem.* **250**, 2182–2188.

Schneider, D. A., Roe, A. L., Mayer, R. J. and Que, L., Jr (1984) Evidence for synergistic anion binding to iron in ovotransferrin complexes from resonance Raman and extended X-ray absorption fine structure analysis. *J. Biol. Chem.* **259**, 9699–9703.

Schrauzer, G. N. and Guth, T. D. (1976) Hydrogen evolving systems. I. The formation of H_2 from aqueous suspensions of $Fe(OH)_2$ and reactions with reducible substrates, including molecular nitrogen. *J. Am. Chem. Soc.* **98**, 3508–3513.

Schwartz, A. W. and Orgel, L. E. (1985) Template-directed polynucleotide synthesis on mineral surfaces. *J. Mol. Evol.* **21**, 299–300.

Seligman, P. A., Schleicher, R. B. and Allen, R. H. (1979) Isolation and characterization of the transferrin receptor from human placenta. *J. Biol. Chem.* **254**, 9943–9946.

Shongwe, M. S., Smith, C. A., Ainscough, E. W., Baker, H. M., Brodie, A. M. and Baker, E. N. (1992) Anion binding by human lactoferrin: Results from crystallographic and physicochemical studies. *Biochemistry* **31**, 4451–4458.

Smith, A. K. and Emery, T. (1982) A novel iron protein from *Desulfovibrio gigas*. *Biochim. Biophys. Acta* **719**, 606–611.

Smith, C. A., Baker, H. M. and Baker, E. N. (1991) Preliminary crystallographic studies of copper(II)- and oxalate-substituted human lactoferrin. *J. Mol. Biol.* **219**, 155–159.

Smith, J. M. A., Ford, G. C. and Harrison, P. M. (1988a) Very-low-resolution structure of a bacterioferritin. *Biochem. Soc. Trans.* **16**, 836–838.

Smith, J. M. A., Quirk, A. V., Plank, R. W. H., Diffin, F. M., Ford, C. and Harrison, P. M. (1988b) The identity of *E. coli* bacterioferritin and cytochrome b1. *Biochem. J.* **255**, 737–740.

Smith, R. M. and Martell, A. M. (1976) *Critical Stability Constants. Volume 4: Inorganic Ligands*, Plenum Press, New York, p. 7.

Spiro, S. and Guest, J. R. (1991) Adaptive responses to oxygen limitation in *E. coli*. *Trends Biochem. Sci.* **16**, 310–314.

Stibler, H. (1991) Carbohydrate-deficient transferrin in serum: A new marker of potentially harmful alcohol consumption reviewed. *Clin. Chem.* **37**, 2029–2037.

Stiefel, E. I. and Watt, G. D. (1979) *Azotobacter* cytochrome$_{557.5}$ is a bacterioferritin. *Nature* **279**, 81–83.

Stratil, A., Bobák, P., Valenta, M. and Tomášek, V. (1983) Partial characterization of transferrins of some species of the family Cyprinidae. *Comp. Biochem. Physiol.* **74B**, 603–610.

Teng, C. T., Pentecost, B. T., Marshall, A. *et al.* (1987) Assignment of the lactotransferrin gene to human chromosome 3 and to mouse chromosome 9. *Somat. Cell Mol. Genet.* **13**, 689–693.

Theil, E. C. (1987) Ferritin: structure, gene regulation, and cellular function in animals, plants and microorganisms. *Annu. Rev. Biochem.* **56**, 289–315.

Tsuji, Y., Miller, L. L., Miller, S. C., Torti, S. V. and Torti, F. M. (1991) Tumor necrosis factor-α and interleukin 1-α regulate transferrin receptor in human diploid fibroblasts. Relationship to the induction of ferritin heavy chain. *J. Biol. Chem.* **266**, 7257–7261.

Vali, H. and Kirschvink, J. L. (1991) Observation of magnetosome organization, surface structure, and iron biomineralization of undescribed magnetic bacteria: evolutionary speculations. In: *Iron Biominerals* (eds R. B. Frankel and R. P. Blakemore), Plenum Press, New York, pp. 97–115.

van der Wal, P. (1991) Structure and formation of the magnetite-bearing cap of Polyplacophorian tricuspid radular teeth. In: *Iron Biominerals* (eds R. B. Frankel and R. P. Blakemore), Plenum Press, New York, pp. 221–229.

van Eijk, H. G. and van Noort, W. L. (1986) A non-random distribution of transferrin iron in fresh human sera. *Clin. Chim. Acta* **157**, 299–304.

Vogel, W., Herold, M., Margreiter, R. and Bomford, A. (1989) Occupancy of the iron-binding sites of human transferrin in sera obtained from different anatomical sites. *Klin. Wochenschr.* **67**, 538–542.

Wade, V. J., Levi, S., Arosio, P., Treffry, A., Harrison, P. M. and Mann, S. (1991) Influence of site-directed modifications on the formation of iron cores in ferritin. *J. Mol. Biol.* **221**, 1443–1452.

Watt, G. D., Frankel, R. B. and Papaefthymiou, G. C. (1985) Reduction of mammalian ferritin. *Proc. Natl. Acad. Sci. USA* **82**, 3640–3643.

Watt, G. D., Frankel, R. B., Papaefthymiou, G. C., Spartalian, K. and Stiefel, E. I. (1986) Redox properties and Mossbauer spectroscopy of *Azotobacter vinelandii* bacterioferritin. *Biochemistry* **25**, 4330–4336.

Webb, J., Macey, D. J. and Mann, S. (1989) Biomineralization of iron in molluscan teeth. In: *Biomineralization: Chemical and Biochemical Perspectives* (eds S. Mann, J. Webb and R. J. P. Williams), VCH Publishers, Weinheim, pp. 345–387.

Williams, J. (1982) The evolution of transferrin. *Trends Biochem. Sci.* **7**, 394–397.

Williams, J. and Moreton, K. (1980) The distribution of iron between the metal-binding sites of transferrin in human serum. *Biochem. J.* **185**, 483–488.

Williams, J., Grace, S. A. and Williams, J. M. (1982) Evolutionary significance of the renal excretion of transferrin half-molecule fragments. *Biochem. J.* **201**, 417–419.

Williams, R. J. P. (1990) Iron and the origin of life. *Nature* **343**, 214–215.

Woese, C. R., Kandler, O. and Wheelis, M. L. (1990) Towards a natural system of organisms: Proposal for the domains Achaea, Bacteria and Eucarya. *Proc. Natl. Acad. Sci. USA* **87**, 4576–4579.

Yamashiro, D. J., Fluss, S. R. and Maxfield, F. R. (1983) Acidification of endocytic vesicles by an ATP-dependent proton pump. *J. Cell Biol.* **97**, 929–934.

Yang, F., Lum, J. B., McGill, J. R. *et al.* (1984) Human transferrin: cDNA characterization and chromosomal localization. *Proc. Natl. Acad. Sci. USA* **81**, 2752–2756.

Yariv, J. (1983) The identity of bacterioferritin and cytochrome b_5. *Biochem. J.* **211**, 527.

Young, S. P., Bomford, A. and Williams, R. (1984) The effect of the iron saturation of transferrin on its binding and uptake by rabbit reticulocytes. *Biochem. J.* **219**, 505–510.

Zak, O. and Aisen, P. (1985) Preparation and properties of a single-sited fragment from the C-terminal domain of human transferrin. *Biochim. Biophys. Acta* **829**, 348–353.

Zak, O. and Aisen, P. (1986) Nonrandom distribution of iron in circulating human transferrin. *Blood* **68**, 157–161.

Zapolski, E. J. and Princiotto, J. V. (1976) Failure of rabbit reticulocytes to incorporate conalbumin or lactoferrin iron. *Biochim. Biophys. Acta* **421**, 80–86.

2. The Red Cell Cycle

G. M. BRITTENHAM

Division of Hematology, Department of Medicine, Case Western Reserve University, Cleveland, Ohio, USA

1. INTRODUCTION

Each day, almost 200 billion red blood cells are produced in the normal adult to replace a like number reaching the end of their life span. Each red cell contains more than a billion atoms of iron, four in each tetrameric molecule of haemoglobin, so that more than 200 quintillion (200×10^{18}) atoms of iron are needed daily for erythropoiesis or almost 20 mg of iron by weight. Human iron metabolism is distinguished by an efficient cycling of iron from recently destroyed to newly formed red cells. Normally, less than 0.05% of the total body iron is acquired or lost each day, making humans unique among animals in the effectiveness with which iron is conserved.

The *erythron* consists of the aggregate of all erythroid elements, including cells at all stages of development, immature and mature, and at all sites within the body, in the marrow, circulation and extravascular space. While iron is an essential nutrient required by every human cell, quantitatively most of the iron in the body is found within the erythron and most of the daily movement of iron cycles through the erythron. Physiologically, iron is carried into the erythron by the transport protein transferrin via a specific receptor located on the surface membrane of developing erythroid cells. Most erythron iron is then incorporated into haemoglobin and enters the circulation within red blood cells dedicated to oxygen transport. Small amounts of iron are used in the haem and non-haem enzymes of developing erythroid cells, sequestered within the iron storage protein ferritin or dissipated during ineffective attempts at red cell production. Red cells at the end of their life span are phagocytised by a select population of macrophages in the bone marrow, liver and spleen which then promptly renders up most of the catabolized iron to transferrin for return to the erythron. After summarizing the overall pattern of iron uptake and utilization by the erythron, this chapter will consider in turn each of the portions of the circuit of iron to and from the red cell and conclude with a discussion of iron studies available for the assessment of erythropoiesis.

2. MOVEMENT OF IRON THROUGH THE RED CELL CYCLE

An inventory of the distribution of iron in the body and a schematic representation of the patterns of iron utilization are shown in Fig. 2.1. The concentration of iron in the human body is normally about 40 mg Fe/kg body weight in women and about 50 mg Fe/kg in men (Brittenham, 1991). Most of this iron is a component of various functional compounds devoted to oxygen transport, delivery, utilization or consumption. The major portion of iron is found in the erythron as haemoglobin iron (28 mg/kg in women, 32 mg/kg in men) dedicated to oxygen transport and delivery. Small amounts of erythron iron (< 1 mg/kg) are also present in haem and non-haem enzymes in developing red cells. The remainder of functional iron is found as myoglobin iron (4 mg/kg in women, 5 mg/kg in men) in muscle and as iron-containing and iron-dependent enzymes (1–2 mg/kg) throughout the cells of the body. Small amounts of iron are deposited within ferritin in erythroid cells but most storage iron (5–6 mg Fe/kg in women, 10–12 mg Fe/kg in men) is held in reserve by hepatocytes and macrophages in the liver, bone marrow, spleen and muscle. The small fraction of transport iron (about 0.2 mg/kg) in the plasma and extracellular fluid is bound to the protein transferrin which carries iron to meet tissue needs throughout the body.

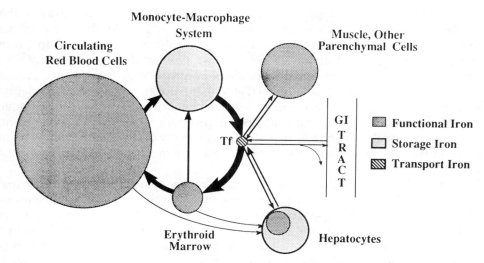

Fig. 2.1 Body iron supply and storage. The figure shows a schematic representation of the routes of iron movement in the adult. The area of each circle is proportional to the amount of iron contained in the compartment and the width of each arrow is proportional to the daily flow of iron from one compartment to another. Transferrin is abbreviated as Tf. Estimates for typical magnitudes of iron flux are provided in the text. The major pathway of internal iron exchange is a unidirectional flow from plasma transferrin to the erythron to the monocyte–macrophage system and back to plasma transferrin. Storage iron in the macrophages of the liver, bone marrow and spleen is derived almost entirely from phagocytosis of senescent erythrocytes or defective developing red cells. The macrophage has a limited ability to take up iron from plasma transferrin while the hepatocyte may either donate iron to or receive iron from plasma transferrin. Normally, the overall magnitude of iron exchange by hepatocytes is only about one-fifth that of macrophages. Other pathways of iron movement involve approximately equal exchanges for iron absorption and losses, for transfer between the plasma and extravascular transferrin compartments, and for movement between extravascular transferrin and parenchymal tissues. The estimates of the size of iron compartments and the magnitude of iron movement shown in the figure are derived from Harris and Kellermeyer, 1970; Bothwell *et al.*, 1979; Finch and Huebers, 1982; and Brittenham, 1991.

This chapter will primarily examine the major pathway of internal iron exchange, shown in Fig. 2.1 as a unidirectional flux from plasma transferrin to the erythron to the macrophage and back to plasma transferrin. In an iron replete 70 kg man, the amount of transferrin iron in the plasma at any given time is only about 3 mg but more than 30 mg of iron moves through this transport compartment each day. Most (about 24 mg Fe/day) of the iron is taken up by erythroid precursors in the marrow. The majority of this iron (17 mg Fe/day) becomes haemoglobin iron in circulating red cells that are subsequently catabolized by specialized macrophages in the marrow, spleen and liver with the iron then released from the haemoglobin and returned to the plasma transferrin. Some of the erythroid marrow iron (7 mg Fe/day) arrives at the macrophage more directly because of phagocytosis of defective erythroid precursors or removal of erythrocyte ferritin, with the result that the macrophage can return to the plasma transferrin an amount of iron (22 mg Fe/day) almost equivalent to that donated to the erythron. The remainder of daily erythron iron turnover is derived from some of the newly absorbed iron from the gastrointestinal tract and from the minor fraction (2 mg Fe/day) of haemoglobin iron that is lost into the plasma with enucleation of normoblasts or from intravascular haemolysis, then bound to haptoglobin or haemopexin and delivered to the hepatocyte for eventual return to plasma transferrin. Movement of iron to and from the erythron accounts for about 80% of the iron flowing through the transferrin compartment each day. The remaining 20% of iron carried by transferrin includes (i) iron exchange with hepatocytes (5 mg Fe/day), (ii) movement between the plasma and extravascular transferrin compartments (about 3 mg Fe/day), (iii) exchange between extravascular transferrin and parenchymal tissues (about 2 mg Fe/day), and (iv) limited external exchange of iron through obligatory losses and absorption of iron from the gastrointestinal tract (about 1 and 1.5 mg Fe per day for men and women, respectively).

Within the body, the supply and storage of iron is mediated by three principal proteins (Table 2.1): (i) *transferrin*, a transport protein which carries iron in the plasma and extracellular fluid to supply tissue needs; (ii) *transferrin receptor*, a glycoprotein on cell membranes which binds the transferrin–iron complex, is internalized in a vesicle where iron is released and then returns to the cell membrane, liberating apotransferrin into the plasma; and (iii) *ferritin*, an iron storage protein which sequesters iron in a presumably non-toxic form while holding it ready for prompt mobilization in time of need. These proteins are described in Chapters 1, 3 and 4; this chapter will describe the integration of their functions within the specific types of cells involved in the red cell cycle. The successive movement of iron from plasma transferrin to the erythron to the macrophage and back to plasma transferrin may now be considered with particular attention to those factors which regulate the flow of iron through the red cell cycle.

2.1. Movement of Iron from Transferrin to the Erythron

The movement of iron from transferrin to the erythron is determined by (i) the aggregate number of transferrin receptors on erythroid precursors in the erythron and on cells in non-erythroid tissues and (ii) the amounts of apo-, mono- and diferric plasma transferrin. This section will describe the pattern of iron uptake and utilization by erythroid cells; control of the supply of iron from macrophages, hepatocytes and enterocytes to transferrin will then be considered. The number of transferrin receptors is a prime determinant of cellular iron supply. Because the number of transferrin receptors in non-erythroid tissues is stable under normal circumstances, the rate of erythropoiesis is the major determinant of the total number of transferrin receptors. As the rate of erythropoiesis increases, greater numbers of erythroid precursors with transferrin receptors are produced, increasing the rate of iron uptake. After considering the interaction of transferrin with transferrin receptors on erythroid cells, the control of iron uptake and utilization for haem synthesis within the erythron will be examined.

2.1.1. *Transferrin-mediated Iron Delivery via the Transferrin Receptor to Erythroid Precursors*

Transferrin (Table 2.1) mediates physiological iron delivery to the erythron (Morgan, 1981; Huebers and Finch, 1987). The total amount of apotransferrin in humans is

Table 2.1 Selected proteins involved in the red cell cycle

Protein	Chromosomal location of gene(s)	M_r	Structure	Function(s)
Transferrin	3q21-qter	79 570	Single-chain glycoprotein with 2 iron-binding sites	Iron transport in plasma and extracellular fluid
Transferrin receptor	3q26.2-qter	185 000	Transmembrane glycoprotein dimer with 2 transferrin-binding sites	Receptor-mediated endocytosis of ferric transferrin; is recycled
Ferritin	H subunit: 11; L subunit: 19; multigene family	440 000	Spherical protein of 24 subunits, binds up to 4500 iron atoms	Iron storage
Iron-responsive element binding protein (IRE-BP)	9	90 000	Member of family of [4 Fe-4 S] cluster proteins; homology with aconitase	Coordinate regulation of translation of ferritin, transferrin receptor and δ-aminolaevulinic acid
Erythropoietin	7pter-q22	34 000	Glycoprotein of 166 amino acids in four antiparallel α-helices with 2 long and 1 short loop connections	Support survival and differentiation of erythroid precursors
Erythropoietin receptor	19p	55 000	Single-chain peptide of 508 amino acids with a single transmembrane domain	Mediate erythroid cell uptake of erythropoietin
Erythroid-specific δ-amino-laevulinic acid synthase	Xp21-q21	59 500	Single-chain peptide of 579 amino acids with presequence of 56 highly basic residues	Catalyses condensation of glycine and succinyl CoA to form δ-amino-laevulinic acid
Haem oxygenase	Not known	32 800	Single-chain peptide of 289 amino acids with hydrophobic region at carboxy terminus	Enzymatic degradation of haem
Haptoglobin	16q22	85 000	α2-glycoprotein	Bind intravascular haemoglobin dimers and transport to hepatocytes
Haptoglobin receptor	Not known	Not known	Membrane glycoprotein	Receptor-mediated endocytosis of haemoglobin–haptoglobin complex
Haemopexin	11p15.4-p15.5	70 000	β-glycoprotein	Bind intravascular haem and transport to hepatocytes
Haemopexin receptor	Not known	85 000	Composed of two subunits of M_r 20 000 and 65 000	Receptor-mediated endocytosis of haem–haemopexin complex; is recycled

about 240 mg/kg, almost equally divided between the plasma and extravascular fluids (Huebers and Finch, 1987). Most apotransferrin is produced by hepatocytes (Aisen, 1984); other potential sources of synthesis are of little importance *in vivo*. Apotransferrin is a true carrier that is not lost in delivering iron so its turnover is unrelated to the plasma iron turnover; the half-life is about 8 days (Awai and Brown, 1963). As discussed in Chapter 1, apotransferrin is a single-chain glycoprotein composed of two homologous N-terminal and C-terminal lobes. Each lobe can independently bind a single ferric ion so the molecule can exist as apotransferrin, as monoferric transferrin with an atom of iron bound in either the N-terminal (Fe_NTf) or C-terminal (Fe_CTf) lobe or as diferric transferrin (Fe_2Tf) (Bali and Aisen, 1991). The lobes are in the shape of prolate ellipsoids and each is further divided into two dissimilar domains. Each iron-binding site is located within the interdomain cleft where the iron is bound by two tyrosines, a histidine and an aspartic acid residue (Bailey *et al.*, 1988). An anion (bicarbonate or carbonate) is bound with each ferric ion, serving as a bridging ligand between the iron and protein, with the remaining coordination site occupied by a water molecule or a hydroxyl ion (Schlabach and Bates, 1975; Chasteen, 1983). Each lobe of transferrin binds ferric iron with high affinity; under physiological conditions the effective stability constant for each is about $10^{24} M^{-1}$ (Aisen and Leibman, 1968). Binding of two atoms of ferric iron by transferrin results in conformational changes making the molecule more compact, more soluble and more resistant to oxidative or tryptic denaturation. The two iron-binding domains differ in their spectroscopic, thermodynamic, kinetic and chemical properties (Zak and Aisen, 1990). A difference in the ability of the two iron-binding sites of transferrin to donate iron to reticulocytes for haemoglobin synthesis was postulated a quarter of a century ago (Fletcher and Huehns, 1968) but the functional physiological importance of the evident physical and chemical differences between the two sites remains uncertain. In fresh sera from healthy individuals, the N-terminal monoferric species (Fe_NTf) is more common than the C-terminal form (Fe_CTf) (Williams and Moreton, 1980; van Eijk and van Noort, 1986; Zak and Aisen, 1990) but so little is known about the manner in which transferrin acquires iron from macrophages and enterocytes (see below) that the significance of this difference remains uncertain.

The transferrin receptor (Table 2.1) not only provides transferrin-bound iron access into the cell but also plays a critical role in the release of iron from transferrin within the cell. Transferrin receptors appear to be expressed on virtually all nucleated cells and are present in large numbers on erythroid precursors. The structure and function of transferrin receptors are discussed in Chapter 3. The number of receptors on the cell surface can be modified to reflect cellular iron requirements as discussed in Chapter 5. Each transferrin receptor can bind two molecules of transferrin; if each transferrin is diferric, the dimeric receptor can carry a total of four atoms of transferrin-bound iron. At a physiologic pH of 7.4, the receptor has very little affinity for apotransferrin, while the affinity for diferric transferrin is more than four-fold greater than for monoferric transferrin (Huebers *et al.*, 1985). Only a single gene for the transferrin receptor has been recognized (Table 2.1), but studies using monoclonal antibodies raised against cultured erythroid cells have suggested the existence of two isoforms of the transferrin receptor: one expressed on all receptor bearing cells and another antigenically distinct form that is preferentially expressed on erythroid precursors (Cotner *et al.*, 1989). The structural basis for this apparently erythroid-specific form of the transferrin receptor has not been determined and functional differences, if any, between the two forms of the receptor have not been characterized.

Iron delivery to an erythroid cell involves the binding of up to two molecules of mono- or diferric transferrin to a transferrin receptor in an energy and temperature dependent process (Jandl and Katz, 1963; Zaman *et al.*, 1980) that is complete within two to three minutes. The efficiency of iron delivery to the cell depends on the amounts of mono- and diferric plasma transferrin available. With normal erythropoiesis and a normal transferrin saturation of about 33%, the higher affinity of the receptor for diferric transferrin results in most of the iron supply to cells being derived from this form, providing four atoms of iron with each cycle. At a transferrin saturation of about 19%, equal amounts of iron are provided by mono- and diferric transferrin while at lower saturations, most of the iron is derived from the monoferric form (Huebers *et al.*, 1985; Huebers and Finch, 1987; Intragumtornchai *et al.*, 1988). Whether mono- or diferric, the fate of transferrin bound to the transferrin receptor is the same. The role of receptor-mediated endocytosis and the acidic endosomal pH (5.6) in releasing the iron is discussed in Chapter 3. Within the endosomes of erythroid cells, iron release is virtually complete from both transferrin sites within two to three minutes (Bomford *et al.*, 1985; Bali *et al.*, 1991). Transferrin receptor binding at endosomal pH seems substantially to enhance both the rate and completeness of iron release from transferrin within the erythroid cell while minimizing differences between the N- and C-terminal sites (Bali and Aisen, 1992) (see Chapters 1 and 3).

The exact form and fate of the iron derived from the endosome are still unknown (Richardson and Baker, 1992) but this newly released iron presumably is available to the mitochondria of the erythroid cell for haem synthesis or to ferritin for storage.

2.1.2. *Erythroid Cell Ferritin*

Iron delivered to developing red cells by the transferrin mechanism that is in excess of erythroid requirements for haem synthesis is sequestered within ferritin. As detailed in Chapters 1 and 4, ferritin is the major iron storage protein, composed of 24 subunits of at least two types: L (or light: M_r 19 700; more acidic with pI 4.5–5.0) and H (or heavy: M_r 21 100; more basic with pI 5.0–5.7) (Ford *et al.*, 1984). Tissues functioning as major iron storage depots, such as liver and spleen, have a preponderance of the L-subunit while tissues which do not normally act as iron storage sites, such as heart, have higher proportions of H-subunits. Within a specific tissue, greater amounts of storage iron are associated with a greater predominance of L-subunits. These patterns have suggested that ferritins enriched in L-subunits may have a long-term iron storage function while ferritins with a predominance of H-subunits may be more active in iron metabolism. Recent studies using site-directed mutagenesis have now found the ferritin H-subunit contains a ferroxidase site lacking from the L-subunit (Broxmeyer *et al.*, 1991; Lawson *et al.*, 1991). Using recombinant human homopolymers, those composed solely of H-subunits have been found to take up iron at a rate several times that of homopolymers composed only of L-subunits (Levi *et al.*, 1988, 1989).

Studies of the erythroid marrow have found that the more immature erythroid precursors, the proerythroblasts and basophilic erythroblasts, contain higher concentrations of intracellular ferritin than mature forms and also have greater proportions of the H-type subunit (Cazzola *et al.*, 1983; Hodgetts *et al.*, 1986; Invernizzi *et al.*, 1990). The physiological role of the iron contained in the H-rich ferritin in erythroid cells has not been established. The possibility that the iron within the H-rich ferritin is stored temporarily before use in haem synthesis was suggested by early studies (Speyer and Fielding, 1979) and has been advocated, along with the suggestion that the L-rich ferritin functions as a more stable reservoir for excess iron (Cazzola *et al.*, 1983; Invernizzi *et al.*, 1990). Other investigations using radiolabelled iron have been unable to demonstrate that erythroid ferritin iron could function as a donor for haem synthesis (Ponka *et al.*, 1982; Adams *et al.*, 1989). In any event, the major determinants of the ferritin content of the erythroid cell appear to be the plasma transferrin saturation, reflecting the iron supply to the erythroblast, and the rate of haemoglobin synthesis, as an indicator of the erythroid iron requirement. Erythroid cell ferritin is decreased in patients with iron deficiency or with severe inflammatory disorders and increased in patients with other conditions where haemoglobin synthesis is reduced, such as thalassaemic disorders or sideroblastic anaemias, or with iron overload (Cazzola and Ascari, 1986).

2.1.3. *Control of Iron and Haem Metabolism during Erythroid Differentiation*

Erythropoiesis is the physiological process of producing and maintaining the haemoglobin–red cell mass. Control of red cell production involves a complex interaction between erythropoietic cells and accessory cells within the microenvironment of the bone marrow together with the interaction of cytokines and growth factors that may support or suppress erythroid proliferation and maturation. The earliest progenitor cells uniquely committed to erythroid maturation are identified as erythroid burst-forming units (BFU-E) which give rise to erythroid colony forming units (CFU-E) which in turn differentiate into the morphologically recognizable erythroid precursors identified as the proerythroblast, the basophilic, the polychromatophilic and the orthochromatic erythroblast and, ultimately, the anucleate reticulocyte. With the synergistic enhancement of c-*kit* ligand, the growth of immature BFU-E is dependent upon the presence of interleukin (IL)-3 and granulocyte colony stimulating factor (G-CSF) or granulocyte–monocyte colony stimulating factor (GM-CSF), while more mature BFU-E undergo a well controlled switch to a dependence on erythropoietin for viability (Krantz, 1991).

Erythropoietin (Table 2.1) acts as the principal humoral regulator of red blood cell production by stimulating the proliferation and differentiation of committed erythroid progenitors (Finch, 1982). Most (85–90%) erythropoietin is produced by peritubular interstitial cells in the kidney in response to hypoxaemia, apparently detected by a haem protein functioning as an oxygen sensor (Goldberg *et al.*, 1988; Krantz, 1991). The remaining 10–15% of plasma erythropoietin is secreted by hepatocytes. Erythropoietin functions by binding to specific erythropoietin receptors on the surface of immature erythroid cells. The erythropoietin receptor has been found to be a member of the haematopoietin receptor superfamily (D'Andrea *et al.*, 1989; Jones *et al.*, 1990) but the structural organization of the receptor, the details of receptor binding to erythropoietin, the roles of high- and low-affinity receptors and the mechanism of signal transduction are still under investigation (Bailey *et al.*, 1991).

The response to erythropoietin is closely correlated with the presence of erythropoietin receptors. BFU-E lack erythropoietin receptors until late in their development when the numbers increase with the emergence of erythropoietin dependency. The number of receptors is highest in CFU-E, with more than 1000 sites per cell, then declines to about 1000 in proerythroblasts, and to 300 or less in early basophilic erythroblasts. As haemoglobin synthesis is established, erythropoietin receptors progressively undergo degradation. Receptors are absent on late basophilic, polychromatophilic and orthochromatic erythroblasts and on reticulocytes; these cells do not require erythropoietin for survival (Jones et al., 1990). Erythropoietin acts to protect erythroid cells, especially CFU-E and proerythroblasts, from apoptosis (programmed cell death), perhaps by preventing DNA cleavage and breakdown (Koury and Bondurant, 1990). Under normal conditions, circulating erythropoietin concentrations permit only a minority of CFU-E to differentiate into mature red cells; most CFU-E do not survive. In response to hypoxia, increases in circulating erythropoietin can quickly rescue additional CFU-E to differentiate into mature red cells. As discussed in Chapter 11, inflammation and inflammatory cytokines may affect erythropoiesis (i) by specifically altering the amounts of erythropoietin produced in response to hypoxia (Faquin et al., 1992), (ii) by diminishing the responsiveness of erythroid progenitors to erythropoietin (Johnson et al., 1989, 1991; Miller et al., 1990), and by altering iron delivery to developing erythroid cells (see below).

The control of the acquisition, utilization and storage of iron seems to differ during the period of erythropoietin dependency from that operative when haemoglobin synthesis is fully established. While the available evidence is fragmentary and incomplete, studies of human bone marrow and of erythroid cell lines in culture have suggested that erythropoietin acts as an inducer for the transcription of messenger ribonucleic acid (mRNA) for the erythroid-specific enzymes δ-aminolaevulinic acid (ALA) synthase and porphobilinogen (PBG) deaminase in the haem biosynthetic pathway (Abraham et al., 1989) and of α- and β-globin mRNA (Nijhof et al., 1987). Repression of haem oxygenase, the enzyme responsible for haem degradation, has been proposed as an initiating event in the differentiation of erythroid progenitors (Abraham, 1991). In erythroblasts, haem enhances the transcription of globin mRNA and acts to increase the stability of globin mRNA (Bonanou-Tzedaki et al., 1984). Other studies, using erythroid cells obtained from chick embryos at early stages of maturation, have found that the transferrin receptor gene is hyperexpressed and regulated at the transcriptional level by mechanisms that are not responsive to the availability of intracellular iron (Chan and Gerhardt, 1992). In the mouse, BFU-E have few transferrin receptors but the number is increased in CFU-E (Lesley et al., 1984). The number of transferrin receptors on the cell surface then progressively increases to about 300 000 per cell at the proerythroblast stage to reach a peak of about 800 000 per cell in basophilic erythroblasts where maximal transferrin and iron uptake occurs (Iacopetta et al., 1982; Iacopetta and Morgan, 1983). Further erythroblast maturation is associated with a fall in the number of receptors to about 100 000 in the circulating reticulocyte. The rate of iron uptake from transferrin during erythroid cell development correlates closely with the number of transferrin receptors. These observations suggest that the level of transferrin receptors is the major factor which determines the rate of iron uptake during erythroid cell development (Iacopetta et al., 1982). The increase in transferrin receptor expression thus follows the increase in the expression of erythropoietin receptors but precedes the onset of haem synthesis (Cox *et al.*, 1990). Using the Friend erythroleukaemia cell model of erythroid differentiation, experimental data have suggested that haem synthesis is required for effective transcription of mRNA for the transferrin receptor (Battistini *et al.*, 1991a) and the H-subunit of ferritin (Coccia *et al.*, 1992). Other studies using the same model have suggested that the increase in haem occurring during erythroid differentiation is required for the optimal transcription of mRNA for globin chains, transferrin receptor and ferritin (Battistini *et al.*, 1991b). After haemoglobin synthesis is fully established in late erythroblasts and reticulocytes, translational control of the expression of transferrin receptor, ferritin and haem seems to become the more important regulatory mechanism.

2.1.4. *Translational Control of Iron Uptake and Storage in Erythroid Precursors*

Overall, the patterns of iron exchange shown schematically in Fig. 2.1 can be considered as the net result of the movement of iron to and from each cell in the body. In turn, a major determinant of the physiological pattern of iron uptake and release seems to be the availability of iron within that cell. The pivotal protein that provides the means for iron to self-regulate its intracellular availability is the *iron-responsive element-binding protein* (IRE-BP) (Leibold and Munro, 1988; Rouault *et al.*, 1988). The IRE-BP is a *trans*-acting cytoplasmic ribonucleic acid (RNA) binding protein that regulates the expression of messenger ribonucleic acids mRNAs containing a *cis*-acting regulatory structure termed the iron-responsive element (IRE) (Hentze *et al.*, 1987). The structure and function of the IRE and IRE-BP are described in Chapter 5. The available evidence suggests that the IRE-BP is an iron-sulfur protein that functions by reversible interconversions between the [3Fe-4S] and [4Fe-4S] states of its Fe-S cluster (Constable *et al.*, 1992; see below). According to this scheme, the reduced [3Fe-4S] form of the IRE-BP is increased when there is less available intracellular iron, and has a high affinity for the IRE. By contrast the oxidized [4Fe-4S] form is increased in the presence of readily available intracellular iron and has a low affinity for the IRE.

In erythroid precursors that are actively synthesizing haemoglobin – erythroblasts and reticulocytes – the IRE-BP provides the means for the coordinate regulation of the physiological uptake and storage of iron by translational control of the synthesis of transferrin receptor and ferritin (Cox *et al.*, 1985; Rouault *et al.*, 1985, 1988; Leibold and Munro, 1988; Harford and Klausner, 1990). Transferrin receptor synthesis is controlled by adjusting the amounts of cytoplasmic transferrin receptor mRNA. The 3' untranslated region (3' UTR) of transferrin receptor mRNA contains five IREs. Binding of IRE-BPs to the IREs in the 3' UTR retards cytoplasmic degradation, increasing the concentration of cytoplasmic transferrin receptor mRNA and the rate of transferrin receptor synthesis. With an increased number of cellular transferrin receptors, iron uptake is enhanced. By contrast, ferritin synthesis is controlled without changes in the amount of ferritin mRNA present by repressing translation of ferritin mRNA. The 5' untranslated region (5' UTR) of ferritin mRNA contains a single IRE. Binding of an IRE-BP to the IRE in the 5' UTR arrests translation of the ferritin mRNA so less ferritin is produced and iron sequestration is diminished. Altogether, the coordinate regulation of intracellular iron availability by the IRE-BP has opposite effects on the synthesis of transferrin receptor and ferritin. These balanced and opposing alterations in iron uptake and storage governed by the IRE-BP serve to maintain consistent physiological iron homeostasis within the developing erythroid cell.

2.1.5. *Erythroid Iron Utilization*

Almost all of the iron taken up by the erythron is used for the synthesis of haem, the prosthetic group of haemoglobin, with small amounts reserved for use in iron-containing enzymes in erythroid cells or sequestered within ferritin. In the adult, the erythron produces over 85% of the total haem synthesized in the body with most of the remainder produced by the liver (Granick and Sassa, 1978). Haem (ferrous protoporphyrin IX) is a planar molecule consisting of an atom of ferrous iron in the centre of a tetrapyrrole ring. Haem is synthesized in eight biochemical steps with the first and final three steps catalysed by mitochondrial enzymes and the four intermediate steps taking place in the cytoplasm. The final synthetic step is the formation of haem from protoporphyrin IX and ferrous iron, catalysed by the mitochondrial enzyme, ferrochelatase.

(a) *Control of haem synthesis*. In human erythroid cells, haem synthesis seems to be controlled at the first step in the production of protoporphyrin IX. Feedback inhibition by haem limits one or more steps which lead to the formation of δ-aminolaevulinic acid, the first committed precursor in the porphyrin pathway (Gardner and Cox, 1988; Gardner *et al.*, 1991). In erythroid cells, this first enzymatic reaction in haem biosynthesis is catalysed by the erythroid-specific form (see below) of 5-aminolaevulinate synthase (ALA synthase) and consists of the condensation of glycine and succinyl CoA to form δ-aminolaevulinic acid, a reaction requiring pyridoxal phosphate. Haem does not affect the level of the mRNA for erythroid-specific ALA synthase and has no evident direct effect on the enzyme. Instead, haem seems to reduce the activity of the erythroid-specific ALA synthase by an indirect cellular process that has not yet been characterized (Cox *et al.*, 1990; Gardner *et al.*, 1991).

The enzymes of the haem biosynthetic pathway must be expressed during the life of each cell in the body to provide for cytochrome and other vital haem enzymes. In addition to these constitutive or 'housekeeping enzymes' produced during the life of all cells, erythroid-specific isozymes have been identified for ALA synthase, which catalyses the first step in the haem biosynthetic pathway, and for porpho-bilinogen deaminase (PBG deaminase), which catalyses the third. In humans, the two isozymes for ALA-synthase are encoded by different genes, with the gene for the constitutive or 'housekeeping' isozyme on chromosome 3p21 and that for the erythroid-specific form on the X chromosome (Xp21-q21) (Sutherland *et al.*, 1988; Bishop *et al.*, 1990; Fujita *et al.*, 1991). Only a single gene for PBG deaminase is present in the human genome but this gene has two overlapping transcription units (Grandchamp *et al.*, 1987). An upstream promoter is active in all cells while the downstream promoter is erythroid-specific (Chretien *et al.*, 1988). Alternative splicing produces two mRNAs which encode the PBG deaminase isozymes (Mignotte *et al.*, 1989a; Raich *et al.*, 1989). Studies of the promoter regions for the erythroid-specific forms of ALA synthase and PBG deaminase have established that both have *cis*-acting control motifs similar to those in the β-globin gene promoters, including both GATA-1 and NF-E2 binding sites (Chretien *et al.*, 1988; Mignotte *et al.*, 1989a,b; Cox *et al.*, 1991). These observations suggest that globin genes and the erythroid-specific forms of both ALA synthase and PBG deaminase are all subject to developmental control by common *trans*-acting factors during erythropoiesis (Cox *et al.*, 1991). These *trans*-acting factors may mediate the effects of erythropoietin on the transcription of mRNAs for globin, ALA synthase and PBG deaminase described above.

The erythroid ALA synthase gene on the X chromosome has also been found to contain an IRE motif in the 5' UTR which is not present in the 'housekeeping' gene on chromosome 3. The available studies provide strong experimental evidence that the corresponding IRE is functional *in vivo* and that, if intracellular iron availability is low, binding of an IRE-BP will prevent translation of the erythroid-specific ALA synthase mRNA (Cox *et al.*, 1991; Dandekar *et al.*, 1991) (see also Chapter 5). The IRE in the 5' UTR of the erythroid-specific ALA synthase mRNA may help coordinate iron uptake and haem synthesis in erythroid cells (Dandekar *et al.*, 1991). The observation that erythroid ALA synthase activity is decreased in erythroblasts from bone marrow obtained from patients with iron deficiency (Houston *et al.*, 1991) is consistent with translational regulation of erythroid ALA synthase mRNA by the IRE-BP. A reduction in erythroid ALA synthase activity in patients with iron deficiency anaemia has been suggested to be a protective mechanism in erythroblasts to prevent the accumulation of porphyrins and porphyrin precursors and the manifestations of acquired porphyria (Houston *et al.*, 1991). Red cell protoporphyrin concentrations do increase with iron deficiency anaemia (Brittenham, 1991) but the magnitude of the increase may be restricted by translational regulation of erythroid ALA synthase activity. The experimental data seem to exclude any involvement of the IRE in the 5' UTR of the mRNA in the feedback inhibition of erythroid ALA synthase by haem (Gardner *et al.*, 1991). Haemin (ferric protoporphyrin IX) has been reported to inactivate the IRE-BP (Lin *et al.*, 1990a,b, 1991; Goessling *et al.*, 1992) but both the specificity of this effect and the physiological relevance of this observation are uncertain (Haile *et al.*, 1990; Eisenstein *et al.*, 1991). Release of iron from haem into the intracellular iron pool may affect iron-regulated systems but this is an effect of the iron derived from haem rather than a direct effect of haem itself (Rouault *et al.*, 1985; Eisenstein *et al.*, 1991). Altogether, the available evidence suggests that regulation of the activity of erythroid-specific ALA synthase and, thereby, of the rate of haem synthesis in erythroid cells, involves (i) developmental *transcriptional* control by erythroid-specific *trans*-acting factors, (ii) feedback inhibition by haem through a still undefined mechanism that does not influence the availability of the mRNA for the enzyme, and (iii) intracellular iron availability through IRE-BP control of the *translation* of the erythroid-specific ALA synthase mRNA.

(b) *Other regulatory roles for iron availability in erythroid precursors.* Iron availability in erythroid cells may not only specifically alter the rates of production of haem, transferrin receptor and ferritin through the IRE-BP but may also have more general effects on the metabolism of the developing erythroid cell. As described in Chapter 5, human IRE-BP has been found to share (Kaptain *et al.*, 1991; Constable *et al.*, 1992) considerable amino acid sequence homology with two iron-sulfur (Fe-S) proteins, aconitase and isopropylmalate isomerase (Hentze and Argos, 1991; Rouault *et al.*, 1991). Aconitase [citrate (isocitrate) hydro-lyase] is an enzyme in the

Krebs cycle that catalyses the interconversion of citrate and isocitrate via dehydration to *cis*-aconitate and subsequent rehydration (Zheng *et al.*, 1992). The 18 active site residues of mitochondrial aconitase and of the IRE-BP are identical. Moreover, purified IRE-BP has been shown to have aconitase activity and may account for some or all of the cytoplasmic aconitase activity in cells (Hentze and Argos, 1991; Kaptain *et al.*, 1991; Rouault *et al.*, 1991). While no formal characterization of the iron-sulfur cluster chemistry of the IRE-BP has yet been reported, the resemblance between IRE-BP and aconitase has led to the suggestion that the IRE-binding and aconitase activities of the IRE-BP are inversely coupled *in vivo* (Constable *et al.*, 1992). According to this hypothesis, with low intracellular iron, the IRE-BP would be in the reduced, high-affinity [3Fe-4S] state with increased binding to IREs. With increased intracellular iron, the IRE-BP would be converted into the oxidized, low-affinity [4Fe-4S] state, detach from IREs and become enzymatically active as an aconitase. Although not yet reported for erythroid cells, the finding of an IRE in the 5' UTR of (pig heart) *mitochondrial* aconitase (Dandekar *et al.*, 1991) raises the possibility of a further role for iron availability in the regulation of cellular metabolism by coupling iron availability and the activity of the Krebs cycle.

(c) *Coordination of haem and globin synthesis.* Haem, in addition to self-regulating its own synthesis, has other regulatory roles in the formation of haemoglobin in developing erythroid cells. Haem also controls the initiation step of globin mRNA translation (London *et al.*, 1987). During the initiation process in reticulocyte lysates, eukaryotic initiation factor (eIF)-2 forms a ternary complex with methionyl-tRNA$_f$ and GTP, catalysing the binding of the initiator tRNA to the 40S ribosomal subunit. Lack of haem activates a protein kinase (called haemin-controlled repressor (HCR) or inhibitor (HCI)) that phosphorylates the smallest, or a, subunit of eIF-2. This phosphorylation of eIF-2a impairs the ability of a 'reversing factor' (eIF-2B) to promote exchange of GTP for GDP bound to eIF-2 and thereby permit eIF-2 to recycle and form a new ternary complex with methionyl-tRNA$_f$. The eIF-2B is bound to the fraction of eIF-2 that is contained in the complex composed of eIF-2, phosphorylated eIF-2a and GDP (London *et al.*, 1987). Inhibition of polypeptide chain initiation is also mediated by the inability to dissociate eIF-2·GDP from the 60S subunit of complete initiation complexes (Gross *et al.*, 1987), further contributing to the block in recycling eIF-2. This translational control mechanism is not restricted to the initiation of globin chain synthesis alone but also affects the production of nonglobin proteins (Lodish and Desalu, 1973).

While sufficient haem is required for efficient protein synthesis, an excess is deleterious (Ranu and London, 1979; Gardner and Cox, 1988) and is avoided by the self-regulation by haem of its own synthesis as described above. Minor imbalances between haem and globin chain biosynthesis in the developing erythroid cell are managed either by adenosine triphosphate (ATP)-dependent proteolysis for globin excess (Haas *et al.*, 1982; Speiser and Etlinger, 1982) or by microsomal haem oxygenase for excess haem (Tenhunen *et al.*, 1970). Once formed, the reaction between haem and globin is rapid (Rose and Olson, 1983) and haem is probably incorporated into the globin chain either during translation or shortly thereafter. Haem-containing α- and β-subunits then combine in an electrostatic, noncovalent, but nearly irreversible, reaction to form an $\alpha\beta$ dimer. Pairs of $\alpha\beta$ dimers then join, in a readily reversible reaction, to form the functioning $\alpha_2\beta_2$-tetramer of haemoglobin A (Bunn, 1987).

Orthochromatic erythroblasts, with nuclei that are unable to synthesize DNA, gradually lose most mitochondria and halt RNA synthesis but continue to produce haemoglobin. The pyknotic nucleus is finally extruded through the erythroblast membrane with the loss of about 5–10% of the haemoglobin that had been synthesized previously. The resultant reticulocyte continues to synthesize haemoglobin for another 2–3 days until the cellular supply of mRNA is exhausted, producing as much as 30% of the total haemoglobin complement of the cell. Eventually the reticulocyte is released from the marrow and remodelled and pitted of siderotic granules and debris within the spleen to emerge as a mature red cell dedicated to oxygen delivery over its lifespan of three to four months.

2.2. Movement of Iron from the Erythron to the Macrophage

The major pathway of iron movement from the erythron is to a specialized population of macrophages in the bone marrow, liver and spleen as red cells reach the end of their lifespan (Fig. 2.1). While the developing erythroid cell is dedicated to the acquisition of iron from transferrin for use in haemoglobin synthesis, these select macrophages are devoted to the extraction of iron from haemoglobin for prompt return to transferrin or, if necessary, for storage for future use. In contrast to the detailed understanding that has been gained about haemoglobin synthesis and red cell production, little information is available about the determinants of the fate of the senescent red cell and its contents. Less is known about the molecular mechanisms underlying the disposition of iron by the macrophage than about any other aspect of iron metabolism (Aisen, 1990). This section of the chapter will briefly consider factors involved in the removal of erythrocytes from the circulation and then examine the processing of the iron derived from the catabolism of red cell haemoglobin. The recycling of this iron to circulating transferrin will be discussed in a subsequent section.

2.2.1. Removal of Senescent Erythrocytes from the Circulation

Senescent or damaged erythrocytes are selectively recognized and removed from the blood stream by a specialized population of macrophages in the bone marrow, liver and especially in the spleen. Macrophages in the bone marrow also have the responsibilities of culling defective immature erythroid cells to prevent their release into the circulation and of removing some deposits of erythrocyte ferritin from developing red cells. During their time in the blood stream, red cells undergo oxidant damage, alterations of membrane proteins and lipids, loss of surface sialic acid and electrostatic charge, decreases in ion gradients and metabolic depletion of glycolytic and other enzymes (Clark, 1988; Danon and Marikovsky, 1988; Thorburn and Beutler, 1991). Hemichrome formation with oxidative damage to membrane transport proteins may produce increased membrane permeability and defective volume regulation (Low et al., 1985). Crosslinking by haemoglobin or hemichromes of membrane band-3 molecules and the formation of 'senescent' antigens have been reported (Kay et al., 1982; Low et al., 1985; Lutz et al., 1988). Aged erythrocytes become dehydrated and lose surface area, with a decrease in cell volume and an increase in intracellular haemoglobin concentration making the cells less deformable

(Waugh *et al.*, 1992). Despite all these known changes in aged red cells, the characteristic or combination of characteristics that is the proximate cause of the removal of senescent erythrocytes from the circulation remains unknown. Under normal circumstances, billions of red cells are eliminated from the circulation each day without any evidence of overt erythrophagocytosis within macrophages, suggesting that some form of erythrocyte fragmentation occurs before ingestion by macrophages (Jandl, 1987).

2.2.2. *Role of the Macrophage in Red Blood Cell Destruction*

The heterogeneity of the monocyte–macrophage system *in vivo* greatly complicates the design and interpretation of studies of their iron metabolism. Normally, a distinct set of macrophages in the liver, spleen and bone marrow, having specialized adaptations not shared by all mononuclear phagocytes, is specifically dedicated to reprocessing haemoglobin iron from senescent erythrocytes. Macrophages are likely to differ in their handling of iron depending upon (i) the specific type of macrophage studied (peritoneal, alveolar, marrow or splenic macrophages; Kupffer cells; peripheral blood monocytes, isolated or in culture; cultured cell lines), (ii) the amount and form in which the iron is presented (including haemoglobin iron within erythrocytes, transferrin-bound iron, lactoferrin iron, iron chelates, iron-containing enzymes, colloidal or particulate iron), (iii) the state of the macrophage (extent of iron-loading; exposure to inflammatory stimuli and cytokines); and (iv) whether studies are carried out *in vivo* or *in vitro*, in short- or long-term culture, with isolated cells or cell lines. These limitations in the available experimental data created by the heterogeneity of the monocyte–macrophage system underlie many uncertainties about the conclusions that can be reached from the investigations described below.

The overall pattern of the metabolism of catabolized haemoglobin in humans has been examined using heat-damaged erythrocytes labelled with radioactive iron (Fillet *et al.*, 1989). After injection of the labelled red cells, a delay of about 40 minutes precedes the appearance of radioiron in the plasma, presumably representing the time needed for phagocytosis of the damaged erythrocytes and catabolism of haem. Radioiron is then released in a biphasic manner, a pattern that has also been observed in dogs (Fillet *et al.*, 1974) and in macrophages in culture (Bassett *et al.*, 1982; Custer *et al.*, 1982; Brock *et al.*, 1984). In normal human volunteers, two-thirds of the administered radioiron reemerges in an early, rapid phase of iron release with a $t_{1/2}$ of slightly more than half an hour; the remaining third is incorporated into macrophage stores and reappears in a late, slow phase with a $t_{1/2}$ of about 6 days (Fillet *et al.*, 1989). With iron deficiency, iron release is derived entirely from the recently catabolized erythrocyte. With increasing iron stores, the proportion of the radioiron derived from ingested red cells declines, especially during the early, rapid phase of iron output. The rate of late release is also influenced by the magnitude of iron stores; the greater the amount of storage iron, the longer the delay in release. In these studies, the macrophage seemed unable to retain more than 80% of the administered radioiron in storage form, even with plasma transferrin fully saturated (Fillet *et al.*, 1989). Inflammation (Noyes *et al.*, 1960; Lipschitz *et al.*, 1971a; Fillet *et al.*, 1989) and ascorbic acid deficiency (Lipschitz *et al.*, 1971b) also increase the proportion of catabolized erythrocyte iron retained within macrophages.

The catabolism of red cells after phagocytosis by macrophages *in vitro* has been examined ultrastructurally in studies of the processing of IgG-coated red blood cells by Kupffer cells (Edwards and Simon, 1970; Munthe-Kass, 1976; Munthe-Kass *et al.*, 1976; Rama *et al.*, 1988). Studies have suggested that each macrophage is able to process fully at least one ingested erythrocyte per hour (Kondo *et al.*, 1988). Ingested antibody-coated erythrocytes are surrounded by projections of the plasma membrane and moved to the perinuclear area. Macrophage lysosomes fuse with the vacuole containing the phagocytozed red cell, forming a network of inter-connecting channels which fragment the erythrocyte as its components are digested (Edwards and Simon, 1970). The erythrocyte membrane is lysed and the haemoglobin within oxidatively precipitated. Almost all the haemoglobin is rapidly catabolized with the globin proteolytically processed to amino acids, releasing haem. The haem is somehow transported to the endoplasmic reticulum of the macrophage to be degraded by haem oxygenase. Erythrophagocytosis has been shown to induce synthesis of haem oxygenase (Clerget and Polla, 1990).

2.2.3. *Catabolism of Haemoglobin Iron*

Haem oxygenase (Table 2.1) is a microsomal enzyme that catalyses the rate-limiting step in the oxidative catabolism of haem. Two isoforms (or isozymes) of haem oxygenase have been recognized in rat liver and testis, and designated as HO-1 and HO-2 (Maines *et al.*, 1986; Trakshel *et al.*, 1986), but studies of the form or forms present in macrophages have not been reported. Recent studies have suggested that the two forms of haem oxygenase may be different gene products (Cruse and Maines, 1988; McCoubrey *et al.*, 1992); only HO-1 seems to be substrate inducible by haem. The process of haem degradation by haem oxygenase has been characterized as a series of autocatalytic oxidations with the reaction intermediates as cofactors (Abraham *et al.*, 1988). A total of three oxygen molecules and six reducing equivalents is required to degrade oxidatively one haem molecule to biliverdin IXα with one iron and one carbon monoxide molecule released. The precise reaction sequence has not been established but a single haem oxygenase binds a single haem and cleaves the α-methane bridge, leaving a biliverdin–iron complex. The α-methane carbon is converted to carbon monoxide, the sole physiological source of carbon monoxide in the body. Iron is then released from the biliverdin–iron complex, generating the linear tetrapyrrole biliverdin IXα which is then reduced by biliverdin reductase to bilirubin IXα (Abraham *et al.*, 1988).

The disposition of iron after release from haem by haem oxygenase is incompletely understood. The fraction of this iron that is retained within the macrophage will be considered here; the portion that is returned to plasma transferrin will be discussed below. Presumably the iron freed from haem enters an intracellular reservoir where the IRE-BP monitors iron availability. The expression and regulation of IRE-BP and of transferrin receptor and ferritin have recently been examined in cultures of human peripheral blood monocytes maturing to macrophages. While peripheral blood monocytes have few transferrin receptors, cultured monocytes and macrophages of a variety of types seem to express surface transferrin receptors and to be able to take up iron by this route (MacSween and MacDonald, 1969; Hirata *et al.*, 1986). By contrast, ferrokinetic investigations in humans have found no evidence for movement of iron from transferrin to the macrophage *in vivo* (Finch *et al.*, 1970), although these studies may be less sensitive than studies of individual cells. Maturation of monocytes to macrophages was associated with marked increases in active (reduced, high affinity) IRE-BP and in both mRNA and protein for transferrin receptor and ferritin, probably as a result of increased gene *transcription* (Testa *et al.*, 1991). Most importantly, exposure of cultured macrophages to iron salts *stimulated* IRE-BP activity and seemed to be associated with a *translationally* mediated *increase* in both transferrin receptor and ferritin synthesis; treatment with the iron chelator desferrioxamine decreased transferrin receptor synthesis (Testa *et al.*, 1991). These results should be contrasted with the findings in erythroid cells where an increase in iron exposure would diminish IRE-BP activity with a resultant decrease in transferrin receptor synthesis and an increase in ferritin synthesis; treatment with an iron chelator would result in an increase in transferrin receptor synthesis. The consequences of these contrasting patterns of response to iron loading would apparently be to maintain a constant and consistent supply of iron for utilization in haem synthesis in the erythroid cell but to increase iron acquisition and storage in the macrophage. Overall, this pattern would serve to move iron to the erythron from the macrophage in times of lack but to store iron within the macrophage system during periods of excess. The molecular bases for the difference in regulation of transferrin receptor and ferritin synthesis in the developing erythroid cell and the macrophage have not yet been determined.

2.2.4. *Storage of Iron within the Macrophage*

Under normal circumstances, the macrophages in the liver, spleen and bone marrow that are dedicated to reprocessing haemoglobin iron from senescent erythrocytes maintain an equilibrium between iron storage and release. Whatever the molecular mechanisms involved, synthesis of ferritin is induced in response to erythrophagocytosis and, in the absence of iron deficiency, a portion of the iron derived from the ingested erythrocyte is retained within the macrophage as ferritin iron. No data are available to indicate whether incorporation into ferritin is an obligatory step during the passage of all iron through the macrophage or whether only that fraction to be stored is incorporated into ferritin. Based on studies with heat-damaged erythrocytes labelled with radioactive iron, the fraction of radio-iron sequestered within the macrophage can vary from virtually none in association with iron deficiency to a maximum of almost 80% in the presence of marrow aplasia and a fully saturated plasma transferrin (Fillet *et al.*, 1989). Within the macrophage, this iron is stored predominantly in ferritin rich L-subunits (Invernizzi *et al.*, 1990). While no data are available for macrophage ferritin, the half-life of hepatic ferritin is about 60 hours (Treffry *et al.*, 1984). Catabolism of cellular ferritin may result from digestion of the protein shell with reutilization of the iron core or in conversion to haemosiderin, an amorphous water insoluble storage compound with a higher iron content and slower turnover than ferritin that is suitable for long-term storage of iron (Wixom *et al.*, 1980; Richter, 1984). With increasing amounts of storage iron within the macrophage, the proportion of iron stored within haemosiderin progressively increases. Ascorbic acid seems to retard ferritin degradation by reducing lysosomal autophagy of the protein (Bridges and Hoffman, 1986; Bridges, 1987), thereby increasing the amount of iron stored in cytoplasmic ferritin. The effects of inflammation on iron storage within the macrophage are detailed in Chapter 11. As will be noted below, ferritin and haemosiderin iron stored within the macrophage remains available for mobilization in time of need.

2.3. Movement of Iron from the Erythron to the Hepatocyte

The remaining pathway of iron movement from the erythron provides a means for haemoglobin iron that is released into the plasma with the enucleation of erythroblasts or as a result of intramedullary or intravascular haemolysis to be delivered to the hepatocyte for eventual return to the plasma transferrin (Fig. 2.1). With normal erythropoiesis this portion of the total iron flux is minor but can increase substantially in disorders with increased ineffective erythropoiesis or intravascular haemolysis. Delivery of haemoglobin iron from the plasma to hepatocytes depends primarily upon two glycoproteins (Table 2.1), (i) haptoglobin for the binding and transport of $\alpha\beta$-dimers of haemoglobin, and (ii) haemopexin for the binding and transport of haem, assisted, if needed, by albumin.

2.3.1. Release of Haemoglobin into the Plasma

Haemoglobin may escape into the plasma with the enucleation of erythroblasts on their transformation into reticulocytes, with the destruction of defective developing red cells within the marrow or with haemolysis in the circulation. At the low plasma concentration of haemoglobin produced by these processes, most of the haemoglobin A dissociates into $\alpha\beta$ dimers. Pairs of $\alpha\beta$ dimers are then quickly bound in a symmetrical fashion to a single molecule of haptoglobin (Table 2.1). The half-life of apohaptoglobin is about five days but that of the haemoglobin–haptoglobin complex is only about 10–30 minutes as the complexes are cleared by specific hepatocyte receptors (Oshiro and Nakajima, 1988). The haemoglobin–haptoglobin complex (M_r 150 000) is too large to be filtered by the kidneys, a feature that helps restrict the renal loss of iron with haemoglobinaemia. After binding to the haptoglobin receptor of the hepatocyte (Table 2.1) the haemoglobin–haptoglobin receptor complex is internalized and dissociated symmetrically by limited proteolysis into two subunits of M_r 82 000 having intact haems. Unlike the transferrin–transferrin receptor complex, the haemoglobin–haptoglobin receptor is degraded and cannot be recycled. The haems are then released to an unidentified carrier and catabolized by haem oxygenase, releasing iron within the hepatocyte (Oshiro and Nakajima, 1988; Okuda et al., 1992). Consumption of haptoglobin does not induce increased hepatic production with the result that sustained haemoglobinaemia produces hypo- or ahaptoglobinaemia. Haptoglobin is a positive acute phase reactant so inflammatory or infectious episodes may increase plasma concentrations.

Haemoglobin leaked into the plasma that is not bound to haptoglobin is soon oxidized to ferrihaemoglobin (methaemoglobin) that in turn can dissociate into globin and ferrihaem (methaem). Ferrihaem can then be bound by haemopexin (Table 2.1); a single haemopexin binds a single ferrihaem (Muller-Eberhard, 1970). The half-life of apohaemopexin is about seven days but that of the haem–haemopexin complex is 7–8 h as the complexes are cleared by specific hepatocyte receptors (Smith and Hunt, 1990; Smith et al., 1991). After binding to the hepatocyte haemopexin receptor (Table 2.1) the haem–haemopexin receptor complex is internalized within clathrin-coated pits. Receptor-mediated endocytosis of the haem–haemopexin results in catabolism of haem but not of the haemopexin or haemopexin receptor which are recycled to the cell surface for reutilization in a manner analogous to the transferrin–transferrin receptor complex (Smith and Hunt, 1990). Delivery of haem into the hepatocyte results in induction of haem oxygenase, which releases the iron from the haem in the cell (Alam and Smith, 1989; Taketani et al., 1990). Despite recycling, haemopexin may become depleted in patients with haemolysis. Each molecule of human albumin contains two binding sites for ferrihaem but these have a much lower affinity than the binding site of haemopexin. Binding of ferrihaem produces methaemalbumin which, after a delay of several days, ultimately also delivers the haem to the hepatocyte where the iron is liberated for reuse (Bunn and Jandl, 1968). The further metabolism of iron by the hepatocyte is described in Chapter 4.

2.4. Movement of Iron from the Macrophage to Transferrin

The final step in the movement of iron through the red cell cycle requires the return of iron derived from the catabolism of senescent erythrocytes to plasma transferrin (Fig. 2.1) for delivery to the erythroid marrow. The outpouring of iron to plasma apotransferrin from macrophages in the bone marrow, liver and spleen normally constitutes the largest single flux of iron from cells in the body. Despite the importance and magnitude of this flow of iron, the mechanisms permitting the exit of iron from the macrophage remain an almost complete mystery. Virtually no definite information is available about (i) the form of iron within the cell before its departure, (ii) the manner in which the iron is able to pass through the plasma membrane, (iii) the form of the iron on its emergence from the cell, (iv) the site and manner of delivery of the iron to plasma apotransferrin, or (v) the physiological relevance and quantitative importance of iron release from the macrophage that is not mediated by transferrin but involves ferritin or other carriers.

2.4.1. Release of Macrophage Iron to Transferrin

As noted above, studies with radiolabelled, heat-damaged erythrocytes in normal volunteers have found a biphasic pattern of release of iron from the macrophage, with an early, rapid phase ($t_{1/2}$ about 30 minutes) and a late, slow phase ($t_{1/2}$ about 6 days) (Fillet et al., 1989). Variations in iron release from the macrophage have been considered to be responsible for diurnal variations in the plasma iron concentration. The amount of the iron released is a function, in part, of the amount delivered to the macrophage. Modest increases in the red cell load to the macrophage without changes in the activity of the erythroid marrow may be matched by similar increases in iron release to the plasma, but with larger amounts an increased proportion of the iron will be stored within the macrophage (Noyes et al., 1960; Fillet et al., 1974). In some manner, iron release from the macrophage also seems to be influenced by erythroid marrow requirements (Bothwell et al., 1979). With iron deficiency, all the iron derived from haemoglobin catabolism is promptly returned to the plasma and none is diverted to macrophage stores (Fillet *et al.*, 1989). With the increase in erythropoiesis associated with acute blood loss, macrophage iron stores are mobilized but the maximal rate of release from this source in the adult is limited to about 40–60 mg iron per day (Hillman and Henderson, 1969). If erythroid marrow activity is increased in association with a sustained haemolytic state in which nonviable cells are returned to the macrophage, as much as 80–160 mg of iron per day may be released from the macrophage to transferrin (Hillman and Henderson, 1969). Decreases in erythropoiesis can be matched by reductions in macrophage iron release to some extent but a minimum of about 20% of the iron load presented to the macrophage must be returned to the plasma daily (Bothwell *et al.*, 1979; Fillet *et al.*, 1989). Iron release from macrophages may be inadequate to meet erythroid marrow needs in inflammatory states (Noyes *et al.*, 1960; Beamish *et al.*, 1971; Lipschitz *et al.*, 1971b; Hershko *et al.*, 1974; Cavill *et al.*, 1977; Fillet *et al.*, 1989) (see also Chapter 11), ascorbate deficiency (Lipschitz *et al.*, 1971a), and copper deficiency. In copper deficiency, hypoferraemia is corrected by the administration of ceruloplasmin but not by copper itself (Ragan *et al.*, 1969; Osaki *et al.*, 1971).

While the overall patterns of iron release from the macrophage in various circumstances have been described, the underlying mechanisms are almost entirely obscure. The release of iron is temperature dependent, with the rate at 4°C less than one-fifth that at 37°C (Custer *et al.*, 1982; Kondo *et al.*, 1988), implying that macrophage processing and release of iron are energy-dependent processes. After the completion of erythrophagocytosis, iron export is not affected by iodoacetate, chloroquine, colchicine, cytochalasin B or cyclohexamide, suggesting the lack of any role in the release process for glycolysis, acidification of an intracellular compartment, microtubule function, microfilament function or protein synthesis (Custer *et al.*, 1982; Kondo *et al.*, 1988). Inflammatory states are associated with delayed processing and release of iron from the macrophage (Deiss, 1983; Alvarez-Hernandez *et al.*, 1986), an effect reproduced when isolated Kupffer cells are incubated with serum from rats with sterile, turpentine-induced abscesses. The exact mediators of this response with the macrophage are uncertain; no influence on the course of iron release from the Kupffer cell was found with interleukin (IL)-1, γ-interferon or tumour necrosis factor (Kondo *et al.*, 1988). In other studies of peritoneal macrophages from mice, incubation with tumour necrosis factor *in vitro* decreased iron release (Brock and Alvarez-Hernandez, 1989; Alvarez-Hernandez *et al.*, 1989) (see also Chapter 11).

Although transferrin acts as the sole physiological means for the transport of iron to the erythroid marrow, a requirement for the presence of unsaturated transferrin for release of iron from the macrophage has not been established. Apotransferrin does not enter the macrophage and accepts iron only after the release of iron from the cell (Saito *et al.*, 1986; Kondo *et al.*, 1988). Studies *in vivo* found that release of iron derived from heat-damaged red cells was unaffected by transferrin saturation (Noyes *et al.*, 1960; Fillet *et al.*, 1974; Siegenberg *et al.*, 1990) and that the injection of apotransferrin did not increase iron release (Lipschitz *et al.*, 1971b; Finch *et al.*, 1982). Experiments in which infused iron seemed to diminish macrophage iron release (Lipschitz *et al.*, 1971b; Bergamaschi *et al.*, 1986) are difficult to interpret because of the possibility that the infused iron not only saturated plasma transferrin but also depleted the capacity of the plasma to bind iron independently of transferrin (Siegenberg *et al.*, 1990). *In vitro*, the presence of apotransferrin has had little or no effect on the magnitude of iron release in most investigations (Esparza and Brock, 1981; Brock *et al.*, 1984; Saito *et al.*, 1986; Kondo *et al.*, 1988) although an enhancement of release has been reported in some studies (Fedorko, 1974; Rama *et al.*, 1988). The explanation for these apparently discrepant findings is not evident. Although apotransferrin may not be required for the exit of iron from the macrophage, much or most of the iron released is nonetheless available for binding by transferrin (Brock *et al.*, 1984; Saito *et al.*, 1986; Rama *et al.*, 1988).

Several studies have now found that much of the iron released from macrophages is in the form of ferritin both in experiments *in vitro* (Saito *et al.*, 1986; Rama *et al.*, 1988; Kondo *et al.*, 1988; Sibille *et al.*, 1988) and *in vivo*, after the administration of heat-damaged red cells to rats (Siimes and Dallman, 1974) but the physiological fate of this released ferritin and its iron remain uncertain (Aisen, 1990). Iron-loaded ferritin released by Kupffer cells after erythrophagocytosis *in vitro* has been shown to be readily taken up by hepatocytes (Kondo *et al.*, 1988; Sibille *et al.*, 1988), possibly by specific hepatocyte ferritin receptors (Mack *et al.*, 1983) (see also Chapter 4). These results have suggested the possibility that ferritin released by Kupffer cells may serve as an intrahepatic carrier of iron to the hepatocyte. Such a mechanism would protect the hepatocyte against iron deficiency but would also create the risk of iron loading with chronic haemolysis (Aisen, 1990).

3. ASSESSMENT OF ERYTHROPOIESIS USING MEASURES OF PLASMA IRON TURNOVER

Having traced the flow of iron through each of the portions of the red cell cycle, this chapter will conclude with a discussion of methods to evaluate erythropoiesis. Ferrokinetic studies for the assessment of erythroid marrow activity began more than 40 years ago with studies in which a plasma sample was obtained from a patient, incubated with radioiron and reinjected into the patient (Huff *et al.*, 1950, 1951). Additional blood samples were obtained over the next several hours to measure the rate of disappearance of the radioiron and again at two weeks to determine the proportion of the radioiron incorporated into red cells. Analysis first used a one-compartment model in which all the iron leaving the plasma was considered to be taken up by the erythroid marrow and incorporated into red blood cells. The *plasma iron turnover* (PIT, expressed as mg iron/dl whole blood/day), was calculated as the plasma iron concentration divided by the plasma iron disappearance rate ($T_{1/2}$). The *red cell utilization* (RCU, expressed as a per cent) was the proportion of injected radioiron incorporated into circulating red cells at two weeks. The *red cell iron turnover* (RCIT, mg iron/dL whole blood/day), calculated as PIT×RCU, was originally considered to represent the portion of the plasma iron turnover that had been used for effective red cell production. Plasma iron turnover (or red cell iron turnover) measurements were then used to evaluate erythroid marrow activity as increased or decreased by comparison with values derived from studies of healthy volunteers.

Both the procedures used and the analysis of the data obtained became increasingly refined as technical pitfalls (e.g. in not using tracer amounts of iron, in failure of binding of the radioiron to transferrin, in artifacts from haemolysis in samples, in fluctuations in plasma iron concentration) were recognized and the complexity of internal iron exchange was appreciated (Bothwell *et al.*, 1979). The plasma radioiron disappearance curve was recognized as being the sum of several components due to the return of radioiron from the extravascular fluid compartment and from erythroid and nonerythroid tissues. A progressive increase in plasma iron turnover with increasing transferrin saturation was observed but not satisfactorily explained (Cook *et al.*, 1970; Bauer *et al.*, 1981; Uchida *et al.*, 1983). Increasingly complex ferrokinetic models were elaborated that provided vital insights into the pathways of iron exchange between tissues (Pollycove and Mortimer, 1961; Garby *et al.*, 1963; Najean *et al.*, 1967; Cook *et al.*, 1970; Finch *et al.*, 1970; Ricketts *et al.*, 1975; Barosi *et al.*, 1978) but all assumed that the plasma iron constituted a single kinetic pool. Subsequently, the existence of two plasma pools of iron was recognized, consisting of the diferric and two monoferric forms of transferrin described earlier (Skarberg *et al.*, 1978). With sufficient transferrin present to maintain receptor saturation, diferric transferrin has a substantially greater capacity to deliver iron to tissue receptors than the monoferric forms (Huebers *et al.*, 1983, 1985). This preferential uptake of diferric transferrin by transferrin receptors was found to explain the increase in plasma iron turnover seen with increasing transferrin saturation. Uptake of the transferrin–transferrin receptor complex into the cell occurs at the same rate whether the transferrin carries one or two atoms of iron but diferric transferrin has both a higher affinity for the receptor and delivers two atoms of iron with each cycle (Cazzola *et al.*, 1985, 1987a).

The *erythron transferrin uptake* (ETU, expressed as μmol transferrin/L whole blood/day) was then devised to provide a measure of erythropoiesis that was independent of plasma iron concentration and transferrin saturation. The plasma iron turnover is converted into the erythron transferrin uptake using the plasma iron turnover, the haematocrit, and the plasma iron and iron-binding capacity by (i) subtracting the extravascular flux (EVF) of iron entering the extravascular space, (ii) converting iron uptake into transferrin uptake by taking account of the proportions of mono- and diferric transferrin, and (iii) subtracting transferrin uptake by nonerythroid tissues (Cazzola *et al.*, 1985). The most important qualification to the use of the erythron transferrin uptake as a measure of erythroid marrow activity is the requirement that the number of iron-bearing transferrin molecules present be sufficient to saturate transferrin receptors. If not, the uptake of iron-bearing transferrin will be reduced to an extent proportional to the degree of unsaturation (Beguin *et al.*, 1988a). This requirement may be a limitation in the evaluation of patients with iron deficiency anaemia or with marked erythroid hyperplasia (Pootrakul *et al.*, 1988). Despite this restriction, the erythron transferrin uptake has been validated as a useful means of assessing erythroid marrow activity in a variety of anaemias (Cazzola *et al.*, 1987a,b; Beguin *et al.*, 1988b; Pootrakul *et al.*, 1988; Hughes *et al.*, 1990; Howarth *et al.*, 1991).

Since the development of the technique for the measurement of the erythron transferrin uptake, another means of assessing erythropoietic activity has become available: the soluble transferrin receptor (Kohgo *et al.*, 1986; Cazzola and Beguin, 1992). The soluble transferrin receptor is a truncated form of the tissue transferrin receptor consisting of the N-terminal cytoplasmic domain that has probably been proteolytically released from the cell membrane (Baynes *et al.*, 1990; Shih *et al.*, 1990). The circulating form seems to be composed of two receptor monomers binding a single molecule of transferrin. Soluble transferrin receptor concentration in the plasma can readily be measured by immunometric assays (Flowers *et al.*, 1989). While much remains to be learned about the origin and fate of the plasma transferrin receptors, most are derived from the erythroid marrow and the concentration of circulating soluble transferrin receptor is primarily determined by erythroid marrow activity (Kohgo *et al.*, 1987; Beguin *et al.*, 1988c; Flowers *et al.*, 1989; Huebers *et al.*, 1990). Iron deficiency also increases soluble transferrin receptor concentrations but it is not clear to what extent this is the result of increased transferrin receptor expression in individual erythroblasts or simply appropriate to the degree of anaemia and associated erythropoietin stimulation (Intragumtornchai *et al.*, 1988; Kohgo *et al.*, 1988; Beguin *et al.*, 1990; Huebers *et al.*, 1990; Skikne *et al.*, 1990). Decreased levels of circulating soluble transferrin receptor are found in patients with erythroid hypoplasia (aplastic anaemia, chronic renal failure) while increased levels are present in patients with erythroid hyperplasia (thalassaemia major, sickle cell anaemia, chronic haemolytic anaemia). Notably, a close correlation has been demonstrated between the plasma concentration of soluble transferrin receptor and the erythron transferrin uptake (Huebers *et al.*, 1990). In a research setting, the erythron transferrin uptake remains the most accurate means now available for the evaluation of erythropoiesis. For clinical evaluation of erythroid marrow activity, measurement of plasma transferrin receptor would now seem to be the method of choice, because of the simplicity and ease of the determination, the avoidance of exposing patients to radioactivity and the ability to carry out serial determinations. It seems fitting that the understanding of internal iron exchange and the red cell cycle, gained through difficult and laborious ferrokinetic investigations, has helped lead to a useful, simple and convenient means for the clinical assessment of erythropoiesis.

ACKNOWLEDGEMENT

Supported in part by research grants from the Cooley's Anemia Foundation, the Food and Drug Administration (FD-U-000532) and the National Institutes of Health (1RO1 HL42824).

REFERENCES

Abraham, N. G. (1991) Molecular regulation – biological role of heme in hematopoiesis. *Blood Rev.* **5**, 19–28.

Abraham, N. G., Lin, J. H. C., Schwartzman, M. L., Levere, R. D. and Shibahara, S. (1988) The physiological significance of heme oxygenase. *Int. J. Biochem.* **20**, 543–558.

Abraham, N. G., Nelson, J. C., Ahmed, T., Konwalinka, G. and Levere, R. D. (1989) Erythropoietin controls heme metabolic enzymes in normal human bone marrow culture. *Exp. Hematol.* **17**, 908–913.

Adams, M. L., Ostapiuk, I. and Grasso, J. A. (1989) The effect of inhibitors of heme synthesis on the intracellular localization of iron in rat reticulocytes. *Biochim. Biophys. Acta* **1012**, 243–253.

Aisen, P. (1984) Transferrin metabolism and the liver. *Semin. Liver Dis.* **4**, 192–206.

Aisen, P. (1990) Iron metabolism in the reticuloendothelial system. In: *Iron Transport and Storage* (eds P. Ponka, H. M. Schulman and R. C. Woodworth), CRC Press, Boca Raton, pp. 281–295.

Aisen, P. and Leibman, A. (1968) The stability constants of the Fe3+ conalbumin complexes. *Biochem. Biophys. Res. Comm.* **3**, 407–413.

Alam, J. and Smith, A. (1989) Receptor-mediated transport of heme by hemopexin regulates gene expression in mammalian cells. *J. Biol. Chem.* **264**, 17637–17640.

Alvarez-Hernandez, X., Feldstein, M. V. and Brock, J. H. (1986) The relationship between iron release, ferritin synthesis and intracellular iron distribution in mouse peritoneal macrophages. Evidence for a reduced level of metabolically available iron in elicited macrophages. *Biochim. Biophys. Acta* **886**, 214–222.

Alvarez-Hernandez, X., Licéaga, J., McKay, I. C. and Brock, J. H. (1989) Induction of hypoferremia and modulation of macrophage iron metabolism by tumour necrosis factor. *Lab. Invest.* **61**, 319–322.

Awai, M. and Brown, E. B. (1963) Clinical and experimental studies of the metabolism of I^{131}-labeled human transferrin. *J. Lab. Clin. Med.* **61**, 363–396.

Bailey, S., Evans, R. W., Garratt, R. C. *et al.* (1988) Molecular structure of serum transferrin at 3.3 Å resolution. *Biochemistry* **27**, 5804–5812.

Bailey, S. C., Spangler, R. and Sytkowski, A. J. (1991) Erythropoietin induces cytosolic protein phosphorylation and dephosphorylation in erythroid cells. *J. Biol. Chem.* **266**, 24121–24125.

Bali, P. K. and Aisen, P. (1991) Receptor-modulated iron release from transferrin: differential effects on N- and C-terminal sites. *Biochemistry* **30**, 9947–9952.

Bali, P. K. and Aisen, P. (1992) Receptor-induced switch in site-site cooperativity during iron release by transferrin. *Biochemistry* **31**, 3963–3967.

Bali, P. K., Zak, O. and Aisen, P. (1991) A new role for the transferrin receptor in the release of iron from transferrin. *Biochemistry* **30**, 324–328.

Barosi, G., Cazzola, M., Morandi, S., Stefanelli, M. and Perugini, S. (1978) Estimation of ferrokinetic parameters by a mathematical model in patients with primary acquired sideroblastic anaemia. *Br. J. Haematol.* **39**, 409–422.

Bassett, M. L., Halliday, J. W. and Powell, L. W. (1982) Ferritin synthesis in peripheral blood monocytes in idiopathic hemochromatosis. *J. Lab. Clin. Med.* **100**, 137–145.

Battistini, A., Marziali, G., Albertini, R. *et al.* (1991a) Positive modulation of hemoglobin, heme, and transferrin receptor synthesis by murine interferon-alpha and -beta in differentiating Friend cells. *J. Biol. Chem.* **266**, 528–535.

Battistini, A., Coccia, E. M., Marziali, G. *et al.* (1991b) Intracellular heme coordinately modulates globin chain synthesis, transferrin receptor number, and ferritin content in differentiating Friend erythroleukemia cells. *Blood* **78**, 2098–2103.

Bauer, W., Stray, S., Huebers, H. and Finch, C. (1981) The relationship between plasma iron and plasma iron turnover in the rat. *Blood* **37**, 239–242.

Baynes, R. D., Bezwoda, W. R., Dajee, D., Lamparelli, R. D. and Bothwell, T. H. (1990) Effects of alpha-interferon on iron-related measurements in human subjects. *S. Afr. Med. J.* **78**, 627–628.

Beamish, M. R., Davies, A. G., Eakins, J. D., Jacobs, A. and Trevett, D. (1971) The measurement of reticuloendothelial iron release using iron dextran. *Br. J. Haematol.* **21**, 617–622.

Beguin, Y., Huebers, H. and Finch, C. A. (1988a) Random distribution of iron among the two binding sites of transferrin in patients with various hematologic disorders. *Clin. Chim. Acta* **173**, 299–304.

Beguin, Y., Stray, S., Cazzola, M., Huebers, H. and Finch, C. A. (1988b) Ferrokinetic measurement of erythropoiesis. *Acta Haematol.*, **79**, 121–126.

Beguin, Y., Huebers, H. A., Josephson, B. and Finch, C. A. (1988c) Transferrin receptors in rat plasma. *Proc. Natl. Acad. Sci. USA* **85**, 637–640.

Beguin, Y., Lipscei, G., Oris, R., Thoumsin, H. and Fillet, G. (1990) Serum immunoreactive erythropoietin during pregnancy and in the early postpartum. *Br. J. Haematol.* **76**, 545–549.

Bergamaschi, G., Eng, M. J., Huebers, H. A. and Finch, C. A. (1986) The effect of transferrin saturation on internal iron exchange. *Proc. Soc. Exp. Biol. Med.* **183**, 66–73.

Bishop, D. F., Henderson, A. S. and Astrim, K. M. (1990) Human delta-aminolevulinate synthase: assignment of the housekeeping gene to 3p21 and the erythroid specific gene to the X-chromosome. *Genomics* **7**, 207–214.

Bomford, A., Young, S. P. and Williams, R. (1985) Release of iron from the two iron-binding sites of transferrin by cultured human cells: modulation by methylamine. *Biochemistry* **24**, 3472–3478.

Bonanou-Tzedaki, S. A., Sohi, M. K. and Arnstein, H. R. (1984) The effect of haemin on RNA synthesis and stability in differentiating rabbit erythroblasts. *Eur. J. Biochem.* **144**, 589–596.

Bothwell, T. H., Charlton, R. W., Cook, J. D. and Finch, C. A. (1979) *Iron Metabolism in Man*, Blackwell Scientific Publications, Oxford.

Bridges, K. R. and Hoffman, K. E. (1986) The effects of ascorbic acid on the intracellular metabolism of iron and ferritin. *J. Biol. Chem.* **261**, 14273–14277.

Bridges, K. R. (1987) Ascorbic acid inhibits lysosomal autophagy of ferritin. *J. Biol. Chem.* **262**, 1–6.

Brittenham, G. M. (1991) Disorders of iron metabolism: deficiency and overload. In: *Hematology: Basic Principles and Practice* (eds R. Hoffman, E. Benz, S. Shattil, B. Furie and H. Cohen), Churchill Livingstone, New York, pp. 327–349.

Brock, J. H. and Alvarez-Hernandez, X. (1989) Modulation of macrophage iron metabolism by tumour necrosis factor and interleukin 1. *FEMS Microbiol. Immunol.* **1**, 309–310.

Brock, J. H., Esparza, I. and Logie, A. C. (1984) The nature of iron released by resident and stimulated mouse peritoneal macrophages. *Biochim. Biophys. Acta* **797**, 105–111.

Broxmeyer, H. E., Cooper, S., Levi, S. and Arosio, P. (1991) Mutated recombinant human heavy-chain ferritins and myelosuppression *in vitro* and *in vivo*: a link between ferritin ferroxidase activity and biological function. *Proc. Natl. Acad. Sci. USA* **88**, 770–774.

Bunn, H. F. (1987) Subunit assembly of hemoglobin: an important determinant of hematologic phenotype. *Blood* **69**, 1–6.

Bunn, H. F. and Jandl, J. H. (1968) Exchange of heme among hemoglobins and between hemoglobin and albumin. *J. Biol. Chem.* **243**, 465–475.

Cavill, I., Ricketts, C., Napier, J. A. F. and Jacobs, A. (1977) Ferrokinetics and erythropoiesis in man: red cell production and destruction in normal and anaemic subjects. *Br. J. Haematol.* **35**, 33–40.

Cazzola, M. and Ascari, E. (1986) Red cell ferritin as a diagnostic tool. *Br. J. Haematol.* **62**, 209–213.

Cazzola, M. and Beguin, Y. (1992) New tools for clinical evaluation of erythron function in man. *Br. J. Haematol.* **80**, 278–284.

Cazzola, M., Dezza, L., Bergamaschi, G. *et al.* (1983) Biologic and clinical significance of red cell ferritin. *Blood* **62**, 1078–1087.

Cazzola, M., Huebers, H. A., Sayers, M. H., MacPhail, A. P., Eng, M. and Finch, C. A. (1985) Transferrin saturation, plasma iron turnover, and transferrin uptake in normal humans. *Blood* **66**, 935–939.

Cazzola, M., Pootrakul, P., Bergamaschi, G., Huebers, H. A., Eng, M. and Finch, C. A. (1987a) Adequacy of iron supply for erythropoiesis: in vivo observations in humans. *J. Lab. Clin. Med.* **110**, 734–739.

Cazzola, M., Pootrakul, P., Huebers, H. A., Eng, M., Eschbach, J. and Finch, C. A. (1987b) Erythroid marrow function in anemic patients. *Blood* **69**, 296–301.

Chan, L. N. L. and Gerhardt, E. M. (1992) Transferrin receptor gene is hyperexpressed and transcriptionally regulated in differentiating erythroid cells. *J. Biol. Chem.* **267**, 8254–8259.

Chasteen, N. D. (1983) The identification of the probable locus of iron and anion binding in the transferrins. *Trends Biochem. Sci.* **8**, 272–275.

Chretien, S., Dubart, A., Beaupain, D. *et al.* (1988) Alternative transcription and splicing of the human porphobilinogen deaminase gene result either in tissue-specific or in housekeeping expression. *Proc. Natl. Acad. Sci. USA* **85**, 6–10.

Clark, M. R. (1988) Senescence of red blood cells: progress and problems. *Physiol. Rev.* **68**, 503–554.

Clerget, M. and Polla, B. S. (1990) Erythrophagocytosis induces heat shock protein synthesis by human monocytes–macrophages. *Proc. Natl. Acad. Sci. USA* **87**, 1081–1085.

Coccia, E. M., Profita, V., Fiorucci, G. *et al.* (1992) Modulation of ferritin H-chain expression in Friend erythroleukemia cells: transcriptional and translational regulation by hemin. *Mol. Cell. Biol.* **12**, 3015–3022.

Constable, A., Quick, S., Gray, N. K. and Hentze, M. W. (1992) Modulation of the RNA-binding activity of a regulatory protein by iron in vitro: switching between enzymatic and genetic function. *Proc. Natl. Acad. Sci. USA* **89**, 4554–4558.

Cook, J. D., Marsaglia, J. W., Eschbach, J. W., Funk, D. D. and Finch, C. A. (1970) Ferrokinetics: a biological model for plasma iron exchange in man. *J. Clin. Invest.* **49**, 197–205.

Cotner, T., Das Gupta, A., Papayannopoulou, Th. and Stamatoyannopoulos, G. (1989) Characterization of a novel form of transferrin receptor preferentially expressed on normal erythroid progenitors and precursors. *Blood* **73**, 214–221.

Cox, T. C., Bawden, M. J., Martin, A. and May, B. K. (1991) Human erythroid 5-aminolevulinate synthase: promoter analysis and identification of an iron-responsive element in the mRNA. *EMBO J.* **10**, 1891–1902.

Cox, T. M., Ponka, P. and Schulman, H. N. (1990) Erythroid cell iron metabolism and heme synthesis. In: *Iron Transport and Storage* (eds P. Ponka, H. M. Schulman and R. C. Woodworth). CRC Press, Boca Raton, pp. 263–279.

Cruse, I. and Maines, M. D. (1988) Evidence suggesting that the two forms of heme oxygenase are products of different genes. *J. Biol. Chem.* **263**, 3348–3353.

Custer, G., Balcerzak, S. and Rinehart, J. (1982) Human macrophage hemoglobin–iron metabolism *in vitro. Am. J. Hematol.* **13**, 23–36.

D'Andrea, A. D., Fasman, G. D. and Lodish, H. F. (1989) Erythropoietin receptor and interleukin-2 receptor β-chain: a new receptor family. *Cell* **58**, 1023–1024.

Dandekar, T., Stripecke, R., Gray, N. K. *et al.* (1991) Identification of a novel iron-responsive element in murine and human erythroid delta-aminolevulinic acid synthase mRNA. *EMBO J.* **10**, 1903–1909.

Danon, D. and Marikovsky, Y. (1988) The aging of the red blood cell. A multifactor process. *Blood Cells* **14**, 7–18.

Deiss, A (1983) Iron metabolism in reticuloendothelial cells. *Semin. Hematol.* **20**, 81–90.

Edwards, V. D. and Simon, G. T. (1970) Ultrastructural aspects of red cell destruction in the normal rat spleen. *J. Ultrastructur. Res.* **33**, 187–201.

Eisenstein, R. S., Garcia-Mayol, D., Pettingell, W. and Munro, H. N. (1991) Regulation of ferritin and heme oxygenase synthesis in rat fibroblasts by different forms of iron. *Proc. Natl. Acad. Sci. USA* **88**, 688–692.

Esparza, I. and Brock, J. H. (1981) Release of iron by resident and stimulated mouse peritoneal macrophages following ingestion and degradation of transferrin–antitransferrin immune complexes. *Br. J. Haematol.* **49**, 603–614.

Faquin, W. C., Schneider, T. J. and Goldberg, M. A. (1992) Effect of inflammatory cytokines on hypoxia-induced erythropoietin production. *Blood* **79**, 1987–1994.

Fedorko, M. E. (1974) Loss of iron from mouse peritoneal macrophages *in vitro* after uptake of [55]Fe ferritin and [55]Fe ferritin rabbit antiferritin complexes. *J. Cell Biol.* **62**, 802–814.

Fillet, G., Cook, J. D. and Finch, C. A. (1974) Storage iron kinetics. VII. A biologic model for reticuloendothelial iron transport. *J. Clin. Invest.* **53**, 1527–1533.

Fillet, G., Beguin, Y. and Baldelli, L. (1989) Model of reticuloendothelial iron metabolism in humans: abnormal behavior in idiopathic hemochromatosis and in inflammation. *Blood* **74**, 844–851.

Finch, C. A. (1982) Erythropoiesis, erythropoietin and iron. *Blood* **60**, 1241–1246.

Finch, C. A. and Huebers, H. (1982) Perspectives in iron metabolism. *New Engl. J. Med.* **306**, 1520–1528.

Finch, C. A., Deubelbeiss, K, Cook, J. D. *et al.* (1970) Ferrokinetics in man. *J. Clin. Invest.* **43**, 17–53.

Finch, C. A., Huebers, H., Eng, M. and Miller, L. (1982) Effect of transfused reticulocytes on iron exchange. *Blood* **59**, 364–369.

Fletcher, J. and Huehns, E. R. (1968) Function of transferrin. *Nature* **218**, 1211–1214.

Flowers, C. H., Skikne, B. S., Covell, A. M. and Cook, J. D. (1989) The clinical measurement of serum transferrin receptor. *J. Lab. Clin. Med.* **114**, 368–377.

Ford, G. C., Harrison, P. M., Rice, D. W., Smith, J. M. A. and Treffry, A. (1984) Ferritin: design and formation of an iron-storage molecule. *Phil. Trans. R. Soc. Lond.* **B304**, 551–565.

Fujita, H., Yamamoto, M., Yamagami, T., Hayashi, N. and Sassa, S. (1991) Erythroleukemia differentiation. Distinctive responses of the erythroid-specific and the nonspecific delta-aminolevulinate synthase mRNA. *J. Biol. Chem.* **266**, 17494–17502.

Garby, L., Schneider, W., Sundquist, O. and Vuille, J. C. (1963) A ferroerythrokinetic model and its properties. *Acta Physiol. Scand.* **59**, suppl **216**, 4–26.

Gardner, L. C. and Cox, T. M. (1988) Biosynthesis of heme in immature erythroid cells. The regulatory step for heme formation in the human erythron. *J. Biol. Chem.* **263**, 6676–6682.

Gardner, L. C., Smith, S. J. and Cox, T. M. (1991) Biosynthesis of delta-aminolevulinic acid and the regulation of heme formation by immature erythroid cells in man. *J. Biol. Chem.* **266**, 22010–22018.

Goessling, L. S., Daniels-McQueen, S., Bhattacharyya-Pakrasi, M., Lin, J. J. and Thach, R. E. (1992) Enhanced degradation of the ferritin repressor protein during induction of ferritin messenger RNA translation. *Science* **256**, 670–673.

Goldberg, M. A., Dunning, S. P. and Bunn, H. F. (1988) Regulation of the erythropoietin gene: evidence that the oxygen sensor is a heme protein. *Science* **242**, 1412–1415.

Grandchamp, B., De Verneuil, H., Beaumont, C., Chretien, S., Walter, O. and Nordmann, Y. (1987) Tissue-specific expression of porphobilinogen deaminase. Two isoenzymes from a single gene. *Eur. J. Biochem.* **162**, 105–110.

Granick, J. L. and Sassa, S. (1978) Hemin control of heme biosynthesis in mouse Friend-virus transformed erythroleukemia cells in culture. *J. Biol. Chem.* **253**, 5402–5406.

Gross, M., Wing, M., Rundquist, C. and Rubino, M. S. (1987) Evidence that phosphorylation of eIF-2(alpha) prevents the eIF-2B-mediated dissociation of eIF-2 X GDP from the 60 S subunit of complete initiation complexes. *J. Biol. Chem.* **262**, 6899–6907.

Haas, A. L., Warms, J. V. B., Hershko, A. and Rose, I. A. (1982) Ubiquitin-activating enzyme: mechanism and role in protein–ubiquitin conjugation. *J. Biol. Chem.* **257**, 2543–2548.

Haile, D. J., Rouault, T. A., Harford, J. B. and Klausner, R. D. (1990) The inhibition of the iron responsive element RNA–protein interaction by heme does not mimic in vivo iron regulation. *J. Biol. Chem.* **265**, 12786–12789.

Harford, J. B. and Klausner, R. D. (1990) Coordinate post-transcriptional regulation of ferritin and transferrin receptor expression: the role of regulated RNA–protein interaction. *Enzyme* **44**, 28–41.

Harris, J. W. and Kellermeyer, R. W. (1970) *The Red Cell. Production, Metabolism, Destruction: Normal and Abnormal*, Harvard University Press, Cambridge, pp. 1–795.

Hentze, M. W. and Argos, P. (1991) Homology between IRE-BP, a regulatory RNA-binding protein, aconitase, and isopropylmalate isomerase. *Nucleic Acids Res.* **19**, 1739–1740.

Hentze, M. W., Caughman, S. W., Rouault, T. A. *et al.* (1987) Identification of the iron-responsive element for the translational regulation of human ferritin mRNA. *Science* **238**, 1570–1573.

Hershko, C., Cook, J. D. and Finch, C. A. (1974) Storage iron kinetics. VI. The effect of inflammation on iron exchange in the rat. *Br. J. Haematol.* **28**, 67–75.

Hillman, R. S. and Henderson, P. A. (1969) Control of marrow production by relative iron supply. *J. Clin. Invest.* **48**, 454–460.

Hirata, T., Bitterman, P. B., Mornex, J. F. and Crysta, R. G. (1986) Expression of the transferrin receptor gene during the process of mononuclear phagocyte maturation. *J. Immunol.* **136**, 1339–1345.

Hodgetts, J., Peters, S. W., Hoy, T. G. and Jacobs, A. (1986) The ferritin content of normoblasts and megaloblasts from human bone marrow. *Clin. Sci.* **70**, 47–51.

Houston, T., Moore, M. R., McColl, K. E. and Fitzsimons, E. (1991) Erythroid 5-aminolaevulinate synthase activity during normal and iron deficient erythropoiesis. *Br. J. Haematol.* **78**, 561–564.

Howarth, J. E., Waters, H. M., Hyde, K., Shanks, D. and Geary, C. G. (1991) Comparative ferrokinetic study with initial and extended iron clearance models. *J. Clin. Pathol.* **44**, 395–399.

Huebers, H. A. and Finch, C. A. (1987) The physiology of transferrin and transferrin receptors. *Physiol. Reviews* **67**, 520–582.

Huebers, H. A., Csiba, E., Huebers, E. and Finch, C. A. (1983) Competitive advantage of diferric transferrin in delivering iron to reticulocytes. *Proc. Natl. Acad. Sci. USA* **80**, 300–304.

Huebers, H., Csiba, E., Huebers, E. and Finch, C. A. (1985) Molecular advantage of diferric transferrin in delivering iron to reticulocytes: a comparative study. *Proc. Soc. Exp. Biol. Med.* **179**, 222–226.

Huebers, H. A., Beguin, Y., Pootrakul, P., Einspahr, D. and Finch, C. A. (1990) Intact transferrin receptors in human plasma and their relation to erythropoiesis. *Blood* **75**, 102–107.

Huff, R. L., Hennessy, T. G., Austin, R. E., Garcia, J. F., Roberts, B. M. and Lawrence, J. H. (1950) Plasma and red cell iron turnover in normal subjects and in patients having various hematopoietic disorders. *J. Clin. Invest.* **29**, 1041–1052.

Huff, R. L., Elmlinger, P. J., Garcia, J. F., Oda, J. M., Cockrell, M. C. and Lawrence, J. H. (1951) Ferrokinetics in normal persons and in patients having various erythropoietic disorders. *J. Clin. Invest.* **30**, 1512–1526.

Hughes, R. T., Cotes, P. M., Pippard, M. J. *et al.* (1990) Subcutaneous administration of recombinant human erythropoietin to subjects on continuous ambulatory peritoneal dialysis: an erythrokinetic assessment. *Br. J. Haematol.* **75**, 268–273.

Iacopetta, B. J. and Morgan, E. H. (1983) Transferrin endocytosis and iron uptake during erythroid cell development. *Biomed. Biochim. Acta* **42**, S182–S186.

Iacopetta, B. J., Morgan, E. H. and Yeoh, G. C. T. (1982) Transferrin receptors and iron uptake during erythroid cell development. *Biochim. Biophys. Acta* **687**, 204–210.

Intragumtornchai, T., Huebers, H. A., Eng, M. and Finch, C. A. (1988) In vivo transferrin–iron receptor relationships in erythron of rats. *Am. J. Physiol.* **255**, R326–331.

Invernizzi, R., Cazzola, M., De Fazio, P., Rosti, V., Ruggeri, G. and Arosio, P. (1990) Immunocytochemical detection of ferritin in human bone marrow and peripheral blood cells using monoclonal antibodies specific for the H and L subunit. *Br. J. Haematol.* **76**, 427–432.

Jandl, J. H. (1987) *Blood: Textbook of Hematology*, Little, Brown and Company, Boston.

Jandl, J. H. and Katz, J. H. (1963) The plasma-to-cell cycle of transferrin. *J. Clin. Invest.* **42**, 314–326.

Johnson, C. S., Keckler, D. J., Topper, M. I., Braunschweiger, P. G. and Furmanski, P. (1989) In vivo hematopoietic effects of recombinant interleukin-1a in mice: stimulation of granulocytic, monocytic, megakaryocytic, and early erythroid progenitors, suppression of late stage erythropoiesis and reversal of erythroid suppression with erythropoietin. *Blood* **73**, 678–682.

Johnson, C. S., Pourbohloul, C. and Furmanski, P. (1991) Negative regulators of in vivo erythropoiesis: interaction of IL-1a and TNF-a and the lack of a strict requirement for T or NK cells for their activity. *Exp. Hematol.* **19**, 101–105.

Jones, S. S., D'Andrea, A. D., Haines, L. L. and Wong, G. G. (1990) Human erythropoietin receptor: cloning expression and biological characteristics. *Blood* **76**, 31–35.

Kaptain, S., Downey, W. E., Tang, C. *et al.* (1991) A regulated RNA binding protein also possesses aconitase activity. *Proc. Natl. Acad. Sci. USA* **88**, 10109–10113.

Kay, M. M. B., Sorensen, K., Wong, P. and Bolton, P. (1982) Antigenicity, storage and aging. Physiologic autoantibodies to cell membrane and serum proteins and the senescent cell antigen. *Mol. Cell. Biochem.* **49**, 65–85.

Kohgo, Y., Nishisato, T., Kondo, H., Tsushima, N., Niitsu, Y. and Urushizaki, I. (1986) Circulating transferrin receptor in human serum. *Br. J. Haematol.* **64**, 277–281.

Kohgo, Y., Niitsu, Y., Kondo, H. *et al.* (1987) Serum transferrin receptor as a new index of erythropoiesis. *Blood* **70**, 1955–1958.

Kohgo, Y., Niitsu, Y., Nishisato, T. *et al.* (1988) Immunoreactive transferrin receptor in sera of pregnant women. *Placenta* **9**, 523–531.

Kondo, H., Saito, K., Grasso, J. P. and Aisen, P. (1988) Iron metabolism in the erythrophagocytosing Kupffer cell. *Hepatology* **8**, 32–38.

Koury, M. J. and Bondurant, M. C. (1990) Erythropoietin retards DNA breakdown and prevents programmed death in erythroid progenitors. *Science* **248**, 273–277.

Krantz, S. B. (1991) Erythropoietin. *Blood* **77**, 419–434.

Lawson, D. M., Artymiuk, P. J., Yewdall, S. J. *et al.* (1991) Solving the structure of human H ferritin by genetically engineering intermolecular crystal contacts. *Nature* **349**, 541–544.

Leibold, E. A. and Munro, H. N. (1987) Characterization and evolution of the expressed rat ferritin light subunit gene and its pseudogene family. Conservation of sequences within noncoding regions of ferritin genes. *J. Biol. Chem.* **262**, 7335–7341.

Lesley, J., Hyman, R., Schulte, R. and Trotter, J. (1984) Expression of transferrin receptor on murine hematopoietic progenitors. *Cell Immunol.* **83**, 14–25.

Levi, S., Luzago, A., Cesarni, G. *et al.* (1988) Mechanism of ferritin iron uptake: activity of the H-chain and deletion mapping of the ferro-oxidase site. A study of iron uptake and ferro-oxidase activity of human liver, recombinant H-chain ferritins, and of two H-chain deletion mutants. *J. Biol. Chem.* **263**, 18086–18092.

Levi, S., Luzzago, A., Franceschinelli, F., Santambrogio, P., Cesareni, G. and Arosio, P. (1989) Mutational analysis of the channel and loop sequences of human ferritin H-chain. *Biochem. J.* **264**, 381–388.

Lin, J. J., Daniels-McQueen, S., Gaffield, L., Patino, M. M., Walden, W. E. and Thach, R. E. (1990a) Specificity of the induction of ferritin synthesis by hemin. *Biochim. Biophys. Acta* **1050**, 146–150.

Lin, J. J., Daniels-McQueen, S., Patino, M. M., Gaffield, L., Walden, W. E. and Thach, R. E. (1990b) Derepression of ferritin messenger RNA translation by hemin in vitro. *Science* **247**, 74–77.

Lin, J. J., Patino, M. M., Gaffield, L., Walden, W. E., Smith, A. and Thach, R. E. (1991) Crosslinking of hemin to a specific site on the 90-kDa ferritin repressor protein. *Proc. Natl. Acad. Sci. USA* **88**, 6068–6071.

Lipschitz, D. A., Bothwell, T. H., Seftel, H. C., Wapnick, A. A. and Charlton, R. W. (1971a) The role of ascorbic acid in the metabolism of storage iron. *Br. J. Haematol.* **20**, 155–163.

Lipschitz, D. A., Simon, M. O., Lynch, S. R., Dugard, J., Bothwell, T. H. and Charlton, R. W. (1971b) Some factors affecting the release of iron from reticuloendothelial cells. *Br. J. Haematol.* **21**, 289–303.

Lodish, H. F. and Desalu, O. (1973) Regulation of synthesis of non-globin proteins in cell-free extracts of rabbit reticulocytes. *J. Biol. Chem.* **248**, 3420–3427.

London, I. M., Levin, D. H., Matts, R. L., Thomas, N. S. B., Petryshyn, R. and Chen, J. J. (1987) Regulation of protein synthesis. In: *The Enzymes* (ed. Boyer, P. D.), Academic Press, New York, pp. 359–367.

Low, P. S., Waugh, S. M., Zinke, K. and Drenckhahan, D. (1985) The role of hemoglobin denaturation and band 3 clustering in red cell aging. *Science* **227**, 531–533.

Lutz, H. U., Fasler, S., Stammler, P., Bussolino, F. and Arese, P. (1988) Naturally occurring anti-band 3 antibodies and complement in phagocytosis of oxidatively-stressed and in the clearance of senescent red cells. *Blood Cells* **14**, 175–203.

Mack, U., Powell, L. W. and Halliday, J. W. (1983) Detection and isolation of a hepatic membrane receptor for ferritin. *J. Biol. Chem.* **258**, 4672–4675.

MacSween, R. N. M. and MacDonald, R. A. (1969) Iron metabolism by reticuloendothelial cells. *In vitro* uptake of transferrin-bound iron by rat and rabbit cells. *Lab. Invest.* **21**, 230–235.

Maines, M. D., Trakshel, G. M. and Kutty, R. K. (1986) Characterization of two constitutive forms of rat liver microsomal heme oxygenase. Only one molecular species of the enzyme is inducible. *J. Biol. Chem.* **261**, 411–419.

McCoubrey, W. K., Ewing, J. F. and Maines, M. D. (1992) Human heme oxygenase-2: characterization and expression of a full-length cDNA and evidence suggesting that the two HO-2 transcripts may differ by choice of polyadenylation signal. *Arch. Biochem. Biophys.* **295**, 13–20.

Mignotte, V., Eleouet, J. F., Raich, N. and Romeo, P. H. (1989a) Cis- and trans-acting elements involved in the regulation of the erythroid promoter of the human porphobilinogen deaminase gene. *Proc. Natl. Acad. Sci. USA* **86**, 6548–6552.

Mignotte, V., Wall, L., deBoer, E., Grosveld, F. and Romeo, P. H. (1989b) Two tissue-specific factors bind the erythroid promoter of the human porphobilinogen deaminase gene. *Nucleic Acids Res.* **17**, 37–54.

Miller, C. B., Jones, R. I., Piantadosi, S., Abeloff, M. D. and Spivak, I. L. (1990) Decreased erythropoietin response in patients with the anemia of cancer. *N. Engl. J. Med.* **322**, 1689–1692.

Morgan, E. H. (1981) Transferrin: biochemistry, physiology and clinical significance. In: *Molecular Aspects of Medicine*, Pergamon, Oxford, pp. 1–123.

Muller-Eberhard, U. (1970) Hemopexin. *N. Engl. J. Med.* **283**, 1090–1094.

Munthe-Kaas, A. C. (1976) Phagocytosis in rat Kupffer cells *in vitro*. *Exp. Cell Res.* **99**, 319–327.

Munthe-Kaas, A. C., Kaplan, G. and Sleljelid, R. (1976) On the mechanism of internalization of opsonized particles by rat Kupffer cells *in vitro*. *Exp. Cell Res.* **103**, 201–212.

Najean, Y., Dresch, C., Ardaillou, N. and Bernard, J. (1967) Iron metabolism – study of different models in normal conditions. *Amer. J. Physiol.* **213**, 533–546.

Nijhof, W., Wierenga, P. K., Sahr, K., Beru, N. and Goldwasser, E. (1987) Induction of globin mRNA transcription by erythropoietin in differentiating erythroid precursor cells. *Exp. Hematol.* **15**, 779–784.

Noyes, W. D., Bothwell, T. H. and Finch, C. A. (1960) The role of the reticuloendothelial cell in iron metabolism. *Br. J. Haematol.* **6**, 43–55.

Okuda, M., Tokunaga, R. and Taketani, S. (1992) Expression of haptoglobin receptors in human hepatoma cells. *Biochim. Biophys. Acta* **1136**, 143–149.

Osaki, S., Johnson, D. A. and Frieden, L. (1971) The mobilisation of iron from the perfused mammalian liver by a serum copper enzyme, ferrioxidase. I. *J. Biol. Chem.* **46**, 3018–3023.

Oshiro, S. and Nakajima, H. (1988) Intrahepatocellular site of the catabolism of heme and globin moiety of hemoglobin–haptoglobin after intravenous administration to rats. *J. Biol. Chem.* **263**, 16032–16038.

Pollycove, M. and Mortimer, R. (1961) The quantitative determination of iron kinetics and hemoglobin synthesis in human subjects. *J. Clin. Invest.* **40**, 753–782.

Ponka, P., Wilczynska, A. and Schulman, H. M. (1982) Iron utilization in rabbit reticulocytes. A study using succinylacetone as an inhibitor of heme synthesis. *Biochim. Biophys. Acta* **720**, 96–105.

Pootrakul, P., Kitcharoen, K., Yansukon, P. *et al.* (1988) The effect of erythroid hyperplasia on iron balance. *Blood* **71**, 1124–1129.

Ragan, H. A., Nacht, S., Lee, G. R., Bishop, C. R. and Cartwright, G. E. (1969) Effect of ceruloplasmin on plasma iron in copper-deficient swine. *Am. J. Physiol.* **217**, 1320–1323.

Raich, N., Mignotte, V., Dubart, A. *et al.* (1989) Regulated expression of the overlapping ubiquitous and erythroid transcription units of the human porphobilinogen deaminase (PBG-D) gene introduced into non-erythroid and erythroid cells. *J. Biol. Chem.* **264**, 10186–10192.

Rama, R., Sánchez, J. and Octave, J. N. (1988) Iron mobilization from cultured rat bone marrow macrophages. *Biochim. Biophys. Acta* **968**, 51–58.

Ranu, R. S. and London, I. M. (1979) Regulation of protein synthesis in rabbit reticulocyte lysates: preparation of efficient protein synthesis lysates and the purification and characterization of the heme-regulated translational inhibitory protein kinase. *Methods Enzymol.* **60**, 459–484.

Richardson, D. R. and Baker, E. (1992) Intermediate steps in cellular iron uptake from transferrin. *J. Biol. Chem.* **30**, 21384–21389.

Richter, G. W. (1984) Studies of iron overload. Rat liver siderosome ferritin. *Lab. Invest.* **50**, 26–35.

Ricketts, C., Jacobs, A. and Cavill, I. (1975) Ferrokinetics and erythropoiesis in man: an evaluation of ferrokinetic measurements. *Br. J. Haematol.* **31**, 65–75

Rose, M. Y. and Olson, J. S. (1983) The kinetic mechanism of heme binding to human apohemoglobin. *J. Biol. Chem.* **258**, 4298–4303.

Rouault, T., Rao, K., Harford, J., Mattia, E. and Klausner, R. D. (1985) Hemin, chelatable iron, and the regulation of transferrin receptor biosynthesis. *J. Biol. Chem.* **260**, 14862–14866.

Rouault, T. A., Hentze, M. W., Caughman, S. W., Harford, J. B. and Klausner, R. D. (1988) Binding of a cytosolic protein to the iron-responsive element of human ferritin messenger RNA. *Science* **241**, 1207–1210.

Rouault, T. A., Stout, C. D., Kaptain, S., Harford, J. B. and Klausner, R. D. (1991) Structural relationship between an iron-regulated RNA-binding protein (IRE-BP) and aconitase: functional implications. *Cell* **64**, 881–883.

Saito, K., Nishisato, T., Grasso, J. A. and Aisen P. (1986) Interaction of transferrin with iron-loaded rat peritoneal macrophages. *Br. J. Haematol.* **62**, 275–286.

Schlabach, M. R. and Bates, G. W. (1975) The synergistic binding of anions and Fe^{3+} by transferrin. *J. Biol. Chem.* **250**, 2182–2188.

Shih, Y. J., Baynes, R. D., Hudson, B. G., Flowers, C. H., Skikne, B. S. and Cook, J. D. (1990) Serum transferrin receptor is a truncated form of tissue receptor. *J. Biol. Chem.* **265**, 19077–19081.

Sibille, J. C., Kondo, H. and Aisen, P. (1988) Interactions between isolated hepatocytes and Kupffer cells in iron metabolism: a possible role for ferritin as an iron carrier protein. *Hepatology* **8**, 296–301.

Siegenberg, D., Baynes, R. D., Bothwell, T. H., MacFarlane, B. J. and Lamparelli, R. D. (1990) Factors involved in the regulation of iron transport through reticuloendothelial cells. *Proc. Soc. Exp. Biol. Med.* **193**, 65–72.

Siimes, M. A. and Dallman, P. R. (1974) New kinetic role for serum ferritin in iron metabolism. *Br. J. Haematol.* **28**, 1–18.

Skarberg, K., Eng, K., Huebers, H., Marsaglia, G. and Finch, C. A. (1978) Plasma radioiron kinetics in man. An explanation for the effect of plasma iron concentration. *Proc. Natl. Acad. Sci. USA* **75**, 1559–1561.

Skikne, B. S., Flowers, C. H. and Cook, J. D. (1990) Serum transferrin receptor: a quantitative measure of tissue iron deficiency. *Blood* **75**, 1870–1876.

Smith, A. and Hunt, R. C. (1990) Hemopexin joins transferrin as representative members of a distinct class of receptor-mediated endocytic transport systems. *Eur. J. Cell Biol.* **53**, 234–245.

Smith, A., Farooqui, S. M. and Morgan, W. T. (1991) The murine haemopexin receptor. Evidence that the haemopexin-binding site resides on a 20 kDa subunit and that receptor recycling is regulated by protein kinase C. *Biochem. J.* **276**, 417–425.

Speiser, S. and Etlinger, J. D. (1982) Loss of ATP-dependent proteolysis with maturation of reticulocytes and erythrocytes. *J. Biol. Chem.* **257**, 14122–14127.

Speyer, B. E. and Fielding, J. (1979) Ferritin as a cytosol iron transport intermediate in human reticulocytes. *Br. J. Haematol.* **42**, 255–267.

Sutherland, G. R., Baer, E., Callen, D. F. *et al.* (1988) 5-Aminolevulinate synthase is a 3p21 and thus not the primary defect in X-linked sideroblastic anemia. *Am. J. Human Genet.* **43**, 331–335.

Taketani, S., Kohno, H., Sawamura, T. and Tokunaga, R. (1990) Hemopexin-dependent down-regulation of expression of the human transferrin receptor. *J. Biol. Chem.* **23**, 13981–13985.

Tenhunen, R., Marver, H. S. and Schmidt, R. (1970) Stimulation of microsomal heme oxygenase by hemin. *J. Lab. Clin. Med.* **75**, 410–421.

Testa, U., Petrini, M., Quaranta, M. T. *et al.* (1989) Iron up-modulates the expression of transferrin receptors during monocyte–macrophage maturation. *J. Biol. Chem.* **264**, 13181–13187.

Testa, U., Petrini, M., Quaranta, M. T., Pelosi, E., Kuhn, L. and Peschle, C. (1991) Differential regulation of iron-responsive element-binding protein in activated lymphocytes versus monocytes–macrophages. *Curr. Stud. Hematol. Blood Transfus.* **58**, 158–163.

Thorburn, D. R. and Beutler, E. (1991) The loss of enzyme activity from erythroid cells during maturation. *Adv. Exp. Med. Biol.* **307**, 15–27.

Trakshel, G. M., Kutty, R. K. and Maines, M. D. (1986) Cadmium-mediated inhibition of testicular heme oxygenase activity: the role of NADPH-cytochrome c (P-450) reductase. *Arch. Biochem. Biophys.* **251**, 175–187.

Treffry, A., Lee, P. J. and Harrison, P. M. (1984) The effect of iron on ferritin turnover. *FEBS Lett.* **165**, 243–246.

Trowbridge, I. S. and Omary, M. B. (1984) Human cell surface glycoprotein related to cell proliferation is the receptor for transferrin. *Proc. Natl. Acad. Sci. USA* **78**, 3039–3043.

Uchida, T., Akitsuki, T., Kimura, H., Tanaka, T., Matsuda, S. and Kariyone, S. (1983) Relationship among plasma iron, plasma iron turnover and reticuloendothelial iron release. *Blood* **61**, 799–802.

van Eijk, H. G. and van Noort, W. L. (1986) A non-random distribution of transferrin iron in fresh human sera. *Clin. Chim. Acta* **157**, 299–303.

Waugh, R. E., Narla, M., Jackson, C. W., Mueller, T. J., Suzuki, T. and Dale, G. L. (1992) Rheologic properties of senescent erythrocytes: loss of surface area and volume with red blood cell age. *Blood* **79**, 1351–1358.

Williams, J. and Moreton, K. (1980) The distribution of iron between the metal-binding sites of transferrin in human serum. *Biochem. J.* **185**, 483–488.

Wixom, R. L., Prutkin, L. and Munro, H. N. (1980) Hemosiderin: nature, formation and significance. *Int. Rev. Exp. Pathol.* **22**, 193–225.

Zak, O. and Aisen, P. (1990) Evidence for functional differences between the two sites of rabbit transferrin: effects of serum and carbon dioxide. *Biochim. Biophys. Acta* **1052**, 24–28.

Zaman, Z., Heynen, M. and Verwilghen, R. L. (1980) Studies on the mechanism of transferrin iron uptake by rat reticulocytes. *Biochem. Biophys. Acta* **632**, 553–561.

Zheng, L., Kennedy, M. C., Beinert, H. and Zalkin, H. (1992) Mutational analysis of active site residues in pig heart aconitase. *J. Biol. Chem.* **267**, 7895–7903.

3. Iron Transport

E. BAKER AND E. H. MORGAN

Department of Physiology, The University of Western Australia, Nedlands, Western Australia 6009

I. INTRODUCTION

The behaviour of iron in aqueous media such as in living organisms is largely determined by oxidation–reduction reactions between Fe(II) and Fe(III) and hydrolysis to form hydroxides which are often insoluble and/or unable to enter metabolic pathways. In the aerobic extracellular environment which exists in most multicellular organisms the more soluble Fe(II) is readily oxidized to the much less soluble Fe(III) which could render it unavailable for cellular needs. This problem has been overcome during evolution by the development of complexing agents which can bind Fe(III) and maintain it in a soluble form which can be utilized by cells. In all vertebrate animals, and some invertebrates, this function is served mainly by the iron-binding protein, transferrin. However, in certain situations other proteins (ferritin, lactoferrin, haemopexin, haptoglobin, albumin and vitellogenin) may also play a role in the extracellular transport of iron, and in states of iron overload when transferrin is saturated with iron the plasma may contain iron which is either not bound or only loosely and non-specifically bound to plasma proteins. Hence, extracellular iron may be divided into three general forms: transferrin-bound iron, specific non-transferrin-bound iron (ferritin, etc.) and non-specific non-transferrin-bound iron. Under normal circumstances extracellular iron transport is dominated by the first of these forms.

In addition to extracellular transport, iron must be carried across cellular membranes and within the intracellular matrix of cells so that it can be incorporated into the many cellular haem and non-haem iron-containing proteins. This raises the questions of how iron is released from transferrin, and the mechanisms by which it is transported across cellular membranes and within the cytosol. An important constituent of the process of cellular acquisition of transferrin-bound iron is the transferrin receptor which is present in nearly all types of cells in vertebrate animals.

This review will be concerned with current knowledge and opinion on the transport of transferrin-bound iron and non-transferrin-bound iron (specific and non-specific) in the extracellular fluid, the mechanism of iron uptake and transport across cellular membranes and iron transport within the cytosol. The major emphasis will be on transferrin-bound iron and, due to space limitations, considerations will be limited to vertebrate animals, mainly mammals. It will be possible to cite only a small proportion of the total literature. For detailed information and more extensive literature surveys readers are referred to the many excellent reviews on transferrin (Aisen and Listowsky, 1980; Morgan, 1981; Brock, 1985; Harris and Aisen, 1989) and the transferrin receptor (Newman et al., 1982; Trowbridge et al., 1984; Testa, 1985; Johnstone, 1989; Forsbeck, 1990). The structure and iron-binding properties of transferrin are described in Chapter 1.

2. EXTRACELLULAR TRANSPORT OF IRON

2.1. Transferrin-bound Plasma Iron

Normally the plasma iron concentration is 10–30 μmole/l (mean about 20 μmole/l) and the plasma transferrin concentration 22–35 μmole/l (mean 30 μmole/l) so that the transferrin is about 30% saturated with iron (range 20–50%). Hence the plasma and interstitial fluid contain considerable iron-free transferrin which is able to bind iron absorbed from the intestine or released from cells elsewhere in the body. The plasma concentrations of iron and transferrin vary from the normal adult values at different stages during the life cycle and in many diseases (Laurell, 1947, 1952). Thus, the plasma iron concentration falls during infancy and pregnancy and in iron deficiency, infections, malignancies, protein–calorie malnutrition, nephrotic syndrome and after trauma. However, whereas the plasma transferrin concentration is elevated in infancy, pregnancy and iron deficiency it is usually diminished in the other conditions. Elevated plasma iron concentrations are found in idiopathic haemochromatosis, secondary haemosiderosis, and in haemolytic, hypoplastic and megaloblastic anaemias. In these conditions the plasma transferrin concentration is usually diminished and the plasma latent iron-binding capacity is small. This is especially the case in conditions with severe iron overload when plasma transferrin may be completely saturated with iron so that iron absorbed from the intestine or released from cells cannot be bound by the specific iron-binding sites of transferrin. Instead it is non-specifically bound to plasma proteins or to other ligands present in plasma, and its availability to tissue cells is quite different from that of iron being transported in the normal manner bound to transferrin (see below).

Transferrin, like the other plasma proteins, is distributed throughout most of the extracellular fluid of the body, with a continuous circulation from plasma to interstitial fluid and then back to the blood via the lymph vessels. Approximately 100% of the plasma transferrin circulates through the lymphatics each day (Wasserman et al., 1964). Iron remains bound to transferrin during passage of the protein from plasma to interstitial fluid (Morgan, 1963). The binding of iron to its transport protein means that the circulation of the metal through the extracellular fluids of the body is limited by the same factors which limit the rate of circulation of plasma proteins. Plasma transferrin and transferrin-bound iron have almost unrestricted access to the cells of liver, spleen and bone marrow because the walls of the sinusoids in these organs contain large fenestrae through which plasma proteins can pass readily. By contrast, transferrin and its iron circulate much more slowly through the interstitial spaces bathing the cells of muscle and skin because the capillaries of these tissues have only limited permeability to plasma proteins.

The circulation of transferrin between intravascular and extravascular compartments of the extracellular fluid has no peculiar features but, as mentioned above, it does limit the availability of iron to certain tissues. An excellent example of this effect is placental transfer of iron (Morgan, 1982). In those species with the haemochorial type of placenta, in which the trophoblast cells of the placenta are bathed in maternal blood, the iron destined for transfer to the fetus is derived from maternal plasma transferrin which binds directly to the placenta. However, in many mammalian species the trophoblast is separated from maternal blood by one or more layers of maternal cells. In these species little maternal transferrin is bound by the placenta and little transferrin-bound iron is transferred to the fetuses. The source of iron for the fetal needs appears to be maternal erythrocytes which are extravasated into the lumen of the uterus and are taken up by phagocytosis by the chorionic epithelial cells. Presumably the epithelial layers between maternal plasma and trophoblast cells in species with non-haemochorial types of placenta prevent the transfer of adequate amounts of transferrin-bound iron to the fetuses.

The major functions of transferrin are to maintain extracellular iron in a soluble form which is suitable for cellular uptake, and to regulate the supply of iron to cells by influencing its distribution within the body and its availability to individual cells. The latter function is determined largely by the cell's complement of transferrin receptors, which varies greatly from cell type to cell type and at various times in the life cycle in any one type of cell. In so doing, under normal conditions transferrin not only ensures an adequate supply of iron to meet the individual needs of different cell types but also restricts the uncontrolled entry of excessive amounts of iron into cells with the resultant risk of cellular damage.

An example of this role of transferrin in regulating the tissue distribution of iron is provided by the condition in which transferrin is absent from the plasma, atransferrinaemia, either in humans (Heilmeyer, 1966; Cáp et al., 1968; Sakata, 1969; Goya, 1972) or in the mouse (Bernstein, 1987; Craven et al., 1987). Affected individuals have extremely low plasma transferrin levels, hypochromic microcytic anaemia and excessive iron deposition in the liver, pancreas, heart and other organs except the bone marrow and spleen. When radioactive iron was administered intravenously or orally to atransferrinaemic mice it was taken up mainly into the liver, very little entering the bone marrow, spleen or circulating erythrocytes. In addition, iron absorption from the intestine was found to be increased above the normal level, but was less than that found in dietary iron deficiency. These studies clearly demonstrate that transferrin is important in directing plasma iron to developing erythroid cells, that it is not required for intestinal iron absorption and that non-specific, non-transferrin-bound plasma iron is largely cleared by the liver and to a lesser extent by other non-erythroid organs.

2.1.1. *Plasma Iron Turnover*

The amount of transferrin-bound iron in the plasma of a normal human is about 3 mg and the plasma iron turnover rate is approximately 30–40 mg per day (Cook et al., 1970; Ricketts et al., 1977; Bothwell et al., 1979; Cazzola et al., 1985, 1987a). Hence, the plasma pool of transport iron is turned over more than 10 times per day. This rate is far greater than that at which transferrin circulates through the lymph (about one plasma pool per day) or at which transferrin is catabolized, approximately 15% of the plasma pool per day (Awai and Brown, 1963). Hence, it must be concluded that most of the plasma iron turnover occurs at sites which are in direct anatomical contact with the plasma and do not require the entry of transferrin into the lymph, and that transferrin is not catabolized during the processes involved in the turnover of plasma iron. In other words, most plasma iron turnover occurs in bone marrow, liver and spleen where the sinusoids are freely permeable to transferrin, and the cells of the body can remove iron from transferrin without damaging the protein. Indeed, in humans approximately 80% of the iron which leaves the plasma is destined for the erythroid bone marrow and then the circulating erythrocytes (Chapter 2). Some of the iron taken up by erythrocyte precursors in the bone marrow is not carried forward into the circulating erythrocytes but is transferred to cells of the reticuloendothelial system when a proportion of the erythroid precursors are prematurely destroyed in the marrow (ineffective erythropoiesis).

The majority of the immature erythroid cells do mature into circulating erythrocytes. Their iron is finally returned to plasma transferrin when they are phagocytosed by reticuloendothelial cells at the end of their life span. Much smaller amounts of iron cycle through the liver which can exchange iron bidirectionally with plasma transferrin, and lesser amounts still with the cells of other tissues, many of which retain iron for relatively long periods of time and exchange relatively little iron with transferrin.

The use of plasma iron turnover or ferrokinetics to quantitate the rate of erythropoiesis has been investigated by many workers, especially by Finch and his colleagues. Their publications should be consulted for the theoretical and experimental background of their analytical methods and for evaluation of ferrokinetic models used by other investigators, and this topic is discussed in more detail in Chapter 2. Finch and co-workers have shown that tissue uptake of iron increases as the plasma iron concentration rises due to the increasing proportion of plasma transferrin which is in the diferric form (Cazzola et al., 1985). Such transferrin has a competitive advantage in supplying iron to cells because of its higher affinity for transferrin receptors than monoferric transferrin, and because it can supply two iron atoms per protein molecule bound by the receptors (Huebers et al., 1983, 1985). Methods of analysis of ferrokinetic data which take this effect into account have been developed and can be used to quantitate erythroid uptake of transferrin as well as erythroid and non-erythroid iron uptake (Cazzola et al., 1987b; Beguin et al., 1988; Intragumtornchai et al., 1988). Total transferrin uptake by erythroid tissue is considered to be a measure of the number of transferrin receptors on the cells and of the number of immature erythroid cells.

2.2. Specific, Non-transferrin-bound Plasma Iron

Several proteins which bind iron or iron-containing compounds are present in the plasma and may play a role in the extracellular transport of iron, especially in abnormal conditions such as iron overload, infections and haemolytic states, and during egg laying in avian species. These proteins are ferritin, lactoferrin, haemopexin, haptoglobin, albumin and vitellogenin. With the exception of vitellogenin, the quantities of iron carried by these proteins are uncertain and are probably quite low relative to that transported by transferrin. They act as scavengers which transport iron in various forms from sites of cellular damage or release to the liver where the iron enters the storage pool or is recycled to plasma transferrin. Thus, they represent a sub-circuit within the major circuit of internal iron turnover via transferrin.

The concentration of ferritin in blood plasma of normal individuals is too low significantly to affect the plasma iron concentration and plasma iron turnover. However, in iron overload and in diseases associated with liver cell damage the plasma concentration of ferritin rises and may make an important contribution to the total plasma iron and iron uptake by the liver in addition to transferrin (Pootrakul et al., 1988). The ferritin is cleared from the plasma by hepatocytes (Unger and Hershko, 1974) by receptor-mediated and non-specific endocytosis (Mack et al., 1983; Adams et al., 1988; Osterloh and Aisen, 1989; Adams and Chan, 1990) followed by lysosomal degradation of the protein and entry of the iron into intracellular iron pools (see Chapter 4). Ferritin receptors have also been demonstrated in guinea-pig reticulocytes (Pollack and Campana, 1981) but are absent from those of rat and rabbit (Blight and Morgan, 1983). Hence, in the guinea-pig, ferritin may represent a source of iron for erythroid cells, but its importance in comparison with transferrin is unknown. Possibly human erythroid precursors can also take up ferritin (Bessis and Breton-Gorius, 1962) but, if such is the case, the amount derived from this source must be small since the rate of incorporation of transferrin-bound iron into these

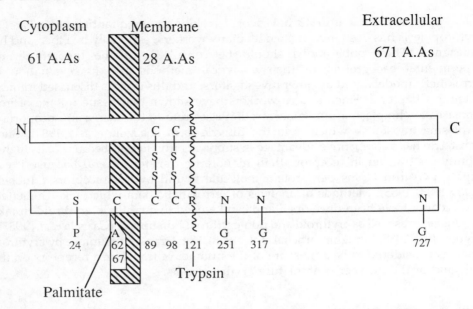

Fig. 3.1 Diagram of the human transferrin receptor, showing its dimeric structure, intracellular, transmembrane and extracellular domains and the amino acid residues (A.As) involved in phosphorylation (P), acylation (A), disulfide bridge formation, glycosylation (G) and the protease sensitive site (Trypsin).

cells is sufficient to account for all of the haemoglobin synthesis which is required for erythropoiesis as calculated from the blood haemoglobin concentration and the red cell life span. There is one known exception to the rule that plasma ferritin is normally only a minor contributor to plasma iron transport, and this is during the larval and metamorphosis stages of the lampreys, *Geotria australis* and *Mardacia mordax* which have very high plasma concentrations of ferritin (Macey *et al.*, 1982, 1985; Smalley *et al.*, 1986).

Lactoferrin is present in the plasma of normal humans at concentrations of 0.1 to 2.6 mg/l and at higher concentrations in lactating women and patients with chronic myeloid leukaemia (Rümke *et al.*, 1971; Bennett and Mohla, 1976). Whether or not plasma lactoferrin plays a role in plasma iron transport is uncertain. If it does the pathway is probably from the mammary glands and inflammatory sites to the liver where it appears to be taken up by hepatocytes, sinusoidal endothelial cells and Kupffer cells (Courtnoy *et al.*, 1984; Debanne *et al.*, 1985; McAbee and Esbensen, 1991).

Haptoglobin can bind haemoglobin, and haemopexin and albumin can bind haem, and transport these iron-containing compounds to the liver where they are taken up by hepatocytes and degraded, releasing the iron to the intracellular iron pools. With haptoglobin and haemopexin, uptake by hepatocytes occurs by receptor-mediated endocytosis, haptoglobin being degraded during this process (Kino *et al.*, 1980; Higa *et al.*, 1981) while haemopexin and its receptor are recycled to the cell membrane (Smith and Morgan, 1978, 1979; Smith and Hunt, 1990). In the case of albumin the haem probably dissociates from the protein before entering hepatocytes and other cells by simple diffusion through the cell membranes. Under normal circumstances the amount of iron transported through the plasma by these proteins is very small

(Garby and Noyes, 1959) but increases in haemolytic states, especially those associated with intravascular haemolysis. The role of haptoglobin and haemopexin in iron recirculation is discussed in Chapter 2.

Vitellogenin is a phospholipoprotein which is synthesized in the liver during the egg-laying period of ovoparous animals such as birds, reptiles and amphibians (Bergink and Wallace, 1974; Clemens, 1974). It carries iron from the liver to the ovaries where the protein is taken up by endocytosis into the developing ova and the iron is deposited in the egg yolk (Ali and Ramsay, 1974; Morgan, 1975). The amount of iron transported by this means can be relatively large, as much as 40% of the plasma iron turnover being directed first to the liver and then via vitellogenin to the eggs in the domestic fowl.

2.3. Non-specific Non-transferrin-bound Iron

Under normal conditions nearly all the non-haem, non-ferritin iron in mammalian blood plasma is bound to transferrin. However, when the plasma transferrin is saturated with iron due to iron overload (e.g. in genetic haemochromatosis, thalassaemia, acute iron poisoning) or atransferrinaemia iron appears in the plasma in a non-specific, non-transferrin bound form. It can be detected and measured by chelation with EDTA or DTPA (diethylenetriaminepentaacetic acid) followed by ultrafiltration (Hershko et al., 1978; Graham et al., 1979) or by the more sensitive bleomycin assay, a method based on the degradation of DNA in the presence of the bleomycin–Fe complex (Gutteridge et al., 1981).

The normal level of non-specific non-transferrin-bound iron in plasma is 0–1 μmole/l (cf. 20 μmole/l for transferrin-bound iron). Much higher levels have been reported in thalassaemia, haemochromatosis and acute iron poisoning (Hershko and Rachmilewitz, 1975; Hershko et al., 1978; Graham et al., 1979; Batey et al., 1980; Fargion et al., 1981; Gutteridge et al., 1985; Hershko and Peto, 1987; Grootveld et al., 1989). In several of these studies the concentration of non-specific iron was found to be correlated with that of plasma ferritin, but it is unlikely to be derived from ferritin since the assay techniques do not measure ferritin iron.

The composition of non-specific plasma iron has been difficult to determine due to the tendency of iron ions to bind to many biological molecules. Much of the iron may be adsorbed non-specifically to plasma proteins since it is not readily dialysable unless a chelator such as EDTA is added to the plasma. Computer simulation studies by May et al. (1980) which took into account the relative concentrations and iron-binding affinities of plasma constituents predicted that the most likely iron complexes in plasma would be with citrate, ascorbate, histidine and other amino acids. Recent studies using nuclear magnetic resonance spectroscopy have demonstrated that 50–70% of the non-specific iron in plasma from haemochromatotic patients is indeed in the form of ferric citrate (Grootveld et al., 1989). It should be noted that iron in this complex would probably be relatively non-toxic since ferric citrate has a low capacity to stimulate the generation of free radicals (Singh and Hider, 1988). Hence, other forms of iron may be the source of the toxic free radical generation which was demonstrated using the plasma of patients with haemochromatosis (Gutteridge et al., 1985).

Non-specific, non-transferrin-bound iron is rapidly cleared from the plasma, mainly by the liver and to a lesser extent by other non-erythroid tissues (Wheby and

Umpierre, 1964; Fawwaz *et al.*, 1967; Craven *et al.*, 1987). As discussed below, studies with the perfused liver indicate that uptake by this organ involves a passive carrier-mediated process (Brissot *et al.*, 1985; Wright *et al.*, 1986). The vulnerability of the liver to iron overload is due to its capacity to take up both specific and non-specific non-transferrin-bound iron and also because absorbed iron is delivered directly to the liver via the portal vein.

3. Cellular Uptake of Iron

3.1. Transferrin-bound Iron

The mechanism by which iron is transported from transferrin into cells is of considerable interest because of the varying iron requirements of different cell types, the extremely high affinity of transferrin for iron and the relative impermeability of cellular membranes to cations. Three stages in the cellular acquisition of transferrin-bound iron, each addressing one of these problems, must therefore be considered. These are (1) recognition and interaction of the transferrin–iron complex with the cell, (2) release of iron from the carrier protein, and (3) iron transport across the cell membrane. The first is mediated by cell membrane receptors for transferrin which are present in nearly all types of cells but vary in number depending on the cell type and its functional state. For example, they are particularly abundant on developing erythroid cells and trophoblast cells of the placenta which have large iron requirements for haemoglobin synthesis or for iron transport to the fetus. The receptors are also involved in iron release from transferrin, by helping to target the iron–transferrin to sites where release can occur as well as possibly by playing a direct role in the release process. Iron transport through cell membranes must occur after its release from transferrin since the protein does not enter the cytosol, and is not retained by the cell or degraded in the process, but is released after it has donated its iron.

3.1.1. *Transferrin Receptor*

The concept that the cellular uptake of transferrin-bound iron involves an interaction with specific cell membrane receptors was proposed some 30 years ago by Jandl and Katz (1963). Subsequent studies have confirmed this hypothesis and have led to isolation, characterization and investigation of the functions of the receptors. Many reviews of this topic have appeared in recent years (Aisen and Listowsky, 1980; Morgan, 1981; Brock, 1985; Harris and Aisen, 1989). The present one will therefore be confined to a brief discussion of the receptor's structure and function. Regulation of its expression is covered in Chapter 5.

(a) *Structure*. The structure of the human transferrin receptor is presented diagrammatically in Fig. 3.1. It is a disulfide-linked dimer of two identical transmembrane subunits, each of approximately 90 000 kDa and containing 760 amino acid residues. Three domains of each subunit can be recognized, an intracellular N-terminus consisting of 61 amino acids, a 28 residue membrane spanning part and a large, extracellular C-terminal domain of 671 residues (Trowbridge and Omary, 1981; Newman *et al.*, 1982; Schneider *et al.*, 1982, 1984; McClelland *et al.*, 1984).

The intracellular domain is necessary for normal endocytosis of the receptor, probably due to the presence of a specific amino acid sequence which is required for interaction with the clathrin lattice of coated pits (Rothenberger *et al.*, 1987; Alvarez *et al.*, 1990a; McGraw and Maxfield, 1990; Gironés *et al.*, 1991; Miller *et al.*, 1991). It contains a phosphorylation site (serine 24). The functional role of phosphorylation is unknown but it does not appear to be essential for endocytosis (Davis and Meisner, 1987; Rothenberger *et al.*, 1987).

The transmembrane domain spans the lipid bilayer once and consists largely of hydrophobic amino acids which function as a membrane anchor for the protein and as the signal peptide for translocation across the rough endoplasmic reticulum membrane during biosynthesis (Zerial *et al.*, 1986, 1987). Also in the transmembrane domain are one or two sites at which post-translational fatty acid acylation, usually with palmitic acid, may occur (Omary and Trowbridge, 1981a; Jing and Trowbridge, 1987; Schneider *et al.*, 1982). The major acylation site (cysteine 62) is close to the intracellular side of the membrane lipid bilayer. The functional significance of the acylation of the receptor is uncertain, but nonacylated mutant receptors are more rapidly endocytosed and mediate more rapid iron uptake than the normal receptor (Alvarez *et al.*, 1990b; Jing and Trowbridge, 1990).

The large extracellular domain contains three N-linked glycosylation sites (asparagines 251, 317 and 727) to which are attached one complex-type and two high mannose-type oligosaccharides (Omary and Trowbridge, 1981b; Schneider *et al.*, 1982, 1984; McClelland *et al.*, 1984). In addition, O-linked glycans have been identified in the receptor from some cell types (Do *et al.*, 1990). Carbohydrate makes up about 15% of the total mass of the receptor. Its function is uncertain but inhibition of glycosylation reduces the rate of translocation to the cell surface (Omary and Trowbridge, 1981b; Enns *et al.*, 1991) and mutant receptors which lack the glycosylation sites show reduced binding of transferrin, disulfide bridge formation and cell surface expression (Williams and Enns, 1991). Hence, the glycans may play a role in the translocation of the receptor to the cell surface and its interaction with transferrin. The transferrin-binding site must be situated on the extracellular domain of the receptor but the location of the interacting sites on either the transferrin or the receptor molecules is unknown. Each receptor dimer can bind two transferrin molecules, probably one to each subunit.

Other features of the extracellular domain are the presence of two disulfide bridges between the monomers, at cysteine 89 which is adjacent to the cell membrane bilayer and at cysteine 98 (Jing and Trowbridge, 1987), and the presence near the cell membrane of a site (arginine 121) which is highly susceptible to cleavage by trypsin and other proteases (Turkewitz *et al.*, 1988). It is uncertain whether the disulfides are required for normal function since mutants which lack them still form dimers in the presence of transferrin and are able to mediate iron uptake by the cell (Alvarez *et al.*, 1989). The presence of a protease-sensitive site may be of biological significance in that it provides one way in which receptors could be shed from cells and enter the circulation. This feature has also been utilized by several investigators to enable the release of the ecto-domain and any bound transferrin from the plasma membrane of various types of cells.

Available evidence indicates that transferrin receptors from different mammalian species have a similar structure to that of the human protein, and that the receptors in different types of human cells are very similar (Stein and Sussman, 1983) but may not be identical since some monoclonal antibodies react with the receptor from one type of cell but not from that of another. However, these different receptors are thought to be the product of a single gene (Cotner *et al.*, 1989).

(b) *Interaction with transferrin.* The interaction between transferrin and its receptor is reversible, pH-dependent and influenced by the iron content of transferrin. At near-neutral pH the receptor has a much higher affinity for diferric transferrin than for apotransferrin and an intermediate affinity for monoferric transferrin (Kornfeld, 1969; Morgan, 1981b; Dautry-Varsat *et al.*, 1983; Klausner *et al.*, 1983; Young *et al.*, 1984). The dissociation constant, Kd, for the binding of diferric transferrin by receptors of various species and cell types has been reported to be 10^{-7} to 10^{-9} M, and that for monoferric transferrin about 10^{-6} M. As a consequence of its higher affinity for the receptor, diferric transferrin has a competitive advantage over monoferric transferrin with respect to binding to the receptor and an even greater advantage in its ability to deliver iron to cells. With reticulocytes this amounts to an 8:1 to 14:1 advantage, depending on the animal species (Huebers *et al.*, 1985). Apotransferrin has little ability to compete with iron–transferrin for binding to the receptor (Morgan, 1981). Hence cells bathed in a mixture of iron–transferrin and apotransferrin, such as in the extracellular fluids of the body, selectively bind iron–transferrin, especially diferric transferrin, and achieve maximal gain from receptor function with respect to iron uptake.

As the pH is lowered below about 6.5 the affinity of receptors for apotransferrin rises and at pH 5–6 is probably as great as that for diferric transferrin at pH 7.4 (Ecarot-Charrier *et al.*, 1980; Dautry-Varsat *et al.*, 1983; Klausner *et al.*, 1983; Morgan, 1983). As a consequence apotransferrin remains bound to the transferrin receptor after it has released its iron at acidic sites within the cell.

(c) *Functions.* The major function of the transferrin receptor and the one which will be considered here is to mediate cellular uptake of transferrin-bound iron. Other proposed functions such as iron release from cells and effects on cell proliferation, growth and differentiation by processes which are independent of iron delivery to cells have been difficult to substantiate.

Two types of mechanisms by which the receptors mediate iron transport into cells have been described. One involves endocytosis and recycling of transferrin and its receptor and the other depends on processes which occur on the outer surface of the plasma membrane. The two mechanisms are not mutually exclusive. Both may operate but to varying degrees in different types of cells. Whatever the mechanism, it is clear that the major determinant of the rate of iron uptake by most cells or tissues is the number of functional transferrin receptors which are present on the cells. The dominant role of the bone marrow in the uptake of plasma iron is a consequence of the large number of transferrin receptors present in immature erythroid cells. In the rat, the total number of erythroid receptors has been shown to change in proportion to the number of erythroid cells when proliferation of these cells is stimulated by induction of haemolytic anaemia (Intragumtornchai *et al.*, 1988). In addition to the erythroid bone marrow, the liver and intestine are tissues in the adult rat which have large numbers of receptors as indicated by the initial distribution of an intravenously injected dose of transferrin-bound radioiron (Fig. 3.2). Other

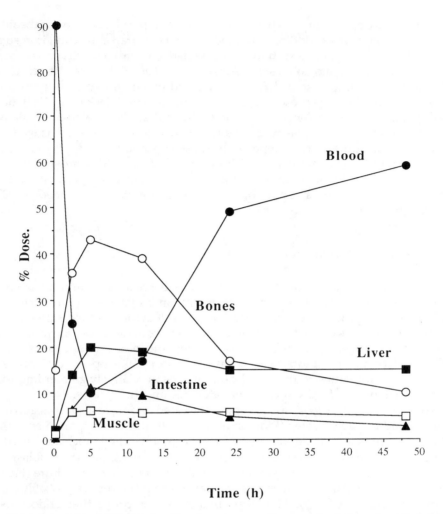

Fig. 3.2 Distribution of ^{59}Fe in the blood and some tissues of adult male rats following intravenous injection of transferrin-bound ^{59}Fe. At the time of sacrifice an exchange transfusion with non-radioactive rat blood was performed to remove intravascular radioactivity from the tissues. Blood radioactivity (●) decreased as iron was transferred from the plasma to the bones (○), liver (■), intestine (▲) and other tissues, and then reappeared in the blood in red blood cells as these cells were released from the bone marrow. Each value is the mean of two animals (Data from Cheney et al., 1967).

tissues such as muscle take up relatively little iron despite their considerable bulk, indicating a paucity of receptors which is compatible with low iron requirements as a result of slow rates of cellular proliferation and iron turnover.

The normal plasma iron and transferrin concentrations in humans are approximately 20 and 30 μmole/l, respectively, and the plasma concentration of diferric transferrin is about 3 μmole/l, higher than the concentration required to saturate transferrin receptors (0.5–1.0 μmole/l). Hence, cellular iron uptake should not be limited by supply of iron from the plasma. However, in iron deficiency when the plasma iron concentration is markedly diminished so that there is very little diferric transferrin and the erythroid marrow is hyperplastic the erythroid cell transferrin receptors are no longer saturated with diferric transferrin and iron supply, mainly in the form of monoferric transferrin at relatively low concentrations, becomes a limiting factor for haemoglobin synthesis (Cazzola *et al.*, 1987a). This is accentuated by the impaired ability of iron-deficient erythroid precursors to take up iron from transferrin even when it is presented as diferric transferrin (Black *et al.*, 1979; Bowen and Morgan, 1987). A similar problem may arise in thalassaemia and in haemolytic anaemias even though the plasma concentration of diferric transferrin is well above that required to saturate the receptors. In these conditions the erythroid marrow is greatly expanded (Langer *et al.*, 1972; Pootrakul *et al.*, 1984; Barosi *et al.*, 1986), and the rate of marrow blood flow, although increased from the normal level, may be insufficient to provide a supply of transferrin adequate for the needs of all the erythroid precursors.

3.1.2. *Iron Release from Transferrin*

Nearly all of the iron transported into cells *in vivo* is released from transferrin after interaction with cell membrane receptors, mainly in immature erythroid cells. Iron release from the protein occurs either within endocytotic vesicles after receptor mediated endocytosis of the iron–transferrin complex or at the cell surface. A small proportion of total iron uptake may occur by fluid-phase endocytosis without involvement of the receptors. The quantity of iron take up by this process is insignificant in immature erythroid cells but may be of relatively greater importance in some other types of cells such as hepatocytes and fibroblasts.

(a) *Receptor-mediated endocytosis*. Receptor-mediated endocytosis of transferrin was first described in reticulocytes (Morgan and Appleton, 1969; Appleton *et al.*, 1971) and subsequently in a wide variety of other cells including nucleated erythroid precursors, hepatocytes, vascular endothelial cells, placental trophoblast cells, myocytes, lymphocytes, fibroblasts and many different cell lines in culture (Hanover and Dickson, 1985). All cells which possess transferrin receptors are probably capable of endocytosing transferrin. However, this does not prove that endocytosis is necessary for iron uptake, nor does it indicate why endocytosis is required for this process. Indeed, some workers still question the importance of endocytosis for iron acquisition by cells.

Many of the experiments designed to determine whether endocytosis is required for iron uptake have been performed in reticulocytes. Using these cells the essential role of receptors in iron uptake has been demonstrated by inactivating them through the use of proteolytic enzymes, calcium chelators, specific antisera and heterologous transferrins, all of which inhibit transferrin endocytosis and iron uptake in proportion to the degree of inhibition of transferrin binding to the receptors (Morgan and Baker, 1988). Evidence that endocytosis is necessary for iron uptake is derived from measurements of the rates of transferrin endocytosis and iron accumulation by the cells under control conditions and when the endocytotic rate is varied by the use of inhibitors, alterations to the cellular environment and incubation temperature. In all such experiments a close correlation was found between the rates of the two processes under each experimental condition, indicating the dependence of iron uptake on endocytosis (Morgan and Baker, 1988).

The most likely answer to the question of why endocytosis is required for iron uptake is that it provides the microenvironment necessary for iron release from transferrin, probably as a consequence of the acidic nature of the endocytic vesicles (Baker, 1977). Support for this hypothesis comes from many experiments in a variety of cells in which vesicular pH was elevated by the use of weak bases, ionophores and mutant cell lines which are incapable of acidifying their vesicles – with resultant loss of iron uptake by the cells (Octave et al., 1979, 1982; Paterson and Morgan, 1980; Morgan, 1981b; Karin and Mintz, 1982; Harding and Stahl, 1983; Klausner et al., 1984).

Several steps in the process by which iron is transported into cells as a result of receptor-mediated endocytosis of transferrin are recognized (Fig. 3.3). The receptors on the cell surface bind transferrin and cluster into coated pits. This is followed by endocytosis, uncoating of the vesicles to form smooth vesicles or endosomes, and acidification of their contents by the action of an ATP-dependent proton pump. In studies with K562 cells and reticulocytes the pH within the endosomes was estimated to be about 5.5 (van Renswoude et al., 1982; Paterson et al., 1984) but higher values (6.0–6.5) have also been reported for other types of cells (Yamashiro et al., 1984; Sipe and Murphy, 1987). The acidification of the vesicles is followed by release of iron from transferrin and its transport across the endosomal membrane into the cytosol. The apotransferrin and the receptors then recycle to the plasma membrane and the apotransferrin is released by exocytosis. Since apotransferrin has a high affinity for the receptor at pH 5–6.5, but low affinity at pH 7.4 it remains bound to the receptor during the whole of the intracellular cycle but is rapidly released once exocytosis has occurred. The receptor is then free to bind iron–transferrin, especially diferric transferrin which has the highest affinity for the receptor at extracellular pH levels. The cycle can then be repeated (Dautry-Varsat et al., 1983; Harding and Stahl, 1983; Klausner et al., 1983; Morgan, 1983).

This is the simplest type of transferrin endocytic cycle. It is found in reticulocytes where the cycle time is quite small, 2–3 minutes (Intragumtornchai et al., 1990; Qian and Morgan, 1992), the endosomal pH is about 5.5, and cycle efficiency is high so that virtually all of the iron endocytosed on transferrin is released from the protein and retained by the cell. At pH 5.5 iron would dissociate from transferrin but probably not at a sufficient rate to allow both iron atoms, especially that at the less acid-labile site, to be released during the intracellular cycle time. Hence other factors in addition to acidification are likely to be involved in the iron release process. One is reduction of the iron, possibly through the action of a transmembrane ferrireductase, as will be discussed below. Although claims in favour of a reductive process have been made by some investigators this has been difficult to substantiate because the evidence in favour of reduction has been acquired through the use of ferrous iron chelators which may themselves catalyse reduction and produce misleading results. A second possible factor involved in iron release is the effect which binding to the receptor has on the conformation of the transferrin molecule. Recent studies indicate that changes in conformation occur and accelerate the release of iron from transferrin at the acid pH present in endosomes (Teeters et al., 1986; Bali and Aisen, 1991; Bali et al., 1991; Sipe and Murphy, 1991). A third possibility is that iron release is mediated by the action of small molecular weight iron chelators which could be derived from the cytosol. However, there is no experimental evidence for this.

The intracellular pathway for endocytosed transferrin may be more complex than the simplest one described above for reticulocytes. Generally, the increase in

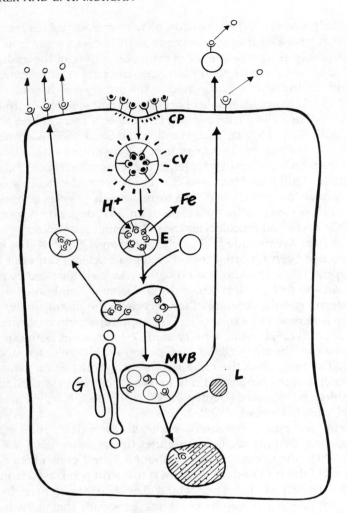

Fig. 3.3 Diagrammatic representation of pathways involved in the endocytosis of transferrin and its receptor in vertebrate cells. The figure shows ferri-transferrin (●), apotransferrin (○), transferrin receptor (Y), coated pit (CP), coated vesicle (CV), endosome (E), multivesicular body (MVB), Golgi complex (G) and lysosome (L). The shorter cycle occurs more frequently than the longer cycle in most types of cells, and fusion with lysosomes occurs infrequently, if at all.

complexity involves the fusion of endocytic vesicles with other intracellular vesicles, passage of the endosomes to the region of the Golgi complex and the formation of multivesicular bodies (Fig. 3.3). Although these processes occur to some degree in reticulocytes they are more prominent in nucleated cells which have far better developed Golgi complexes. The more complex cycles lead to the possibility of loss of receptors from the cell by exocytosis of multivesicular bodies as illustrated in Fig. 3.3 and even to transferrin and receptor degradation by fusion with lysosomes. The exocytotic loss of receptors is probably one of the mechanisms by which they are shed from reticulocytes during their transformation into mature erythrocytes

(Pan and Johnstone, 1983; Harding *et al.*, 1984; Pan *et al.*, 1985). Proteolytic cleavage from the cell surface, as mentioned above, may also be involved in this process. Such mechanisms are probably the source of cell-free transferrin receptors which have been found in the blood plasma and are being advocated as useful in assessing the rate of erythropoiesis and the presence of iron deficiency (Kohgo *et al.*, 1987; Flowers *et al.*, 1989; Skikne *et al.*, 1990; see also Chapters 7 and 14). However, it should be noted that the circulating receptor is reported to consist of amino acid residues 100–760 (Shih *et al.*, 1990), while the sensitive site for proteolytic cleavage is at arginine-121 (Turkewitz *et al.*, 1988).

It is generally assumed that the continued binding of transferrin to its receptor during the intracellular cycle protects the transferrin from degradation. A comparison of the rates of turnover of plasma iron and plasma transferrin indicate that this must be true for the vast majority of cycles, especially in erythroid precursors. In humans the plasma iron is turned over more than 10 times per day, about 80% of the turnover being directed to erythroid tissue, while only about 15% of the plasma transferrin is catabolized per day (Awai and Brown, 1963). However, transferrin catabolism is believed to occur more in the liver and other tissues than in the erythron. Hence, it is possible that a small proportion of transferrin taken up by receptor-mediated endocytosis in non-erythroid cells is directed to the lysosomes and is degraded (as suggested in Fig. 3.3). Alternatively, transferrin degradation may occur only as a consequence of fluid-phase endocytosis, a process which accounts for very little iron uptake in erythroid cells, but may be of greater significance in other types of cells.

Some consequences of the binding of transferrin to its receptor and the changes in affinity which occur with alterations of pH and the iron content of transferrin are of great functional importance and deserve emphasis. They are that diferric transferrin, as distinct from monoferric transferrin and apotransferrin, is preferentially taken up by cells, thus optimizing iron uptake, that transferrin is recycled undegraded and that the interaction with the receptor probably aids iron release from transferrin. Another to be discussed below is the hypothesis that transferrin and the receptor may together form an iron channel through which the iron released from transferrin can pass into the cytosol. In addition, there is the question as to whether the binding of transferrin to the receptor triggers endocytosis. Although claims that this is the case have been published (Larrick *et al.*, 1985) more recent evidence suggests that receptor endocytosis and recycling is probably a constitutive process which proceeds independently of the presence of transferrin (Watts, 1985; Ajioka and Kaplan, 1986; Stein and Sussman, 1986) although the rates of endocytosis and exocytosis may be accelerated by its presence (Gironés and Davis, 1989).

(b) *Iron release at the plasma membrane*. Despite earlier objections and criticisms it is now generally agreed that one of the mechanisms of iron transport into animal cells involves receptor-mediated endocytosis of transferrin. As discussed above and elsewhere (Morgan and Baker, 1988; Thorstensen and Romslo, 1990) current information supports the conclusion that it is the major, if not the only, mode of uptake of transferrin-bound iron by immature erythroid cells which are the dominant participants in iron uptake from plasma transferrin in the living animal. However, in the liver which also has a quantitatively important role in internal iron metabolism there is evidence that some of the iron taken up from transferrin results from processes which take place at the plasma membrane. This includes the observations that hydrophilic as well as hydrophobic iron chelators block iron uptake from transferrin, that weak bases and ionophores which raise endosomal pH produce only a small degree of inhibition of iron uptake, and that hepatocytes have a high capacity to take up non-specific non-transferrin-bound iron (Grohlich *et al.*, 1979; Page *et al.*, 1984; Brissot *et al.*, 1985; Wright *et al.*, 1986; Thorstensen, 1988; Thorstensen and Romslo, 1988).

It has been proposed that iron uptake by hepatocytes and some other types of cells is dependent on reductive iron release from transferrin at the cell membrane. Several oxidoreductive enzymes in the plasma membranes of animal cells have been described (Crane *et al.*, 1985; Löw *et al.*, 1990). The one most likely to be involved in iron release from transferrin is a NADH:acceptor transplasma membrane oxidoreductase. It has been identified in the membrane of many types of cells as an enzyme capable of reducing several extracellular electron acceptors, including ferricyanide, ferric salts, ferric chelates and transferrin-bound iron. Evidence in favour of the concept that this enzyme mediates iron uptake from transferrin by hepatocytes and other types of cells is that iron uptake is inhibited by ferricyanide and other membrane-impermeable electron acceptors and is stimulated by low oxygen concentrations (Thorstensen, 1988; Thorstensen and Romslo, 1988). The hypothesis has been criticized on the basis that the reduction potential of transferrin-bound iron is considerably lower than that of NADH so that reduction of the iron by NADH is not possible (Thorstensen and Aisen, 1990). This assessment is based on consideration of the properties of transferrin–iron in aqueous solution at neutral pH. However, the NADH-dependent transplasma membrane electron flow is accompanied by release of protons at the cell surface (Sun *et al.*, 1987, 1988), which could lower the pH of the microenvironment of transferrin bound to the cell membrane. This, plus conformational changes induced in transferrin as a result of interaction with its receptor, may raise the reduction potential of transferrin–iron to a level which would allow it to be reduced by NADH. Further work is required to investigate this possibility.

The protagonists of the membrane release hypothesis generally assume that the process involves interaction of transferrin with its receptors. However, this is not supported by studies of the effects of monoclonal antibodies to the transferrin receptor, and measurements of the Km for transferrin–iron reduction. Antibodies which bind to the high affinity transferrin binding sites of the receptor did not inhibit the reduction of ferric iron by HeLa cells, while antibodies which bind elsewhere on the receptor were inhibitory (Toole-Simms *et al.*, 1991). Also, the Km for reduction of the iron was found to be about 2×10^{-5} M, far higher than the Kd for transferrin binding to the high affinity receptor (5×10^{-7} M) (Löw *et al.*, 1987). These results raise the possibility that low affinity transferrin-binding sites, either on the receptor or elsewhere on the cell membrane, could be involved in iron release from transferrin and its uptake by cells. This is of interest, particularly with respect to hepatocytes because these cells have been shown to take up iron from transferrin by a low affinity adsorptive process which becomes apparent when the diferric transferrin concentration is raised above that required to saturate the high affinity binding sites of the receptors (Cole and Glass, 1983; Page *et al.*, 1984; Thorstensen and Romslo, 1984a,b; Trinder *et al.*, 1986). Since this process appears to discriminate between transferrin and albumin (Morgan *et al.*, 1986) it may be a consequence of the presence of low affinity sites on transferrin receptors. In any case, the evidence obtained by subcellular fractionation of the intact liver or isolated hepatocytes is that this process involves endocytosis of transferrin rather than being restricted to the outer cell membrane (Young *et al.*, 1985; Morgan *et al.*, 1986; Goldenberg *et al.*, 1988, 1991; Jackle *et al.*, 1991).

Our assessment of current evidence is that hepatocytes and several cell lines do possess a plasma membrane NADH oxidoreductase which can reduce transferrin-bound iron. However, it is uncertain whether this activity is required for iron uptake by the cells. Possibly the transplasma membrane redox system is more involved with the control of cell proliferation than with iron acquisition. It should also be remembered that a membrane redox system may be present in endosomal membranes as well as the outer cell membrane since these are derived, at least in part, from the plasma membrane. Hence, such a system could play a part in the reduction of iron released from transferrin in the endosome and aid the release reaction.

(c) *Iron uptake by hepatocytes*. The liver is second only to the erythroid marrow in its capacity to take up transferrin-bound iron. This iron is directed very largely to the hepatocytes (Hershko *et al.*, 1973). However, whereas the mechanism of iron uptake by erythroid cells is well understood and appears to occur largely or completely as a result of receptor mediated endocytosis of transferrin, there are many uncertainties and discrepancies in the literature with respect to iron uptake by the liver. Several of these questions have been dealt with elsewhere, so that they will only be briefly summarized here.

The major unsettled question is the quantitative and functional importance of transferrin receptors and receptor-mediated endocytosis of transferrin as a means of iron assimilation by hepatocytes when compared with plasma membrane mediated uptake processes, low affinity adsorptive endocytosis and fluid phase endocytosis. Even though some investigators failed to detect transferrin receptors on hepatocytes (Sibille *et al.*, 1982; Soda and Tavassoli, 1984; Sharma and Grant, 1991) others have been more successful (Young and Aisen, 1980, 1981; Cole and Glass, 1983; Thorstensen and Romslo, 1984b; Trinder *et al.*, 1986; Vogel *et al.*, 1987; Muller-Eberhard *et al.*, 1988; Rudolph *et al.*, 1988). There is also convincing evidence that the receptors mediate iron uptake by hepatocytes, especially at low concentrations of transferrin–iron (Trinder *et al.*, 1988). At concentrations above those which saturate the receptors iron uptake is probably the result of a low affinity, high capacity process unlike that which would be expected of the high affinity receptors (Cole and Glass, 1983; Morgan *et al.*, 1986; Trinder *et al.*, 1986, 1988). Yet, in an interspecies study *in vivo* several heterologous transferrins which cannot donate iron to erythroid tissue (where iron uptake is believed to be entirely receptor mediated) also failed to donate iron to the liver (Morgan, 1991). This suggests that iron uptake was mediated only by the specific transferrin receptors, and that receptor-independent processes do not have a significant role. Possibly, as suggested by the experiments with monoclonal antibodies to the transferrin receptor mentioned earlier, hepatic transferrin receptors have high and low affinity binding sites both of which show species specificity. The results obtained with the heterologous transferrins indicate that receptor-independent processes, such as non-specific adsorptive endocytosis or fluid-phase endocytosis, are unlikely to be major contributors to the total iron uptake by hepatocytes even at physiological iron–transferrin concentrations.

Whether or not hepatocyte iron uptake depends on plasma membrane or endocytic processes is uncertain. Possibly both types co-exist. There is a wealth of conflicting evidence, due in part to the use of different cell preparations (freshly isolated hepatocytes, cultured hepatocytes, perfused liver and the liver in the intact animal), different culture conditions, and different ways of assessing endocytosis. In general, the results from experiments which have used subcellular fractionation to measure endocytosis support the concept that endocytosis is important in iron uptake while experiments with freshly isolated cells are more in keeping with plasma membrane-mediated processes.

Another question of some concern is whether hepatic sinusoidal endothelial cells are involved in the mechanism of iron uptake from hepatocytes. Tavassoli and his colleagues have proposed that plasma transferrin is first endocytosed by the endothelial cells, desialated and then passed on to the neighbouring hepatocytes, presumably after passing across the space of Dissé (Tavassoli, 1988). This hypothesis ignores the observations that hepatic sinusoids have discontinuous walls which are believed to be freely permeable to plasma proteins, that hepatocytes have receptors for transferrin (as well as for asialoglycoproteins), that ^{125}I-labelled transferrin molecules are found mainly in hepatocytes, not endothelial cells, within 1–2 min after intravenous injection (Morgan and Baker, 1986; Morgan et al., 1986) and that exogenous transferrin taken up by the liver is in the fully sialylated form (Goldenberg et al., 1988). Hence, it is unlikely that the sinusoidal endothelial cells play an essential role in transferrin–iron uptake by hepatocytes although they probably possess transferrin receptors and are able to endocytose the protein.

3.2. Transmembrane Transport

Whether or not iron is released from transferrin within endosomes or at the outer cell membrane it must traverse a cellular membrane before entering the cytosol. The mechanism by which this occurs is still obscure but current research using reticulocytes, hepatocytes and other types of cells is helping to clarify the picture. Generally, the studies with these cells have used non-transferrin-bound iron in various forms as model systems in order to determine iron transport mechanisms. These should be applicable to the transport of iron derived from transferrin as well as to non-specific non-transferrin-bound iron.

3.2.1. Reticulocytes

Although transferrin is the normal source of iron for haem synthesis in reticulocytes many other ligands can donate iron to the cell for this purpose. These include pyridoxal isonicotinoyl hydrazone (PIH) and other aroyl hydrazones, penicillamine, citrate, ascorbate and sucrose (Ponka et al., 1982; Egyed, 1988; Fuchs et al., 1988; Morgan, 1988). Several lines of evidence show that the iron uptake from these sources is independent of transferrin endocytosis, e.g. depletion of endogenous transferrin, receptor inactivation with antisera or proteolytic enzymes and the use of incubation conditions which inhibit endocytosis. Hence, iron uptake from the non-transferrin ligands probably occurred at the plasma membrane and the use of these complexes may provide a means of determining how iron is transported across cellular membranes. Only with the ascorbate and sucrose complexes has this possibility been pursued. The results from both sets of experiments provide evidence for carrier-mediated iron transport.

Iron uptake from ascorbate by reticulocytes incubated in NaCl buffered at pH 7.4 showed saturation kinetics with a Km of 8.8×10^{-6} M (Egyed, 1988). Mature erythrocytes could not take up ascorbate–iron. It was concluded that reticulocytes possess a carrier-mediated iron transport system. In later studies with this system iron uptake was found to be stimulated if the NaCl in the medium was replaced by LiCl or KCl, or the intracellular Na^+ concentration was raised (Egyed, 1991). To account for these and other results it was proposed that iron is transported into the cells by a Na^+/Fe^{2+} exchange system.

Reticulocytes can also take up iron when incubated with $FeSO_4$ dissolved in isotonic sucrose (Morgan, 1988). The process is efficient and leads to even greater iron uptake and incorporation into haem than is seen with transferrin-bound iron. It is saturable with a Km of approximately 0.2×10^{-6} M, has a pH maximum of 6.4–6.5, and is inhibited by low concentrations of other divalent metals (Mn, Co, Ni, Zn, Pb) and by an increase in the ionic strength of the solution. It is also inhibited by metabolic inhibitors, and the rate of iron uptake varies in proportion to the cellular ATP concentration. Hence it has many of the characteristics of an active, carrier mediated transport process. Iron uptake disappears as reticulocytes mature, very closely paralleling the disappearance of the transferrin receptors (Qian and Morgan, 1990, 1991, 1992). This raises the possibility that the putative iron carrier is the transferrin receptor or that it is associated with the receptor in the cell membrane so that they are lost simultaneously during maturation of the cells. However, recent studies have shown that iron uptake by reticulocytes in isotonic sucrose can still occur after removal of transferrin receptors by proteolysis (Morgan, 1993). This may be dependent on reduction of iron to the ferrous state and active transport across the cell membrane by an iron carrier that normally functions in the membrane lining the endosomes.

Iron ascorbate and iron sucrose are not physiological compounds and iron transport into the cytosol of reticulocytes occurs in the endosomal membrane, not the plasma membrane. Hence, the physiological relevance of the above observations may be queried. However, they do provide sound evidence for the presence of an iron carrier in the plasma membrane and this is the source of some if not all of the endosomal membrane. The same carrier could therefore also be present in the endosomes. The apparently unphysiological nature of iron uptake from sucrose solution at pH 6.4–6.5 also requires explanation. One may speculate that iron does not enter the aqueous phase within the endosomes after it is released from transferrin but remains within the glycocalyx of the membrane before traversing the membrane. Possibly the sucrose mimics this step by presenting the iron to the membrane iron-binding component while it is on the outer cell membrane, and most effectively at an acid pH similar to that found in the endosomes. In this context it should be noted that there is evidence that iron released from transferrin within reticulocyte endosomes is transiently bound by a membrane protein with an apparent molecular weight of 450 000 (Nunez et al., 1989). This may be the putative iron carrier.

The presence of an iron carrier in the reticulocyte endosomal and plasma membranes is also indicated by investigation of the cause of the anaemia of the Belgrade laboratory rat. These animals have a severe hypochromic microcytic anaemia which is inherited as an autosomal recessive trait. The underlying defect appears to be impaired transport of iron across the endosomal membrane after it has been released from transferrin (Edwards *et al.*, 1980, 1986; Bowen and Morgan, 1987). This suggests that the genetic abnormality leads to the expression of a defective iron carrier protein in the reticulocyte endosomal membrane. The transport of iron from sucrose solution across the plasma membrane is also impaired (Farcich and Morgan, 1992a), which supports the concept that the same iron carrier is present in both plasma and endosomal membranes. In addition, defective iron uptake from transferrin was observed in the intestine, placenta, brain and fibroblasts from homozygous animals (Farcich and Morgan, 1992b). Hence, the carrier may be present in the membranes of many or all different types of cells.

3.2.2. *Hepatic and Other Cell Types*

It has long been known that liver cells *in vivo* and hepatocytes *in vitro* will take up non-specific non-transferrin-bound iron added to plasma or iron bound to various chelates (Wheby and Umpierre, 1964; Fawwaz *et al.*, 1967; Zimelman *et al.*, 1977; Grohlich *et al.*, 1979; Page *et al.*, 1984). More recently the mechanisms involved have been investigated in detail using the isolated rat liver perfused with solutions containing Fe(II) or Fe(III) maintained in solution through the use of ascorbate and various other iron complexing agents (Brissot *et al.*, 1985; Wright *et al.*, 1986, 1988). Iron uptake, mainly by hepatocytes as determined by autoradiography, was saturable with an apparent Km of about 2×10^{-5} M, and was temperature sensitive but unaffected by metabolic inhibitors. It appeared to be responsive to the membrane potential difference and was inhibited by Zn, Co and Mn. The results were interpreted as evidence for a transport process for the uptake of non-transferrin-bound iron but whether it is also responsible for the uptake of transferrin–iron and its relationship with the reticulocyte carrier are yet to be determined.

Evidence for saturable uptake of iron bound to chelators (citrate, nitrilotriacetate, ascorbate) has also been obtained using a variety of cultured cells, small intestinal fragments and small intestine brush border membrane vesicles (Simpson and Peters, 1985; Bassett *et al.*, 1986; Raja *et al.*, 1987; Stremmel *et al.*, 1987; Teichmann and Stremmel, 1990; Kaplan *et al.*, 1991; Seligman *et al.*, 1991). Hence, in these systems there is also evidence for the presence of iron carrier mechanisms.

3.2.3. *Membrane Iron Carrier*

The mounting evidence for the presence of facilitated iron transport across the membranes of a variety of cells has led to the search for carrier proteins. Only with intestinal mucosal cells has this met with any success. Iron-binding proteins in addition to transferrin and ferritin have been isolated from these cells by two groups of investigators. One was solubilized from rat and human microvillous membranes (Stremmel *et al.*, 1987; Teichmann and Stremmel, 1990). It is a 160 000 kDa glycoprotein which consists of three 50 kDa subunits. The other protein, of molecular mass 56 kDa, was isolated from rat and human duodenal mucosa (Conrad *et al.*, 1990, 1992). However, since it appears to be derived from the cytosol it is uncertain whether it is related to the protein isolated from the microvillus membrane. The putative role of these proteins in iron absorption is discussed in Chapter 6.

One may ask why carrier proteins have not been isolated from other types of cells such as reticulocytes, which have a high iron transport capacity. Possibly it is through lack of endeavour. Alternatively it may be because the iron carrier function is served by a well recognized protein, the transferrin receptor, as proposed by Singer (1989). He suggested that four transferrin molecules and two receptor molecules (four monomers) may interact to produce a complex which acts as a transmembrane carrier of iron. Iron released from the transferrin molecules would not enter the lumen of the endosome but would travel through a channel formed from the receptor tetramer.

Singer based his model for iron transport on the putative structure of several bacterial periplasmic transport systems which consist of periplasmic ligand binding proteins (cf. transferrin) and transmembrane proteins (cf. transferrin receptor). Crystallographic studies have demonstrated the very close structural similarity between lactoferrin and transferrin on the one hand, and periplasmic ligand-binding proteins on the other, a single lobe of transferrin corresponding to the whole molecule of the periplasmic proteins which have only one ligand-binding site (Anderson et al., 1987; Baker et al., 1987).

This hypothesis is highly speculative but deserves further consideration and investigation for several reasons. It is compatible with the observations that receptor monomers can form non-disulfide linked dimers in the presence of transferrin (Alvarez et al., 1989), and that the transferrin–receptor complex isolated from rat erythroid cell membranes has an apparent molecular weight of 580 000 and, therefore, could consist of four receptor monomers and four transferrin molecules (Intragumtornchai et al., 1988). Also, it could explain why the membrane transport of non-transferrin-bound iron decreases at the same rate as the number of transferrin receptors during maturation of reticulocytes, and is accelerated by incubation of the cells with an antibody to the transferrin receptor (Qian and Morgan, 1992).

3.2.4. Non-transferrin-bound Iron

Specific non-transferrin-bound iron in the form of ferritin, haem–haemopexin and haemoglobin–haptoglobin are removed from the plasma by hepatocytes, and vitellogenin by the ova, by receptor mediated endocytosis as mentioned in Section 2.2. Available information on the mechanism involved in the membrane transport of non-specific non-transferrin-bound iron has also been summarized above (Section 3.2.1).

3.3. Regulation of Membrane Transport

3.3.1. Transferrin-bound Iron

The main determinant of the capacity of cells to assimilate transferrin-bound iron is their complement of transferrin receptors. This is exemplified by measurements of receptor numbers and iron uptake in developing erythroid cells (Iacopetta and Morgan, 1983), maturing reticulocytes (Nunez et al., 1977; Qian and Morgan, 1992) and the placenta at different stages of fetal development (McArdle and Morgan, 1982). In each of these situations there is a very close parallel between receptor numbers and iron transport into cells. There is no evidence that other possible regulatory mechanisms such as changes in the affinity of receptors for transferrin, alterations of their cycling rate and efficiency of iron release have any physiological significance.

As discussed in Chapter 5 and elsewhere (Kuhn *et al.*, 1990), the main determinants of the rate of transferrin receptor synthesis and receptor numbers on cells are believed to be the level of iron supply and the rate of proliferation of the cells. Possibly the effects of proliferative rate are a consequence of increased iron requirements and are therefore another manifestation of the regulation of receptor synthesis through iron availability. Virtually all of the experiments which have delineated the mechanisms involved in the regulation of transferrin receptor synthesis have been performed *in vitro* using various cell lines. It is therefore necessary to ask to what extent the same mechanisms operate *in vivo* and how they affect iron metabolism.

The major iron transporting tissue of the body is the erythroid bone marrow. Transferrin receptor numbers and iron uptake by developing erythroid cells are maximal at the basophilic normoblast stage of development and decline thereafter as the cells cease dividing and mature to the reticulocyte and, finally, to the circulating erythrocyte stages when all receptors have disappeared. Are the receptor numbers influenced by iron supply? There is no evidence that iron overload leads to a reduction, but iron deficiency is associated with an increase (Muta *et al.*, 1987; Intragumtornchai *et al.*, 1988). Hence, iron supply may be a regulator of receptor synthesis leading to an increase above a certain relatively high basal level which is characteristic of the erythroid cell lineage. It may also be involved in the decrease in receptor numbers which occurs as the cells mature. Using mouse erythroleukaemic cells Hradilek *et al.* (1992) have acquired evidence that the low cellular non-haem iron concentration which results from the requirements of haem synthesis maintains the high level of transferrin receptor synthesis in erythroid cells after the cessation of cell division. Declining rates of haem synthesis during cell maturation may allow the non-haem iron pool to increase, thereby reducing receptor synthesis. This is compatible with observations that during reticulocyte maturation haem synthesis decreases at a greater rate than do transferrin receptor numbers (Qian and Morgan, 1992). However, the loss of protein synthesis capacity plus shedding of receptors by mechanisms which are not regulated by iron are probably the main contributors to the disappearance of the receptors by the time that the mature red cell stage is reached.

Changes in transferrin receptor expression *in vivo* as a consequence of iron deficiency and iron overload have also been reported for the liver and other tissues of humans and rats (Lombard *et al.*, 1989; Lu *et al.*, 1989; Sciot *et al.*, 1989). Generally, these studies have employed immunohistochemical staining of the receptors and are therefore only semiquantitative. However, in the liver and the brain of the rat there is quantitative data from transferrin binding studies that receptor numbers are increased in iron deficiency, and in the brain that they decrease in iron overload (Holmes and Morgan, 1989; Taylor *et al.*, 1991). These changes were associated with expected alterations in the rate of iron uptake by these tissues.

The rate of cell proliferation probably affects receptor expression and iron uptake *in vivo* just as it does *in vitro*. For instance, receptor numbers are usually high in rapidly proliferating tumour cells, and they increase in hepatectomy (Tei *et al.*, 1984). Possibly, also, the high rate of proliferation of erythroid precursors is a factor which contributes to their high receptor numbers and proliferation of intestinal mucosal cells to the rate of iron uptake by the intestine (Fig. 3.2). If this is true one would expect cellular receptor numbers and iron uptake to be elevated in fetal and post-natal life when cell proliferation and tissue growth is rapid. Little information on this issue is available. However, it has been noted that transferrin binding and iron uptake by brain capillary endothelial cells is maximal during the suckling period of the rat when brain growth is occurring most rapidly and declines to low levels as the animals age and brain growth declines (Taylor and Morgan, 1990).

3.3.2. *Non-transferrin-bound Iron*

No information is available concerning regulatory mechanisms which may affect the cellular uptake of specific non-transferrin-bound iron. In the case of non-specific non-transferrin-bound iron there is evidence that iron loading of cells increases their capacity to take up further iron. Pre-exposure of several types of cultured cell lines to inorganic iron (ferric ammonium citrate, ferrous sulfate) led to enhanced uptake of ^{59}Fe bound to nitrilotriacetate, citrate or ascorbate (Kaplan *et al.*, 1991). This raises the possibility that the presence of transferrin-free extracellular iron may induce the activity of membrane transporters of iron and thus accelerate the clearance of potentially toxic iron complexes from the plasma. It is of interest to note that preincubation of melanoma cells with ferric ammonium citrate also caused an increase in the non-receptor-mediated uptake of iron from transferrin while decreasing receptor-mediated uptake (Richardson and Baker, 1992).

4. CYTOSOLIC TRANSPORT

After iron has traversed the endosomal or plasma membranes of cells it is transported to sites where it is incorporated into haem, ferritin and other non-haem iron proteins. Numerous studies have demonstrated the presence of low molecular weight iron or radioiron in the cytosol of a variety of cells and tissues (Greenough *et al.*, 1962; Primosigh and Thomas, 1968; Pollack and Campana, 1980; Mulligan *et al.*, 1986). This iron is generally considered to be the transit or labile iron pool which acts as a means of intracellular iron transport between cell membranes and intracellular organelles (e.g. endosomes, mitochondria, lysosomes) and iron–protein complexes (Jacobs, 1977). It may be part of the chelatable pool of intracellular iron which is transiently available to exogenous chelators (Baker *et al.*, 1980; Pippard *et al.*, 1982) (see also Chapter 12) but is not likely to be identical, since the chelators will alter equilibria between intracellular iron complexes.

The chemical nature of the cytosolic iron transport pool has been difficult to determine, possibly because of the low concentrations and transient nature of the iron complexes. Ferritin has been proposed as one component of this pool (Speyer and Fielding, 1979), but other investigators have shown that the rate of turnover of ferritin iron is far too slow for it to act as the hypothetical carrier (Zail *et al.*, 1964; Grasso *et al.*, 1984). Recent studies have concentrated attention on lower molecular weight iron complexes with reported molecular weights varying from a few hundred to 56 000. Two proteins with putative cytosolic iron transport functions have been isolated. One, a 56 kDa protein from intestinal mucosal cells was mentioned above (p. 82). The other, a 16 kDa protein from rat liver has iron-binding properties but appears to be localized mainly in the microsomes and may not have cytosolic functions (Furukawa *et al.*, 1991). The role of proteins as cytosolic iron carriers therefore remains in doubt. Possibly a variety of intracellular compounds which can bind iron, such as pyrophosphate, nucleotides, amino acids, ascorbate and citrate, act as the carriers. In the case of reticulocytes, ATP-Fe and AMP-Fe have been isolated from the cytosolic low molecular weight iron pool (Weaver and Pollack, 1989). Since these compounds can donate iron to mitochondria (Konopka and Romslo, 1980) they may act as the iron carrier between endosomal membranes and mitochondrial ferrochelatase. Whether they can transport iron to the sites of incorporation into other iron complexes, or function as iron carriers in non-erythroid cells is yet to be determined. The use of non-invasive techniques such as Mossbauer spectroscopy may prove to be of value for the characterization of cytosolic iron transport complexes in future investigations (St Pierre *et al.*, 1992).

REFERENCES

Adams, P. C. and Chan, L. A. (1990) Hepatic ferritin uptake and hepatic iron. *Hepatology* **11**, 805–808.

Adams, P. C., Powell, L. W. and Halliday, J. W. (1988) Isolation of a human hepatic ferritin receptor. *Hepatology* **8**, 719–721.

Aisen, P. and Listowsky, I. (1980) Iron transport and storage proteins. *Ann. Rev. Biochem.* **49**, 357–393.

Ajioka, R. S. and Kaplan, J. (1986) Intracellular pools of transferrin receptors result from constitutive internalization of unoccupied receptors. *Proc. Natl. Acad. Sci. USA* **83**, 6445–6449.

Ali, K. E. and Ramsay, W. N. M. (1974) Phosphoprotein bound iron in the blood plasma of the laying hen. *Quart. J. Exp. Physiol.* **59**, 159–165.

Alvarez, E., Gironés, N. and Davis, R. J. (1989) Intermolecular disulfide bonds are not required for the expression of the dimeric state and functional activity of the transferrin receptor. *EMBO J.* **8**, 2231–2240.

Alvarez, E., Gironés, N. and Davis, R. J. (1990a) A point mutation in the cytoplasmic domain of the transferrin receptor inhibits endocytosis. *Biochem. J.* **267**, 31–35.

Alvarez, E., Gironés, N. and Davis, R. J. (1990b) Inhibition of receptor mediated endocytosis of diferric transferrin is associated with the covalent modification of the transferrin receptor with palmitic acid. *J. Biol. Chem.* **265**, 16644–16655.

Anderson, B. F., Baker, H. M., Dodson, E. J. *et al.* (1987) Structure of human lactoferrin at 3.2-Å resolution. *Proc. Natl. Acad. Sci. USA* **84**, 1769–1773.

Appleton, T. C., Morgan, E. H. and Baker, E. (1971) A morphological study of transferrin uptake by reticulocytes. In: *The Regulation of Erythropoiesis and Haemoglobin Synthesis* (eds T. Trávenicèk and J. Neuwirt), University Karlova, Praha, pp. 310–315.

Aruoma, O. I., Bomford, A., Polson, R. J. and Halliwell, B. (1988) Nontransferrin-bound iron in plasma from hemochromatosis patients: effects of phlebotomy therapy. *Blood* **72**, 1416–1419.

Awai, M. and Brown, E. B. (1963) Studies of the metabolism of I[131]-labelled human transferrin. *J. Lab. Clin. Med.* **63**, 363–396.

Baker, E. N., Rumball, S. V. and Anderson, B. F. (1987) Transferrins: insights into structure and function from studies of lactoferrin. *Trends Biochem. Sci.* **12**, 350–353.

Baker, E. (1977) General Discussion II. In: *Iron Metabolism: Ciba Foundation Symposium 51 (new series)* (eds R. Porter and D. W. Fitzsimons), Elsevier, Amsterdam, pp. 364–369.

Baker, E., Morton, A. G. and Tavill, A. S. (1980) The regulation of iron release from the perfused rat liver. *Br. J. Haematol.* **45**, 607–620.

Bali, P. K. and Aisen, P. (1991) Receptor-modulated iron release from transferrin: differential effects on N- and C-terminal sites. *Biochemistry* **30**, 9947–9952.

Bali, P. K., Zak, O. and Aisen, P. (1991) A new role for the transferrin receptor in the release of iron from transferrin. *Biochemistry* **30**, 324–328.

Barosi, G., Zanella, A., Berziuni, A. *et al.* (1986) Iron supply to erythropoiesis in hereditary spherocytosis: study of relative iron deficiency. *Blood* **68**, 43a.

Bassett, P., Quesneau, Y. and Zwiller, J. (1986) Iron-induced L1210 cell growth: evidence of a transferrin-independent iron transport. *Cancer Res.* **46**, 1644–1647.

Batey, R. G., Fong, P. L. C., Shamir, S. and Sherlock, S. (1980) A non-transferrin-bound serum iron in idiopathic hemochromatosis. *Dig. Dis. Sci.* **25**, 340–346.

Beguin, Y., Stray, S. M., Cazzola, M., Huebers, H. and Finch, C. A. (1988) Ferrokinetic measurements of erythropoiesis. *Acta Haematol.* **79**, 121–126.

Bennett, R. M. and Mohla, C. (1976) A solid-phase radioimmunoassay for the measurement of lactoferrin in human plasma: variation with age, sex and disease. *J. Lab. Clin. Med.* **88**, 156–166.

Bernstein, S. E. (1987) Hereditary hypotransferrinemia with hemosiderosis, a murine disorder resembling human atransferrinemia. *J. Lab. Clin. Med.* **110**, 690–705.

Bergink, E. W. and Wallace, R. A. (1974) Precursor–product relationship between amphibian vitellogenin and the yolk proteins, lipovitellin and phosvitin. *J. Biol. Chem.* **249**, 2897–2903.

Bessis, M. C. and Breton-Gorius, J. (1962) Iron metabolism in the bone marrow as seen by electron microscopy: a critical review. *Blood* **19**, 635–663.

Black, C. B., Glass, J., Nunez, M. T. and Robinson, S. H. (1979) Transferrin binding and iron transport in iron-deficient and iron-replete rat reticulocytes. *J. Lab. Clin. Med.* **93**, 645–651.

Blight, G. D. and Morgan, E. H. (1983) Ferritin and iron uptake by reticulocytes. *Br. J. Haematol.* **55**, 59–71.

Bothwell, T. H., Charlton, R. W., Cook, J. D. and Finch, C. A. (1979) *Iron Metabolism in Man*, Blackwell, Oxford.

Bowen, B. J. and Morgan, E. H. (1987) Anemia of the Belgrade rat: evidence for defective membrane transport of iron. *Blood* **70**, 38–44.

Brissot, P., Wright T. L., Ma, W.-L. and Weisiger, R. A. (1985) Efficient clearance of non-transferrin-bound iron by rat liver. *J. Clin. Invest.* **76**, 1463–1470.

Brock, J. H. (1985) *Transferrins in Metalloproteins* (ed. P. Harris), Macmillan Press, London, pp 183–262.

Cáp, J., Lehotska, V. and Mayerova, A. (1968) Congenital atransferrinemia in an eleven-month-old baby. *Cesk. Pediat.* **23**, 1020–1025.

Cazzola, M., Huebers, H. A., Sayers, M. H., MacPhail, A. P., Eng, M. and Finch, C. A. (1985) Transferrin saturation, plasma iron turnover and transferrin uptake in normal humans. *Blood* **66**, 935–939.

Cazzola, M., Pootrakul, P., Bergamaschi, G., Huebers, H. A., Eng, M. and Finch, C. A. (1987a) Adequacy of iron supply for erythropoiesis: in vivo observations in humans. *J. Lab. Clin. Med.* **110**, 734–739.

Cazzola, M., Pootrakul, P., Huebers, H. A., Eng, M., Esbach, J. and Finch, C. A. (1987b) Erythroid marrow function in anemic patients. *Blood* **69**, 296–301.

Cheney, B. A., Lothe, K., Morgan, E. H., Sood, S. K. and Finch, C. A. (1967) Internal iron exchange in the rat. *Am. J. Physiol.* **212**, 376–380.

Clemens, M. J. (1974) The regulation of egg yolk protein synthesis by steroid hormones. *Progr. Biophys. Molec. Biol.* **28**, 69–108.

Cole, E. S. and Glass, J. (1983) Transferrin binding and iron uptake in mouse hepatocytes. *Biochim. Biophys. Acta* **762**, 102–110.

Conrad, M. E., Umbreit, J. N. and Moore, E. G. (1990) A newly identified iron binding protein in duodenal mucosa of rats. Purification and characterization of mobiliferrin. *J. Biol. Chem.* **265**, 5273–5279.

Conrad, M. E., Umbreit, J. N., Moore, E. G. and Rodning, C. R. (1992) Newly identified iron-binding protein in human duodenal mucosa. *Blood* **79**, 244–247.

Cook, J. D., Marsaglia, G., Eschbach, J. W., Funk, D. D. and Finch, C. A. (1970) Ferrokinetics: a biologic model for iron exchange in man. *J. Clin. Invest.* **49**, 197–205.

Cotner, T., Gupta, A. D., Papayannopoulou, Th. and Starmatoyannopoulos, G. (1989) Characterization of a novel form of transferrin receptor preferentially expressed on normal erythroid progenitors and precursors. *Blood* **73**, 214–221.

Courtnoy, P. J., Moguilevsky, N., Retequi, L. A., Castracane, C. E. and Massan, P. L. (1984) Uptake of lactoferrin by the liver II. Endocytosis by sinusoidal cells. *Lab. Invest.* **50**, 329–334.

Crane, F. L., Sun, I. L., Clark, M. G., Grebing, C. and Löw, H. (1985) Transplasma-membrane redox systems in growth and development. *Biochim. Biophys. Acta* **811**, 233–264.

Craven, C. M., Alexander, J., Eldridge, M., Kushner, J. P., Bernstein, S. and Kaplan, J. (1987). Tissue distribution and clearance kinetics of non-transferrin-bound iron in the hypotrans-ferrinemic mouse: a rodent model for hemochromatosis. *Proc. Natl. Acad. Sci. USA* **84**, 3457–3461.

Dautry-Varsat, A., Ciechanover, A. and Lodish, H. F. (1983) pH and the recycling of transferrin during receptor-mediated endocytosis. *Proc. Natl. Acad. Sci. USA* **80**, 2258–2262.

Davis, R. J. and Meisner, H. (1987) Regulation of transferrin receptor cycling by protein kinase C is independent of receptor phosphorylation at serine 24 in Swiss 3T3 fibroblasts. *J. Biol. Chem.* **262**, 16041–16047.

Debanne, M. T., Regoeczi, E., Sweeney, G. D. and Krestynski, F. (1985) Interaction of human lactoferrin with the liver. *Am. J. Physiol.* **248**, G463–G469.

Do, S.-I., Enns, C. and Cummings, R. D. (1990) Human transferrin receptor contains O-linked oligosaccharides. *J. Biol. Chem.* **265**, 114–125.

Ecarot-Charrier, B., Grey, V. L., Wilczynska, A. and Schulman, H. M. (1980) Reticulocyte membrane transferrin receptors. *Canad. J. Biochem.* **58**, 418–426.

Edwards, J. A., Sullivan, A. L. and Hoke, J. E. (1980) Defective delivery of iron to the developing red cells of the Belgrade laboratory rat. *Blood* **55**, 645–648.

Edwards, J. A., Huebers, H., Kunzler, C. and Finch, C. A. (1986) Iron metabolism in the Belgrade rat. *Blood* **67**, 623–628.

Egyed, A. (1988) Carrier mediated iron transport through erythroid cell membrane. *Br. J. Haematol.* **68**, 483–486.

Egyed, A. (1991) Na$^+$ modulates carrier-mediated Fe^{2+} transport through the erythroid cell membrane. *Biochem. J.* **275**, 635–638.

Enns, C. A., Clinton, E. M., Reckhow, C. L., Root, B. J., Do, S.-I. and Cook, C. (1991) Acquisition of the functional properties of the transferrin receptor during its biosynthesis. *J. Biol. Chem.* **266**, 13272–13277.

Farcich, E. A. and Morgan, E. H. (1992a) Uptake of transferrin-bound and nontransferrin-bound iron by reticulocytes from Belgrade laboratory rat: comparison with Wistar rat transferrin and reticulocytes. *Am. J. Hematol.* **39**, 9–14.

Farcich, E. A. and Morgan, E. H. (1992b) Diminished iron acquisition by cells and tissues of Belgrade laboratory rats. *Am. J. Physiol.* **262**, R220–R224.

Fargion, S., Cappellini, M. D., Sampietro, M. and Fiorelli, G. (1981) Non-specific iron in patients with beta-thalassemia trait and chronic active hepatitis. *Scand. J. Haemat.* **26**, 161–167.

Fawwaz, R. A., Winchell, H. S., Pollycove, M. and Sargent, T. (1967) Hepatic iron deposition in humans. I. First-pass hepatic deposition of intestinally absorbed iron in patients with low plasma latent iron-binding capacity. *Blood* **30**, 417–424.

Flowers, C. H., Skikne, B. S., Covell, A. M. and Cook, J. D. (1989) The clinical measurement of serum transferrin receptor. *J. Lab. Clin. Med.* **114**, 368–377.

Forsbeck, K. (1990) The transferrin receptor and iron accumulation in erythroid cells. In: *Blood Cell Biochemistry Vol. 1 Erythroid Cells*, (ed. J. R. Harris), Plenum: New York, pp. 403–427.

Fuchs, O., Borová, J., Hradilek, A. and Neuwirt, J. (1988) Non-transferrin donors of iron for heme synthesis in immature erythroid cells. *Biochem. Biophys. Acta* **969**, 158–165.

Furukawa, T., Taketani, S., Kohno, H. and Tokunaga, R. (1991) A newly identified iron-binding protein in rat liver: purification and characterization. *Biochem. Biophys. Res. Comm.* **181**, 409–415.

Garby, L. and Noyes, W. D. (1959) Studies on the hemoglobin metabolism. I. The kinetic properties of the plasma hemoglobin pool in normal man. *J. Clin. Invest.* **38**, 1479–1486.

Gironés, N. and Davis, R. J. (1989) Comparison of the kinetics of cycling of the transferrin receptor in the presence or absence of bound diferric transferrin. *Biochem. J.* **264**, 36–46.

Gironés, N., Alvarez, E., Seth, A., Lin. I.-M., Latour, D. A. and Davis, R. J. (1991) Mutational analysis of the cytoplasmic tail of the human transferrin receptor. Identification of a subdomain that is required for rapid endocytosis. *J. Biol. Chem.* **266**, 19006–19012.

Goldenberg, H., Eder, M., Pumm, R., Wallner, E., Retzek, H. and Hüttinger, M. (1988) Uptake and subcellular distribution of injected transferrin in rat liver. *Biochim. Biophys. Acta* **968**, 331–339.

Goldenberg, H., Seelos, C., Chatwani, S., Chegini, S. and Pumm, R. (1991) Uptake and endocytic pathway of transferrin and iron in perfused rat liver. *Biochim. Biophys. Acta* **1067**, 145–152.

Goya, N., Miyazaki, S., Kodate, S. and Ushio, B. (1972) A family of congenital atransferrinemia. *Blood* **40**, 239–245.

Graham, G., Bates, G. W., Rachmilewitz, E. A. and Hershko, C. (1979) Nonspecific serum iron in thalassemia: quantitation and chemical reactivity. *Am. J. Hemat.* **6**, 207–217.

Grasso, J. A., Hillis, T. J. and Mooney-Frank, J. A. (1984) Ferritin is not a required intermediate for iron utilization in heme synthesis. *Biochim. Biophys. Acta* **797**, 247–255.

Greenough, W. B., Peters, T. and Thomas, E. D. (1962) An intracellular protein intermediate for hemoglobin formation. *J. Clin. Invest.* **41**, 1116–1124.

Grohlich, D., Morley, C. G. and Bezkorovainy, A. (1979) Some aspects of iron uptake by hepatocytes in suspension. *Int. J. Biochem.* **10**, 797–802.

Grootveld, M., Bell, J. D., Halliwell, B., Aruoma, O. I., Bomford, A. and Sadler, P. J. (1989) Non-transferrin-bound iron in plasma or serum from patients with idiopathic hemochromatosis. *J. Biol. Chem.* **264**, 4417–4422.

Gutteridge, J. M. C., Rowley, D. A. and Halliwell, B. (1981) Superoxide-dependent formation of hydroxy radicals in the presence of iron salts. Detection of 'free' iron in biological systems by using bleomycin-dependent degradation of DNA. *Biochem. J.* **199**, 263–265.

Gutteridge, J. M. C., Rowley, D. A., Griffiths, E. and Halliwell, B. (1985) Low-molecular-weight iron complexes and oxygen radical reactions in idiopathic haemochromatosis. *Clin. Sci.* **68**, 463–467.

Hanover, J. A. and Dickson, R. B. (1985) Transferrin: receptor-mediated endocytosis and iron delivery. In: *Endocytosis* (eds I. Pastan and M. C. Willingham), Plenum Press: New York, pp. 131–161.

Harding, C. and Stahl, P. (1983) Transferrin cycling in reticulocytes: pH and iron are important determinants of ligand binding and processing. *Biochem. Biophys. Res. Comm.* **113**, 650–658.

Harding, C., Heuser, J. and Stahl, P. (1984) Endocytosis and intracellular processing of transferrin and colloidal gold–transferrin in rat reticulocytes: demonstration of a pathway for receptor shedding. *Eur. J. Cell. Biol.* **35**, 256–263.

Harris, D. C. and Aisen, P. (1989) Physical biochemistry of the transferrins. In: *Iron Carriers and Iron Proteins* (ed. T. M. Loehr), VCH: New York, pp. 239–371.

Heilmeyer, L. (1966) Dix Atransferrinamien. *Acta Haematol.* **36**, 40–49.

Hershko, C. and Peto, T. E. A. (1987) Non-transferrin plasma iron. *Br. J. Haematol.* **66**, 149–151.

Hershko, C. and Rachmilewitz, E. A. (1975) Non-transferrin plasma iron in patients with transfusional iron overload. In: *Proteins of Iron Storage and Transport in Biochemistry and Medicine* (ed. R. R. Crichton), North-Holland: Amsterdam, pp. 427–432.

Hershko, C., Cook, J. D. and Finch, C. A. (1973) Storage iron kinetics. III. Study of desferrioxamine action by selective radioiron labels of RE and parenchymal cells. *J. Lab. Clin. Med.* **81**, 876–886.

Hershko, C., Graham, G., Bates, G. W. and Rachmilewitz, E. A. (1978) Non-specific serum iron in thalassemia: an abnormal serum iron fraction of potential toxicity. *Br. J. Haematol.* **40**, 255–263.

Higa, Y., Oshiro, S., Kino, K., Tsunoo, H. and Nakajima, H. (1981) Catabolism of globin–haptoglobin in liver cells after intravenous administration of hemoglobin–haptoglobin to rats. *J. Biol. Chem.* **256**, 12322–12328.

Holmes, J. M. and Morgan, E. H. (1989) Uptake and distribution of transferrin and iron in perfused iron deficient rat liver. *Am. J. Physiol.* **256**, G1022–G1027.

Hradilek, A., Fuchs, O. and Neuwirt, J. (1992) Inhibition of heme synthesis decreases transferrin receptor expression in mouse erythroleukemia cells. *J. Cell. Physiol.* **150**, 327–333.

Huebers, H. and Finch, C. A. (1987) The physiology of transferrin and transferrin receptors. *Physiol. Rev.* **67**, 520–582.

Huebers, H, Csiba, E., Huebers, E. and Finch, C. A. (1983) Competitive advantage of diferric transferrin in delivering iron to reticulocytes. *Proc. Natl. Acad. Sci. USA* **80**, 300–304.

Huebers, H., Csiba, E., Huebers, E. and Finch, C. A. (1985) Molecular advantage of diferric transferrin in delivering iron to reticulocytes: a comparative study. *Proc. Soc. Exp. Biol. Med.* **179**, 222–226.

Iacopetta, B. J. and Morgan, E. H. (1983) Transferrin endocytosis and iron uptake during erythroid cell development. *Biomed. Biochim. Acta* **42**, S182–S186.

Intragumtornchai, T., Huebers, H. A., Eng, M. and Finch, C. A. (1988) In vivo transferrin–iron receptor relationships in erythron of rats. *Am. J. Physiol.* **255**, R326–R331.

Intragumtornchai, T., Huebers, H. A. and Finch, C. A. (1990) Transferrin–reticulocyte cycle time in rat reticulocytes. *Blut* **60**, 249–252.

Jackle, S., Runquist, E. A., Miranda-Brady, S. and Havel, R. J. (1991) Trafficking of the epidermal growth factor receptor and transferrin in three hepatocyte endosomal fractions. *J. Biol. Chem.* **266**, 1396–1402.

Jacobs, A. (1977) Low molecular weight intracellular iron transport compounds. *Blood* **50**, 433–439.

Jandl, J. H. and Katz, J. H. (1963) The plasma-to-cell cycle of transferrin. *J. Clin. Invest.* **42**, 314–326.

Jing, S. and Trowbridge, I. S. (1987) Identification of the intermolecular disulfide bonds of the human transferrin receptor and its lipid-attachment site. *EMBO J.* **6**, 327–331.

Jing, S. and Trowbridge, I. S. (1990) Nonacylated human transferrin receptors are rapidly internalized and mediate iron uptake. *J. Biol. Chem.* **265**, 11555–11559.

Johnstone, R. M. (1989) The transferrin receptor. In: *Red Blood Cell Membranes* (eds P. Agre and J. C. Parker), Marcel Dekker: New York, pp. 325–365.

Kaplan, J., Jordan, I. and Sturrock, A. (1991) Regulation of the transferrin-independent iron transport system in cultured cells. *J. Biol. Chem.* **266**, 2997–3004.

Karin, M. and Mintz, B. (1981) Receptor mediated endocytosis of transferrin in developmentally totipotent mouse teratocarcinoma stem cells. *J. Biol. Chem.* **256**, 3245–3252.

Kino, K., Tsumoo, H., Higa, Y., Takami, M., Hamaguchi, H. and Nakajima, H. (1980) Hemoglobin–haptoglobin receptor in rat liver plasma membrane. *J. Biol. Chem.* **255**, 9616–9620.

Klausner, R. D., Ashwell, G., van Renswoude, J., Harford, J. and Bridges, K. (1983) Binding of apotransferrin to K562 cells: explanation of the transferrin cycle. *Proc. Natl. Acad. Sci. USA* **80**, 2263–2266.

Klausner, R. D., van Renswoude, J., Kempf, C., Rao, K., Bateman, J. L. and Robbins, A. R. (1984) Failure to release iron from transferrin in a Chinese hamster ovary cell mutant pleiotropically defective in endocytosis. *J. Cell. Biol.* **98**, 1098–1101.

Kohgo, Y., Nütsu, Y. and Kondo, H. (1987) Serum transferrin receptor as a new index of erythropoiesis. *Blood* **70**, 1955–1958.

Konopka, K. and Romslo, I. (1980) Uptake of iron from transferrin by isolated rat-liver mitochondria mediated by phosphate compounds. *Eur. J. Biochem.* **107**, 433–439.

Kornfeld, S. (1969) The effect of metal attachment to human apotransferrin on its binding to reticulocytes. *Biochim. Biophys. Acta* **194**, 25–33.

Kuhn, L., Schulman, H. M. and Ponka, P. (1990) Iron–transferrin requirements and transferrin receptor expression in proliferating cells. In: *Iron Storage and Transport* (eds P. Ponka, H. M. Schulman and R. C. Woodworth), CRC Press: Boca Raton, pp. 149–191.

Langer, E. E., Haining, R. G., Labbe, R. F., Jacobs, P., Crosby, E. F. and Finch, C. A. (1972) Erythrocyte protoporphyrin. *Blood* **40**, 1121–1128.

Larrick, J. W., Enns, C., Raubitschek, A. and Weintraub, H. (1985) Receptor-mediated endocytosis of human transferrin and its cell surface receptor. *J. Cell. Physiol.* **124**, 283–287.

Laurell, C.-B. (1947) Studies on the transportation and metabolism of iron in the body with special reference to the iron-binding component of human plasma. *Acta Med. Scand.* **14**, Suppl. 46, 1–129.

Laurell, C.-B. (1952) Plasma iron and the transport of iron in the organism. *Pharm. Rev.* **4**, 371–395.

Lombard, M., Bomford, A., Hynes, M. *et al.* (1989) Regulation of hepatic transferrin receptor in hereditary hemochromatosis. *Hepatology* **9**, 1–5.

Löw, H., Grebing, C., Lindgren, A., Tally, M., Sun, I. L. and Crane, F. L. (1987) Involvement of transferrin in the reduction of iron by the transplasma membrane electron transport system. *J. Bioenerg. Biomemb.* **19**, 535–549.

Löw, H., Crane, F. L., Morré, D. J. and Sun, I. L. (1990) Oxidoreductase enzymes in the plasma membrane. In: *Oxidoreduction at the Plasma Membrane: Relation to Growth and Transport. Vol. 1, Animals*, CRC Press, Boca Raton, pp. 30–65.

Lu, U.-P., Hayashi, K. and Awai, M. (1989) Transferrin receptor expression in normal, iron-deficient and iron-overloaded rats. *Acta Path. Jpn.* **39**, 759–764.

McAbee, D. D. and Esbensen, K. (1991) Binding and endocytosis of apo- and holo-lactoferrin by isolated rat hepatocytes. *J. Biol. Chem.* **266**, 23624–23631.

McArdle, H. J. and Morgan, E. H. (1982) Transferrin and iron movements in the rat conceptus during gestation. *J. Reprod. Fertil.* **66**, 529–536.

McClelland, A., Kuhn, L. C. and Ruddle, F. H. (1984). The human transferrin receptor gene: genomic organization, and the complete primary structure of the receptor deduced from a cDNA sequence. *Cell* **39**, 267–274.

McGraw, T. E. and Maxfield, F. R. (1990) Human transferrin receptor internalization is partly dependent upon an aromatic amino acid on the cytoplasmic domain. *Cell Regulation* **1**, 369–377.

Macey, D. J., Webb, J. and Potter, I. C. (1982) Iron levels and major iron binding proteins in the plasma of ammocoetes and adults of the southern hemisphere lamprey *Geotria australis*. *Gray. Comp. Biochem. Physiol.* **72A**, 307–312.

Macey, D. J., Smalley, S. R., Potter, I. C. and Cake, M. H. (1985) The relationship between total non-haem ferritin and haemosiderin iron in larvae of southern hemisphere lampreys (*Geotria australis* and *Mordacia mardax*). *J. Comp. Physiol. B.* **156**, 269–276.

Mack, V., Powell, L. W. and Halliday, J. W. (1983) Detection and isolation of a hepatic membrane receptor for ferritin. *J. Biol. Chem.* **258**, 4672–4675.

May, P. M., Williams, D. R., and Linder, P. W. (1980) The biological significance of low molecular weight Fe Complexes. In: *Metal Ions in Biological Systems*, (ed. H. Sigel), Marcel Decker Inc.: New York, pp. 29–76.

Miller, K., Shipman, M., Trowbridge, I. S. and Hopkins, C. R. (1991) Transferrin receptors promote the formation of clathrin lattices. *Cell* **65**, 621–632.

Morgan, E. H. (1963) Exchange of iron and transferrin across endothelial surfaces in the rat and rabbit. *J. Physiol.* **169**, 339–352.

Morgan, E. H. (1975) Plasma iron transport during egg laying and after oestrogen administration in the domestic fowl (*Gallus domesticus*). *Quart. J. Exp. Physiol.* **60**, 233–247.

Morgan, E. H. (1981a) Inhibition of reticulocyte iron uptake by NH_4Cl and methylamine. *Biochim. Biophys. Acta* **642**, 119–134.

Morgan, E. H. (1981b) Transferrin, biochemistry, physiology and clinical significance. *Mol. Aspects Med.* **4**, 1–123.

Morgan, E. H. (1982) Placental transfer of iron. *Proc. Aust. Physiol. Pharmacol. Soc.* **13**, 11–17.

Morgan, E. H. (1983) Effect of pH and iron content of transferrin on its binding to reticulocyte receptors. *Biochim. Biophys. Acta* **762**, 498–502.

Morgan, E. H. (1988) Membrane transport of non-transferrin-bound iron by reticulocytes. *Biochim. Biophys. Acta* **943**, 428–439.

Morgan, E. H. (1991) Specificity of hepatic iron uptake from plasma transferrin in the rat. *Comp. Biochem. Physiol.* **99A**, 91–95.

Morgan, E. H. (1993) Receptor-independent uptake of transferrin-bound iron by reticulocytes. Abstract, 11th International Conference on Iron and Iron Proteins, Jerusalem, p. 40.

Morgan, E. H. and Appleton, T. C. (1969) Autoradiographic localization of ^{125}I-labelled transferrin in rabbit reticulocytes. *Nature* **223**, 1371–1372.

Morgan, E. H. and Baker, E. (1986) Iron uptake and metabolism by hepatocytes. *Fed. Proc.* **45**, 2810–2816.

Morgan, E. H. and Baker, E. (1988) Role of transferrin receptors and endocytosis in iron uptake by hepatic and erythroid cells. *Ann. NY Acad. Sci.* **256**, 65–82.

Morgan, E. H., Smith, G. D. and Peters, T. J. (1986) Uptake and subcellular processing of ^{59}Fe and ^{125}I-transferrin by rat liver. *Biochem. J.* **237**, 163–173.

Muller-Eberhard, V., Liem, H. H., Grasso, J. A., Giffhorn-Katz, S., de Falco, M. G. and Katz, N. R. (1988) Increase in surface expression of transferrin receptors on cultured hepatocytes of adult rats in response to iron deficiency. *J. Biol. Chem.* **263**, 14753–14756.

Mulligan, M., Althaus, B. and Linder, M. C. (1986) Non-ferritin, non-heme iron pools in rat tissues. *Int. J. Biochem.* **18**, 791–798.

Muta, K., Nishimura, J., Ideguchi, H., Umemura, T. and Ibayashi, H. (1987) Erythroblast transferrin receptors and transferrin kinetics in iron deficiency and various anemias. *Am. J. Hemat.* **25**, 155–163.

Newman, R., Schneider, C., Sutherland, R., Vodinelich, L. and Greaves, M. (1982) The transferrin receptor. *Trends Biochem. Sci.* **1**, 397–400.

Nunez, M. T., Glass, J., Fischer, S., Lavidor, L. M., Lenk, E. M. and Robinson, S. H. (1977) Transferrin receptors in developing murine erythroid cells. *Br. J. Haematol.* **36**, 519–526.

Nunez, M. T., Pinto, I. and Glass, J. (1989) Assay and characteristics of the iron binding moiety of reticulocyte endocytic vesicles. *J. Memb. Biol.* **107**, 129–135.

Octave, J.-N., Schneider, Y.-J., Hoffman, P., Trouet, A. and Crichton, R. R. (1979) Transferrin protein and iron uptake by cultured rat fibroblasts. *FEBS Lett.* **108**, 127–130.

Octave, J.-N., Schneider, Y.-J., Hoffman, P., Trouet, A. and Crichton, R. R. (1982) Transferrin uptake by cultured rat embryo fibroblasts. The influence of lysomotropic agents, iron chelators and colchicine on the uptake of iron and transferrin. *Eur. J. Biochem.* **123**, 235–240.

Omary, M. B. and Trowbridge, I. S. (1981a) Covalent binding of fatty acid to the transferrin receptor in cultured human cells. *J. Biol. Chem.* **256**, 4715–4718.

Omary, M. B. and Trowbridge, I. S. (1981b) Biosynthesis of the human transferrin receptor in cultured cells. *J. Biol. Chem.* **256**, 12888–12892.

Osterloh, K. and Aisen, P. (1989) Pathways in the binding and uptake of ferritin by hepatocytes. *Biochim. Biophys. Acta* **1011**, 40–45.

Page, M. A., Baker, E. and Morgan, E. H. (1984) Transferrin and iron uptake by rat hepatocytes in culture. *Am. J. Physiol.* **246**, G26–G33.

Pan, B.-T. and Johnstone, R. M. (1983) Fate of the transferrin receptor during maturation of sheep reticulocytes in vitro: selective externalization of the receptor. *Cell* **33**, 967–977.

Pan, B.-T., Teng, K., Wu, C., Adam, M. and Johnstone, R. M. (1985) Electron microscopic evidence for externalization of the transferrin receptor in vesicular form in sheep reticulocytes. *J. Cell. Biol.* **101**, 942–948.

Paterson, S. and Morgan, E. H. (1980) Effect of changes in the ionic environment of reticulocytes on the uptake of transferrin-bound iron. *J. Cell. Physiol.* **105**, 484–502.

Paterson, S., Armstrong, N. J., Iacopetta, B. J., McArdle, H. J. and Morgan, E. H. (1984) Intravesicular pH and iron uptake by immature erythroid cells. *J. Cell. Physiol.* **120**, 225–232.

Pippard, M. J., Johnson, D. K. and Finch, C. A. (1982) Hepatocyte iron kinetics in the rat explored with an iron chelator. *Br. J. Haematol.* **52**, 211–224.

Pollack, S. and Campana, T. (1980) Low molecular weight nonheme iron and a highly labelled heme pool in the reticulocyte. *Blood* **55**, 564–566.

Pollack, S. and Campana, T. (1981) Immature red cells have ferritin receptors. *Biochem. Biophys. Res. Comm.* **100**, 1667–1672.

Ponka, P., Schulman, H. M. and Wilczynska, A. (1982) Ferric pyridoxal isonicotinoyl hydrazone can provide iron for heme synthesis in reticulocytes. *Biochim. Biophys. Acta* **718**, 151–156.

Pootrakul, P., Wattanasaree, J., Anuwatanakulchai, M. and Wasi, P. (1984) Increased red blood cell protoporphyrin in thalassemia: a result of relative iron deficiency. *Am. J. Clin. Path.* **82**, 289–293.

Pootrakul, P., Josephson, B., Huebers, H. A. and Finch, C. A. (1988) Quantitation of ferritin iron in plasma, an explanation of non-transferrin iron. *Blood* **71**, 1120–1123.

Primosigh, J. V. and Thomas, E. D. (1968) Studies on the partition of iron in bone marrow cells. *J. Clin. Invest.* **47**, 1473–1482.

Qian, Z. M. and Morgan, E. H. (1990) Effect of lead on the transport of transferrin-free and transferrin-bound iron into rabbit reticulocytes. *Biochem. Pharmacol.* **40**, 1049–1054.

Qian, Z. M. and Morgan, E. H. (1991) Effect of metabolic inhibitors on uptake of non-transferrin-bound iron by reticulocytes. *Biochim. Biophys. Acta* **1073**, 456–462.

Qian, Z. M. and Morgan, E. H. (1992) Changes in the uptake of transferrin-free and transferrin-bound iron during reticulocyte maturation in vivo and in vitro. *Biochim. Biophys. Acta* **1135**, 35–43.

Raja, K. B., Bjarnason, I., Simpson, R. J. and Peters, T. J. (1987) *In vitro* measurement and adaptive response of Fe^{3+} uptake by mouse intestine. *Cell Biochem. Funct.* **5**, 69–76.

Richardson, D. and Baker, E. (1992) Two mechanisms of iron uptake from transferrin by melanoma cells. The effect of desferrioxamine and ferric ammonium citrate. *J. Biol. Chem.* **267**(20), 13972–13979.

Ricketts, C., Cavill, I., Napier, J. A. F. and Jacoby, A. (1977) Ferrokinetics and erythropoiesis in man: an evaluation of ferrokinetic measurements. *Br. J. Haematol.* **35**, 41–47.

Rothenberger, S., Iacopetta, B. J. and Kuhn, L. C. (1987) Endocytosis of the transferrin receptor requires the cytoplasmic domain but not its phosphorylation site. *Cell* **49**, 423–431.

Rudolph, J. R., Regoeczi, E. and Southward, S. (1988) Quantitation of rat-hepatocyte transferrin receptors with poly- and monoclonal antibodies and protein A. *Histochemistry* **88**, 187–192.

Rümke, P. L., Visser, D., Kiva, H. G. and Hast, A. A. M. (1971) Radio-immunoassay of lactoferrin in blood plasma of breast cancer patients, lactating and normal women; prevention of false high levels caused by leakage from neutrophil leukocytes *in vitro*. *Folia Med. Neerl.* **14**, 156–168.

Sakata, T. (1969) A case of congenital atransferrinemia. *Shonika Shinryo* **32**, 1523–1529.

Schneider, C., Sutherland, R., Newman, R. and Greaves, M. (1982) Structural features of the cell surface receptor for transferrin that is recognized by the monoclonal antibody OKT9. *J. Cell. Biol.* **257**, 8516–8522.

Schneider, C., Owen, M. J., Banville, D. and Williams, J. G. (1984) Primary structure of human transferrin receptor deduced from the mRNA sequence. *Nature* **311**, 675–678.

Sciot, R., van Eyken, P., Facchetti, F., Callea, F., van der Steen, K., van Dijck, H. *et al.* (1989) Hepatocellular transferrin receptor expression in secondary siderosis. *Liver* **9**, 52–61.

Seligman, P. A., Kovar, J., Schleicher, R. B. and Gelfand, E. W. (1991) Transferrin-independent iron uptake supports B-lymphocyte growth. *Blood* **78**, 1526–1531.

Sharma, R. J. and Grant, D. A. W. (1991) Fe_2^{3+}-transferrin and Fe_2^{3+}-asialotransferrin deliver iron to hepatocytes by an identical mechanism. *Eur. J. Biochem.* **195**, 137–143.

Shih, Y. J., Baynes, R. D., Hudson, B. G., Flowers, C. H., Skikne, B. S. and Cook, J. D. (1990) Serum transferrin is a truncated form of tissue transferrin receptor. *J. Biol. Chem.* **265**, 19077–19081.

Sibille, J.-C., Octave, J.-N., Schneider, Y.-J., Trouet, A. and Crichton, R. R. (1982) Transferrin protein and iron uptake by cultured hepatocytes. *FEBS Lett.* **150**, 365–369.

Simpson, R. J. and Peters, T. J. (1985) Fe^{2+} uptake by intestinal brush border membrane vesicles from normal and hypoxic mice. *Biochim. Biophys. Acta* **814**, 381–388.

Singer, S. J. (1989) On the structure and function of endocytic transport systems. *Biol. Cell.* **65**, 1–5.

Singh, H. and Hider, R. C. (1988) Colorimetric detection of the hydroxyl radical and comparison of hydroxyl-radical-generating ability of various iron complexes. *Anal. Biochem.* **171**, 42–54.

Sipe, D. M. and Murphy, R. F. (1987) High-resolution kinetics of transferrin acidification in BALB/c3T3 cells: exposure to pH 6 followed by temperature-sensitive alkalinization during recycling. *Proc. Natl. Acad. Sci. NY* **84**, 7119–7123.

Sipe, D. M. and Murphy, R. F. (1991) Binding to cellular receptors results in increased iron release from transferrin at mildly acidic pH. *J. Biol. Chem.* **266**, 8002–8007.

Skikne, B. S., Flowers, C. H. and Cook, J. D. (1990) Serum transferrin receptor: a quantitative measure of tissue iron deficiency. *Blood* **75**, 1870–1876.

Smalley, S. R., Macey, D. J. and Potter, I. C. (1986) Changes in the amount of nonhaem iron in the plasma, whole body, and selected organs during post larval life of the lamprey *Geotria australis*. *J. Exp. Zool.* **237**, 149–157.

Smith, A. and Hunt, R. C. (1990) Hemopexin joins transferrin as representative members of a distinct class of receptor-mediated endocytic transport systems. *Eur. J. Cell. Biol.* **53**, 234–245.

Smith, A. and Morgan, W. T. (1978) Transport of heme by hemopexin to the liver: evidence for receptor-mediated uptake. *Biochem. Biophys. Res. Comm.* **84**, 151–157.

Smith, A. and Morgan, W. T. (1979) Haem transport to the liver by haemopexin. Receptor-mediated uptake with recycling of the protein. *Biochem. J.* **182**, 47–54.

Soda, R. and Tavassoli, M. (1984) Liver endothelium and not hepatocytes or Kupffer cells have transferrin receptors. *Blood* **63**, 270–276.

Speyer, B. E. and Fielding, J. (1979) Ferritin as a cytosol iron transport intermediate in human reticulocytes. *Br. J. Haematol.* **42**, 255–267.

Stein, B. S. and Sussman, H. H. (1983) Peptide mapping of the human transferrin receptor in normal and transformed cells. *J. Biol. Chem.* **258**, 2668–2673.

Stein, B. S. and Sussman, H. H. (1986) Demonstration of two distinct transferrin receptor recycling pathways and transferrin-independent receptor internalization in K562 cells. *J. Biol. Chem.* **261**, 10319–10331.

St Pierre, T. G., Richardson, D. R., Baker, E. and Webb, J. (1992) A low-spin iron complex in human melanoma and rat hepatoma cells and a high-spin iron (II) complex in rat hepatoma cells. *Biochim. Biophys. Acta* **1135**, 154–158.

Stremmel, W., Lotz, G., Niederau, C., Teschke, R. and Strohmeyer, G. (1987) Iron uptake by rat duodenal microvillous membrane vesicles: evidence for a carrier mediated transport system. *Eur. J. Clin. Invest.* **17**, 136–145.

Sun, T. L., Garcia-Canero, R., Liu, W. *et al.* (1987) Diferric transferrin reduction stimulates the Na$^+$/H$^+$ antiport of HeLa cells. *Biochem. Biophys. Res. Comm.* **145**, 467–473.

Sun, I. L., Toole-Sims, W., Crane, F. L., Morré, D. J., Löw, H. and Chou, J. Y. (1988) Reduction of diferric transferrin by S.V.40 transformed pineal cells stimulates Na$^+$/H$^+$ antiport activity. *Biochim. Biophys. Acta* **938**, 17–23.

Tavassoli, M. (1988) The role of liver endothelium in the transfer of iron from transferrin to the hepatocyte. *Ann. NY Acad. Sci.* **526**, 83–92.

Taylor, E. M. and Morgan, E. H. (1990) Developmental changes in transferrin and iron uptake by the brain in the rat. *Devel. Brain Res.* **55**, 35–42.

Taylor, E. M., Crowe, A. and Morgan, E. H. (1991) Transferrin and iron uptake by the brain: effects of altered iron status. *J. Neurochem.* **57**, 1584–1592.

Teeters, C. L., Lodish, H. F., Ciechanover, A. and Wallace, B. A. (1986) Transferrin and apotransferrin: pH-dependent conformational changes associated with receptor-mediated uptake. *Ann. NY Acad. Sci.* **463**, 403–407.

Tei, I., Makino, Y., Kadofuku, T., Kanamaru, I. and Konno, K. (1984) Increase of transferrin receptors in regenerating rat liver cells after partial hepatectomy. *Biochem. Biophys. Res. Comm.* **121**, 717–721.

Teichmann, R. and Stremmel, W. (1990) Iron uptake by human upper small intestine microvillous membrane vesicles. Indication for a facilitated transport mechanism mediated by a membrane iron-binding protein. *J. Clin. Invest.* **86**, 2145–2153.

Testa, V. (1985) Transferrin receptors: structure and function. *Curr. Topics Hemat.* **5**, 127–161.

Thorstensen, K. (1988) Hepatocytes and reticulocytes have different mechanisms for the uptake of iron from transferrin. *J. Biol. Chem.* **263**, 16837–16841.

Thorstensen, K. and Aisen, P. (1990) Release of iron from diferric transferrin in the presence of rat liver plasma membranes: no evidence of a plasma membrane diferric transferrin reductase. *Biochem. Biophys. Acta* **1052**, 29–35.

Thorstensen, K. and Romslo, I. (1984a) Uptake of iron from transferrin by isolated hepatocytes. *Biochim. Biophys. Acta* **804**, 200–208.

Thorstensen, K. and Romslo, I. (1984b) Albumin prevents nonspecific binding and iron uptake by isolated hepatocytes. *Biochim. Biophys. Acta* **804**, 393–397.

Thorstensen, K. and Romslo, I. (1988) Uptake of iron from transferrin by isolated rat hepatocytes. A redox-mediated plasma membrane process. *J. Biol. Chem.* **263**, 8844–8850.

Thorstensen, K. and Romslo, I. (1990) The role of transferrin in the mechanism of cellular iron uptake. *Biochem. J.* **271**, 1–10.

Toole-Simms, W., Sun, I. L., Faulk, W. P. *et al.* (1991) Inhibition of transplasma membrane electron transport by monoclonal antibodies to the transferrin receptor. *Biochem. Biophys. Res. Comm.* **176**, 1437–1442.

Trinder, D., Morgan, E. H. and Baker, E. (1986) The mechanisms of iron uptake by fetal rat hepatocytes in culture. *Hepatology* **6**, 852–858.

Trinder, D., Morgan, E. H. and Baker, E. (1988) The effects of an antibody to the rat transferrin receptor and of rat serum albumin on the uptake of diferric transferrin by rat hepatocytes. *Biochim. Biophys. Acta* **943**, 440–446.

Trowbridge, I. S. and Omary, M. B. (1981) Human cell surface glycoprotein related to cell proliferation is the receptor for transferrin. *Proc. Natl. Acad. Sci. USA* **78**, 3039–3043.

Trowbridge, I. S., Newman, R. A., Domingo, D. L. and Sauvage, C. (1984) Transferrin receptor: structure and function. *Biochem. Pharmacol.* **33**, 925–932.

Turkewitz, A. P., Amatruda, J. F., Borhani, D., Harrison, S. C. and Schwartz, A. L. (1988) A high yield purification of the human transferrin receptor and properties of its major extracellular fragment. *J. Biol. Chem.* **263**, 8316–8325.

Unger, A. and Hershko, C. (1974) Hepatocellular uptake of ferritin in the rat. *Br. J. Haematol.* **28**, 169–179.

van Renswoude, J., Bridges, K. R., Harford, J. B. and Klausner, R. D. (1982) Receptor-mediated endocytosis of transferrin and the uptake of Fe in K562 cells: identification of a nonlysosomal acidic compartment. *Proc. Natl. Acad. Sci. USA* **79**, 6186–6190.

Vogel, W., Bomford, A., Young, S. and Williams, R. (1987) Heterogeneous distribution of transferrin receptors on parenchymal and nonparenchymal liver cells: biochemical and morphological evidence. *Blood* **69**, 264–270.

Wasserman, L. R., Sharney, L., Gevirtz, N. R. *et al.* (1964) The exchange of iron with interstitial fluid. *Proc. Soc. Exp. Biol. Med.* **115**, 817–820.

Watts, C. (1985) Rapid endocytosis of the transferrin receptor in the absence of bound transferrin. *J. Cell. Biol.* **100**, 633–637.

Weaver, J. and Pollack, S. (1989) Low-M_r iron isolated from guinea pig reticulocytes as AMP-Fe and ATP-Fe complexes. *Biochem. J.* **261**, 787–792.

Wheby, M. S. and Umpierre, G. (1964) Effect of transferrin saturation on iron absorption in man. *New Eng. J. Med.* **271**, 1391–1395.

Williams, A. M. and Enns, C. A. (1991) Mutated transferrin receptor lacking asparagine-linked glycosylation sites shows reduced functionality and an association with binding immunoglobulin protein. *J. Biol. Chem.* **266**, 17648–17654.

Wright, T. L., Brissot, P., Ma, W.-L. and Weisiger, R. A. (1986) Characterization of non-transferrin-bound iron clearance by rat liver. *J. Biol. Chem.* **261**, 10909–10914.

Wright, T. L., Fitz, J. G. and Weisiger, R. A. (1988) Non-transferrin-bound iron uptake by rat liver. Role of membrane potential difference. *J. Biol. Chem.* **263**, 1842–1847.

Yamashiro, D. J., Tycho, B., Fluss, S. R. and Maxfield, F. R. (1984) Segregation of transferrin to a mildly acidic (pH 6.5) para-Golgi compartment in the recycling pathway. *Cell* **37**, 789–800.

Young, S. P. and Aisen, P. (1980) The interaction of transferrin with isolated hepatocytes. *Biochim. Biophys. Acta* **633**, 145–153.

Young, S. P. and Aisen, P. (1981) Transferrin receptors and the uptake and release of iron by isolated hepatocytes. *Hepatology* **1**, 114–119.

Young, S. P., Bomford, A. and Williams, R. (1984) The effect of the iron saturation of transferrin on its binding and uptake by rabbit reticulocytes. *Biochem. J.* **219**, 505–510.

Young, S. P., Roberts, S. and Bamford, A. (1985) Intracellular processing of transferrin and iron by isolated rat hepatocytes. *Biochem. J.* **232**, 819–823.

Zail, S. S., Charlton, R. W., Torrance, J. D. and Bothwell, T. H. (1964) Studies on the formation of ferritin in red cell precursors. *J. Clin. Invest.* **43**, 670–680.

Zerial, M., Melancon, P., Schneider, C. and Garoff, H. (1986) The transmembrane segment of the human transferrin receptor functions as a signal peptide. *EMBO J.* **5**, 1543–1550.

Zerial, M., Huylebroek, D. and Garoff, H. (1987) Foreign transmembrane peptides replacing the internal signal sequence of transferrin receptor allow its translocation and membrane binding. *Cell* **48**, 147–155.

Zimelman, A. P., Zimmerman, H. J., McLean, R. and Weintraub, L. R. (1977) Effect of iron saturation of transferrin on hepatic iron uptake: an in vitro study. *Gastroenterology* **72**, 129–131.

4. Cellular Iron Processing and Storage: The Role of Ferritin

J. W. HALLIDAY[1], G. A. RAMM[2] AND L. W. POWELL[1]

[1]*Liver Unit, Queensland Institute of Medical Research and The University of Queensland, The Bancroft Centre, Brisbane, Queensland, Australia 4029*
[2]*Department of Internal Medicine, Division of Gastroenterology and Hepatology, St Louis University Medical Center, St Louis, MO 63110-0250, USA*

In comparison with the mechanisms of cellular iron uptake, relatively little is known of the subsequent intracellular pathways of iron, through which it is incorporated into functional iron compounds (including haem proteins and iron-sulfur enzymes) or storage compounds (ferritin and haemosiderin). Cellular function clearly influences the destination of the iron. Thus, in addition to the normal 'housekeeping' cellular iron enzymes, the developing erythroid precursors need iron mainly for the synthesis of haemoglobin (Chapter 2). Intestinal mucosal cells and macrophages of the reticuloendothelial system have a primary function of releasing their iron, taken up from the gut contents and from senescent red cells respectively, to the plasma for distribution to other iron-demanding tissues, including erythroid precursors and hepatocytes. In all cells iron taken up in excess of current metabolic requirements is incorporated into ferritin. In the intestinal mucosal cells this applies to iron which is not absorbed, and such iron is lost as the cells are sloughed off the mucosa. This plays an important role in maintaining body iron stores within 'normal' limits (Chapter 6). However, macrophages and hepatocytes are adapted for iron storage, excess iron being retained as a reserve to be called on in times of increased body iron needs. The hepatocyte, being able to take up iron in a variety of different forms and also acting as a major site of available iron stores, has a central 'buffering' role in internal iron exchange. In addition, within the liver the possibility exists of excretion of substances into the bile.

   This chapter will discuss intracellular iron movements with particular reference to ferritin iron uptake and release, and the metabolic pathways followed by ferritin and ferritin iron. The role of the macrophage in processing haemoglobin iron, in iron storage, and in recycling the iron to circulating transferrin has been discussed in Chapter 2. The present chapter will therefore concentrate on discussion of cellular iron processing by the liver.

I. THE LIVER AND NORMAL IRON METABOLISM

The liver is a major iron storage organ and synthesizes ferritin for this purpose. In addition the synthesis of the iron transport protein, transferrin, occurs in the liver. Approximately one-third of the body iron is present in the iron stores in normal subjects and approximately one-third of this storage iron is found in the liver. In normal individuals, liver iron is predominantly found in the hepatocytes (approximately 0.4 g) with smaller quantities located in the Kupffer cells of the reticuloendothelial system: the latter contain 1.5% of total liver iron in normal rats (Van Wyk *et al.*, 1971). The liver is second only to the erythron in terms of iron usage for essential proteins, such as the cytochromes. Because of its role as a storage organ and the need for release of this iron in times of need, such as in states of increased erythropoiesis, the liver must participate in the bi-directional traffic of iron both into and out of the cells. In addition the liver is made up of several different cell types of which parenchymal cells (hepatocytes) predominate. Hepatocytes in culture, derived from normal rats, have been shown to release approximately 40 000 iron atoms per cell per minute to apotransferrin in the medium (Young and Aisen, 1988). The release of iron from hepatocytes is not limited by the availability of iron sites on transferrin, since even in the absence of protein in the external milieu iron leaves hepatocytes. In *in vitro* studies such iron release is largely abolished at 4°C which would indicate that active cellular metabolism is necessary for it to occur. Kupffer cells may process more than 10^7 iron atoms per minute (Kondo *et al.*, 1988). Such an iron traffic, if it occurred under *in vivo* conditions would be approximately ten times faster than that which crosses the membranes of immature erythroid cells which are actively synthesizing haemoglobin.

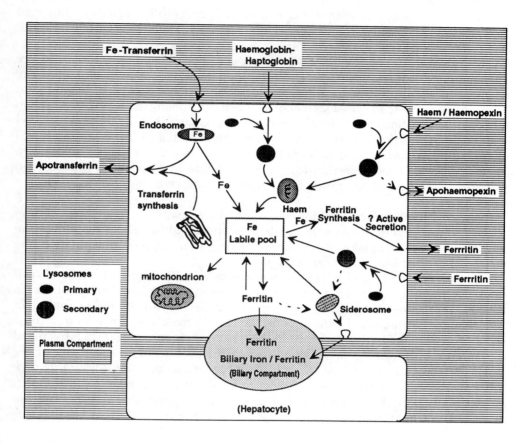

Fig. 4.1 Pathways of normal hepatic iron metabolism. The hypothetical pathways of receptor mediated iron uptake are indicated. The possible uptake via non-transferrin bound iron is omitted as it is believed to be important only in the presence of iron-overload.

Hepatocyte iron is found associated with several different molecules including ferritin, haemosiderin, transferrin and haem. In normal hepatocytes, large deposits of ferritin have been demonstrated in the cytosol and in lysosomes, with smaller quantities observed in the rough and smooth endoplasmic reticulum. Haemosiderin, thought to be derived from ferritin, has been demonstrated to be predominantly localized in the secondary lysosomes of the reticuloendothelial cells and deposits are occasionally observed in normal hepatocytes (Richter, 1978; Parmley et al., 1981; McClain et al., 1991).

As discussed in Chapter 3, iron enters the hepatocyte in several different forms and via several different pathways, as iron bound to transferrin (Bomford and Munro, 1985; Morgan and Baker, 1988; Thorstensen and Romslo, 1990), in haemoglobin bound to haptoglobin (Hershko et al., 1972; Kino et al., 1980), in haem bound to haemopexin (Smith and Morgan, 1981), as circulating low molecular weight chelates of iron (Brissot et al., 1985; Wright et al., 1986; Wright and Lake, 1990) and as iron bound to tissue ferritin (Kondo *et al.*, 1988; Sibille *et al.*, 1988). This tissue ferritin iron may be derived from Kupffer cells (see later) or from leakage from damaged cells in iron-rich tissues. (Unger and Hershko, 1974; Halliday *et al.*, 1979; Mack *et al.*, 1983, 1985) (Fig. 4.1).

Circulating levels of the relatively iron-poor glycosylated serum ferritin are low in normal individuals (female 10–150 μg/l; male 20–200 μg/l) and therefore true serum ferritin is not considered to provide a major source of hepatic iron even in iron-overload diseases such as haemochromatosis, where the serum ferritin concentrations are often elevated to levels greater than 1000 μg/l (Worwood *et al.*, 1976). In contrast, tissue ferritins have the potential to carry vast quantities of iron. In 1983, Mack and colleagues described a specific receptor mechanism for the removal of tissue ferritin from the circulation by isolated rat hepatocytes, thereby providing another potentially important source of entry of iron into the liver.

The route of iron uptake may influence its ultimate pathway. The uptake of iron in the form of haem appears to result in a similar ultimate destination of the iron to that of the uptake of transferrin bound iron, namely the putative low molecular weight iron pool (see below).

The form of iron bound to iron-containing or iron-binding proteins is of considerable importance. Iron bound to haem in haemoglobin is in the ferrous form essential for the oxygen-carrying capacity of the molecule. Iron bound to transferrin is in the ferric form as is the iron within the ferritin molecule; however iron must be taken up into the ferritin molecule in the ferrous form and appears to be oxidized to the ferric form during its passage through the channels into the centre of the molecule (Harrison *et al.*, 1986) where it is incorporated into the ferrihydrite core (Chapter 1). The interconversion of ferrous to ferric iron thus appears to be essential, but such reactions have the potential to generate highly toxic free radicals, as discussed in Chapter 10.

1.1. The Intracellular Iron Pool

The low molecular weight chelatable form of iron or 'intracellular transit pool' (Cavill *et al.*, 1975; Jacobs, 1977; Young and Aisen, 1982), is postulated to play an important role in intermediary iron metabolism. This pool of intracellular iron has not as yet been adequately characterized, although it has been proposed at various times that the iron is bound to some or all of a variety of different compounds including aconitase, adenosine triphosphate, guanosine triphosphate, adenosine diphosphate, citrate, ascorbic acid, glutathione, pyrophosphates, riboflavin, cysteine, glucose, lactose, fructose and 2,3-diphosphoglycerate (Bacon and Tavill, 1984). It has been suggested that the size of this iron pool 'regulates' iron pathways since it will reflect the available iron stores within the cell (Cavill *et al.*, 1975). Iron is released from transferrin within endosomes probably accompanied by reduction from ferric to ferrous iron and the iron is then taken up by cytosolic ferritin; thus transport across the endosome membrane must occur, though the mechanism remains speculative (Chapter 3).

2. THE MAJOR IRON-BINDING PROTEINS AND THEIR RELATIONSHIP TO THE LIVER

2.1. Transferrin

The transferrins comprise a group of closely related proteins including serum transferrin, lactoferrin and melanotransferrin. Serum transferrin and lactotransferrin possess the ability to bind reversibly two ferric ions per molecule. Their structure, iron binding and receptors are discussed in Chapters 1 and 3.

As discussed in Chapter 1, the major site of transferrin synthesis is the liver, though smaller quantities are produced in other tissues such as the brain, heart, spleen, kidney, muscle (Aldred et al., 1987), testis (Lee et al., 1986), mammary gland (Lee et al., 1987) and thymus (Lum, 1987). Hepatic transferrin synthesis is upregulated by iron deficiency, but synthesis by other tissues appears to be unaffected by decreased iron availability (Idzerda et al., 1986). Transferrin-receptors have been identified on many cells, especially on dividing cells. In human liver they have been identified immunohistochemically on both hepatocytes and Kupffer cells (Gatter et al., 1983).

The principal function of transferrin is the delivery of iron to the cells that require it. These cells express a transmembrane glycoprotein receptor which consists of two identical disulfide-bonded 90 kDa subunits. Iron uptake by these cells occurs by receptor-mediated endocytosis. The role of the transferrin receptor in iron uptake by hepatocytes is discussed in Chapter 3.

The expression of transferrin receptors on the plasma membrane of cells appears to depend on the iron status of the cell. In experiments using cultured cell lines Rouault and colleagues (1985) have demonstrated that transferrin receptors are up-regulated in the presence of desferrioxamine and down-regulated in the presence of excess iron. In the human genetic disease haemochromatosis (HC), where vast quantities of hepatic iron may accumulate, Bjorn-Rasmussen et al. (1985) using monocytes derived from patients with HC, demonstrated an increase in transferrin receptors relative to control subjects. Other investigators have however obtained conflicting results, which suggest that transferrin receptor expression may also depend on cell type. Transferrin receptor number and function have been shown to be similar in a number of studies using cultured skin fibroblasts isolated from haemochromatosis subjects and normal individuals (Ward et al., 1981, 1984). Sciot and colleagues (1987) demonstrated a decrease in the expression of hepatic transferrin receptors in genetic haemochromatosis, which suggested that transferrin receptors are not involved in the primary defect of the disease.

Recently Tavassoli (1988) demonstrated a predominance of transferrin receptors on endothelial cells compared with hepatocytes. In this study Tavassoli (1988) observed that following the receptor-mediated endocytosis of transferrin-bound iron by endothelial cells, transferrin is desialylated and released into the space of Disse, where it is subsequently bound by the hepatocyte asialoglycoprotein receptor. As mentioned these results conflict with other reports where three times the number of transferrin receptors have been shown on hepatocytes compared with nonparenchymal cells (Vogel et al., 1987). These studies are discussed in more detail in Chapter 3.

2.2. Ferritin

The ferritin molecule has an important role in the overall physiology of iron metabolism as a result of (i) its ability to maintain iron in a soluble, non-toxic and biologically useful form and (ii) its capacity to sequester vast quantities of iron.

Ferritin is composed of an apoprotein shell (MW approximately 480 kDa) which surrounds a core of up to 4500 atoms of iron in the form of the mineral ferrihydrite (Harrison et al., 1987). The ferritin molecule is composed of 24 subunits of two structurally distinct subunit types. The heavy or H-subunit has a more acid pI and has a molecular weight of approximately 21 kDa. The light or L-subunit is more basic than the H subunit and has a molecular weight of approximately 19 kDa. Different proportions of each subunit in a ferritin molecule give rise to isoferritins which have characteristic isoelectric points and specific tissue distributions. Isoferritins with a higher number of L-subunits are predominantly found in the liver, spleen and placenta. Bomford and colleagues (1981) have demonstrated that the administration of iron results in a preferential synthesis of L-subunits, thereby favouring the assembly of L-rich isoferritins in iron-overload conditions. Isoferritins with an increased percentage of H-subunits are found in tissues such as the heart (Powell et al., 1974, 1975), red blood cells (Peters et al., 1983), lymphocytes and monocytes (Jones et al., 1983) and HeLa cells (Arosio et al., 1976, 1977), which are not primarily involved in iron storage.

2.3. Haemosiderin

Haemosiderin is the major iron storage protein present when excessive iron accumulates in the tissues of patients with genetic haemochromatosis or iron overload secondary to anaemia – as in thalassaemia. While both the protein shell and the iron complex of ferritin have been studied extensively, the chemical and structural nature of haemosiderin is less well understood. In contrast to the water-soluble crystalline ferritin, haemosiderin is observed as an amorphous deposit. Haemosiderin thus appears to consist of degraded ferritin protein and ferric hydroxide polymers or cores of varying size (O'Connell et al., 1988; Ward et al., 1988, 1989), which are found in micelles approximately 70 Å in diameter (Bacon and Tavill, 1984). In normal liver, ferritin is the major iron–protein detected, but in conditions of iron overload, haemosiderin has been shown to predominate. Histological and also immunological studies (O'Connell et al., 1988) have demonstrated a close relationship between ferritin and haemosiderin. Thus antisera raised against ferritin react with haemosiderin indicating that the major peptide in haemosiderin is derived from ferritin. Haemosiderin is also seen in the liver in animal models of iron overload, e.g. after injection of iron dextran (Andrews et al., 1988). Again the presence of peptides cross-reacting with anti-ferritin antisera and the similarities in the structure of the iron cores is consistent with the view that rat liver haemosiderin arises by degradation of ferritin polypeptides.

It has been suggested that haemosiderin may play an important role, either direct or indirect, in iron toxicity and hence a number of studies of the structure of the iron cores of ferritin and haemosiderin have recently been carried out.

The structural identification of haemosiderin iron cores derived from patients with genetic haemochromatosis and from multiply transfused subjects with β-thalassaemia has now been reported (Mann et al., 1988; Ward et al., 1988, 1989). Detailed Mossbauer spectroscopy studies have revealed that the iron cores of haemosiderins appear to be disease specific and significant differences have been reported between haemosiderins from thalassaemic and haemochromatotic livers. Such disease specific differences could clearly play an important role in iron availability as well as potential toxicity. In thalassaemic subjects who have been transfused and treated with iron chelators in attempts to reduce the iron burden, the iron core structures are those of crystalline goethite (Mann et al., 1988; Ward et al., 1988). However in untreated thalassaemia (Webb et al., personal communication) and in genetic haemochromatosis, the iron cores are relatively disordered and their structure is consistent with that of ferrihydrite as is found in the associated liver ferritin. The goethite-like deposits appear to be less labile and hence are theoretically less accessible to chelation therapy than the ferrihydrite model. The peptide structures of these haemosiderins have also been shown to differ (Ward et al., 1989). It may be that the treatment of thalassaemic patients has contributed in some way to the observed differences but their significance remains to be finally elucidated particularly in relation to the development of new orally active iron chelating agents.

3. FERRITIN-IRON UPTAKE

The specific configuration of subunits making up the apoferritin shell of the ferritin molecule results in the formation of a number of channels, approximately 0.5 nm wide, through which iron is able to pass in or out (Ford et al., 1984). Iron is generally taken up as the ferrous (FeII) form, which is oxidized to the ferric (FeIII) form at the surface and channelled into the molecule where it is subsequently incorporated into the ferrihydrite core (Bakker and Boyer, 1986). The nature of the sites where oxidation is initiated is unclear. A number of investigators using spectroscopic, crystallographic and chemical modification studies, have suggested that carboxylic acid residues, which are highly conserved along the hydrophilic channels of the apoferritin molecule, may be directly involved in the initiation process (Wetz and Crichton, 1976; Rice et al., 1983; Harrison et al., 1986; Yang et al., 1987). Carboxylate groups are known to ligate a variety of different metal ions and therefore may provide appropriate anchorage for iron to form oxo or hydroxo bridges to neighbouring iron atoms in the initiation of the polynuclear core formation (Rice et al., 1983; Harrison et al., 1986).

The mechanisms of iron storage in the protein shell of ferritin have recently been investigated by several different methods including Mossbauer spectroscopic techniques, UV difference spectroscopy and site-directed mutagenesis of the ferritin subunits (Bauminger et al., 1991; Treffry et al., 1991; Levi et al., 1991).

Lawson et al. (1991) have described a 'ferroxidase centre' on ferritin which was not located in the threefold channels as previously suggested. This centre is conserved in ferritins of vertebrates, invertebrates and of plants. Bauminger and colleagues (1991) using Mossbauer spectroscopy have confirmed that the catalysis of Fe(II) oxidation is associated with a residue situated only on ferritin H-chains and that

Table 4.1 Ferritin subunit functions studied by site-directed mutagenesis

Ferritin Mutants	Mutations	Ferroxidase Activity	Receptor Binding	Myelosuppressive Activity
HrHF	Wild type	+	+	+
HrLF	Wild type	−	−	−
HrHF-222	Four helix bundle	−	+	−
HrHF-115	N-terminus	+	+	+
HrHF-9cd	Loop	+	+	+
HrHF-174	Hydrophilic channel	+	+	+
HrHF-91	Hydrophobic channel	+	+	+

HrHF = human recombinant H-ferritin.
HrLF = human recombinant L-ferritin.

this activity is located at the 'ferroxidase centre' described by Lawson and colleagues (1991). Levi and colleagues (1991) have studied the sequences involved in ferritin iron incorporation by making alanine mutations of acidic residues on recombinant H-ferritin (r-HF) and also on a mutant H-ferritin which was shown to be devoid of ferroxidase activity (HrHF-222). They concluded that it is the number of negative charges in the cavity that drives ferritin iron incorporation and also that ferroxidase activity overrides the cavity effect. The reported myelosuppressive effects of H-ferritins (Broxmeyer, 1989) also appear to be related to the ferroxidase activity (Broxmeyer et al., 1991) (Table 4.1).

4. FERRITIN-IRON RELEASE

The release of iron from the ferritin molecule *in vitro*, requires reducing agents such as thioglycollate, dithionite or reduced flavins (Crichton, 1973; Harrison et al., 1974; Harrison, 1977; Funk et al., 1985; Bonomi and Pagani, 1986) or free radicals (Thomas and Aust, 1986). Release has also been shown to be enhanced by low pH (Watt et al., 1985). Iron release *in vivo* is thought to occur in lysosomes or endosomes with acid pH. Green and Mazur (1957) suggested that xanthine oxidase may directly catalyse the reduction of ferric iron to ferrous iron. Since this time, other investigators have suggested that the flavins may offer a more plausible explanation of the reduction of ferric iron. The maximum rate of iron release brought about by reduced riboflavin for example, may exceed 100 atoms per minute per molecule of ferritin (Sirivech et al., 1974). Therefore, the average load of a ferritin molecule (approximately 1200 atoms) could be mobilized in under 60 minutes to accommodate an acute iron shortage. An NADH-FMNH$_2$-dependent enzyme system has been shown to remove iron from ferritin (Osaki and Sirivech, 1971), as have FADH$_2$ and FMNH$_2$ (Sirivech et al., 1974; Crichton et al., 1980). The formation of the superoxide free radical by FMNH$_2$ has been suggested by McCord and Day (1978), to play an important role in the free radical catalysed reduction of ferric iron via the Haber–Weiss reaction. This reaction could therefore provide the mechanism by which xanthine oxidase, using either $NADH_2$ or $FADH_2$, could facilitate the release of iron from ferritin (Mazur et al., 1958; Topham et al., 1982). Thomas and colleagues (1985) demonstrated that oxygen free radicals produced by xanthine oxidase, release iron from ferritin at a rate comparable with that observed in vivo. It has also been suggested that the degradation of ferritin may be necessary for the release of its iron. The precise mechanisms remain to be elucidated.

5. FERRITIN SYNTHESIS

Ferritin synthesis in the liver occurs primarily on free polyribosomes in hepatocytes, with approximately 15% synthesized on the rough endoplasmic reticulum (Konijn and Hershko, 1977; Doolittle and Richter, 1981). The rate of ferritin synthesis is sensitive to the presence of iron and the iron status of the cell.

Iron appears to stimulate ferritin synthesis at the translational level rather than at transcription (Chapter 5). This was originally demonstrated by Drysdale and Munro (1965), who observed that pretreatment of the liver with actinomycin D, which suppresses mRNA formation, had no effect on the iron-inducible effect on ferritin synthesis, and has since been confirmed in a number of other studies including that of Shull and Theil (1982), who observed a 40- to 50-fold iron-inducible increase in ferritin protein synthesis in tadpole reticulocytes, without a concomitant increase in messenger RNA (mRNA) levels.

Brown and colleagues (1983) have shown that L-subunits are the predominant ferritin subunit synthesized upon iron stimulation. With the entry of iron into the cell, ferritin L-subunits appear to be synthesized from an intracellular storage pool of ferritin mRNA, which is activated and channelled through polysomes, where translation of the message is completed (Zahringer et al., 1976). This phenomenon of early ferritin translation may therefore provide DNA with a protective mechanism against the toxicity of iron, before excess iron has entered the cell (Shull and Theil, 1982). Hepatic ferritin levels are also elevated in conditions of inflammation where excess iron does not appear to be a contributing factor (Halliday and Powell, 1984). In this situation, ferritin may be acting as an acute phase reactant possibly under hormonal control (Drysdale, 1983). (See also Chapter 11.)

Changes in ferritin content are also observed during both myeloid and erythroid differentiation (Drysdale et al., 1985; Louache et al., 1985). Chou and colleagues (1986), using human pro-myelocytic HL60 cells, demonstrated that during differentiation the ratio of ferritin H- to L-subunit mRNA varies markedly. This variance in mRNA is mirrored by a proportional alteration in subunit ratios, indicating a transcriptional rather than translational control of ferritin biosynthesis. Thus, the biosynthesis of ferritin appears to be under the control of multiple factors and the regulatory mechanisms involved may vary according to the metabolic state, the degree of differentiation and the iron status of the cell.

Recent investigations (described more fully in Chapter 5) by a number of different groups have demonstrated a specific regulatory mechanism for the translation of ferritin mRNA through an iron-regulatory element (IRE) located at the 5' untranslated region of the ferritin mRNA molecule. A group of similar structures is located in the 3′ untranslated region of the transferrin receptor mRNA. An IRE-binding protein (IRE-BP) appears to regulate concurrently the translation of the ferritin and transferrin receptor mRNAs by binding both to the ferritin mRNA-IRE, which acts to repress translation, and also to one or more of the four functional IRE structures on the transferrin receptor mRNA (Rouault et al., 1988; Haile et al., 1989; Koeller et al., 1989; Müllner et al., 1989), which protects the transferrin receptor mRNA from degradation and allows translation to occur. This mechanism can now explain the coordinate regulation of ferritin and the transferrin receptor.

6. SERUM FERRITIN AND IRON HOMEOSTASIS

The concentration of ferritin in the plasma of normal subjects (15–300 μg/l) remains remarkably constant, providing a reliable reflection of the body iron stores of the individual (Walters et al., 1973). Patients with serum ferritin levels < 15 μg/l were therefore classified as iron deficient and iron-overloaded subjects had ferritin levels > 300 μg/l (Jacobs et al., 1972). Ferritin levels are elevated in patients with liver damage or inflammatory diseases and therefore serum ferritin is not a good indicator of iron status in these subjects (Worwood, 1986). This subject is discussed in detail in Chapter 14.

The origin of serum ferritin remains unclear, with several investigators postulating a number of potential sources. Cragg and colleagues (1980) suggested that serum ferritin is probably ferritin released from cells of the reticuloendothelial system. However, ferritin levels in the serum are also related to hepatocyte iron stores. In haemochromatosis, where iron is stored primarily in hepatocytes, the serum ferritin concentration is elevated above the normal range well before there is an increase in Kupffer cell iron (Bassett et al., 1986), implying that parenchymal cells may be a source of serum ferritin.

Unlike tissue ferritin, serum ferritin from both normal and iron-loaded subjects has a low iron content (Arosio et al., 1977). Another difference between tissue and serum ferritin is the fact that a significant proportion of serum ferritin is glycosylated, which suggests that serum ferritin may be actively secreted from cells rather than being released by leakage (Halliday and Powell, 1979; Worwood et al., 1979, 1980).

In addition to the ferritin H- and L-subunits found in the tissues and plasma of normal, iron-overloaded and iron deficient animals, another subunit has been identified in ferritin from the plasma of patients with iron overload. This subunit, called the G-subunit, appears to contain carbohydrate and has a molecular weight of approximately 23 kDa (Cragg et al., 1981). Its function in iron homeostasis is not known.

7. THE PLASMA HALF-LIFE OF SERUM AND TISSUE FERRITINS

The plasma half-life of tissue ferritin has been reported to be approximately 3–30 minutes, with ferritin removed from the circulation by the liver (Hershko et al., 1973;

Siimes and Dallman, 1974; Unger and Hershko, 1974; Pollock et al., 1978; Halliday et al., 1979; Cragg et al., 1983). The removal of serum ferritin from the plasma is not as efficient with a half-life of up to 30 hours (Halliday et al., 1979; Worwood et al., 1982; Cragg et al., 1983). This prolonged half-life appears to be related to the presence of carbohydrate on the serum ferritin molecule (Halliday et al., 1979; Worwood et al., 1980; Worwood 1986). The rapid clearance of tissue ferritin from the circulation by the liver has led us to postulate the existence of a specific hepatocyte mechanism for the uptake of ferritin from the circulation (see below).

8. THE FERRITIN RECEPTOR

Tissue ferritins characteristically carry iron, up to 4500 atoms per molecule, in iron-loaded tissues. Hence such ferritin could theoretically provide an important source of iron if taken up into other body tissues. Tissue ferritin injected intravenously into rats is taken up virtually exclusively by the liver (Lipschitz et al., 1971; Halliday et al., 1979), specifically by the hepatocytes (Hershko et al., 1973; Unger and Herskho, 1974; Mack et al., 1983, 1985). Until 1983, the precise mechanism by which the liver takes up ferritin was unknown. The most plausible explanation was the existence of a ferritin receptor on the hepatocyte plasma membrane. In studies conducted by Sasaki and Wagner (1979), the uptake of fluorescent-labelled ferritin by isolated rat hepatocytes was shown to be consistent with a receptor-mediated endocytic process. Other investigators were able to demonstrate an association of ferritin with plasma membrane upon liver homogenization or detergent solubilization of the membrane (Sargent and Munro, 1975; Zuyderhoudt et al., 1979).

A hepatic membrane receptor for rat ferritin was detected and isolated by Mack et al. (1983). Using Scatchard analysis, they demonstrated the specific binding of ^{125}I-ferritin to rat hepatocytes, with a binding association constant (Ka) of $1.1 \times 10^8 \, mol^{-1}l$ and 3.2×10^4 binding sites/hepatocyte. These authors further purified a suspension of insolubilized ferritin receptor and verified the binding studies. Scatchard analysis of the binding of ferritin to the insolubilized ferritin receptor revealed a Ka of $2.7 \times 10^8 \, mol^{-1}l$. The same group also demonstrated that the rat hepatic ferritin receptor was specific for ferritin and did not bind human asialoorosomucoid, bovine serum albumin or rat transferrin (Mack et al., 1983) (Fig. 4.2). Further characterization of the binding of ferritin to the rat hepatic ferritin receptor revealed that the receptor binds ferritin derived from rat spleen, heart and kidney, human liver, guinea-pig liver and horse spleen with the same affinity as rat liver ferritin (Mack et al., 1985). They also observed a significantly lower binding affinity for serum ferritin, which could account for the increased half-life of serum ferritin. Several authors have previously proposed that the binding of ferritin to its receptor may be carbohydrate-mediated (Worwood et al., 1977; Halliday et al., 1979). In the study by Mack and colleagues (1985), glycosidase treatment of tissue ferritins had no effect on their receptor-binding capabilities, suggesting that the binding of ferritin to the receptor was not carbohydrate-mediated. However neuraminidase treatment of both human and rat serum ferritin resulted in an increase in their binding affinity to the rat hepatic ferritin receptor, to a level equal to that of tissue ferritins.

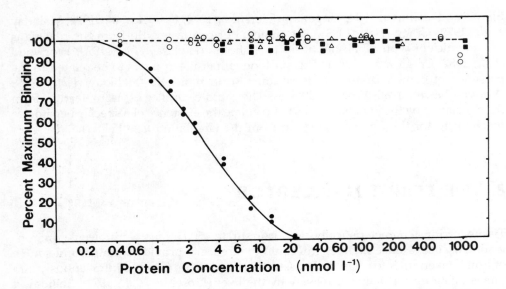

Fig. 4.2 Specificity of binding of 1 μg ^{125}I-labelled rat liver ferritin to insolubilized ferritin receptor in the presence of increasing concentrations of bovine serum albumin (○---○), human asialoorosomucoid (■---■), rat transferrin (△ --- △) and rat liver ferritin (●—●). From Mack *et al.* (1983) with permission.

This phenomenon is not restricted to rats as was demonstrated by Cragg and colleagues (1983), who observed hepatic ferritin uptake in man. Neither is it restricted to hepatocytes. In 1981 Pollack and Campana, observed that tissue ferritin binds to the membranes of guinea-pig reticulocytes *in vitro*. Blight and Morgan (1983) took this work a step further when they demonstrated that ferritin was internalized by guinea-pig reticulocytes and that the ferritin iron was utilized for the synthesis of haem. Simon and colleagues (1987) have since confirmed these findings using ferritin doubly labelled with ^{59}Fe and ^{125}I injected intravenously into normal, phenylhydrazine-treated and scorbutic guinea-pigs, *in vivo*. A hepatic ferritin receptor has also been described in humans (Adams *et al.*, 1988a) and in pigs (Adams *et al.*, 1988b).

8.1. The Receptor-mediated Endocytosis of Ferritin

Until recently, the precise physiological function of the ferritin receptor and, more particularly, the manner by which ferritin is removed from the circulation by its receptor, remained unclear. However, Ramm *et al.* (1990) demonstrated for the first time that the receptor-mediated endocytosis of exogenous tissue ferritin was inhibited by the administration of the microtubule-inhibiting drug colchicine to normal and iron-loaded rats *in vivo*. This observation indicated that the clearance of ferritin by the hepatic ferritin receptor is a microtubule-dependent process. Further studies using another microtubule-inhibiting agent vinblastine have confirmed the microtubule-dependent pathway of ferritin uptake by the liver as shown schematically in Fig. 4.1 (Ramm, 1993).

9. VESICULAR LOCALIZATION OF INTERNALIZED FERRITIN

The fate of ferritin taken up by the hepatic ferritin receptor has only recently been investigated. Using electron microscopic techniques, Blight and Morgan (1987) utilized the natural electron density of ferritin and transferrin coupled to colloidal gold, to examine the endocytosis of transferrin and ferritin in guinea-pig reticulocytes. They observed a common endocytic pathway for their clearance from the circulation. After the initial binding at 37°C, ferritin was internalized along with transferrin, via coated pits and endocytic vesicles. After 5 minutes, ferritin began to disappear from these endocytic vesicles and was observed bound to the membranes of larger, so-called multivesicular endosomes (MVE). Ferritin remained in the MVE compartment for up to 60 minutes after initial binding. At this point, some of the ferritin had dissociated from its receptor, unlike transferrin, where virtually all of the ligand remained bound to its receptor.

Zuyderhoudt et al. (1982) studied the role of rat liver lysosomes in the catabolism of intravenously injected rat liver ferritin in rats made anaemic by orbital punctures and iron-restricted food. Anaemic rats were used, as anaemia was previously reported to stimulate the catabolism of intravenously injected ferritin (Hershko et al., 1973) and was thought to cause a decrease in the levels of endogenous liver ferritin. It was found that ferritin accumulated in liver lysosomes approximately 60 minutes after intravenous injection into rats and that lysosomes accumulated ferritin for up to 4 hours after ferritin administration, with a peak in accumulation after 2 hours. They also reported that after the lysosomal levels of ferritin decreased (after 24 hours), no ferritin was detectable in the mitochondrial fraction and there was no evidence of ferritin in the bile. Therefore it appears that in anaemic rats, ferritin is taken up by lysosomes and is totally degraded by these organelles.

10. INTRACELLULAR DEGRADATION OF FERRITIN

10.1. The Passage of Ferritin From Vesicle to Lysosome

The mechanism by which endogenous ferritin enters the lysosomal compartment is unclear. Trump et al. (1975) suggested one of two possibilities. The first is that ferritin follows the route taken by lysosomal hydrolases after synthesis on membrane-bound polysomes, i.e. rough endoplasmic reticulum – Golgi – Golgi vesicle – secondary lysosome. This pathway however, was not favoured by Trump et al. as ferritin appeared to be primarily synthesized on free polysomes and the major part of the tissue ferritin did not appear to be glycosylated. The Golgi apparatus has been shown to contain a series of glycosyl transferases and many proteins known to be glycosylated pass through this organelle (Whaley et al., 1972). Worwood et al. (1979) have demonstrated that approximately 60% of ferritin from normal serum binds to the lectin concanavalin A, implying that it is glycosylated, which suggests that serum ferritin, at least, may pass through the Golgi complex at some stage in its intracellular transit. It also implies that ferritins of different subunit composition may follow separate intracellular pathways.

The second possibility and more feasible explanation is that ferritin undergoes autophagocytosis, that is endogenous cytoplasmic ferritin is engulfed by membranes of the smooth endoplasmic reticulum and these vesicles then fuse with the membranes of the lysosome, forming a secondary lysosome.

10.2. Cellular Differences in Ferritin Degradation

A significant feature of ferritin metabolism is that certain cells are able to degrade ferritin to haemosiderin with greater ease than others. Van Wyk and colleagues (1971) observed that hepatocytes in rat livers respond to iron loading with increased deposits of ferritin, whereas Kupffer cells from the same iron-loaded livers deposit haemosiderin, with very little ferritin detectable. Other investigators have found similar results using injections of iron dextran into rats, where iron was preferentially deposited as ferritin in the secondary lysosomes of hepatocytes, compared with Kupffer cell lysosomes which retained iron in the form of haemosiderin (Arborgh et al., 1974).

The catabolic pathways taken by ferritin appear to be determined according to the type of cell, i.e. hepatocyte or reticuloendothelial cell. Hepatocytes contain fewer lysosomes than cells of the reticuloendothelial system, and most of the degradation of ferritin occurs in the cytosol by proteolytic enzymes. In reticuloendothelial cells (with an increased number of lysosomes) ferritin is catabolized by the fusion of vesicles derived from receptor-mediated endocytosis or of autophagic vacuoles with a primary lysosome, thus forming the secondary lysosome (Bacon and Tavill, 1984).

10.3. The Fate of Lysosomal Ferritin

After the formation of the secondary lysosome, the digestion of ferritin then takes place through the action of hydrolytic enzymes, which degrade the protein component of ferritin, leaving behind the stable ferric hydroxide core and the partial degradation product haemosiderin (Trump et al., 1973; Munro and Linder, 1978; Wixom et al., 1980). In normal human hepatocytes, only very small amounts of ferritin–iron particles can be observed in the cytoplasm or lysosomes (Beaumont et al., 1980; Selden et al., 1980). Bacon and Tavill (1984) have suggested that this may indicate a possible enhancement of lysosomal degradative pathways as a consequence of increased intracellular ferritin levels.

Ferritin is more resistant than most proteins to lysosomal degradation (Coffey and De Duve, 1968; Rhodes, 1971), therefore one might expect to see undigested ferritin in secondary lysosomes for longer periods. Trump et al. (1973) have suggested that the final fate of lysosomal ferritin and haemosiderin may be either expulsion from the cell through the fusion of the secondary lysosomal membrane with the sinusoidal cell membrane, or continued accumulation in cellular lysosomes containing accumulated undigested ferritin, haemosiderin and iron. Bradford et al. (1969) observed clusters of membrane-bound organelles in the pericanalicular region of hepatocytes from iron-loaded rats, an observation later verified by others (Hultcrantz *et al.*, 1980; Park *et al.*, 1987). Bradford *et al.* (1969) also demonstrated that the contents of siderosomes and lysosomes from iron-loaded animals could be detected in the biliary canaliculus and in bile.

10.4. The Biliary Excretion of Ferritin and Iron

Iron deposits have been reported in bile duct epithelial cells of patients with iron-overload diseases (Scheuer, 1977) and other investigators have demonstrated a correlation between the amount of liver ferritin and ferritin protein in the bile of iron-loaded rats (Zuyderhoudt *et al.*, 1983).

Cleton and colleagues (1986) demonstrated the localization of ferritin particles inside the lumina of the bile canaliculus in liver biopsies from patients with varying degrees of iron overload (including genetic haemochromatosis and sideroblastic anaemia). Ferritin-containing lysosomes were found in cells bordering a bile canaliculus or duct and they reported that ferritin was present in the lumen of the canaliculus regardless of the cause of iron overload or the degree of fibrosis. This work in iron-loaded human subjects confirmed the earlier experiments on iron-loaded rats (Bradford *et al.*, 1969) and baboons (Iancu *et al.*, 1985). These findings are consistent with the involvement of the biliary system in iron excretion and indicate that biliary ferritin excretion may be an integral part of the excretion of this iron in hepatic parenchymal cells. LeSage *et al.* (1986) showed that the release of iron in iron-overloaded subjects is augmented by the administration of the microtubular inhibitor colchicine.

Based on the work of several investigators, Cleton *et al.* (1986) proposed two different theories for the excretion of ferritin-iron into bile: (a) excretion of iron into bile by transmembrane movement of ferritin particles (Iancu *et al.*, 1977; Parmley *et al.*, 1981) and (b) the expulsion of ferritin, haemosiderin and iron by fusion of secondary lysosomes with the biliary canalicular membrane (Bradford *et al.*, 1969). This latter theory has some support as 'lysosomal defaecation' or 'exocytosis' has been reported by other investigators in different cell systems using alternative ligands (Kerr, 1970; Douglas *et al.*, 1971; Kramer and Geuze, 1974; LaRusso and Fowler, 1979; LeSage *et al.*, 1986). The same investigators also demonstrated coated vesicles in the pericanalicular region of the parenchymal cells and coated pits between the microvilli bordering the canalicular lumen. They claim to have observed ferritin in these coated vesicles and hypothesized the existence of a direct shuttle mechanism for certain molecules, including ferritin, and hence also ferritin-iron taken up from the blood by receptor-mediated endocytosis and transported to the bile canaliculus for excretion.

Although providing morphological evidence of ferritin in the bile canaliculus, this study did not present any direct evidence of 'lysosomal exocytosis' of ferritin. Hultcrantz *et al.* (1989) demonstrated the presence of both iron and ferritin in the bile of patients with genetic haemochromatosis. They also postulated that ferritin is excreted into bile by lysosomal exocytosis. Recent studies by Ramm (1993) have provided some support for this hypothesis.

Ferritin has been detected in the bile of both iron-loaded animals and humans and it is evident that cells release ferritin molecules into the blood, as increased levels of serum ferritin are indicative of iron overload (Beamish *et al.*, 1974; Lipschitz *et al.*, 1974). However it is not known whether cells of the liver parenchyma or reticuloendothelial system are the source of increased levels of circulating ferritin (Worwood, 1986). It is also not known whether the biliary excretion of ferritin-iron is of quantitative importance in these disease states. The mechanisms involved in siderosomal accumulation, biliary excretion and sinusoidal release of ferritin, haemosiderin and iron are discussed below.

II. MECHANISMS OF FERRITIN RELEASE

The origin of serum ferritin and biliary ferritin has been a subject of conjecture for some years. Many questions remain unanswered: are serum and biliary ferritin actively secreted? How and why does serum or tissue ferritin traverse the cell, bound for extracellular release? Does internalized ferritin follow the same intracellular pathways of catabolism and/or release as endogenous ferritin?

In recent studies (Ramm, 1993) the lysosomotropic agent chloroquine and the microfilament inhibitor cytochalasin D were used to demonstrate that the release of endogenous ferritin into the plasma of normal rats is facilitated by a system of chloroquine-sensitive vesicles that are dependent on the normal functioning of the microfilamentous system of the liver cell cytoplasm. This was the first demonstration of an organized secretion of ferritin into the circulation of normal animals, which may help to dispel the theories of a passive leaking of ferritin from normal liver parenchyma.

In contrast the serum ferritin concentration of iron-loaded rats did not appear to be affected by either chloroquine or cytochalasin D, which suggested a possible difference in the intracellular metabolism of ferritin in iron-overloaded animals. In the same study the excretion of biliary ferritin in iron-loaded rats was shown to be facilitated by the same chloroquine-sensitive, microfilament-dependent mechanism as observed with the release of endogenous ferritin into the serum of normal rats.

The observations using chloroquine are similar to those of several investigators who have demonstrated that the secretion of very-low-density lipoproteins (VLDL) from isolated rat hepatocytes is inhibited by chloroquine (Nossen *et al.*, 1984; Rustan *et al.*, 1985, 1987). These studies suggested that the secretion of VLDL from hepatocytes is facilitated via a system of Golgi-derived vesicles involving a pathway that is disrupted by both chloroquine and the carboxylic ionophore monensin.

12. IRON EXCRETION AND IRON CHELATORS

The excretory pathways for iron in the human body are limited and therefore when excess iron is presented to the liver, it accumulates. This emphasizes the importance of understanding the possible pathways of ferritin and haemosiderin iron excretion, so that these pathways may be enhanced for treatment of subjects with iron-overload.

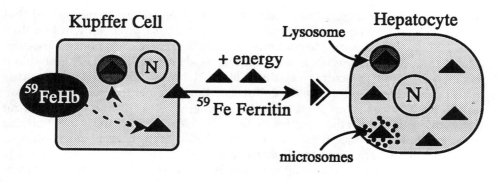

Fig. 4.3 Ferritin redistribution in the liver: a schematic representation of the postulated metabolic pathways by which ferritin and ferritin iron are exchanged between Kupffer cells and hepatocytes.

Parenterally administered chelators such as desferrioxamine have been used with some success in the treatment of iron-overload diseases (see Chapter 9).

Enhanced biliary iron excretion is observed with a variety of iron chelators, including desferrioxamine, in both animal and human studies. Such biliary iron excretion may result from chelation of iron either directly from hepatocellular ferritin at one or more points in its metabolic pathways, or after the iron has been released from its ferritin protein shell, perhaps within lysosomes. The nature and source of chelatable iron are discussed further in Chapter 12, together with the possibility of modifying chelators to remove iron selectively from particular liver cell types (hepatocytes and Kupffer cells).

13. FERRITIN AS AN IRON TRANSPORT PROTEIN

A large proportion of the research into ferritin and iron metabolism has focused on the uptake, intracellular transport and release of ferritin and/or iron by hepatocytes of both normal and iron-loaded liver. However, the mechanism of transfer of iron between cells in close proximity is also of interest.

The Kupffer cell has been shown to be extremely dynamic in its ingestion and subsequent digestion of immunosensitized erythrocytes (Munthe-Kaas, 1976). Young and Aisen (1982) reported that the normal rat macrophage appears capable of processing one ingested erythrocyte per hour. The Kupffer cell is capable of ingesting 12 or more immunosensitized erythrocytes at a time, *in vivo* (Mellman et al., 1983) or *in vitro* (Kondo et al., 1988). Thus the fate of iron released from the erythro-phagocytosing Kupffer cell and the subsequent involvement of ferritin and/or transferrin is an area that requires much more investigation (see also Chapter 2).

Kondo et al. (1988) immunosensitized ^{59}Fe-labelled erythrocytes with rabbit antierythrocyte antibodies and incubated them with adherent Kupffer cells in culture, according to the method of Saito and colleagues (1986). They demonstrated that when the average number of erythrocytes ingested per Kupffer cell was less than 1.5, the viability of the macrophages remained at 95% for at least 24 hours. However, the cells continually released ^{59}Fe, with approximately 40% of the total ingested iron being released into the culture medium after 24 hours. The addition of either transferrin or desferrioxamine to the culture medium augmented the release of iron from the Kupffer cell, consistent with the augmentation of iron release from rat hepatocytes using both of these agents (Baker *et al.*, 1985). Neither the lysosomotropic agent chloroquine, the microtubular inhibitor colchicine or the microfilament inhibitor cytochalasin B had any effect on iron release.

Kondo *et al.* (1988) found that approximately one-half of the iron released from the macrophages following *in vitro* ingestion of ^{59}Fe-labelled erythrocytes was present in the culture medium as ferritin. This was presumed by the authors to be a normal physiological process and not a result of ferritin leakage from the cell as there was no evidence of haemoglobin leakage into the culture medium. These findings are consistent with the results of Siimes and Dallman (1974) who demonstrated the presence of labelled ferritin in the serum of rats injected with ^{59}Fe-labelled, heat-damaged erythrocytes.

Sibille *et al.* (1988) followed up this study and demonstrated that ^{59}Fe, derived from the erythrophagocytosis of ^{59}Fe-labelled red blood cells, was released from Kupffer cells as ^{59}Fe-labelled ferritin in an energy-dependent process and not as a result of cell leakage. Using isokinetic sucrose-gradient ultracentrifugation they were also able to show that the released ferritin behaved more like tissue ferritin than serum ferritin, with approximately 2400 atoms of iron per molecule of ferritin. They then reincubated the Kupffer cell-released ^{59}Fe-labelled ferritin with isolated hepatocytes and demonstrated the rapid clearance of this ferritin from the culture medium, presumably via the hepatic ferritin receptor described by Mack *et al.* (1983). They observed the subsequent localization of ^{59}Fe in various compartments of the hepatocyte, with approximately 47% detected in the heavy and light mitochondrial (lysosome-rich) fraction, 10% in the microsomal fraction and the remainder in the nuclear fraction and cytoplasm.

Based on the results of Kondo *et al.* (1988) and their own observations, Sibille and colleagues (1988) hypothesized that as well as performing the function of an intracellular iron storage protein, ferritin may act as an intrahepatic iron transport protein, shunting iron between Kupffer cells and hepatocytes. The authors also proposed that as erythrophagocytosis also takes place in the spleen and the bone marrow with ferritin acting as the likely 'iron-sink', the liver would be bathed by a constant supply of ferritin via the portal circulation. This would therefore suggest that ferritin may play a more significant role in the delivery of iron to the hepatocyte than has previously been recognized, perhaps even more significant than the delivery of iron by transferrin (Fig. 4.3).

There is little understanding of the relationship between the Kupffer cell and the hepatocyte in iron metabolism and the role of ferritin in this association. Ferritin has been shown to possess the capacity to transfer approximately 160 000 atoms of iron per hepatocyte per minute *in vitro*, from Kupffer cell erythrophagocytosis alone (Sibille *et al.*, 1988). Therefore, a greater understanding of the normal metabolic pathways of uptake, intracellular transport and release of ferritin and iron is of paramount importance, particularly when attempting to understand the pathways of altered iron metabolism in disease states such as genetic haemochromatosis and the iron-loading anaemias, including thalassaemia.

REFERENCES

Adams, P. C., Powell, L. W. and Halliday, J. W. (1988a) Isolation of a human hepatic ferritin receptor. *Hepatology* **9**, 719–721.

Adams, P. C., Mack, U., Powell, L. W. and Halliday, J. W. (1988b) Isolation of a porcine hepatic ferritin receptor. *Comp. Biochem. Physiol. (B)* **90**, 837–841.

Aldred, A. R., Dickson, P. W., Marley, P. D. and Schreiber, G. (1987) Distribution of transferrin synthesis in brain and other tissues in the rat. *J. Biol. Chem.* **262**, 5293–5297.

Andrews, S. C., Brady, M. C., Treffry, A. *et al.* (1988) Studies on haemosiderin and ferritin from iron-loaded rat liver. *Biol. Metals* **1**, 33–42.

Arborgh, B. A. M., Glaumann, H. and Ericsson, J. L. E. (1974) Studies on iron loading of rat liver lysosomes: effects on the liver and distribution and fate of iron. *Lab. Invest.* **30**, 664–673.

Arosio, P., Yokota, M. and Drysdale, J. W. (1976) Structural and immunological relationships of isoferritins in normal and malignant cells. *Cancer Res.* **36**, 1–5.

Arosio, P., Yokota, M. and Drysdale, J. W. (1977) Characterization of serum ferritin in iron overload: possible identity to natural apoferritin. *Br. J. Haematol.* **36**, 199–207.

Bacon, B. R. and Tavill, A. S. (1984) Role of the liver in normal iron metabolism. *Sem. Liver Dis.* **4**, 181–192.

Baker, E., Page, M. and Morgan, E. H. (1985) Transferrin and iron release from rat hepatocytes in culture. *Am. J. Physiol.* **248**, G93–G97.

Bakker, G. R. and Boyer, R. F. (1986) Iron incorporation into apoferritin. The role of apoferritin as a ferroxidase. *J. Biol. Chem.* **261**, 13182–13185.

Bassett, M. L., Halliday, J. W. and Powell, L. W. (1986) Value of hepatic iron measurements in early haemochromatosis and determination of the critical iron level associated with fibrosis. *Hepatology* **6**, 24–29.

Bauminger, E. R., Harrison, P. M., Hechel, D., Nowik, I. and Treffry, A. (1991) Mossbauer Spectroscopic Investigation of Structure–Function Relations in Ferritins. Proceedings of the 10th International Conference on Iron and Iron Proteins, Oxford, UK.

Beamish, M. R., Walker, R., Miller, F. *et al.* (1974) Transferrin iron, chelatable iron and ferritin in idiopathic haemochromatosis. *Br. J. Haematol.* **27**, 219–228.

Beaumont, C., Simon, M., Smith, P. M. and Worwood, M. (1980) Hepatic and serum ferritin concentrations in patients with idiopathic haemochromatosis. *Gastroenterology* **79**, 877–883.

Bjorn-Rasmussen, E., Hageman, J., Van Den Dungen, P., Prowitz-Ksiazek, A. and Biberfeld, P. (1985) Transferrin receptors on circulating monocytes in hereditary haemochromatosis. *Scand. J. Haematol.* **34**, 308–311.

Blight, G. D. and Morgan, E. H. (1983) Ferritin and iron uptake by reticulocytes. *Br. J. Haematol.* **55**, 59–71.

Blight, G. D. and Morgan, E. H. (1987) Receptor-mediated endocytosis of transferrin and ferritin by guinea-pig reticulocytes. Uptake by a common endocytic pathway. *Eur. J. Cell Biol.* **43**, 260–265.

Bomford, A. B. and Munro H. N. (1985) Transferrin and its receptor: Their roles in cell function. *Hepatology* **5**, 870–875.

Bomford, A. B., Conlon-Hollingshead, C. and Munro, H. N. (1981) Adaptive responses of rat tissue isoferritins to iron administration. Changes in subunit synthesis, isoferritin abundance and capacity for iron storage. *J. Biol. Chem.* **256**, 948–955.

Bonomi, F. and Pagani, S. (1986) Removal of ferritin-bound iron by DL-dihydrolipoate and DL-dihydrolipoamide. *Eur. J. Biochem.* **155**, 295–300.

Bradford, W. D., Elchlepp, J. G. and Arstila, A. U. (1969) Iron metabolism and cell membranes. I. Relation between ferritin and haemosiderin in bile and biliary excretion of lysosome contents. *Am. J. Pathol.* **56**, 201–228.

Brissot, P., Wright, T. L., Ma, W.-L. and Weisiger, R. A. (1985) Efficient clearance of non-transferrin-bound iron by rat liver. *J. Clin. Invest.* **76**, 1463–1470.

Brown, A. J. P., Leibold, E. A. and Munro, H. N. (1983) Isolation of cDNA clones for the light subunit of rat liver ferritin: evidence that the light subunit is encoded by a multigene family. *Proc. Natl. Acad. Sci. USA* **80**, 1265–1269.

Broxmeyer, H. E. (1989) Iron-binding proteins and the regulation of haematopoietic cell proliferation/differentiation. In: *Iron in Immunity, Cancer and Inflammation* (eds M. De Sousa and J. H. Brock), Wiley, Chichester, pp. 199–221.

Broxmeyer, H. E., Cooper, S., Levi, S. and Arosio, P. (1991) Mutated recombinant human heavy-chain ferritins and myelosuppression *in vitro* and *in vivo*: a link between ferritin ferroxidase activity and biological function. *Proc. Natl. Acad. Sci. USA* **88**, 770–774.

Cavill, I., Worwood, M. and Jacobs, A. (1975) Internal regulation of iron absorption. *Nature* **256**, 328–329.

Chou, C.-C., Gatti, R. A., Fuller, M. L. *et al.* (1986) Structure and expression of ferritin genes in a human promyelocytic cell line that differentiates *in vitro*. *Mol. Cell. Biol.* **6**, 566–573.

Cleton, M. I., Sindram, J. W., Rademakers, L. H. P. M., Zuyderhoudt, F. M. J., Bruijn, W. C. and Marx, J. M. (1986) Ultrastructural evidence for the presence of ferritin–iron in the biliary system of patients with iron overload. *Hepatology*, **6**, 30–35.

Coffey, J. W. and de Duve, C. (1968) Digestive action of lysosomes. I. The digestion of proteins by extracts of rat liver lysosomes. *J. Biol. Chem.* **243**, 3255–3263.

Cragg, S. J., Wagstaff, M. and Worwood, M. (1980) Sialic acid and microheterogeneity of human serum ferritin. *Clin. Sci.* **58**, 259–262.

Cragg, S. J., Wagstaff, M. and Worwood, M. (1981) Detection of a glycosylated subunit in human serum ferritin. *Biochem. J.* **199**, 565–571.

Cragg, S. J., Covell, A. M., Burch, A., Owen, G. M., Jacobs, A. and Worwood, M. (1983) Turnover of ^{131}I-human spleen ferritin in plasma. *Br. J. Haematol.* **55**, 83–92.

Crichton, R. R. (1973) Ferritin. Structure and bonding. *Struct. Bonding Berlin* **17**, 67–134.

Crichton, R. R., Roman, F. and Roland, F. (1980) Iron mobilization from ferritin by chelating agents. *J. Inorg. Chem.* **13**, 305–316.

Doolittle, R. L. and Richter, G. W. (1981) Isoferritins in rat Kupffer cells, hepatocytes and extrahepatic macrophages. Biosynthesis in cell suspensions and cultures in response to iron. *Lab. Invest.* **45**, 567–574.

Douglas, W. W., Nagasawa, J. and Schulz, R. (1971) Electron microscopic studies on the mechanism of posterior pituitary hormones and the significance of microvesicles ('synaptic vesicles'): evidence of secretion by exocytosis and formation of microvesicles as a byproduct of this process. In: *Subcellular Organization and Function in Endocrine Tissues* (eds H. Heller and R. Lederis), University, Cambridge, pp. 353–378.

Drysdale, J. W. (1983) Regulation of ferritin biosynthesis. In: *Structure and Function of Iron Storage and Transport Proteins* (eds I. Urushizaki, P. Aisen, I. Listowski and J. W. Drysdale), Elsevier, Amsterdam, pp. 81–88.

Drysdale, J. W., Jain, S. K., Boyd, D. *et al.* (1985) Human ferritin: Genes and proteins. In: *Proteins of Iron Storage and Transport* (ed. G. Spik), Elsevier, Amsterdam, pp. 343–347.

Drysdale, J. W. and Munro, H. N. (1965) Failure of actinomycin to prevent induction of liver apoferritin after iron administration. *Biochim. Biophys. Acta* **103**, 185–188.

Ford, G. C., Harrison, P. M., Rice, D. W. *et al.* (1984) Ferritin: design and information of an iron storage molecule. *Phil. Trans. R. Soc. London Ser. B.*, **304**, 551–565.

Funk, F., Lenders, J.-P., Crichton, R. R. and Schneider, W. (1985) Reductive mobilisation of ferritin iron. *Eur. J. Biochem.* **152**, 167–172.

Gatter, K. C., Brown, G., Trowbridge, I. S., Woolstone, R. E. and Mason, D. Y. (1983) Transferrin receptors in human tissue: their distribution and possible clinical relevance. *J. Clin. Pathol.* **36**, 539–545.

Green, S. and Mazur, A. (1957) Uric acid metabolism and the mechanism of iron release from hepatic ferritin. *Science* **124**, 1149–1150.

Haile, D. J., Hentze, M. W., Rouault, T. A., Harford, J. B. and Klausner, R. D. (1989) Regulation of interaction of the iron-responsive element binding protein with iron-responsive RNA elements. *Mol. Cell. Biol.* **9**, 5055–5061.

Halliday, J. W. and Powell, L. W. (1979) Serum ferritin and isoferritins in clinical medicine. *Prog. Haematol.* **11**, 229–266.

Halliday, J. W. and Powell, L. W. (1984) Ferritin metabolism and the liver. *Sem. Liver Dis.* **4**, 207–216.

Halliday, J. W., Mack, U. and Powell, L. W. (1979) The kinetics of serum and tissue ferritins: relation to carbohydrate content. *Br. J. Haematol.* **42**, 535–546.

Harrison, P. M. (1977) Ferritin: an iron storage molecule. *Sem. Haematol.* **14**, 55–70.

Harrison, P. M., Clegg, G. A. and May, K. (1980) Ferritin structure and function. In: *Iron in Biochemistry and Medicine, II* (eds A. Jacobs and M. Worwood), Academic Press, London, pp. 131–171.

Harrison, P. M., Hoare, R. J., Hoye, T. G. and Macara, I. G. (1974) Ferritin and haemosiderin. In: *Iron in Biochemistry and Medicine* (eds A. Jacobs and M. Worwood), Academic Press, New York, pp. 73–114.

Harrison, P. M., Ford, G. C., Rice, D. W., Smith, J. M. A., Treffry, A. and White, J. L. (1986) The three dimensional structure of apoferritin: a framework controlling ferritin's iron storage and release. In: *Frontiers in Bioinorganic Chemistry* (ed. A. V. Xavier), VCH, Weinheim, pp. 268–277.

Harrison, P. M., Ford, G. C., Rice, D. W., Smith, J. M. A., Treffry, A. and White, J. L. (1987) Structural and functional studies on ferritins. *Biochem. Soc. Trans.* **15**, 744–748.

Hershko, C., Cook, J. D. and Finch, C. A. (1972) Storage iron kinetics. II. The uptake of hemoglobin iron by hepatic parenchymal cells. *J. Lab. Clin. Med.* **80**, 624–634.

Hershko, C., Cook, J. D. and Finch, C. A. (1973) Storage iron kinetics. III. Study of desferrioxamine action by selective radioiron labels of RE and parenchymal cells. *J. Lab. Clin. Med.* **81**, 876–886.

Hultcrantz, R., Arborgh, B., Wroblewski, R. and Ericsson, J. L. (1980) Studies on the rat liver following iron overload. *Acta Pathol. Microbiol. Scand. A* **88A**, 341–353.

Hultcrantz, R., Angelin, B., Björn-Rasmussen, E., Ewerth, S. and Einarsson, K. (1989) Biliary excretion of iron and ferritin in idiopathic hemochromatosis. *Gastroenterology* **96**, 1539–1545.

Iancu, T. C., Neustein, H. B. and Landing, B. H. (1977) The liver in thalassaemia major: ultrastructural observations. In: *Iron Metabolism* (Ciba Foundation Symposium 51) (eds R. Porter and D. W. Fitzsimons), Elsevier, Amsterdam, pp. 293–316.

Iancu, T. C., Rabinowitz, H., Brissot, P., Guillouzo, A., Deugnier, Y. and Bourel, M. (1985) Iron overload of the liver in the baboon – an ultrastructural study. *J. Hepatol.* **1**, 261–275.

Idzerda, R. L., Huebers, H., Finch, C. A. and McKnight, G. S. (1986) Rat transferrin gene expression: tissue-specific regulation by iron deficiency. *Proc. Natl. Acad. Sci. USA* **83**, 3723–3727.

Jacobs, A. (1977) Low molecular weight intracellular iron transport compounds. *Blood* **50**, 433–439.

Jacobs, A., Millar, F., Worwood, M., Beamish, M. R. and Wardrop, C. A. (1972) Ferritin in the serum of normal subjects and patients with iron deficiency and iron overload. *Br. Med. J.* **4**, 206–208.

Jones, B. M., Worwood, M. and Jacobs, A. (1983) Isoferritins in normal leucocytes. *Br. J. Haematol.* **55**, 73–81.

Kerr, J. F. R. (1970) Liver cell defaecation: an electron microscope study of the discharge of lysosomal residual bodies in the cellular space. *J. Pathol.* **100**, 99–103.

Kino, K., Tsunoo, H., Higa, Y., Takami, M., Hamaguchi, H. and Nakagima, H. (1980) Hemoglobin–haptoglobin receptor in rat liver plasma membranes. *J. Biol. Chem.* **255**, 9616–9620.

Koeller, D. M., Casey, J. L., Hentze, M. W. *et al.* (1989) A cytosolic protein binds to structural elements within the iron regulatory region of the transferrin receptor mRNA. *Proc. Natl. Acad. Sci. USA* **86**, 3574–3578.

Kondo, H., Saito, K., Grasso, J. P. and Aisen, P. (1988) Iron metabolism in the erythrophagocytosing Kupffer cell. *Hepatology* **8**, 32–38.

Konijn, A. M. and Hershko, C. (1977) Ferritin synthesis in inflammation I. Pathogenesis of impaired iron release. *Br. J. Haematol.* **37**, 7–16.

Kramer, M. F. and Geuze, J. J. (1974) Redundant cell-membrane regulation in the exocrine pancreas after pilocarpine stimulation of secretion. In: *International Symposium on Cell Biology and Cytopharmacology* (eds B. Ceccarelli, F. Clementi and J. Meldolesi), Raven, New York, pp. 87–97.

La Russo, N. F. and Fowler, S. (1979) Coordinate secretion of acid hydrolases in rat bile. Hepatocyte exocytosis of lysosomal protein. *J. Clin. Invest.* **64**, 948–954.

Lawson, D. M., Artymiuk, P. J., Yewdall, S. J. *et al.* (1991) Solving the structure of human H ferritin by genetically engineering intermolecular crystal contacts. *Nature* **349**, 541–544.

Lee, N. T., Chae, C. B. and Kierzenbaum, A. L. (1986) Contrasting levels of transferrin gene activity in cultured rat Sertoli cells and intact seminiferous tubules. *Proc. Natl. Acad. Sci. USA* **83**, 8177–8181.

Lee, EY. H., Barcellos-Hoff, M. H., Chen, L. H., Parry, G. and Bissell, M. J. (1987) Transferrin is a major mouse milk protein and is synthesized by mammary epithelial cells. *In Vitro Cell Dev. Biol.* **23**, 221–226.

LeSage, G. D., Kost, L. J., Barham, S. S. and LaRusso, N. F. (1986) Biliary excretion of iron from hepatocyte lysosomes in the rat. *J. Clin. Invest.* **77**, 90–97.

Levi, S., Cozzi, A., Santambrogio, P. and Arosio, P. (1991) Study of the sequences involved in ferritin iron incorporation. Proceedings of the 10th International Conference on Iron and Iron Proteins, Oxford, UK.

Lipschitz, D. A., Dugard, J., Simon, M. O., Bothwell, T. H. and Charlton, R. W. (1971) The site of action of desferrioxamine. *Br. J. Haematol.* **20**, 395–404.

Lipschitz, P. A., Cook, J. P. and Finch, C. A. (1974) A clinical evaluation of serum ferritin. *N. Engl. J. Med.* **290**, 1213–1216.

Louache, F., Testa, U., Titeux, M. and Rochant, H. (1985) Expression of transferrin receptors and intracellular ferritin during differentiation of two human leukaemic cell lines HL-60 and U 937. In: *Proteins of Iron Storage and Transport* (ed. G. Spik), Elsevier, Amsterdam, pp. 365–368.

Lum, J. B. (1987) Role of transferrin in cellular proliferation. Ph.D. Thesis, University of Texas Graduate School of Biomedical Science, San Antonio.

Mack, U., Powell, L. W. and Halliday, J. W. (1983) Detection and isolation of a hepatic membrane receptor for ferritin. *J. Biol. Chem.* **258**, 4672–4675.

Mack, U., Storey, E. L., Powell, L. W. and Halliday, J. W. (1985) Characterization of the binding of ferritin to the rat hepatic ferritin receptor. In: *Proteins of Iron Storage and Transport* (eds G. Spik, J. Montreuil, R. R. Crichton and J. Mazurier), Elsevier, Amsterdam, pp. 203–206.

Mann, S., Wade, V. J., Dickson, D. P. *et al.* (1988) Structural specificity of haemosiderin iron cores in iron overload diseases. *FEBS Letters* **234**, 69–72.

Mazur, A., Green, S., Saha, A. and Carleton, A. (1958) Mechanisms of release of ferritin iron in vivo by xanthine oxidase. *J. Clin. Invest.* **37**, 1809–1817.

McClain, C. J., Marsano, L., Burk, R. F. and Bacon, B. R. (1991) Trace metals in liver disease. *Sem. Liver Dis.* **11**, 321–339.

McCord, J. M. and Day, E. D., Jr. (1978) Superoxide-dependent production of hydroxyl radical catalysed by iron-EDTA complex. *Fed. Eur. Biochem. Soc. Letters* **86**, 139–142.

Mellman, I. S., Plutner, H., Steinman, R. M., Unkeless, J. C. and Cohn, Z. A. (1983) Internalization and degradation of macrophage Fc receptors during receptor-mediated phagocytosis. *J. Cell Biol.* **96**, 887–895.

Morgan, E. H. and Baker, E. (1988) Role of transferrin receptors and endocytosis in iron uptake by hepatic and erythroid cells. *Ann. NY Acad. Sci.* **526**, 65–82.

Müllner, E. W., Neupert, B. and Kühn, L. C. (1989) A specific mRNA binding factor regulates the iron-dependent stability of cytoplasmic transferrin receptor mRNA. *Cell* **58**, 373–382.

Munro, H. N. and Linder, M. C. (1978) Ferritin: structure, biosynthesis and role in iron metabolism. *Physiol. Rev.* **58**, 317–396.

Munthe-Kaas, A. C. (1976) Phagocytosis in rat Kupffer cells in vitro. *Exp. Cell Res.* **99**, 319–327.

Nossen, J. Ø., Rustan, A. C., Barnard, T. and Drevon, C. A. (1984) Inhibition by chloroquine of the secretion of very low density lipoproteins by cultured rat hepatocytes. *Biochim. Biophys. Acta* **803**, 11–20.

O'Connell, M. J., Ward, R. J., Baum, H., Treffry, A. and Peters, T. J. (1988) Evidence of a biosynthetic link between ferritin and haemosiderin. *Biochem. Soc. Trans.* **16**, 828–829.

Osaki, S. and Sirivech, S. (1971) Identification and partial purification of a ferritin reducing enzyme in liver (abstr). *Fed. Proc.* **30**, 1292.

Park, C. H., Bacon, B. R., Brittenham, G. M. and Tavill, A. S. (1987) Pathology of dietary carbonyl iron overload in rats. *Lab. Invest.* **57**, 555–563.

Parmley, R. T., May, M. E., Spicer, S. S., Buse, M. G. and Alvarez, C. J. (1981) Ultrastructural distribution of inorganic iron in normal and iron-loaded hepatic cells. *Lab. Invest.* **44**, 475–485.

Peters, S. W., Jacobs, A. and Fitzsimmons, E. (1983) Erythrocyte ferritin in normal subjects and patients with abnormal iron metabolism. *Br. J. Haematol.* **30**, 47–55.

Pollack, S. and Campana, T. (1981) Immature red cells have ferritin receptors. *Biochem. Biophys. Res. Commun.* **100**, 1667–1672.

Pollock, A. S., Lipschitz, D. A. and Cook, J. D. (1978) The kinetics of serum ferritin. *Proc. Soc. Exp. Biol. Med.* **157**, 481–485.

Powell, L. W., Alpert, E., Drysdale, J. W. and Isselbacher, K. J. (1974) Abnormality in tissue isoferritins in idiopathic hemochromatosis. *Nature* **250**, 333–335.

Powell, L. W., Alpert, E., Isselbacher, K. J. and Drysdale, J. W. (1975) Human isoferritins: organ specific iron and apoferritin distribution. *Br. J. Haematol.* **30**, 47–55.

Ramm, G. A. (1993) Pathways of ferritin metabolism in the liver: Effects of lysosomotropic agents. Ph.D. Thesis, The University of Queensland.

Ramm, G. A., Powell, L. W. and Halliday, J. (1990) Effect of colchicine on the clearance of ferritin in vivo. *Am. J. Physiol.* **258**, G707–G713.

Rhodes, J. M. (1971) In vitro studies on the fate of antigen. I. The digestion of human serum albumin and ferritin by extracts of mouse spleen. *Acta Pathol. Microbiol. Scand. Sect. B*, **79**, 153–162.

Rice, D. W., Ford, G. C., White, J. L., Smith, J. M. A. and Harrison, P. M. (1983) Recent advances in the three dimensional structure of ferritin. In: *Structure and Function of Iron Storage and Transport Proteins* (eds I. Urushizaki, P. Aisen, I. Listowsky and J. W. Drysdale), Elsevier, Amsterdam, pp. 11–16.

Richter, G. W. (1978) The iron-loaded cell – the cytopathology of iron storage. *Am. J. Pathol.* **91**, 363–396.

Rouault, T. A., Rao, K., Harford, J., Mattia, E. and Klausner, R. D. (1985) Hemin, chelatable iron and the regulation of transferrin biosynthesis. *J. Biol. Chem.* **259**, 14862–14866.

Rouault, T. A., Hentze, M. W., Caughman, S. W., Harford, J. B. and Klausner, R. D. (1988) Binding of a cytosolic protein to the iron-responsive element of human ferritin messenger RNA. *Science* **241**, 1207–1210.

Rustan, A., Nossen, J. Ø., Berg, T. and Drevon, C. A. (1985) The effects of monensin on secretion of very-low-density lipoprotein and metabolism of asialofetuin by cultured rat hepatocytes. *Biochem. J.* **227**, 529–536.

Rustan, A., Nossen, J. Ø., Tefre Toril, T. and Drevon, C. A. (1987) Inhibition of very-low-density lipoprotein secretion by chloroquine, verapamil and monensin takes place in the Golgi complex. *Biochim. Biophys. Acta* **930**, 311–319.

Saito, K., Nishisato, T., Grasso, J. A. and Aisen, P. (1986) Interaction of transferrin with iron-loaded rat peritoneal macrophages. *Br. J. Haematol.* **62**, 275–286.

Sargent, K. S. and Munro, H. N. (1975) Association of ferritin with liver cell membrane fractions. *Exp. Cell Res.* **93**, 15–22.

Sasaki, A. W. and Wagner, R. C. (1979) Endocytosis of fluorescent-labelled ferritin by isolated rat hepatocytes (abstr). *Gastroenterology* **77**, A38.

Scheuer, P. J. (1977) *Liver Biopsy Interpretation*, 2nd edn. Baillière, Tindall and Cassell, London.

Sciot, R., Paterson, A. C., Van den Oord, J. J. and Desmet, V. J. (1987) Lack of hepatic transferrin receptor expression in haemochromatosis. *Hepatology* **7**, 831–837.

Selden, C., Owen, M., Hopkins, J. M. O. and Peters, T. J. (1980) Studies on the concentration and intracellular localization of iron proteins in liver biopsy specimens from patients with iron overload with special reference to their role in lysosomal disruption. *Br. J. Haematol.* **44**, 593–603.

Shull, G. E. and Theil, E. C. (1982) Translational control of ferritin synthesis by iron in embryonic reticulocytes of the bull-frog. *J. Biol. Chem.* **257**, 14187–14191.

Sibille, J. C., Kondo, H. and Aisen, P. (1988) Interactions between isolated hepatocytes and Kupffer cells in iron metabolism: a possible role for ferritin as an iron carrier protein. *Hepatology* **8**, 296–301.

Siimes, M. and Dallman, P. R. (1974) New kinetic role for serum ferritin in iron metabolism. *Br. J. Haematol.* **28**, 7–18.

Simon, M., MacPhail, P., Bothwell, T., Lyons, G., Baynes, R. and Torrance, J. (1987) The fate of intravenously administered hepatic ferritin in normal, phenylhydrazine-treated and scorbutic guinea-pigs. *Br. J. Haematol.* **65**, 239–243.

Sirivech, S., Freiden, E. and Osaki, S. (1974) The release of iron from horse spleen ferritin by reducing flavins. *Biochem. J.* **143**, 311–315.

Smith, A. and Morgan, W. T. (1981) Hemopexin-mediated transport of heme into isolated rat hepatocytes. *J. Biol. Chem.* **256**, 10902–10909.

Tavassoli, M. (1988) The role of liver endothelium in the transfer of iron from transferrin to the hepatocyte. *Ann NY Acad. Sci.* **526**, 83–92.

Thomas, C. E. and Aust, S. D. (1986) Reductive release of iron from ferritin by cation free radicals of paraquat and other bipyridyls. *J. Biol. Chem.* **261**, 13064–13070.

Thomas, C. E., Morehouse, L. E. and Aust, S. D. (1985) Ferritin and superoxide-dependent lipid peroxidation. *J. Biol. Chem.* **260**, 3275–3280.

Thorstensen, K. and Romslo, I. (1990) The role of transferrin in the mechanisms of cellular iron uptake. *Biochem. J.* **271**, 1–10.

Topham, R. W., Walker, M. C. and Calisch, M. P. (1982) Liver xanthine dehydrogenase and iron mobilization. *Biochem. Biophys. Res. Commun.* **109**, 1240–1246.

Treffry, A., Hirzmann, J., Hodson, N. W. and Harrison, P. M. (1991) Binding of iron and other metals to recombinant apoferritins studies by UV-difference spectroscopy. Proceedings of the 10th International Conference on Iron and Iron Proteins, Oxford, UK.

Trump, B. F., Valigorsky, J. M., Arstila, A. U., Mergner, W. J. and Kinney, T. D. (1973) The relationship of intracellular pathways of iron metabolism to cellular iron overload and the iron storage diseases. *Am. J. Pathol.* **72**, 295–324.

Trump, B. F., Arstila, A. U., Valigorsky, J. M. and Barret, L. A. (1975) Subcellular aspects of ferritin metabolism. In: *Proteins of Iron Storage and Transport in Biochemistry and Medicine* (ed. R. R. Crichton), North-Holland, Amsterdam, pp. 343–350.

Unger, A. and Hershko, C. (1974) Hepatocellular uptake of ferritin in the rat. *Br. J. Haematol.* **28**, 169–179.

Van Wyk, C. P., Linder-Horowitz, M. and Munro, H. N. (1971) Effect of iron loading on non-heme iron compounds in different liver cell populations. *J. Biol. Chem.* **246**, 1025–1031.

Vogel, B. W., Bomford, A. and Young, S. (1987) Heterogenous distribution of transferrin receptors on parenchymal and nonparenchymal liver cells: Biochemical and morphological evidence. *Blood* **69**, 264–270.

Walters, G. O., Millar, F. M. and Worwood, M. (1973) Serum ferritin concentration and iron stores in normal subjects. *J. Clin. Pathol.* **26**, 770–772.

Ward, J. H., Kushner, J. P. and Kaplan, J. (1981) Fibroblast transferrin receptors in normal human subjects and in patients with haemochromatosis (abstr.). *Clin. Res.* **29**, 352A.

Ward, J. H., Kushner, J. P., Ray, F. A. and Kaplan, J. (1984) Transferrin receptor function in hereditary haemochromatosis. *J. Lab. Clin. Med.* **103**, 246–254.

Ward, R. J., O'Connell, M. J., Dickson, D. P. E. *et al.* (1989) Biochemical studies of the iron cores and polypeptide shells of haemosiderin isolated from patients with primary or secondary haemochromatosis. *Biochim. Biophys. Acta* **993**, 131–133.

Ward, R. J., O'Connell, M. J., Mann, S. *et al.* (1988) Heterogeneity of the iron cores in hepatic haemosiderins from primary and secondary haemochromatosis. *Biochem. Soc. Trans.* **16**, 830–831.

Watt, G. D., Frankel, R. B. and Papefthymiou, G. C. (1985) Reduction of mammalian ferritin. *Proc. Natl. Acad. Sci. USA* **82**, 3640–3643.

Wetz, K. and Crichton, R. R. (1976) Chemical modification as a probe of the topography and reactivity of horse-spleen apoferritin. *Eur. J. Biochem.* **61**, 545–550.

Whaley, W. G., Dauwalder, M. and Kephart, J. E. (1972) Golgi apparatus: influence on cell surfaces. *Science* **175**, 596–599.

Wixom, R. L., Prutkin, L. and Munro, H. N. (1980) Haemosiderin: nature, formation and significance. *Int. Rev. Exp. Pathol.* **22**, 193–225.

Worwood, M. (1986) Serum ferritin. *Clin. Sci.* **70**, 215–220.

Worwood, M. (1990) Ferritin. *Blood Rev.* **4**, 259–269.

Worwood, M., Dawkins, S., Wagstaff, M. and Jacobs, A. (1976) The purification and properties of ferritin from human serum. *Biochem. J.* **157**, 97–103.

Worwood, M., Wagstaff, M., Jones, B. M., Dawkins, S. and Jacobs, A. (1977) Biochemical and immunological properties of human isoferritins. In: *Proteins of Iron Metabolism* (eds E. B. Brown, P. Aisen, J. Fielding and R. R. Crichton), Grune and Stratton, New York, p. 79.

Worwood, M., Cragg, S. J., Wagstaff, M. and Jacobs, A. (1979) Binding of human serum ferritin to concanavalin A. *Clin. Sci.* **56**, 83–87.

Worwood, M., Cragg, S. J., Jacobs, A., McLaren, C., Ricketts, C. and Economidou, J. (1980) Binding of serum ferritin to concanavalin A: patients with homozygous β-thalassaemia and transfusional iron overload. *Br. J. Haematol.* **46**, 409–416.

Worwood, M., Cragg, S. J., Williams, A. M., Wagstaff, M. and Jacobs, A. (1982) The clearance of ^{131}I-human plasma ferritin in man. *Blood* **60**, 827–833.

Wright, T. L., Brissot, P., Ma, W. L. and Weisiger, R. A. (1986) Characterization of non-transferrin-bound iron clearance by rat liver. *J. Biol. Chem.* **261**, 10909–10914.

Wright, T. L. and Lake, J. R. (1990) Mechanisms of transport of non-transferrin-bound iron in basolateral and canalicular rat liver plasma membrane vesicles. *Hepatology*, **12**, 498–504.

Yang, C. Y., Meagher, A., Huynh, B. H., Sayers, D. E. and Theil, E. C. (1987) Fe(III) clusters bound to horse-spleen apoferritin: an X-ray absorption (EXAFS) and Mossbauer spectroscopy study which shows that iron core nuclei can form on the protein. *Biochemistry* **26**, 497–503.

Young, S. P. and Aisen, P. (1982) The liver and iron. In: *The Liver: Biology and Pathobiology* (eds I. M. Arias, H. Popper, D. Shafritz and W. Jakoby), Raven, New York.

Young, S. P. and Aisen, P. (1988) The liver and iron. In: *The Liver: Biology and Pathology*, 2nd edn (eds I. M. Arias, W. B. Jakoby, H. Popper, D. Schachter and D. A. Shafritz), Raven, New York, pp. 535–550.

Zahringer, J., Baliga, B. S. and Munro, H. N. (1976) Novel mechanism for translational control in regulation of ferritin synthesis by iron. *Proc. Natl. Acad. Sci. USA* **73**, 857–861.

Zuyderhoudt, F. M. J., Willekens, F. L. A. and Schreuder, W. O. (1979) Annotations on the measurement of liver ferritin, especially in the rat. *Anal. Biochem.* **98**, 204–207.

Zuyderhoudt, F. M. J., Uiterdijk, H. G. and Jörning, G. G. A. (1982) On the role of rat liver lysosomes in the catabolism of intravenously injected rat liver ferritin. In: *The Biochemistry and Physiology of Iron* (eds P. Saltman and J. Hegenauer), Elsevier, Amsterdam, pp. 479–483.

Zuyderhoudt, F. M. J., Vos, P., Jörning, G. G. A. and Van Gool, J. (1983) Ferritin in liver, plasma and bile of the iron-loaded rat. In: *Structure and Function of Iron Storage and Transport Proteins* (eds I. Urushizaki, P. Aisen, I. Listowski and J. W. Drysdale), Elsevier, Amsterdam, pp. 215–216.

5. The Control of Cellular Iron Homeostasis

J. B. HARFORD[1], T. A. ROUAULT AND R. D. KLAUSNER

Cell Biology and Metabolism Branch, National Institute of Child Health and Development, National Institutes of Health, Bethesda, MD 20892, USA

I. OVERVIEW OF CELLULAR IRON HOMEOSTASIS

The ability to regulate the expression of particular genes is central to all life forms. In unicellular organisms, gene regulation is utilized to respond to environmental conditions in the quest for nutrients and in defence against toxic substances. In addition, distinct genes are expressed during different phases of the life cycle of the organism. In multicellular organisms, gene regulation is critical to the establishment of specialized cellular functions during developmental differentiation. In common with lower organisms, cells of higher eukaryotes also respond to their environment by altering gene expression. These environmental stimuli include molecules like hormones and growth factors, but may also include nutrients and toxic substances. Iron falls into both of these latter categories.

With but a few notable exceptions, all organisms require a nearly continuous source of environmental iron for growth and the maintenance of a wide range of metabolic pathways (Neilands, 1974; Stubbe, 1990). Iron's flexible coordination chemistry and favourable redox potential are responsible for the fact that the metal is utilized as a

[1]Present address: RiboGene, Inc., 21375 Cabot Boulevard, Hayward, CA 94545, USA.

cofactor for a variety of both structural and metabolic functions (Crichton, 1991). However, iron in conjunction with oxygen becomes a source of dangerous toxicity as a generator of hydroxyl radicals which has a variety of toxic effects on cells (Gutteridge, 1989). Thus, much of the current efforts to understand cellular iron metabolism is aimed at understanding how cells obtain iron from the environment, how they detoxify excess iron, and how they regulate these processes in a way that balances critical metabolic needs with the toxicity of iron. The emphasis of this chapter will be on the regulation of gene expression in response to iron scarcity or abundance. The remainder of this book deals with the details as to why such regulation is necessary and these issues will be discussed but briefly here.

In the dividing cells of higher eukaryotes, iron is acquired via the transferrin cycle involving the serum iron-carrying protein transferrin (Tf) and the membrane-associated transferrin receptor (TfR). In addition to the coverage afforded the transferrin cycle in Chapter 3 of this text, there have appeared several reviews that have dealt with various aspects of the biochemistry and cell biology of the TfR and with its involvement in cellular iron metabolism (Hanover and Dickson, 1985; Crichton and Charloteaux-Wauters, 1987; Huebers and Finch, 1987; Kühn, 1989; Harford et al., 1990). Here, major emphasis will be placed on the regulation of the expression of the TfR that occurs in response to alterations in iron availability.

Protection from the harmful effects of iron plus oxygen is in large measure accomplished through the process of iron sequestration. Other chapters of this text cover iron toxicity and iron sequestration at some length (Chapters 4 and 10). The protein that subserves the function of sequestering intracellular iron in the cytoplasm of higher eukaryotes is ferritin (Munro and Linder, 1978; Theil, 1987). Different cell types differentially express members of the ferritin gene family and ferritin expression may be regulated by factors other than iron. The post-transcriptional regulation of ferritin biosynthesis by iron will be discussed here in detail. Lesser emphasis will be placed on the body of evidence indicating that ferritin expression is also regulated in other ways and by other agents or circumstances. Together with the post-transcriptional regulation of TfR expression, ferritin post-transcriptional regulation allows the cells of higher eukaryotes to balance their need for iron and their aversion to iron's toxicity (Klausner and Harford, 1989; Harford and Klausner, 1990; Theil, 1990; Kühn and Hentze, 1992; Klausner et al., 1993).

2. REGULATION OF CELLULAR IRON HOMEOSTASIS

It has been known since the 1940s that ferritin levels vary directly with the amount of iron given to an individual (Granick, 1946). Beginning in the mid-1970s, Munro and colleagues presented evidence indicating that this regulation took place at the translational level (Zahringer et al., 1976; Munro and Linder, 1978; Rogers and Munro, 1987). Deletion analysis of the ferritin mRNA localized the region responsible for translational control to about 30 nucleotides of the 212 nucleotides 5' untranslated region (UTR) of human H-chain ferritin mRNA (Hentze et al., 1986, 1987b). Examination of these 30 nucleotides revealed that they could be folded into a moderately stable stem-loop structure (Fig. 5.1) that was similar to potential stem-loop structures present in the 5'UTR of the other ferritin genes that had been cloned

Examples of IREs

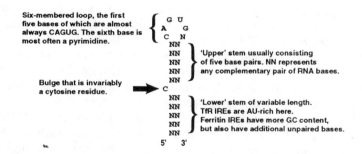

Human Ferritin H-Chain mRNA	Rat Ferritin L-Chain mRNA	Bullfrog Ferritin H-Chain mRNA	Human TfR mRNA

Consensus IRE

Fig. 5.1 The sequence and proposed structures of IREs. Sequences of IREs from the 5′UTRs of mRNAs encoding human ferritin H-chain, rat ferritin L-chain, and bullfrog ferritin H-chain are shown along with IREs from the human TfR mRNA (labelled A–E as described by Casey *et al.*, 1988a). Nucleotides indicated by arrows in the TfR mRNA IREs are bases that are different in the corresponding motifs of the chicken TfR mRNA (Chan *et al.*, 1989; Koeller *et al.*, 1989). Based on the sequences of the IREs of all known ferritin mRNAs and those of all known TfR mRNAs, a consensus IRE motif is depicted. Features of the IRE consensus are indicated.

at the time (Hentze *et al.*, 1988). This sequence element, when placed in the 5′UTR of heterologous mRNAs, conferred iron-dependent translational control to these transcripts. The sequence element from the human ferritin H-chain mRNA that was both necessary and sufficient for iron-dependent translational control was termed an iron-responsive element or IRE (Hentze *et al.*, 1987a). At about the same time, Munro and colleagues (Aziz and Munro, 1987; Leibold and Munro, 1987, 1988) demonstrated that a corresponding sequence element from rat ferritin L-chain mRNA also functioned as a translational control element. Thus both H-chain and L-chain ferritins are regulated at the level of translation mediated by very similar RNA elements (the IREs) within their 5′UTR. Change of a single nucleotide within the H-chain IRE could completely ablate the ability of the sequence to result in translational control; when the first C of the loop was removed, the IRE failed to function (Hentze et al., 1987a). Similarly, when alterations in sequence were made that disrupted the upper stem, IRE function was lost (Hentze et al., 1987a; Leibold et al., 1990; Bettany et al., 1992). The hairpin nature of the RNA corresponding to the IREs from two bull-frog ferritin mRNAs has been confirmed by direct in vitro structural analysis (Wang et al., 1990).

The expression of the TfR is also regulated. Within populations of proliferating cells the expression of TfR is modulated by iron availability with fewer receptors expressed when iron is abundant (Pelicci et al., 1982; Ward et al., 1982; Mattia et al., 1984). Quantitative immunoprecipitation of TfR translated in vitro from RNA isolated from iron-treated and chelator-treated K562 cells indicated that the iron-dependent alterations in TfR biosynthesis were a reflection of alterations in the level of TfR mRNA (Mattia et al., 1984; Rao et al., 1985). The availability of a molecular probe for the TfR mRNA (McClelland et al., 1984) allowed the direct quantitation of TfR mRNA. The steady-state level of TfR mRNA was found to be increased after cells were treated with an iron chelator and decreased after exogenous iron was supplied (Rao et al., 1986). The predominant locus of iron regulation of TfR expression lies not in the promoter but in sequences corresponding to the 3′UTR of the TfR mRNA (Owen and Kühn, 1987; Casey et al., 1988a,b). The 3′UTR of the TfR mRNA was shown to be sufficient to confer iron regulation to the expression of a chimeric transcript encoding HLA-A2 (Müllner and Kühn, 1988) or human growth hormone (Casey et al., 1988a).

The region within the 3′UTR of the TfR mRNA that is the predominant locus of iron regulation has been defined as being within a fragment of 678 nucleotides (Casey et al., 1988a). Examination of the sequence of the critical 678 nucleotides fragment revealed that a high degree of RNA secondary structure is possible within this region that is very similar to a possible secondary structure that can be adopted by corresponding sequences within the 3′UTR of the chicken TfR mRNA (Chan et al., 1989; Koeller et al., 1989). Perhaps the most interesting insight resulting from inspection of the possible secondary structure of the regulatory region of the TfR mRNA was the discovery of five stem-loop structures within the TfR 3′UTR that bore striking similarity to the IRE found within the 5′UTR of mRNAs encoding ferritin (Casey et al., 1988a; Fig. 5.1). Although the IREs of ferritins and the TfR can be fit to a consensus motif, the IREs contained in the TfR mRNA have distinct sequences from those of known ferritins in the bases that make up the stems of the IRE stem-loops.

3. THE IRON-RESPONSIVE ELEMENT-BINDING PROTEIN AS THE MEDIATOR OF CELLULAR IRON HOMEOSTASIS

RNA secondary structure within the 5′UTR of an mRNA can directly influence translation (Pelletier and Sonenberg, 1985; Kozak, 1986). However, the predicted stability of the ferritin IRE stem loop (< 10 kcal/mol) is insufficient to be likely to impede translation on its own. In fact, evidence has been presented suggesting that the IRE alone is a positive effector of ferritin translation (Dix et al., 1992). Using rodent cell lysates, Leibold and Munro (1988) first reported the demonstration of a cellular factor that specifically interacted with an RNA transcript containing an IRE. This demonstration was accomplished by a modification of the gel electrophoretic mobility shift or band shift assay first utilized for demonstrating specific DNA–protein interactions. With similar methodology, Rouault et al. (1988) demonstrated that human cell lysates contained an IRE-binding protein (IRE-BP). It was noted that there was increased binding activity present in the cytosol of cells that had been treated with the iron chelator, desferrioxamine, as compared with lysates of cells exposed to normal levels of iron in culture. It has been shown by 'footprinting' that interaction of the IRE-BP with bullfrog ferritin mRNA in vitro is confined to the region of the IRE (Harrell et al., 1991).

All available data are consistent with the IRE-BP being an iron-regulated repressor of ferritin translation in vivo (Caughman et al., 1988). Other terms including p90 (Harrell et al., 1991) and iron regulatory factor or IRF (Müllner et al., 1989) have also been used for this protein. The protein's interaction with the IRE has also been directly shown to inhibit specifically the in vitro translation of ferritin mRNA, and as such it has also been termed 'ferritin repressor protein' or 'FRP' (Walden et al., 1988, 1989). Given that ferritin mRNAs are not the only transcripts that contain one or more IREs and that all functions involving gene regulation are associated with binding to IREs, we prefer and will use the more generic name IRE-BP.

Analysis of gel shift data from human cell lysates demonstrated a high affinity ($K_d = 10$–30 pM) binding site for IREs (Haile et al., 1989). All data are consistent with cellular iron homeostasis being accomplished through changes in the number of high affinity IRE-BP molecules (referred to as IRE-BP$_{on}$ in Fig. 5.3). The induction in IRE-BP activity that occurs upon treatment of human RD-4 cells with desferrioxamine did not require new protein synthesis since puromycin treatment was without effect (Hentze et al., 1989). IRE-binding activity could be abolished by the treatment of lysates with alkylating agents such as N-ethylmaleimide (Hentze et al., 1989). Moreover, when the human cellular lysates were simply treated with either 2-mercaptoethanol or dithiothreitol, a large increase in the number of high affinity binding sites was observed. IRE-BP activity has been detected in cell lysates from other species including birds, amphibians, fish and insects (Rothenberger et al., 1990), and post-translational interconversion of pools of IRE-BP by redox reagents is a feature seen in all species examined to date (Haile et al., 1989; Hentze et al., 1989; Barton et al., 1990; Rothenberger et al., 1990; Yu et al., 1992). The IRE-BP is expressed to varying degrees in a broad spectrum of tissues where its RNA binding activity appears to be determined by both the level of its mRNA and the protein's activation state (Müllner et al., 1992; Patino and Walden, 1992).

The human IRE-BP has been isolated from liver by RNA affinity chromatography, molecularly cloned and successfully expressed by transfection in mouse cells (Rouault et al., 1989, 1990; Kaptain et al., 1991). A very similar protein has also been isolated from rabbit liver (Walden et al., 1989). The deduced amino acid sequence of the human IRE-BP is greater than 90% identical to the corresponding protein purified from other species including mouse (Philpott et al., 1991), rabbit (Rouault et al., 1989; Patino and Walden, 1992), and rat (Yu et al., 1992).

Insight into the possible mechanism by which the IRE-BP might sense changes in iron has come from the discovery that the human IRE-BP amino acid sequence is >30% identical to that of mitochondrial aconitases from porcine heart and yeast with >50% of the aligned amino acids being similar or identical (Hentze and Argos, 1991; Rouault et al., 1991). Aconitase is an iron-sulfur (Fe-S) protein whose crystal structure is known (Robbins and Stout, 1989a, b). Aconitase is an enzyme of the citric acid cycle catalyzing the conversion of citrate to isocitrate. Purified aconitase exists in an enzymatically active [4Fe-4S] state and in enzymatically inactive forms that have less than four iron atoms (Beinert, 1990). Thus, aconitase provides a paradigm for a way in which the activity of a protein might be responsive to changes in iron availability since when iron is abundant the [4Fe-4S] state would be more likely. The IRE-BP has been shown directly to possess aconitase activity that is dependent upon the addition of iron (Kaptain et al., 1991). In vitro manipulation of IRE-BP under conditions that are known to affect the Fe-S centre of aconitase modulate RNA binding (Constable et al., 1992; Haile et al., 1992a). The reciprocal modulation of aconitase activity and RNA binding in vitro has been demonstrated directly (Haile et al., 1992a). Moreover, when cells are treated with haemin, the IRE-BP of these cells possesses high aconitase activity and is a poor RNA binder, whereas in chelator-treated cells the opposite is true (Haile et al., 1992a).

Reports have appeared indicating that haem rather than iron per se is the regulator of IRE-BP activity (Lin et al., 1990, 1991). It is clear that haem addition in vitro can inactivate the IRE-BP (Haile et al., 1990; Lin et al., 1990), but it is not clear that this inactivation is specific for the IRE-BP or related to cellular regulation of the IRE-BP (Eisenstein and Munro, 1990; Haile et al., 1990). Indeed, data has been presented indicating that iron released from haemin by the catabolic enzyme haem oxygenase is essential to derepression of ferritin synthesis (Eisenstein and Munro, 1990; Eisenstein et al., 1991). As an alternative to the regulation of iron through reversible alteration of an iron–sulfur centre, it has been suggested that a specific triggering of the degradation of the IRE-BP may result (Goessling et al., 1992) from formation of a covalent adduct of haem with the IRE-BP (Lin et al., 1991). This conclusion would not appear to be consistent with the numerous observations that lysates from haemin- or iron-treated cells displaying low IRE-BP activity can be reactivated in vitro by addition of reducing agents (Haile et al., 1989; Hentze et al., 1989; Barton et al., 1990; Neupert et al., 1990; Rothenberger et al., 1990). Clearly, if the IRE-BP were degraded to any significant degree in cells treated with an iron source, such loss would not be reversed by reducing agents in vitro. The reversible activation/reactivation with redox active agents would appear to favour strongly a post-translational regulation of IRE-BP activity. More recently, the level of IRE-BP along with its rate of biosynthesis and degradation have been compared in haemin- and chelator-treated cells with no differences detected (Tang et al., 1992). The reconciliation of the apparent discrepancy between these findings and those of Goessling et al. (1992) awaits further investigation.

Recent evidence suggests that nitric oxide, a metabolite of L-arginine which can liberate iron from iron–sulfur proteins (Chapter 11), may induce conversion of the IRE-BP to the high-affinity form (Drapier et al., 1993; Weiss et al., 1993). This may provide a mechanism for post-transcriptional regulation of cellular iron homeostasis in conditions such as inflammation where there is no overall change in total iron levels.

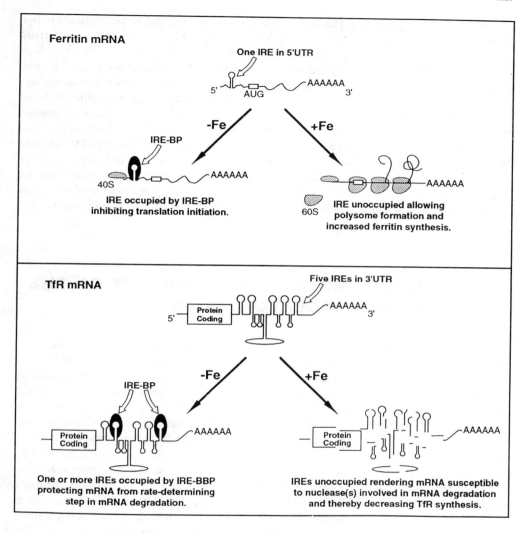

Fig. 5.2 Iron regulation of ferritin mRNA translation (upper panel) and TfR mRNA stability (lower panel). When iron is scarce (–Fe), the IRE-BP interacts with the IRE in the 5′UTR of ferritin mRNA and prevents the translation initiation such that polysomes containing ferritin mRNA are not formed. Ferritin polysomes are formed and ferritin produced when iron is abundant since under these conditions the IRE is not engaged by the high affinity IRE-BP. The conditions under which the IRE-BP associates with one or more of the IREs in the 3′UTR of the TfR mRNA are the same as in the case of ferritin (i.e. –Fe). This interaction inhibits the degradation of the TfR mRNA. When iron is abundant (+Fe) the absence of IRE-BP allows degradation to proceed. The fragmented TfR mRNA shown is for diagrammatic purposes and is not intended to convey information regarding mechanism of degradation nor sites of nuclease attack.

The details of the mechanism by which the interaction between ferritin mRNA and the high affinity form of the IRE-BP represses ferritin translation remain to be elucidated. It is known that this interaction prevents the formation of ferritin mRNA polysomes (Rogers and Munro, 1987). It would appear that this inhibition of polysome formation is accomplished via an interference in translation initiation involving the 5' cap of the mRNA, since there is a position dependence for IRE function in translational regulation (Fig. 5.2, upper panel). If the IRE is moved from its normal position (20–40 nucleotides from the cap) downstream in the 5'UTR of the mRNA, translational regulation is lost (Goossen et al., 1990; Goossen and Hentze, 1992). This finding would suggest that the IRE-BP interaction with the transcript is not acting by preventing scanning of the translational pre-initiation complex since the scanning complex would be required to move through the IRE/IRE-BP complex irrespective of the position of the IRE in the 5'UTR. While it has been suggested that sequences just 5' and just 3' of the IRE (so-called 'flanking sequences') participate in translational regulation (Harrell et al., 1991), other data indicate that these sequences can be deleted without effect (Goossen and Hentze, 1992). It is also clear that the human ferritin H-chain IRE without flanking sequences is a very powerful regulator of the translation of heterologous mRNAs into which it is placed (Caughman et al., 1988; Koeller et al., 1991).

4. THE RAPID TURNOVER DETERMINANT OF THE TRANSFERRIN RECEPTOR mRNA

The regulation of TfR expression is also mediated by the interaction of the iron-regulated IRE-BP with IREs. Here, as in the case of ferritin regulation, the IRE-BP interacts with the IRE RNA structures when iron is scarce (e.g. in desferrioxamine-treated cells in culture). In contrast to the relatively simple regulation of ferritin expression wherein a single IRE is the necessary and sufficient cis-acting RNA element required, regulation of TfR expression requires a rapid turnover determinant that is distinct from the IRE (although perhaps overlapping with the IRE motif). Interestingly, the regulatory region of the TfR mRNA contains five copies of the IRE sequence/structure motif rather than the single copy found in ferritin mRNAs. In the context of the 3'UTR of the TfR mRNA, the IRE/IRE-BP interaction impedes degradation of the TfR mRNA (Casey et al., 1989; Koeller et al., 1991). Comparison of the model for ferritin regulation (Fig. 5.2, upper panel) with that for TfR regulation (Fig. 5.2, lower panel) makes clear the explanation for the opposite directions of the changes in ferritin and TfR biosynthesis in response to the common environmental stimulus of a change in iron availability. Although the rates of biosynthesis of ferritin and the TfR move in opposite directions in response to changes in iron, both RNAs are engaged by the IRE-BP under similar conditions (low iron), and the effect of the interaction is in both instances inhibitory.

The availability of TfR sequences from two relatively distant vertebrate species (human and chicken) allowed prediction of structure of the regulatory region of the mRNA based on phylogenetic comparison. Both transcripts contain five IRE consensus motifs. Only five single nucleotide differences exist within the 143 nucleotides that encode the five IREs, and all of these differences are non-disruptive of the IRE structure motif (Casey et al., 1988a; Chan et al., 1989; Koeller et al., 1989; Fig. 5.1). The comparison of human and chicken mRNA sequences also supports the prediction that other structural motifs within the regulatory region may be critical. Several small non-IRE stem-loop structures and a long base paired structure lying between IREs B and C are contained in the transcripts of both species. Some of these non-IRE sequence/structure motifs have been shown to be necessary for iron regulation (Casey et al., 1989). The sequence of a portion of the 3'UTR of the rat TfR mRNA has also been determined (Roberts and Griswold, 1990). It too contains IREs and, within the previously defined regulatory region, is very similar in sequence (and potential secondary structure) to the human and chicken mRNAs. Evidence has been presented that indicates that as many as four molecules of IRE-BP are capable of interacting with an IRE molecule containing five IREs (Müllner et al., 1989). Despite the fact that each of the TfR IREs compete with a ferritin IRE for binding of the IRE-BP (Koeller et al., 1989) and their striking similarity to the corresponding elements of the chicken mRNA, IREs A and E can be removed from the human TfR mRNA without apparent effect on iron regulation (Casey et al., 1989). Based on extensive deletion analysis of the region, it was concluded that iron-dependent regulation of the TfR mRNA half-life could be conferred by a 250 nucleotide synthetic sequence element termed TRS-1 (Casey et al., 1989). In cells treated with the iron source haemin, an mRNA containing the TRS-1 element as its 3'UTR displayed a half-life of 45–60 minutes, whereas in cells treated with the iron chelator desferrioxamine the TRS-1-containing mRNA displays a half-life of considerably greater than 3 hours (Koeller et al., 1991).

Removal of the 100 nucleotides corresponding to the three IREs of TRS-1 produced an unregulated construct termed TRS-3 (Casey et al., 1989). The level of expression in cells transiently transfected with TRS-3 was found to be relatively high (using a co-transfected plasmid to normalize) and completely unregulated. In contrast, removal of three selected cytosine residues (one from each of the three IRE stem-loops) yielded a construct termed TRS-4 which also exhibited no iron regulation but gave rise to relatively low levels of expression in the transient transfections. The finding of a low level of TRS-4 mRNA in transfections was interpreted as indicating that this mRNA contained an intact rapid turnover determinant that could not be stabilized by interaction with the IRE-BP since removal of the three cytosines eliminates IRE-BP interaction. In contrast, the regulatory 'phenotype' of TRS-3 was interpreted as indicating that the nucleotides of the IREs overlap with those of the rapid turnover determinant. Direct measurement of mRNA stability in stable transformants revealed that the TRS-3 mRNA is indeed intrinsically stable and that the TRS-4 mRNA is intrinsically unstable (Koeller et al., 1991). In contrast to TRS-1 mRNA, the stabilities of TRS-3 and TRS-4 mRNAs were not affected by manipulation of cellular iron availability. The difference in the two types of 'mutants' of the TfR mRNAs can be explained by a model envisioning the regulatory region as containing both a rapid turnover determinant and an element (or elements) that modulate the activity of the rapid turnover determinant (Casey et al., 1989). Although these components of the region may be physically overlapping, their functions can be individually ablated. In 'high and unregulated' mRNAs the rapid turnover determinant activity is altered. For this class of altered mRNAs, binding or not binding the IRE-BP is irrelevant since the rapid turnover determinant is non-functional. For the 'low and unregulated' TRS-4 mRNA, the rapid turnover determinant function is intact, but the transcript cannot be protected because high affinity binding of the IRE-BP does not occur. This perspective of a rapid turnover determinant that is functionally distinct from the protein binding site provided by the IRE also explains why there is no iron regulation of the half-life of the mRNA encoding ferritin – it contains the protein-binding site (the IRE) but lacks the rapid turnover determinant function.

5. THE STRUCTURE OF THE TfR mRNA REGULATORY REGION

In contrast to DNA-binding proteins, the interaction of proteins with RNA is likely to depend on the secondary and tertiary structures formed by intrastrand base-pairing. The regulatory region of the TfR mRNA is capable of forming not only the five IRE stem-loops but also other elements of secondary structure (Koeller *et al.*, 1989). Deletional analysis of the regulatory region of the TfR mRNA (Casey *et al.*, 1988a) revealed that there were non-overlapping deletions that each independently eliminated iron regulation. Subsequently, it was shown that deletion of either of two small non-IRE sequence elements each independently abolished regulation giving rise to a 'high and unregulated phenotype' (Casey *et al.*, 1989). Thus, both of these elements were necessary and neither was sufficient for rapid turnover when iron was present. Moreover the two elements were separated from one another by over 300 nucleotides in the native TfR mRNA. One possibility is that the rapid turnover determinant of the TfR mRNA is a relatively complex structure in three dimensions. Primary or secondary sequence elements that are distant in the primary sequence of the mRNA may be brought into proximity by RNA folding. Together they may form the recognition determinant for the cellular machinery of degradation. In such a model, it would be envisioned that adjacent to or in the midst of this recognition determinant are positioned one or more of the IREs. Binding by the IRE-BP represses the activity of the recognition determinant perhaps by sterically preventing interaction with other components of the mRNA degradation system of the cell.

Owing to the palindromic nature of the IRE primary sequences and the presence of multiple IREs within the TfR mRNA, alternative secondary structures are possible. Indeed, an alternative secondary structure for a portion of the TfR mRNA has been proposed based on a computer algorithm for RNA folding and the results of certain deletions on iron regulation of TfR expression (Müllner and Kühn, 1988). The secondary structure of the portion of the TfR mRNA responsible for the regulation of the transcript's half-life has now been deduced by ribonuclease H cleavage directed by antisense oligodeoxyribonucleotides as well as with other ribonucleases sensitive to RNA secondary structure (Horowitz and Harford, 1992). These data indicate that the synthetic 252 nucleotides of TRS-1 RNA and the comparable portion of the 2.7 kb cellular TRS-1 mRNA each contain all three of their IREs as individual hairpin stem-loops. Moreover, this secondary structure appears to be relatively static with little inter-conversion with other possible structures involving longer range base pairing. The predominance of the structure containing three IRE stem-loops may relate to the importance of more short-range structure elements in determining RNA secondary structure (Abrahams *et al.*, 1990). TRS-4 RNA was shown to adopt a similar, if not identical, secondary structure to that of the TRS-1 RNA. Taken collectively, all of these data suggest that the secondary structure deduced for TRS-1 and TRS-4 represents that of the TfR rapid turnover determinant (Horowitz and Harford, 1992).

6. THE MECHANISM OF TfR mRNA DECAY

When the affinity of the IRE-BP for an IRE is decreased by iron, the TfR mRNA is destroyed. Virtually nothing is known concerning the nuclease(s) involved, but a similar lack of details characterizes most eukaryotic systems wherein genes are regulated at the level of mRNA stability. Detailed study of the nucleases involved remains an important objective. The simplest model for regulation of TfR mRNA expression would envision the IRE-BP as a steric protector of the transcript. Such a model would not necessitate that the nuclease(s) involved in the degradation of the TfR mRNA be iron-regulated, nor would the nuclease(s) be required to have the TfR mRNA as its only substrate.

As is also true for most RNA turnover, a large number of breakdown products of the TfR mRNA have not been observed. This failure to detect breakdown intermediates is thought to be the result of a rate-limiting initial event that is followed by very rapid destruction of the products of this event. One smaller RNA band has been seen on northern blot analysis of samples from murine cells expressing the intrinsically unstable TRS-4 mRNA irrespective of iron treatment (Koeller et al., 1991). An apparently identical RNA is observed in murine cells expressing the TRS-1 mRNA upon haemin treatment of the cells. This smaller RNA species may represent a breakdown product since its presence correlates with rapid turnover of the TfR mRNA. A similar phenomenon involving the endogenous 4.9 kb TfR mRNA of a human cell line has been noted (Harford et al., 1988). Each of these smaller transcripts appear to represent truncations of the full-length transcripts such that they are missing the poly A tail along with significant portions of their 3'UTRs. The 3' ends of these transcripts map within or near the IRE-containing region of each transcript. These truncations are thought to reflect the primary site of cleavage by an endonuclease or a relatively stable pause in the processive action of a 3' to 5' exonuclease.

When transfectants expressing the intrinsically unstable TRS-4 mRNA were treated with cycloheximide (Chx), which inhibits translation elongation but leaves ribosomes on the mRNA, a marked increase in the level of TRS-4 mRNA was seen (Koeller et al., 1991). It has also been reported that the human TfR mRNA expressed in mouse L cells is stabilized by Chx (Müllner and Kühn, 1988). A similar effect on TRS-4 mRNA level was observed when cells were treated with puromycin, which causes premature release of the peptide chain and ribosomes. Thus, the TRS-4 mRNA level is increased by inhibition of protein synthesis irrespective of whether ribosomes are present. As would be anticipated for a long-lived mRNA, no comparable effect on the intrinsically stable TRS-3 mRNA was seen. In cells expressing the iron-regulated TRS-1 mRNA, an effect of Chx on the TRS-1 mRNA level was observed in cells that had been pretreated with the iron source haemin but not in cells treated with the iron chelator desferrioxamine. No effect on an unrelated mRNA (encoding actin) was seen under any regimen of iron treatment.

There exist a number of examples in which levels of rapidly degraded mRNAs are markedly increased in cells treated with inhibitors of protein synthesis. This phenomenon has been seen with several proto-oncogenes including c-myc (Linial et al., 1985; Cole, 1986), c-myb (Thompson et al., 1986), c-fos (Rahmsdorf et al., 1987) and c-jun (Ryseck et al., 1988). These increases in mRNA levels appear to be the result of substantial stabilization of the mRNAs by the protein synthesis inhibitors, and are seen with a variety of types of inhibitors (i.e. both inhibitors of translation initiation and of elongation that act by distinct mechanisms).

The mechanism by which protein synthesis inhibitors stabilize certain mRNAs remains obscure. It is thought that either a highly unstable protein is involved in the degradation of these mRNAs (a so-called *trans*-effect), or that translation of the mRNAs themselves is required for their decay (a *cis*-effect). These two possibilities are not necessarily mutually exclusive and each may be applicable in certain instances. The major difficulty in distinguishing between a *cis*- and a *trans*-effect of protein synthesis inhibitors is that inhibition of global protein synthesis will, by its nature, inhibit both the translation of the mRNA in question and the synthesis of the putative short-lived, *trans*-acting protein. However, the IRE/IRE-BP system has provided a means to distinguish between *cis*- and *trans*-effects of inhibition of protein synthesis. When an IRE exists in the 5′UTR of an mRNA (as in ferritin mRNAs) the translation of the mRNA is regulated by iron such that more translation occurs when iron is abundant and less when iron is scarce. When cells are treated with an iron source, the ferritin mRNA is found associated with polysomes, whereas ferritin mRNA exists as a lower density ribonucleoprotein in chelator-treated cells (Rogers and Munro, 1987). This effect is specific for the mRNA containing an IRE in its 5′UTR, and global protein synthesis is not affected by the experimental manipulations of iron availability. Thus, for an mRNA with an IRE in its 5′UTR, iron chelation can be used to attenuate translation in a way that is completely specific for IRE-containing mRNAs. If a short-lived mRNA contained a properly positioned IRE and were stabilized by global inhibition of protein synthesis, iron chelation should have a similar stabilizing effect only if translation of the mRNA iself were a requirement for mRNA degradation. If instead, a short-lived protein were a necessary component of the degradation of the mRNA and the disappearance of this protein accounted for the effect of global protein synthesis inhibition, then iron manipulation would be predicted to be without effect since the synthesis of this putative short-lived protein would not be expected to be affected by manipulation of cellular iron status.

Several constructs were designed to test whether iron could be used to regulate selectively the translation of a short-lived mRNA (Koeller et al., 1991). Some constructs encoded mRNAs that contained a ferritin IRE within its 5′UTR and a rapid turnover determinant in its 3′UTR. All constructs utilized the TfR protein coding region. In one construct (termed 5′IRE-TR-*fos*), the 3′UTR consisted of a 250 nucleotide segment of the human c-*fos* gene. This segment encodes the AU-rich region that functions as one of the instability determinants in c-*fos* mRNA (Shyu et al., 1989). When transferred to β-globin mRNA, the AU-rich region of c-*fos* mRNA confers a rapid degradation rate (Shaw and Kamen, 1986; Shyu et al., 1989). The c-*fos* element also destabilized the chimeric TfR mRNA irrespective of the presence of an IRE within the 5′UTR (Koeller et al., 1991).

When cells transfected with the 5′IRE-TR-*fos* construct were treated with Chx, a marked increase in the level of the encoded mRNA was seen. This effect was similar to that seen with the TRS-4 construct or the TRS-1 construct in iron-treated cells and was shown to be the result of mRNA stabilization. Treatments of the cells expressing the 5′IRE-TR-*fos* mRNA with an iron source or an iron chelator had a dramatic and specific effect ($\geq$20-fold) on the translation of this mRNA but a negligible effect on the steady-state level of the mRNA. Moreover, direct measurement of the 5′IRE-TR-*fos* mRNA half-life revealed that the transcript was short-lived (half-life = 45–60 minutes) both in cells treated with haemin, where it is well translated, and in cells treated with desferrioxamine, where it is poorly translated (Koeller et al., 1991). The level of mRNA encoded by the construct 5'IRE-TRS-4 that contains, in addition to an IRE in the 5'UTR, the TfR rapid turnover determination rather than that of c-fos was also not affected by iron manipulations despite a 20-fold regulation of its translation. The results of these experiments support the conclusion that the effect of global protein synthesis inhibitors on the stability of mRNAs containing the rapid turnover determinant of the TfR mRNA or the AU-rich element of c-fos is due to a short-lived protein participant(s) in the decay of these transcripts rather than a requirement for the translation of these transcripts per se. The fact that many short-lived mRNAs are similarly stabilized by treatment with protein synthesis inhibitors suggests that the protein(s) responsible for this phenomenon may be common to the degradation pathways of several mRNAs. This important, short-lived protein remains to be characterized.

7. OTHER mRNAs CONTAINING IREs

As first noted by Dierks (1990), a sequence resembling an IRE is contained in the 5'UTR of the mRNA encoding the erythroid form of 5-aminolaevulinate synthase (eALAS) (Dierks, 1990; Cox et al., 1991; Dandekar et al., 1991). IRE-like sequences have also been found in the 5'UTRs of Drosophila toll mRNA (Dandekar et al., 1991) and porcine heart aconitase mRNA (Dandekar et al., 1991; Kaptain et al., 1991). While there is no obvious connection between Drosophila toll, a maternal effect gene (Hashimoto et al., 1988) and cellular iron metabolism, the IRE in the eALAS mRNA is particularly intriguing given that the encoded protein is the first enzyme in the pathway of haem biosynthesis (Ponka et al., 1990; see also Chapter 2). There is evidence indicating that this enzyme is rate-limiting (Bottomly and Müller-Eberhard, 1988; Gardner and Cox, 1988; Ponka et al., 1988) and could thereby serve as the control point for the regulation of haem synthesis. The presence of an IRE in the 5'UTR of the eALAS mRNA suggests that this important enzyme may be translationally controlled by iron in a fashion analogous to ferritin, i.e. more translation when iron is abundant. Translational control of eALAS biosynthesis, suggested by earlier studies (Elferink et al., 1988; Dierks, 1990) has now been confirmed (Melefors et al., 1993), and evidence has been presented that iron uptake limits haem production (Gardner and Cox, 1988; Ponka et al., 1988). The isolated IRE-like segment of the eALAS mRNA is specifically recognized by the IRE-BP in vitro (Dandekar et al., 1991), and can confer iron-regulated translational control to a reporter mRNA (Melefors et al., 1993).

Very recently an IRE-like sequence has been reported in the 5' untranslated region of transferrin mRNA (Cox and Adrian, 1993). It differs somewhat from the IREs in transferrin receptor and ferritin mRNAs, and despite being present in the 5' untranslated region, binding of IRE-BP enhances rather than inhibits translation. However, these findings suggest that transferrin may be regulated translationally as well as transcriptionally (see p. 139 and Chapter 1).

The possibility that mitochondrial aconitase might also be regulated translationally by iron is suggested by the presence of an IRE capable of interaction with the IRE-BP within its mRNA's 5'UTR (Dandekar *et al.*, 1991; Kaptain *et al.*, 1991). This is of particular interest given the striking similarity between the IRE-BP and the cytosolic form of aconitase (Hentze and Argos, 1991; Rouault *et al.*, 1991) and the direct demonstration that the IRE-BP possesses aconitase activity (Kaptain *et al.*, 1991). Moreover, IRE-BP activity and aconitase activity have been shown to be reciprocally regulated by iron *in vitro* and *in vivo* (Haile *et al.*, 1992a). Thus the cytosolic aconitase is both functionally regulated by iron and capable of itself translationally regulating IRE-containing mRNAs including mitochondrial aconitase. Both types of regulation would be predicted to increase activity of both forms of aconitase where iron is abundant. Based on comparison of several characteristics of cellular IRE-BP with spectroscopically defined forms of the protein, it was found that the 4Fe to 3Fe conversion, while sufficient to abolish aconitase enzyme activity, did not result in the activation of RNA binding activity. Instead, the form of the protein produced by cells in response to iron deprivation seemed more closely to resemble the apo-protein form of the IRE-BP (Haile *et al.*, 1992b). Conditions used to interconvert various forms of the IRE-BP *in vitro* involve treatments that are markedly non-physiologic (e.g. high pH, high concentrations of reducing or oxidizing agents, etc.). It is clear that cells must possess distinct means to accomplish these interconversions. The enzymology related to a regulated assembly/disassembly of Fe-S clusters is likely to become a fruitful area of study.

8. OTHER MEANS OF REGULATING THE PROTEINS OF CELLULAR IRON METABOLISM

Thus far, emphasis has been given to the post-transcriptional regulation of the expression of ferritin and the TfR by iron. Two factors account for this emphasis. Firstly, IRE-mediated regulation of ferritin translation and TfR mRNA stability is of a greater magnitude than that reported for other means of regulating these genes (at least in animal cells). Secondly, considerably more is known concerning the molecular details of IRE-mediated regulation. Nonetheless, there is a significant body of evidence indicating that iron and other stimuli also regulate the expression of the proteins of cellular iron metabolism by means distinct from the IRE-mediated regulatory events discussed above.

It is well established that different tissues express the H-chain and L-chain of ferritin in distinctive proportions (Theil, 1987). It is also known that the tissue isoferritins accumulate and release iron differently (Wagstaff *et al.*, 1978) and possess other metabolic differences including distinct ferroxidase activities (Andrews *et al.*, 1992). In rats, the administration of iron results in differential effects on H-chain and L-chain expression in liver resulting in dramatic increases in the L/H ratio (Bomford *et al.*, 1981). The tissue variation in expression of ferritin isoforms is a reflection of the levels of the mRNAs encoding the H- and L-chains, and these differences are, at least in part, due to transcriptional regulation of ferritin mRNA expression in response to iron (White and Munro, 1988). In liver, iron was shown to increase both H- and L-chain translation but to increase preferentially L-chain mRNA levels accounting for the earlier observations related to L/H ratio (Bomford *et al.*, 1981).

Transcriptional control of ferritin expression in response to iron has also been observed in adult erythroid and liver cells from the mouse (Beaumont *et al.*, 1989) and in human HeLa cells (Cairo *et al.*, 1985). In Friend cells, the transcriptional regulation observed upon the addition of the iron source haemin was also seen with protoporphyrin IX (haemin lacking iron) indicating that the porphyrin entity rather than iron per se might be responsible for ferritin transcriptional regulation (Coccia *et al.*, 1992). No changes in ferritin mRNA was observed in this study. In plant cells, it appears that the major regulatory mechanism for control of ferritin biosynthesis by iron is transcriptional (Lescure *et al.*, 1991).

The accumulation of isoferritin mRNAs in animal cells may also be influenced by the stabilities of the mRNAs. H-chain mRNA is transcribed at a similar rate in liver and in Friend erythroleukaemia cells induced to differentiate with dimethyl sulfoxide, but five times more H-chain mRNA accumulates in the Friend cells indicating a difference in mRNA stability (Beaumont *et al.*, 1989). In contrast to the study cited above involving Friend erythroleukaemia cells (Coccia *et al.*, 1992), in human K562 erythroleukaemia cells, two- to -five-fold differences in ferritin mRNA levels were observed after prolonged manipulation of iron availability without corresponding changes in the rate of ferritin mRNA transcription (Mattia *et al.*, 1989, 1990). These differences were ascribed to alterations in the stability of the ferritin mRNA.

In addition to iron, ferritin expression has been reported to be altered by a number of other agents and circumstances. Differentiation of HL-60, a premyelocytic leukaemia cell, by dimethyl sulfoxide results in preferential increase in H-chain mRNA (Chou *et al.*, 1986). Elevated H-chain mRNA expression has also been reported in differentiating smooth muscle cells undergoing growth arrest and may occur through a pathway involving cAMP (Liau *et al.*, 1991). Ferritin H-chain mRNA synthesis is also induced by tumour necrosis factor (Torti *et al.*, 1988) and by the acute phase cytokine interleukin 1 (Wei *et al.*, 1990). Interestingly, interleukin 1 has also been shown to affect translation of both ferritin H- and L-chains (Rogers *et al.*, 1990). A preferential transcriptional suppression of H-chain mRNA occurs when mouse L cells are transfected with the adenovirus E1A oncogene (Tsuji *et al.*, 1993). Moreover, the ferritin H-chain promoter confers upon a heterologous gene this EIA suppression. It has been suggested that ferritin transcription by agents other than iron may be controlled by the binding of the transcription factor NF-$\varkappa$B (Drysdale *et al.*, 1991).

The effects on cellular or whole body iron metabolism of the various agents or circumstances leading to altered ferritin expression have not been explored in detail. These issues may be of considerable importance given the reports linking ferritin expression to malignancy (Jones *et al.*, 1980; Cazzola *et al.*, 1990; Bomford and Munro, 1992).

The level of TfR expression is also related to the proliferative state of the cells (Larrick and Cresswell, 1979; Trowbridge and Omary, 1981; Chitambar *et al.*, 1983) as well as to the induction of differentiation (Hu *et al.*, 1977; Omary *et al.*, 1980; Delia *et al.*, 1982). Resting lymphocytes express few, if any, TfR on their surface but a rapid and dramatic increase in TfR expression occurs following lymphocyte activation (Galbraith and Galbraith, 1981; Sutherland *et al.*, 1981; Neckers and Cossman, 1983). Transcriptional down modulation of TfR mRNA levels has been observed in cultured T cells treated with phorbol esters that decreases proliferation and induces differentiation (Alcantara *et al.*, 1989). These changes are thought to reflect the increased need for iron in dividing cells. Cells of the erythroid lineage have high requirements for iron in the production of haemoglobin. In developing chicken embryos, the level of TfR mRNA is greater than 200 times higher in erythroid cells than in non-erythroid tissues (Chan and Gerhardt, 1992). Nuclear run-off experiments indicated that this hyperexpression in differentiating erythroid cells is transcriptional.

Both α- and γ-interferons (Hamilton et al., 1984; Bourgeade et al., 1992) inhibit expression of the TfR. When WISH cells are stimulated to proliferate, they too exhibit an increase in the steady state level of TfR mRNA. Interestingly, this increase is blocked by interferon-γ (Bourgeade et al., 1992). Nuclear run-off experiments indicate that this effect is apparently not attributable to an increase in TfR mRNA transcription, nor is the effect apparently due to an alteration of the stability of the TfR mRNA. The decrease in TfR mRNA caused by interferon-γ is already reflected in the nuclear TfR mRNA levels. These results suggest that a post-transcriptional mechanism for TfR regulation is operative in the nucleus. Earlier work had indicated that a post-transcriptional mechanism for growth regulation of TfR mRNA expression was distinct from that utilized for iron regulation since deletions is the 3'UTR that eliminated iron regulation did not affect growth-dependent regulation of the TfR (Owen and Kühn, 1987).

Nuclear run-off assays have also been used to assess the effect of manipulation of cellular iron levels on transcription of the TfR gene. Nuclei from cells treated with the iron chelator desferrioxamine incorporate more $[\alpha\text{-}^{32}P]$UTP into TfR RNA than do nuclei from cells treated with haemin, an iron source (Rao et al., 1986). These results suggested that at least a portion of the iron regulation of TfR mRNA levels was occurring at the level of gene transcription. Interestingly, in developing chicken embryos, neither TfR transcription nor TfR mRNA stability appear to be influenced by iron with TfR expression being transcriptionally regulated by as yet undefined developmental and tissue specific mechanisms (Chan and Gerhardt, 1992).

The transcription rate of the TfR gene has also been assessed by nuclear run-off experiments in activated T cells (Kronke et al., 1985) and in HL60 cells induced to differentiate toward monocytes with dibutyryl cAMP (Trepel et al., 1987). Activation of T cells leads to increased TfR expression, whereas cAMP treatment of HL60 results in decreased TfR expression. The corresponding changes in nuclear run-offs that were observed in both instances are consistent with a transcriptional component to these regulations of TfR gene expression.

Attempts to study the transcriptional regulation of the TfR have focused on the characterization of the promoter region of the TfR gene. Genomic DNA corresponding to sequences 5' of the transcription start site of the TfR gene have been isolated using portions of pcD-TR1 and the promoter region has been partially characterized (Miskimins et al., 1986; Owen and Kühn, 1987; Casey et al., 1988b,c). The TfR promoter contains a TATA box approximately 30 bp upstream of the transcription start site. There are several GC-rich regions upstream of the TATA box including several that have sequences resembling the consensus binding site for the transcription factor termed Sp1 (Briggs et al., 1986; Kadonaga et al., 1986). Evidence has been presented for protein binding to the TfR promoter region (Miskimins et al., 1985, 1986; Miskimins, 1992). The activity and/or amount of these proteins has been reported to increase prior to the increase in TfR mRNA levels that occurs upon serum stimulation of quiescent 3T3 cells (Miskimins et al., 1986). DNase I footprinting has indicated that there are several sites for protein binding including a sequence having similarity to a portion of the upstream sequences of the mouse gene for dihydrofolate reductase (DHFR) and a putative Sp1 site (Miskimins *et al.*, 1986). However, this putative Sp1 site has been replaced in the promoter region without affecting the ability of the TfR promoter to drive chloramphenicol acetyl transferase (CAT) expression in transfected human cells.

Progressive 5' to 3' deletions as well as internal sequence substitutions have implicated another upstream sequence element as being critical to full activity of the TfR promoter (Casey *et al.*, 1988b). This critical element bears striking similarity to a portion of the enhancer of polyoma virus. Substitution by unrelated linker sequences reduced the promoter's activity in constructs by more than 90% (Casey *et al.*, 1988b).

The sequence element at $-80/-66$ of the TfR promoter region lies adjacent to the aforementioned DHFR-like sequence and may form part of a protein binding site detected by DNase I protection (Miskimins *et al.*, 1986; Miskimins, 1992). The similar sequence element of polyoma is contained in a portion of the viral enhancer that has been identified as containing sites for the binding of two DNA-binding proteins termed PEA1 and PEA2 (Piette and Yaniv, 1987). A binding site within the TfR promoter region for a transcription factor like PEA1 may account for the DNase I protection and for the functional importance of the $-80/-60$ nucleotides.

In addition to the regulation of ferritin and TfR, the expression of transferrin itself is regulated transcriptionally (Zakin, 1992). As discussed in more detail in Chapter 1, this expression is tissue specific with liver being the main site of Tf synthesis, although several other cell types also express low levels of Tf (Idzerda *et al.*, 1986). Tf mRNA expression is also developmentally programmed (Kahn *et al.*, 1987). Steroid hormones increase Tf mRNA transcription in chicken liver (McKnight *et al.*, 1980b) and in transgenic mice expressing the chicken Tf gene (Hammer *et al.*, 1986). Nutritional iron deficiency also increases transcription of the Tf gene in chicken and rat liver (McKnight *et al.*, 1980a; Idzerda *et al.*, 1986). Deletion analysis of the Tf promoter region and expression in transfected cells and transgenic animals have implicated several critical sequence elements (Idzerda *et al.*, 1989; Schaeffer *et al.*, 1989; Adrian *et al.*, 1990). Moreover several DNA-binding proteins have been identified that interact with the Tf promoter region (Brunel *et al.*, 1988; Mendelzon *et al.*, 1990; Petropoulos *et al.*, 1991). To date, the nature of the interactions that regulate Tf expression in response to nutritional iron have not been characterized although the -622 to $+46$ region has been implicated (Adrian *et al.*, 1990).

9. SUMMARY AND PERSPECTIVES

The proteins involved in cellular iron metabolism are highly regulated. This control includes events at both the transcriptional and post-transcriptional levels. The best understood of these mechanisms is the coordinate post-transcriptional regulation of ferritin translation and of TfR mRNA stability in response to changes in iron availability. A variety of other agents and circumstances have also been reported to alter the expression of genes encoding the proteins involved in cellular uptake and intracellular sequestration of iron.

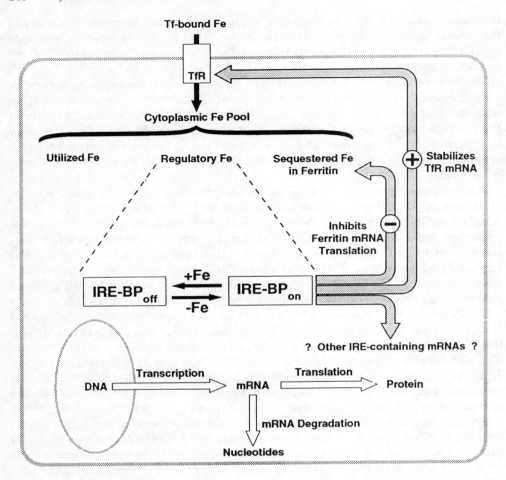

Fig. 5.3 Cellular iron homeostasis is regulated post-transcriptionally through iron-dependent changes in the IRE-BP. Iron enters dividing cells of higher eukaryotes via the TfR. Once inside the cell the iron may be considered to be in one of three pools, although overlap and interchange between these pools may occur. Iron is utilized in a variety of metabolic processes, or iron may be sequestered in ferritin. Intracellular iron also serves to regulate the IRE-BP such that when iron is abundant (e.g. in haemin-treated cells) the IRE-BP is in its 4Fe-4S state which has high aconitase enzymatic activity but low affinity for IREs (IRE-BP$_{off}$). When iron is scarce (e.g. in desferrioxamine-treated cells), the IRE-BP is in its high affinity state for RNA binding (IRE-BP$_{on}$) with negligible aconitase activity. The IRE-BP$_{on}$ state results in decreased translation of ferritin mRNA and increased stability of the TfR mRNA by binding to the IREs contained in these transcripts. The IRE-BP system may also regulate other IRE-containing mRNAs (e.g. mRNAs encoding eALAS and mitochondrial aconitase).

Cells utilize a common *cis*-acting RNA element (the IRE) and a common *trans*-acting protein (the IRE-BP) to modulate at least two genes involved in cellular iron homeostasis. The translation of the mRNA encoding ferritin is attenuated by iron deprivation as is the degradation of the mRNA encoding the TfR. To date, this is the only known example of this sort of overlap in post-transcriptional regulation of the expression of two genes although it may be reminiscent of transcriptional regulation wherein common promoter elements and common transcription factors participate in regulation of distinct genes. Although the levels of expression of ferritin and the TfR are modulated in opposite directions by changes in iron availability, the IRE-BP serves as an iron-regulatable repressor in both instances. Clues as to how the IRE-BP might sense changes in cellular iron status have come from the observation that the IRE-BP is structurally similar to the mitochondrial enzyme, aconitase (Hentze and Argos, 1991; Rouault et al., 1991) and possesses iron-dependent aconitase activity (Kaptain et al., 1991; Haile et al., 1992a). When cellular iron is scarce, the IRE-BP is envisioned as being in a state (referred to as IRE-BP$_{on}$ in Fig. 5.3) where it is a more avid binder of the IREs, and therefore an effective repressor of ferritin mRNA translation and TfR mRNA degradation.

In the TfR mRNA, the IREs are adjacent to (probably overlapping with) a rapid turnover determinant. The simplest view of the action of the IRE-BP is that it sterically blocks accessibility to this rapid turnover determinant. The rapid turnover determinant may be the site of an endonucleolytic cleavage, or it may in some way activate 3' to 5' exonucleolytic destruction of the TfR mRNA. For transfected human TfR mRNAs expressed in mouse cells as well as the endogenous human TfR mRNA, truncated transcripts with properties expected of a degradation intermediate have been observed (Harford et al., 1988; Koeller et al., 1991). It is noteworthy that only one such intermediate is apparent in each case, and that the 3' end of the population of this putative intermediate appears to be relatively uniform. These features are equally consistent with a specific endonucleolytic cleavage or a well-defined pause in the procession of a 3' to 5' exonuclease. In either case, it would appear that even smaller intermediates are extremely unstable.

It is possible that the structure of the mRNA that is recognized by the cellular degradative machinery is a complex entity in three-dimensional space. Deletion analyses are consistent with it being comprised of RNA sequence/structure elements that are well separated in the primary sequence of the RNA. This finding raises the possibility that elements implicated in a deletion analysis of an mRNA are not directly involved in interactions with trans-acting factors but instead play a role in bringing other elements into proper spatial juxtaposition. It is clear that there is much more to be learned about the TfR mRNA and its iron-regulated turnover. A critical goal in this endeavour is the establishment of a cell-free system that accurately reflects cellular turnover of this mRNA. This would need to be sensitive to rather subtle alterations in the mRNA known to affect regulation in vivo (Casey et al., 1989), inhibitable by interaction of the RNA with the high affinity form of the IRE-BP, and involve a short-lived protein (at least in mouse L cells). Such an in vitro turnover system would provide an avenue by which other components of the TfR mRNA degradative machinery might be identified and characterized.

Finally, the finding of IRE-like structures in other mRNAs suggests that iron may regulate expression of these genes. At least two such genes (eALAS and mitochondrial aconitase) have a known connection with iron in that one is the rate limiting step in haem biosynthesis and the other is an iron-sulfur enzyme. It remains to be determined whether yet other genes might utilize the IRE system to control gene expression in response to alterations in iron.

ACKNOWLEDGEMENT

We wish to acknowledge all of our past and present colleagues in the Cell Biology and Metabolism Branch for their experimental and conceptual contributions.

REFERENCES

Abrahams, J. P., van den Berg, M., van Batenburg, E. and Pleij, C. (1990) Prediction of RNA secondary structure, including pseudoknotting, by computer simulation. *Nucleic Acids Res.* **18**, 3035–3044.

Adrian, G. S., Bowman, B. H., Herbert, D. C. *et al.* (1990) Human transferrin: Expression and iron modulation of chimeric genes in transgenic mice. *J. Biol. Chem.* **265**, 13344–13350.

Alcantara, O., Denham, C. A., Phillips, J. L. and Boldt, D. H. (1989) Transcriptional regulation of transferrin receptor expression by cultured lymphoblastoid T cells treated with phorbol esters. *J. Immunol.* **142**, 1719–1726.

Andrews, S. C., Arosio, P., Bottke, W. *et al.* (1992) Structure, function, and evolution of ferritins. *J. Inorg. Biochem.* **47**, 161–181.

Aziz, N. and Munro, H. N. (1987) Iron regulates ferritin mRNA translation through a segment of its 5' untranslated regulated region. *Proc. Natl. Acad. Sci. USA* **84**, 8478–8482.

Barton, H. A., Eisenstein, R. S., Bomford, A. and Munro, H. N. (1990) Determinants of the interaction between the iron-responsive element-binding protein and its binding site in rat L-ferritin mRNA. *J. Biol. Chem.* **265**, 7000–7008.

Beaumont, C., Dugast, F., Renaudie, M., Souroujon, M. and Grandchamp, B. (1989) Transcriptional regulation of ferritin H and L subunits in adult erythroid and liver cells from the mouse: Unambiguous identification of mouse ferritin subunits and in vitro formation of the ferritin shells. *J. Biol. Chem.* **264**, 7498–7504.

Beinert, H. (1990) Recent developments in the field of iron–sulfur proteins. *FASEB J.* **4**, 2483–2491.

Bettany, A. J. E., Eisenstein, R. S. and Munro, H. N. (1992) Mutagenesis of the iron-regulatory element further defines a role for RNA secondary structure in the regulation of ferritin and transferrin receptor expression. *J. Biol. Chem.* **267**, 16531–16537.

Bomford, A. B. and Munro, H. N. (1992) Ferritin gene expression in health and malignancy. *Pathobiol. 1992*, **60**, 10–18.

Bomford, A., Conlon-Hollingshead, C. and Munro, H. N. (1981) Adaptive response of rat tissue isoferritins to iron administration: Changes in subunit synthesis, isoferritin abundance and capacity for iron storage. *J. Biol. Chem.* **256**, 948–955.

Bottomly, S. and Müller-Eberhard, U. (1988) Pathophysiology of heme synthesis. *Semin. Hematol.* **25**, 282–302.

Bourgeade, M.-F., Silbermann, F., Kühn, L. *et al.* (1992) Post-transcriptional regulation of transferrin receptor mRNA by IFNγ. *Nucleic Acids Res.* **20**, 2997–3003.

Briggs, M. R., Kadonaga, J. T., Bell, S. P. and Tjian, R. (1986) Purification and biochemical characterization of the promoter-specific transcription factor Sp1. *Science* **234**, 47–52.

Brunel, F., Ochoa, A., Schaeffer, E. *et al.* (1988) Interactions of DNA-binding proteins with the 5' region of the human transferrin gene. *J. Biol. Chem.* **263**, 10180–10185.

Cairo, G., Bardella, L., Schiaffonati, P., Arosio, P., Levi, S. and Zazzera, A. B. (1985) Multiple mechanisms of iron-induced ferritin synthesis in HeLa cells. *Biochem. Biophys. Res. Commun.* **133**, 314–321.

Casey, J. L., Hentze, M. W., Koeller, D. M. *et al.* (1988a) Iron-responsive elements: regulatory RNA sequences that control mRNA levels and translation. *Science* **240**, 924–928.

Casey, J. L., Di Jeso, B., Rao, K., Klausner, R. D. and Harford, J. B. (1988b) Two genetic loci participate in the regulation by iron of the gene for the human transferrin receptor. *Proc. Natl. Acad. Sci. USA* **85**, 1787–1791.

Casey, J. L., Di Jeso, B., Rao, K. K., Rouault, T. A., Klausner, R. D. and Harford, J. B. (1988c) Deletional analysis of the promoter region of the human transferrin receptor gene. *Nucleic Acids Res.* **16**, 629–646.

Casey, J. L., Koeller, D. M., Ramin, V. C., Klausner, R. D. and Harford, J. B. (1989) Iron regulation of transferrin receptor mRNA levels requires iron-responsive elements and a rapid turnover determinants in the 3′ untranslated region of the mRNA. *EMBO J.* **8**, 3693–3699.

Caughman, S. W., Hentze, M. W., Rouault, T. A., Harford, J. B. and Klausner, R. D. (1988) The iron responsive element is the single element responsible for iron-dependent translational regulation of ferritin biosynthesis: Evidence for function as the binding site for a translational repressor. *J. Biol. Chem.* **263**, 19048–19052.

Cazzola, M., Bergamaschi, G., Dezza, L. and Arosio, P. (1990) Manipulations of cellular iron metabolism for modulating normal and malignant cell proliferation: Achievements and prospects. *Blood* **75**, 1903–1919.

Chan, L.-N. L. and Gerhardt, E. M. (1992) Transferrin receptor gene is hyperexpressed and transcriptionally regulated in differentiating erythroid cells. *J. Biol. Chem.* **267**, 8254–8259.

Chan, L.-N. L., Grammatikakis, N., Banks, J. M. and Gerhardt, E. M. (1989) Chicken transferrin receptor gene: conservation 3′ noncoding sequences and expression in erythroid cells. *Nucleic Acids Res.* **17**, 3763–3771.

Chitamber, C. R., Massey, E. J. and Seligman, P. A. (1983) Regulation of transferrin receptor expression on human leukemic cells during proliferation and induction of differentiation. *J. Clin. Invest.* **72**, 1314–1325.

Chou, C. C., Gatti, R. A., Fuller, M. L. *et al.* (1986) Structure and expression of ferritin genes in a human promyelocytic cell line that differentiates in vitro. *Mol. Cell. Biol.* **6**, 566–573.

Coccia, E. M., Profita, V., Fiorucci, G. *et al.* (1992) Modulation of ferritin H-chain expression in Friend erythroleukemia cells: Transcriptional and translational regulation by hemin. *Mol. Cell. Biol.* **12**, 3015–3022.

Cole, M. D. (1986) The myc oncogene: its role in transformation and differentiation. *Annu. Rev. Genet.* **20**, 361–384.

Constable, A., Quick, S., Gray, N. K. and Hentze, M. W. (1992) Modulation of the RNA-binding activity of a regulatory protein by iron in vitro: switching between enzymatic and genetic functions? *Proc. Natl. Acad. Sci. USA* **89**, 4554–4558.

Cox, L. A. and Adrian, G. S. (1993) Posttranscriptional regulation of chimeric human transferrin genes by iron. *Biochemistry* **32**, 4738–4745.

Cox, T. C., Bawden, M. J., Martin, A. and May, B. K. (1991) Human erythroid 5-aminolevulinate synthase: promoter analysis and identification of an iron-responsive element in the mRNA. *EMBO J.* **10**, 1891–1902.

Crichton, R. R. (1991) *Inorganic Biochemistry of Iron Metabolism*, Ellis Horwood, New York.

Crichton, R. R. and Charloteaux-Wauters, M. (1987) Iron transport and storage. *Eur. J. Biochem.* **164**, 485–506.

Dandekar, T., Stripecke, R., Gray, N. *et al.* (1991) Identification of a novel iron-responsive element in murine and human erythroid delta-aminolevulinic acid synthase mRNA. *EMBO J.* **10**, 1903–1909.

Delia, D., Greaves, M. F., Newman, R. A. *et al.* (1982) Modulation of T leukaemic cell phenotype with phorbol esters. *Int. J. Cancer* **29**, 23–31.

Dierks, P. (1990) Molecular biology of eukaryotic 5-aminolevulinate synthase. In: *Biosynthesis of Heme and Chlorophylls* (ed. H. A. Dailey), McGraw-Hill, New York, pp. 201–233.

Dix, D. J., Lin, P.-N., Kimata, Y. and Theil, E. C. (1992) The iron regulatory region of ferritin mRNA is also a positive control element for iron-dependent translation. *Biochemistry* **31**, 2818–2822.

Drapier, J.-C., Hirling, H., Wietzerbin, J., Kaldy, P. and Kühn, L. C. (1993) Biosynthesis of nitric oxide activates iron regulatory factor in macrophages. *EMBO J.* **12**, 3643–3649.

Drysdale, J., Dugast, I., Papadopoulos, P. and Zappone, E. (1991) Intracellular iron metabolism. *Curr. Stud. Hematol. Blood Transf.* **58**, 148–152.

Eisenstein, R. S. and Munro, H. N. (1990) Translational regulation of ferritin synthesis by iron. *Enzyme* **44**, 42–58.

Eisenstein, R. S., Garcia-Mayol, D., Pettingell, W. and Munro, H. N. (1991) Regulation of ferritin and heme oxygenase synthesis in fibroblasts by different forms of iron. *Proc. Natl. Acad. Sci. USA* **88**, 688–692.

Elferink, C. J., Sassa, S. and May, B. K. (1988) Regulation of 5-aminolevulinate synthase in mouse erythroleukemic cells is different from that of liver. *J. Biol. Chem.* **263**, 13012–13016.

Galbraith, R. M. and Galbraith, G. M. (1981) Expression of transferrin receptors on mitogen-stimulated peripheral blood lymphocytes: Relation to cellular activation and related metabolic events. *Immunology* **44**, 703–710.

Gardner, L. C. and Cox, T. M. (1988) Biosynthesis of heme in immature erythroid cells: The regulatory step for heme formation in the human erythron. *J. Biol. Chem.* **263**, 6676–6682.

Goessling, L. S., Daniels-McQueen, S., Bhattacharyya-Pakrasi, M., Lin, J.-J. and Thach, R. E. (1992) Enhanced degradation of ferritin repressor protein during induction of ferritin messenger RNA translation. *Science* **256**, 670–673.

Goossen, B. and Hentze, M. W. (1992) Position is the critical determinant for function of iron-responsive elements as translational regulators. *Mol. Cell. Biol.* **12**, 1959–1966.

Goossen, B., Caughman, S. W., Harford, J. B., Klausner, R. D. and Henze, M. W. (1990) Translational repression by a complex between the iron-responsive element of ferritin mRNA and its specific cytoplasmic binding protein is position dependent in vivo. *EMBO J.* **9**, 4127–4133.

Granick, S. (1946) Ferritin: Its properties and significance for iron metabolism. *Chem. Rev.* **38**, 379–395.

Gutteridge, J. M. C. (1989) Iron and oxygen: a biologically damaging mixture. *Acta Pediatr. Scan. Suppl.* **361**, 78–85.

Haile, D. J., Henzte, M. W., Rouault, T. A., Harford, J. B. and Klausner, R. D. (1989) Regulation of interaction of the iron-responsive element binding protein with iron-responsive RNA elements. *Mol. Cell. Biol.* **9**, 5055–5061.

Haile, D. J., Rouault, T. A., Harford, J. B. and Klausner, R. D. (1990) The inhibition of the iron responsive element RNA–protein interaction by heme does not mimic in vivo iron regulation. *J. Biol. Chem.* **265**, 12786–12789.

Haile, D. J., Rouault, T. A., Tang, C. K., Chin, J., Harford, J. B. and Klausner, R. D. (1992a) Reciprocal control of RNA binding and aconitase activity in the regulation of the iron-responsive element binding protein: Role of the iron-sulfur cluster. *Proc. Natl. Acad. Sci. USA* **89**, 7536–7540.

Haile, D. J., Rouault, T. A., Harford, J. B. *et al.* (1992b) Cellular regulation of the iron-responsive element binding protein: Disassembly of the cubane iron–sulfur cluster results in high affinity RNA binding. *Proc. Natl. Acad. Sci. USA* **89**, 11735–11739.

Hamilton, T. A., Gray, P. W. and Adams, D. O. (1984) Expression of the transferrin receptor on murine peritoneal macrophages is modulated by in vitro treatment with interferon gamma. *Cell. Immunol.* **89**, 478–488.

Hammer, R. E., Idzerda, R. L., Brinster, R. L. and McKnight, G. S. (1986) Estrogen regulation of the avian transferrin gene in transgenic mice. *Mol. Cell. Biol.* **6**, 1010–1014.

Hanover, J. A. and Dickson, R. B. (1985) Transferrin: Receptor-mediated endocytosis and iron delivery. In: *Endocytosis* (eds I. Pastan and M. C. Willingham), Plenum Press, New York, pp. 131–161.

Harford, J. B. and Klausner, R. D. (1990) Coordinate post-transcriptional regulation of ferritin and transferrin receptor expression: The role of regulated RNA–protein interaction. *Enzyme* **44**, 28–41.

Harford, J., Koeller, D., Casey, J., Hentze, M., Rouault, T. and Klausner, R. D. (1988) Iron-responsive elements within the 3′ untranslated region of the transferrin receptor mRNA (abstract). *J. Cell Biol.* **107**(3), 12a.

Harford, J. B., Casey, J. L., Koeller, D. M. and Klausner, R. D. (1990) In: *Intracellular Trafficking of Proteins* (eds C. J. Steer and J. A. Hanover), Cambridge University Press, Cambridge, pp. 302–334.

Harrell, C. M., McKenzie, A. R., Patino, M. M., Walden, W. E. and Theil, E. C. (1991) Ferritin mRNA: interactions of iron regulatory element with translational regulator P-90 and the effect of base-paired flanking regions. *Proc. Natl. Acad. Sci. USA* **88**, 4166–4170.

Hashimoto, C., Hudson, K. L. and Anderson, K. V. (1988) The Toll gene of *Drosophila*, required for dorsal–ventral embryonic polarity, appears to encode a transmembrane protein. *Cell* **52**, 269–279.

Hentze, M. W. and Argos, P. (1991) Homology between IRE-BP, a regulatory RNA-binding protein, aconitase, and isopropylmalate isomerase. *Nucleic Acids Res.* **19**, 1739–1740.

Hentze, M. W., Keim, S., Papadopoulos, P. *et al.* (1986) Cloning, characterization, expression, and chromosomal localization of a human ferritin heavy-chain gene. *Proc. Natl. Acad. Sci. USA* **83**, 7226–7230.

Hentze, M. W., Caughman, S. W., Rouault, T. A. *et al.* (1987a) Identification of the iron-responsive element for the translational regulation of human ferritin mRNA. *Science* **238**, 1570–1573.

Hentze, M. W., Rouault, T. A., Caughman, S. W., Dancis, A., Harford, J. B. and Klausner, R. D. (1987b) A cis-acting element is necessary and sufficient for translational regulation of human ferritin expression in response to iron. *Proc. Natl. Acad. Sci. USA* **84**, 6730–6734.

Hentze, M. W., Caughman, S. W., Casey, J. L. *et al.* (1988) A model for the structure and functions of iron-responsive elements. *Gene* **72**, 201–208.

Hentze, M. W., Rouault, T. A., Harford, J. B. and Klausner, R. D. (1989) Oxidation–reduction and the molecular mechanism of a regulatory RNA–protein interaction. *Science* **244**, 357–359.

Horowitz, J. A. and Harford, J. B. (1992) The secondary structure of the regulatory region of the transferrin receptor mRNA deduced by enzymatic cleavage. *New Biol.* **4**, 330–338.

Hu, H. Y., Gardner, J. and Aisen, P. (1977) Inducibility of transferrin receptors on friend erythroleukemic cells. *Science* **197**, 559–561.

Huebers, H. A. and Finch, C. A. (1987) The physiology of transferrin and transferrin receptors. *Physiol. Rev.* **67**, 520–582.

Idzerda, R. L., Heubers, H. A., Finch, C. A. and McKnight, G. S. (1986) Rat transferrin gene expression: Tissue specificity and regulation in iron deficiency. *Proc. Natl. Acad. Sci. USA* **83**, 2723–2727.

Idzerda, R. L., Behringer, R. R., Theisen, M., Huggenvik, J. I., McKnight, G. S. and Brinster, R. L. (1989) Expression from the transferrin gene promoter in transgenic mice. *Mol. Cell. Biol.* **9**, 5154–5162.

Jones, B. M., Worwood, M. and Jacobs, A. (1980) Serum ferritin in patients with cancer: Determination with antibodies to HeLa cell and spleen ferritin. *Clin. Chim. Acta* **106**, 203–214.

Kadonaga, J. T., Jones, K. A. and Tjian, R. (1986) Promoter-specific activation of RNA polymerase II transcription by Sp1. *Trends Biochem. Sci.* **11**, 20–23.

Kahn, A., Levin, M. J., Zakin, M. M. and Bloch, B. (1987) The transferrin gene. In: *Oncogenes, Genes, and Growth Factors* (ed. G. Guroff), Wiley–Interscience, New York, pp. 277–309.

Kaptain, S., Downey, W. E., Tang, C. *et al.* (1991) A regulated RNA binding protein also possesses aconitase activity. *Proc. Natl. Acad. Sci. USA* **88**, 10109–10113.

Klausner, R. D. and Harford, J. B. (1989) Cis–trans models for post-transcriptional gene regulations. *Science* **246**, 870–872.

Klausner, R. D., Rouault, T. A. and Harford, J. B. (1993) Regulating the fate of mRNA: The control of cellular iron metabolism. *Cell* **72**, 19–28.

Koeller, D. M., Casey, J. L., Hentze, M. W. *et al.* (1989) A cytosolic protein binds to structural elements within the iron regulatory region of the transferrin receptor mRNA. *Proc. Natl. Acad. Sci. USA* **86**, 3574–3578.

Koeller, D. M., Horowitz, J. A., Casey, J. L., Klausner, R. D. and Harford, J. B. (1991) Translation and the stability of mRNAs encoding the transferrin receptor and c-fos. *Proc. Natl. Acad. Sci. USA* **88**, 7778–7782.

Kozak, M. (1986) Influences of mRNA secondary structure on initiation by eukaryotic ribosomes. *Proc. Natl. Acad. Sci. USA* **83**, 2850–2854.

Kronke, M., Leonard, W. J., Depper, J. M. and Greene, W. C. (1985) Sequential expression of genes involved in human T lymphocyte growth and differentiation. *J. Exp. Med.* **161**, 1593–1598.

Kühn, L. C. (1989) The transferrin receptor: A key function in iron metabolism. *Schweiz. Med. Wochenschr.* **119**, 1319–1326.

Kühn, L. C. and Hentze, M. W. (1992) Coordination of cellular iron metabolism by post-transcriptional gene regulation. *J. Inorg. Biochem.* **47**, 183–195.

Larrick, J. W. and Cresswell, P. (1979) Modulation of cell surface iron transferrin receptors by cell density and state of activation. *J. Supramol. Struct.* **11**, 579–586.

Leibold, E. A. and Munro, H. N. (1987) Characterization and evolution of the expressed rat ferritin light subunit gene and its pseudogene family: Conservation of sequences within noncoding regions of ferritin genes. *J. Biol. Chem.* **262**, 7335–7341.

Leibold, E. A. and Munro, H. N. (1988) Cytoplasmic protein binds in vitro to a highly conserved sequence in the 5′ untranslated region of ferritin heavy- and light-subunit mRNAs. *Proc. Natl. Acad. Sci. USA* **85**, 2171–2175.

Leibold, E. A., Laudano, A. and Yu, Y. (1990) Structural requirements of iron-responsive elements for binding of the protein involved in both transferrin receptor and ferritin mRNA post-transcriptional regulation. *Nucleic Acids Res.* **18**, 1819–1824.

Lescure, A.-M., Proudhon, D., Pesey, H., Ragland, M., Theil, E. C. and Briat, J.-F. (1991) Ferritin gene expression is regulated by iron in soybean cell cultures. *Proc. Natl. Acad. Sci. USA* **88**, 8222–8226.

Liau, G., Chan, L. M. and Feng, P. (1991) Increased ferritin gene expression is both promoted by cAMP and a marker for growth arrest in rabbit vascular smooth muscle cells. *J. Biol. Chem.* **266**, 18819–18826.

Lin, J.-J., Daniels-McQueen, S., Patino, M. M., Gaffield, L., Walden, W. E. and Thach, R. E. (1990) Derepression of ferritin messenger RNA translation by hemin in vitro. *Science* **247**, 74–77.

Lin, J.-J., Patino, M. M., Gaffield, L., Walden, W. E., Smith, A. and Thach, R. E. (1991) Crosslinking of hemin to a specific site on the 90-kDa ferritin repressor protein. *Proc. Natl. Acad. Sci. USA* **88**, 6068–6071.

Linial, M. N., Gunderson, N. and Groudine, M. (1985) Enhanced transcription of c-myc in bursal lymphoma cells requires continuous protein synthesis. *Science* **230**, 1126–1132.

Mattia, E., Rao, K., Shapiro, D. S., Sussman, H. H. and Klausner, R. D. (1984) Biosynthetic regulation of the human transferrin receptor by desferrioxamine in K562 cells. *J. Biol. Chem.* **259**, 2689–2692.

Mattia, E., den Blaauwen, J., Ashwell, G. and van Renswoude, J. (1989) Multiple post-transcriptional regulatory mechanisms in ferritin gene expression. *Proc. Natl. Acad. Sci. USA* **86**, 1801–1805.

Mattia, E., den Blaauwen, J. and van Renswoude, J. (1990) Role of protein synthesis in the accumulation of ferritin mRNA during exposure of cells to iron. *Biochem. J.* **267**, 553–555.

McClelland, A., Kühn, L. C. and Ruddle, F. H. (1984) The human transferrin receptor gene: Genomic organization and complete primary structure of the receptor deduced from a cDNA sequence. *Cell* **39**, 267–274.

McKnight, G. S., Lee, D. C., Hammaplandh, D., Finch, C. A. and Palmiter, R. D. (1980a) Transferrin gene expression: Effect of nutritional iron deficiency. *J. Biol. Chem.* **255**, 144–147.

McKnight, G. S., Lee, D. C. and Palmiter, R. D. (1980b) Transferrin gene expression: Regulation of mRNA transcription in chick liver by seroid hormones and iron deficiency. *J. Biol. Chem.* **255**, 148–153.

Melefors, Ö., Goossen, B., Johansson, H. E., Stripecke, R., Gray, N. K. and Hentze, M. W. (1993) Translational control of 5-aminolevulinate synthase mRNA by iron-responsive elements in erythroid cells. *J. Biol. Chem.* **268**, 5974–5978.

Mendelzon, D., Boissier, F. and Zakin, M. M. (1990) The binding site for the liver-specific transcription factor Tf-LF1 and the TATA box of the human transferrin gene promoter are the only elements necessary to direct liver-specific transcription in vitro. *Nucleic Acids Res.* **18**, 5717–5721.

Miskimins, W. K. (1992) Interaction of multiple factors with a GC-rich element within the mitogen responsive region of the human transferrin receptor gene. *J. Cell Biochem.* **49**, 349–356.

Miskimins, W. K., Roberts, M. P., McClelland, A. and Ruddle, F. H. (1985) Use of a protein blotting procedure and a specific DNA probe to identify nuclear proteins that recognize the promoter region of the transferrin receptor gene. *Proc. Natl. Acad. Sci. USA* **82**, 6741–6744.

Miskimins, W. K., McClelland, A., Roberts, M. P. and Ruddle, F. H. (1986) Cell proliferation and expression of the transferrin receptor gene: Promoter homologies and protein interactions. *J. Cell Biol.* **103**, 1781–1788.

Müllner, E. W. and Kühn, L. C. (1988) A stem-loop in the 3′ untranslated region mediates iron-dependent regulation of transferrin receptor mRNA stability in the cytoplasm. *Cell* **53**, 815–825.

Müllner, E. W., Neupert, B., and Kühn, L. C. (1989) A specific mRNA binding factor regulates the iron-dependent stability of cytoplasmic transferrin receptor mRNA. *Cell* **58**, 373–382.

Müllner, E. W., Rothenberger, S., Müller, A. M. and Kühn, L. C. (1992) In vivo and in vitro modulation of the mRNA-binding activity of iron regulatory factor: Tissue distribution and effects of cell proliferation, iron levels and redox state. *Eur. J. Biochem.* **208**, 597–605.

Munro, H. N. and Linder, M. C. (1978) Ferritin: Structure, biosynthesis, and role in iron metabolism. *Physiol. Rev.* **58**, 317–396.

Neckers, L. M. and Cossman, J. (1983) Transferrin receptor induction in mitogen-stimulated human T lymphocytes is required for DNA synthesis and cell division and is regulated by interleukin 2. *Proc. Natl. Acad. Sci. USA* **80**, 3494–3498.

Neilands, J. B. (1974) In: *Microbial Iron Metabolism* (ed. J. B. Neilands), Academic Press, New York, pp. 3–34.

Neupert, B., Thompson, N. A., Meyer, C. and Kühn, L. C. (1990) A high yield affinity purification method for specific RNA binding proteins: isolation of the iron regulatory factor from human placenta. *Nucleic Acids Res.* **18**, 51–55.

Omary, M. B., Trowbridge, I. S. and Minowada, J. (1980) Human cell surface glycoprotein with unusual properties. *Nature (London)* **286**, 888–891.

Owen, D. and Kühn, L. C. (1987) Noncoding 3′ sequences of the transferrin receptor gene are required for mRNA regulation by iron. *EMBO J.* **6**, 1287–1293.

Patino, M. M. and Walden, W. E. (1992) Cloning of a functional cDNA for the rabbit ferritin mRNA repressor protein: Demonstration of a tissue specific pattern of expression. *J. Biol. Chem.* **267**, 19011–19016.

Pelicci, P. G., Tabillio, A., Thomopoulos, P. *et al.* (1982) Hemin regulates the expression of transferrin receptors in human hematopoietic cell lines. *FEBS Lett.* **145**, 350–354.

Pelletier, J. and Sonenberg, N. (1985) Insertion mutagenesis to increase secondary structure within the 5′ noncoding region of a eukaryotic mRNA reduces translational efficiency. *Cell* **40**, 515–526.

Petropoulous, I., Auge-Gouillou, C. and Zakin, M. M. (1991) Characterization of the active part of the human transferrin gene enhancer and purification of two liver nuclear factors interacting with the TGTTTGC motif present in the region. *J. Biol. Chem.* **266**, 24220–24225.

Philpott, C. C., Rouault, T. A. and Klausner, R. D. (1991) Sequence and expression of the murine iron-responsive element binding protein. *Nucleic Acids Res.* **19**, 6333.

Piette, J. and Yaniv, M. (1987) Two different factors bind to the alpha domain of the polyoma virus enhancer, one of which also interacts with the SV40 and c-fos enhancer. *EMBO J.* **6**, 1331–1337.

Ponka, P., Schulman, H. M. and Martinez-Medellin, J. (1988) Haem inhibits iron uptake subsequent to endocytosis of transferrin in reticulocytes. *Biochem. J.* **251**, 105–109.

Ponka, P., Schulman, H. M. and Cox, T. M. (1990) In: *Biosynthesis of Heme and Chlorophylls* (ed. H. A. Dailey), McGraw-Hill, New York, pp. 393–434.

Rahmsdorf, H. J., Schönthal, A., Angel, P., Litfin, M., Rüther, U. and Herrlich, P. (1987) Post-transcriptional regulation of c-fos mRNA expression. *Nucleic Acids Res.* **15**, 1643–1659.

Rao, K. K., Shapiro, D., Mattia, E., Bridges, K. and Klausner, R. (1985) Effects of alterations in cellular iron on biosynthesis of the transferrin receptor in K562 cells. *Mol. Cell. Biol.* **5**, 595–600.

Rao, K., Harford, J. B., Rouault, T., McClelland, A., Ruddle, F. H. and Klausner, R. D. (1986) Transcriptional regulation by iron of the gene for the transferrin receptor. *Mol. Cell. Biol.* **6**, 236–240.

Robbins, A. H. and Stout, C. D. (1989a) The structure of aconitase. *Proteins* **5**, 289–312.

Robbins, A. H. and Stout, C. D. (1989b) Structure of activated aconitase: formation of the [4Fe-4S] cluster in the crystal. *Proc. Natl. Acad. Sci. USA* **86**, 3639–3643.

Roberts, K. P. and Griswold, M. D. (1990) Characterization of rat transferrin receptor complementary DNA: The regulation of transferrin receptor mRNA in testes and in Sertoli cells in culture. *Mol. Endocrinol.* **4**, 531–542.

Rogers, J. and Munro, H. N. (1987) Translation of ferritin light and heavy subunits mRNAs is regulated by intracellular chelatable iron levels in rat hepatoma cells. *Proc. Natl. Acad. Sci. USA* **84**, 2277–2281.

Rogers, J. T., Bridges, K. R., Durmowicz, G. P., Glass, J., Auron, P. E. and Munro, H. N. (1990) Translational control during acute phase response: Ferritin synthesis in response to interleukin-1. *J. Biol. Chem.* **265**, 14572–14578.

Rothenberg, S., Müllner, E. W. and Kühn, L. C. (1990) The mRNA-binding protein which controls ferritin and transferrin receptor expression is conserved during evolution. *Nucleic Acids Res.* **18**, 1175–1179.

Rouault, T. A., Hentze, M. W., Caughman, S. W., Harford, J. B. and Klausner, R. D. (1988) Binding of a cytosolic protein to the iron-responsive element of human ferritin messenger RNA. *Science* **241**, 1207–1210.

Rouault, T. A., Hentze, M. W., Haile, D. J., Haile, D. J., Harford, J. B. and Klausner, R. D. (1989) The iron-responsive element binding protein: A method for the affinity purification of a regulatory RNA-binding protein. *Proc. Natl. Acad. Sci. USA* **86**, 5768–5772.

Rouault, T. A., Tang, C. K., Kaptain, S. *et al.* (1990) Cloning of the cDNA encoding an RNA regulatory protein: The human iron responsive elements binding protein. *Proc. Natl. Acad. Sci. USA* **87**, 7958–7962.

Rouault, T. A., Stout, C. D., Kaptain, S., Harford, J. B. and Klausner, R. D. (1991) Structural relationship between an iron-regulated RNA-binding protein (IRE-BP) and aconitase: functional implications. *Cell* **64**, 881–883.

Ryseck, R. P., Hirai, S. I., Yaniv, M. and Bravo, R. (1988) Transcriptional activation of c-jun during the G0/G1 transition in mouse fibroblasts. *Nature (London)* **334**, 535–537.

Schaeffer, E., Boisser, F., Py, M. C., Cohen, G. N. and Zakin, M. M. (1989) Cell type specific expression of the human transferrin gene. *J. Biol. Chem.* **264**, 7153–7160.

Shaw, G. and Kamen, R. (1986) A conserved AU sequence from the 3' untranslated region of GM-CSF mRNA mediates selective mRNA degradation. *Cell* **46**, 659–667.

Shyu, A.-B., Greenberg, M. E. and Belasco, J. G. (1989) The c-fos transcript is targeted for rapid decay by two distinct mRNA degradation pathways. *Genes Dev.* **3**, 60–72.

Stubbe, J. (1990) Ribonucleotide reductase. *Adv. Enzymol. Relat. Areas Mol. Biol.* **63**, 349–419.

Sutherland, R., Delia, D., Schneider, C., Newman, R., Kemshead, J. and Greaves, M. (1981) Ubiquitous cell surface glycoprotein on tumor cells is proliferation-associated receptor for transferrin. *Proc. Natl. Acad. Sci. USA* **78**, 4515–4519.

Tang, C. K., Chin, J., Harford, J. B., Klausner, R. D. and Rouault, T. A. (1992) The regulation of the iron responsive element binding protein RNA binding activity occurs post-translationally. *J. Biol. Chem.* **267**, 24466–24470.

Theil, E. C. (1987) Ferritin: Structure, gene regulation, and cellular function in animals, plants, and microorganisms. *Annu. Rev. Biochem.* **56**, 289–315.

Theil, E. C. (1990) Regulation of ferritin and transferrin receptor mRNAs. *J. Biol. Chem.* **265**, 4771–4774.

Thompson, C. B., Challoner, P. B., Neiman, P. E. and Groudine, M. (1986) Expression of the c-myb proto-oncogene during cellular proliferation. *Nature* **319**, 374–380.

Torti, S. V., Kwak, E. L., Miller, S. C. *et al.* (1988) The molecular cloning and characterization of murine ferritin heavy chain, a tumor necrosis factor-inducible gene. *J. Biol. Chem.* **263**, 12638–12644.

Trepel, J. B., Colamonici, O. R., Kelly, K. *et al.* (1987) Transcriptional inactivation of c-myc and the transferrin receptor in dibutyryl cyclic AMP-treated HL60 cells. *Mol. Cell. Biol.* **7**, 2644–2648.

Trowbridge, I. S. and Omary, M. B. (1981) Human cell surface glycoprotein related to cell proliferation is the receptor for transferrin. *Proc. Natl. Acad. Sci. USA* **78**, 3039–3043.

Tsuji, Y., Kwak, E., Saika, T., Torti, S. V. and Torti, F. M. (1993) Preferential repression of the H subunit of ferritin by adenovirus E1A in NIH3T3 mouse fibroblasts. *J. Biol. Chem.* **268**, 7270–7275.

Wagstaff, M., Worwood, M. and Jacobs, A. (1978) Properties of human tissue isoferritins. *Biochem. J.* **173**, 969–977.

Walden, W. E., Daniels-McQueen, S., Brown, P. H. *et al.* (1988) Translational repression in eukaryotes: Partial purification and characterization of a repressor of ferritin mRNA translation. *Proc. Natl. Acad. Sci. USA* **85**, 9503–9507.

Walden, W. E., Patino, M. M. and Gaffield, L. (1989) Purification of a specific repressor of ferritin mRNA translation from rabbit liver. *J. Biol. Chem.* **264**, 13765–13769.

Wang, Y.-H., Sczekan, S. R. and Theil, E. C. (1990) Structure of the 5' untranslated regulatory region of ferritin mRNA studied in solution. *Nucleic Acids Res.* **18**, 4463–4468.

Ward, J. H., Kushner, J. P. and Kaplan, J. (1982) Regulation of HeLa cell transferrin receptors. *J. Biol. Chem.* **257**, 10317–10323.

Wei, Y., Miller, S. C., Tsuji, Y., Torti, S. V. and Torti, F. M. (1990) Interleukin-1 induces ferritin heavy chain in human muscle cells. *Biochem. Biophys. Res. Commun.* **169**, 289–296.

Weiss, G., Goossen, B., Doppler, W. *et al.* (1993) Translational regulation via iron-responsive elements by the nitric oxide/NO synthase pathway. *EMBO J.* **12**, 3651–3657.

White, K. and Munro, H. N. (1988) Induction of ferritin synthesis by iron is regulated at both transcriptional and translational levels. *J. Biol. Chem.* **263**, 8938–8942.

Yu, Y., Radisky, E. and Leibold, E. A. (1992) The iron-responsive element binding protein: Purification, cloning, and regulation in rat liver. *J. Biol. Chem.* **267**, 19005–19010.

Zahringer, J., Baliga, B. S. and Munro, H. N. (1976) Novel mechanism for translational control in regulation of ferritin synthesis by iron. *Proc. Natl. Acad. Sci.* **73**, 857–861.

Zakin, M. M. (1992) Regulation of transferrin gene expression. *FASEB J.* **6**, 3253–3258.

6. Iron Absorption

B. SKIKNE AND R. D. BAYNES

Division of Hematology, University of Kansas Medical Center, 3901 Rainbow Boulevard, Kansas City, KS 66160, USA

The gastrointestinal tract plays a pivotal role in maintaining iron balance. Control manifests at the level of the mucosal cells of the upper small intestine where the majority of food iron absorption occurs. Significant progress in understanding the biochemical mechanisms and factors affecting control of iron absorption and the determinants of food iron bioavailability has occurred during the past 20 years. However, the precise mechanisms of control and their modulation remain important, incompletely understood issues.

I. METHODS USED TO DETERMINE IRON ABSORPTION

Because radioisotopic evaluations of iron uptake are limited in human volunteers, a number of alternative methods have been utilized to assess iron absorption. These include *in vitro* techniques and animal models using haemoglobin repletion, iron balance and isotopic markers. Studies in humans have included iron balance, haemoglobin repletion and plasma iron tolerance methodologies. Recently, stable isotopes have been evaluated as an alternative.

In vitro methods simulating the *in vivo* absorptive process give a general prediction of food iron bioavailability and provide insight into iron solubility from a particular compound or food. These also allow examination of the effect of promotory and inhibitory ligands in modulating the amount of iron available for absorption (Miller *et al.*, 1981; Chidambaram *et al.*, 1989; Whittaker *et al.*, 1989a). Single food types and complex food mixtures can be evaluated. Methods simulating gastrointestinal digestion include acid hydrolysis, proteolytic digestion by pepsin and pancreatin, and finally, the addition of bile acids. The released soluble low molecular weight iron is then measured. An advantage of *in vitro* methods is the elimination of variations in iron absorption which occur *in vivo* due to differences in iron status and day-to-day variability. In most cases, *in vitro* bioavailability measurements provide an estimate of non-haem iron bioavailability in man. While superior to the rat model (Schricker *et al.*, 1981; Forbes *et al.*, 1989), they do not fully simulate the *in vivo* absorptive process (Hurrell *et al.*, 1988, 1989). Their major use is in predicting trends rather than absolute levels of iron absorption.

The growing rat has been extensively utilized for assessing iron bioavailability using haemoglobin repletion methods (Whittaker *et al.*, 1984; Forbes *et al.*, 1989). Radioisotopes are commonly employed for direct absorption measurements. Intestinal loops have been extensively used to study mechanisms of iron absorption. Significant disparities in absorption from iron salts and food iron have been noted between rats and humans with absorption rates being significantly higher from identical meals in rats (Reddy and Cook, 1991). Dietary enhancers and inhibitors that have profound effects on non-haem absorption in man elicit blunted responses in rats, making this model unsuitable for predicting absorption in man.

Prior to the widespread use of radioisotopes, iron balance techniques were used to evaluate iron bioavailability in man. These methods require stool collections over long periods and are cumbersome to perform. Because of the small amounts of iron absorbed daily, these techniques are insensitive and prone to error and are no longer used in human studies. Measurement of plasma iron tolerance after iron ingestion is only useful for assessing absorption from pharmacological doses of iron since food iron absorption is usually too low to produce appreciable changes in plasma iron. This method is highly variable in part because plasma iron measurement at any interval after iron ingestion reflects a transient plasma iron phase. Iron enters the circulating plasma iron pool after absorption and is simultaneously cleared by the bone marrow and other acceptor sites. Since entry and clearance may occur at variable rates, variable measurements may result. Approximate measurements of absorption from pharmacological doses of iron can, however, be determined.

Because of concern regarding the use of radioisotopes in human subjects, especially in children and pregnant women, stable isotopes have recently been evaluated as an alternative. The stable isotopes of iron include ^{54}Fe, ^{56}Fe, ^{57}Fe and ^{58}Fe. These occur with a natural abundance of 5.6%, 91.9%, 2.2% and 0.3%, respectively. Improved methodology allows measurement of the less abundant ones namely ^{54}Fe, ^{57}Fe and ^{58}Fe. These techniques are still in their infancy and require expensive, sophisticated laboratory instrumentation. Large quantities of expensive isotope are required for absorption studies based on their incorporation into circulating red blood cells (Woodhead *et al.*, 1988; Fomon *et al.*, 1989; Whittaker *et al.*, 1989b). Stable isotopes are unsuitable for iron absorption measurements in situations where incorporation into red cells is unpredictable. At present, it seems unlikely that this methodology will replace more conventional isotopic determinations other than in pregnant women and children.

The major progress in understanding iron absorption during the past 30 years has resulted from the use of ^{59}Fe and ^{55}Fe radioisotopes. Absorption is estimated from the amount of radioiron incorporated into circulating red blood cells two to three weeks after ingesting the radioactive label. Incorporation of absorbed radioiron is approximately 80% or greater in normal subjects and patients with iron deficiency. Whole body counters allow measurement of the total assimilated iron including that not incorporated into red cells. This approach is necessary where red cell incorporation is impaired as in inflammation. Early studies examining iron absorption used hydroponically labelled foods of vegetable origin and biosynthetically labelled tissue of animal origin. A disadvantage of intrinsically labelled food is that it limits the number of food constituents that can be evaluated at any one time, since a single food is not eaten alone but as part of a composite meal. The most significant advance in food iron absorption methodology was the demonstration that extrinsic radioiron added to food has essentially the same absorption as the food's intrinsic iron. This was shown for both non-haem and haem iron absorption (Layrisse *et al.*, 1973). Extensive studies led to the pool concept (Layrisse *et al.*, 1973; Hallberg, 1980). Solubilized non-haem iron present in the different constituents of a composite meal enters a common non-haem iron pool in the gastrointestinal tract lumen. Absorption occurs from this pool and different factors present in the particular meal such as the combination of enhancers and inhibitors influence the amount of iron available to the mucosal cell. Similarly, haem iron present in different food constituents enters a common pool from which haem iron is absorbed. The enhancing and inhibiting factors influencing absorption from the non-haem iron pool are, for the most part, without effect on the haem iron pool. These findings allow iron absorption studies to be performed without the need for biosynthetically labelled food.

Because of the desirability of comparing iron absorption results from different studies and the significant variation in absorption between individuals, it is customary to measure absorption from a standard reference dose of inorganic radioiron containing 3 mg iron as ferrous ascorbate (Layrisse et al., 1969; Hallberg, 1981). The ratio of absorption from a given meal to absorption from the reference dose can then be used as a measure of the relative bioavailability of the non-haem iron in the meal. A more concrete measure of the latter is obtained by standardizing the test measurement to a reference value of 40%, the mean absorption value in subjects who are borderline iron deficient (Hallberg, 1980; Magnusson et al., 1981). A disadvantage of the single reference dose is that it is influenced by the day-to-day variability in absorption which commonly occurs in an individual subject. Since serum ferritin concentration is as good a predictor of food iron absorption as the reference salt absorption (Baynes et al., 1987), measurements of serum ferritin during absorption studies to correct for variations in iron status, reduces the observed variability noted with the reference dose method (Cook et al., 1991a). An obvious advantage of serum ferritin correction is that it eliminates the need for the reference salt absorption (Cook et al., 1991a).

2. HAEM IRON ABSORPTION

Foods derived from animal tissues are the major sources of haem iron. Haemoglobin and myoglobin are the main precursor proteins from which haem iron is derived. Haem iron forms an important source of dietary iron intake because of its high bioavailability. In industrial countries haem iron constitutes approximately 10–15% of ingested iron, but because of its high bioavailability, may account for about one-third of the iron absorbed (Cook et al., 1982; Bezwoda et al., 1983).

2.1. Influence of Dose

When haemoglobin is ingested without other food constituents, a decreasing proportion of iron absorption from the haemoglobin occurs with increasing haemoglobin doses (Gabbe et al., 1979; Wheby and Spyker, 1981). Increasing the haemoglobin dose results in an increase in the absolute amount of haem iron absorbed, although the percentage absorbed declines. The relationship between the dose ingested and per cent absorption of haemoglobin iron is linear. When physiological amounts of haem iron, ranging from 0.25 mg to 6 mg, are eaten with food, however, per cent absorption remains constant despite increasing haem iron content of the food (Hallberg et al., 1979; Bezwoda et al., 1983). This results in a linear increase in the absolute amount of haem iron absorbed.

2.2. Intraluminal Factors and Bioavailability

Haemoglobin is converted in the bowel to haem. This conversion occurs relatively rapidly with 70% of a specific haemoglobin dose being converted to haem by 30 minutes in a dog model and 85% within 3 hours (Wheby and Spyker, 1981).

When haem iron is taken with food its absorption is not dependent on the food composition to the same extent as non-haem iron which is significantly affected by inhibitory and promotory ligands. Food composition does affect haem iron absorption in so far as pure haem iron is relatively poorly absorbed, probably because of the formation of non-absorbable haem polymers (Conrad et al., 1966). That haemoglobin iron is better absorbed with food, an effect which is particularly marked with either meat or soy protein (Lynch et al., 1985), suggests that other protein and protein degradation products may preserve haem in the monomeric state. Since pure haem is not ingested, these considerations are of mechanistic rather than practical importance. Because haem iron is well-absorbed relatively independently of the components of the diet, it has been evaluated as an alternative iron fortificant of weaning food by adding it to extruded rice flour (Calvo et al., 1989) and in a school lunch programme by baking it into cookies (Stekel, 1981).

2.3. Mucosal Uptake and Transfer of Haem Iron

Haem is taken up by the mucosal cell via a pathway different from non-haem iron. This has been shown to involve binding to a specific haem receptor (Grasbeck et al., 1979, 1982). Haem iron, as the unchanged porphyrin ring, rapidly enters the mucosal cell. Autoradiographic studies and diaminobenzidine staining of mucosal cells in dogs indicate that haem iron is endocytosed in microendocytic vesicles best observed at the base of microvilli and as tubulovesicular structures in the apical cytoplasm of mucosal cells (Parmley et al., 1981). Haem oxygenase contained in the intestinal mucosal cell breaks down the haem molecule. This intramucosal haem splitting process appears to be the rate limiting step in haem iron absorption (Wheby and Spyker, 1981). After cleavage from the haem molecule, iron enters the same intracellular pool as that of non-haem iron. Large doses of haem iron inhibit absorption of non-haem iron and large doses of non-haem iron inhibit absorption of haem iron (Hallberg et al., 1979). Parenteral administration of desferrioxamine blocks absorption of both forms of iron (Levine et al., 1988) suggesting the existence of a common chelatable cellular iron pool and a shared transcellular, interstitial and intravascular transport pathway.

2.4. Effects of Iron Status

Absorption of haem iron is increased in patients with iron deficiency compared with normal subjects (Gabbe et al., 1979) and the well-known relationship between body iron stores and non-haem iron absorption also applies to haem iron (Lynch et al., 1989b). This relationship is, however, less pronounced for haem iron. At any given serum ferritin level, per cent haem iron absorption is greater than non-haem iron absorption (Fig. 6.1). Inhibition of haem iron absorption is less pronounced at higher storage iron levels than absorption of non-haem iron, with regression slopes of -0.358 and -0.936, respectively (Fig. 6.1). Absolute haem iron absorption from a standard meal is four-fold higher than non-haem iron absorption at a serum ferritin of 100 μg/l. At a serum ferritin of 30 μg/l, absorption of haem iron is approximately two-fold higher and only when iron deficiency is present does non-haem iron

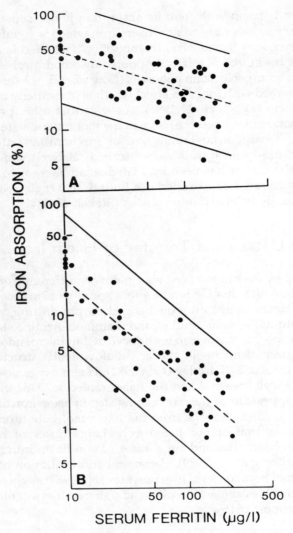

Fig. 6.1 Relationship between serum ferritin and haem (A) and non-haem (B) iron absorption in normal subjects (Lynch *et al.*, 1989b).

absorption exceed, in absolute terms, the amount of iron absorbed from haem. A two-fold decrease in the amount of iron absorbed from haem occurs between a serum ferritin level of 10 μg/l and 100 μg/l, while a nine-fold decrease in non-haem iron is seen (Lynch *et al.*, 1989b).

These data have important ramifications in terms of iron nutrition. Clearly, iron deficiency will be least likely in haem iron consuming regions. Conversely, iron overload is likely to manifest where haem iron consumption is highest. Indeed, while an inverse relationship between stores and absorption is evident for non-haem iron in haemochromatosis, the loss of this relationship for haem iron gives certain insights as to where the metabolic basis of the disease may be localized (see p. 175).

3. NON-HAEM IRON ABSORPTION

3.1. The Role of the Stomach and Luminal Factors

Patients with achlorhydria or gastrectomy develop iron deficiency anaemia due to diminished ability to absorb non-haem dietary iron (Bothwell *et al.*, 1979). The hydrochloric acid content of gastric juice is important for solubilization of non-haem iron. This occurs rapidly with most of the iron being in solution within five minutes (Bezwoda *et al.*, 1978). A significant relationship exists between the ability to solubilize non-haem iron in an individual's gastric juice, the pH of that gastric juice, and non-haem iron absorption from a standard meal (Bezwoda *et al.*, 1978). At gastric juice pH >2.5, iron solubilization is significantly reduced. Absorption of ferric iron salts is more affected by achlorhydria than absorption of ferrous iron salts (Jacobs *et al.*, 1968). Ferrous iron remains in solution at a higher pH than does ferric iron. Upon entry to the duodenum the pH rise results in rapid precipitation of ferric iron due to the formation of ferric oxyhydroxide. This is emphasized by a study of patients with achlorhydria, where absorption of ferrous iron salts improved two-fold when administered with hydrochloric acid as compared with a four-fold improvement in absorption from ferric iron salts. A two-fold increase in absorption from bread occurred after the addition of normal gastric juice to a meal in achlorhydrics (Cook *et al.*, 1964) and neutralization of added gastric acid reduced that response (Cook *et al.*, 1964; Jacobs and Owen, 1969). Using an H_2 receptor blocker, a selective inhibitor of gastric acid secretion, reduction of gastric acid output by 60–80% produced a modest 28% reduction in non-haem food iron absorption. Further reduction in gastric acid output with increasing doses of H_2-receptor blocker led to a 42–65% reduction in absorption suggesting that non-haem food iron absorption is only significantly reduced when acid secretion is markedly reduced (Skikne *et al.*, 1981). Increasing gastric acid output using pentagastrin (Skikne *et al.*, 1981) or addition of gastric juice from patients with normal acid output to normal subjects does not increase non-haem iron absorption further (Jacobs *et al.*, 1967), suggesting that under normal circumstances the acid output in response to a meal is sufficient to ensure adequate absorption of the available iron.

The physical form of ingested food and the retention time in the stomach may play a role in solubilizing iron from food. This may not relate to the duration of exposure to acid since iron is relatively rapidly solubilized. Studies in man examining the gastric emptying rate from a standard meal failed to show a correlation between emptying rate and absorption of non-haem and haem iron (Skikne *et al.*, 1983). Homogenization of the meal, however, led to a 31% increase in the gastric emptying rate. Unexpectedly, this was accompanied by a 22% and 42% increase in non-haem and haem iron absorption, respectively. It is possible that quicker gastric emptying allows less time for pH buffering by pancreatic secretions and less time for binding by inhibitory ligands to occur, thus improving the ability of solubilized iron to be taken up by acceptor sites on the mucosal cell. This does not explain the observed increase in haem iron absorption. The changes in absorption related to gastric emptying rate are small, and how they relate to day-to-day variability seen in iron absorption is uncertain.

The low pH of the gastric content is neutralized to a pH >4 within five to six minutes of its arrival in the duodenum (Hungerford and Linder, 1983). The iron loses solubility under these conditions. Concomitant with the changing pH in the duodenum, iron absorption begins. Uptake into the mucosal cell occurs rapidly, the greatest proportion taking place within the first five minutes. After this time, the uptake reaches a plateau. With addition of an iron chelator, such as ascorbic acid, to the gastrointestinal contents, absorption continues to increase into the mucosal cell without plateau, despite the pH remaining unchanged. Thus, if iron is maintained in a water soluble state, absorption continues despite the pH status within the bowel lumen.

Ascorbic acid and other ligands play an important role in maintaining ferric iron in solution. The enhancing effect of bile on iron absorption may or may not relate to its ascorbic acid content (Conrad and Schade, 1968; Jacobs and Miles, 1970) and to its premicellar taurocholate content which increases iron solubility within the intestinal lumen (Sanyal et al., 1990). Pancreatic secretions also influence non-haem iron absorption. Bicarbonate secretion and the resultant rise in pH reduces non-haem iron solubility and pancreatic enzymes themselves may have an inhibitory effect on non-haem iron absorption (Zemspky et al., 1989). Pancreatic insufficiency has been associated with increased iron absorption although this is controversial (Bothwell et al., 1979). The extent to which variability of bile and pancreatic secretion rates may contribute to day-to-day variability of iron absorption remain to be defined.

3.2. The Effect of Dose

The percentage absorption from therapeutic iron decreases with increasing dosage but the overall amount of iron increases. Fatalities from ingestion of excess medicinal iron are well established. There is a linear relationship between the dose of administered ferrous and ferric iron salts (50–400 mg) and the amount absorbed (Bothwell et al., 1979). The slope, however, is steeper for the ferrous iron salts. In contradistinction to increased therapeutic iron absorption with increasing dose, the absolute amount of non-haem iron absorbed from food does not increase significantly with increasing non-haem iron content of food. Within a physiological range of food non-haem iron varying between 1.5 mg to 5.7 mg, per cent absorption decreases with increasing amounts of iron. This results in little variation in the overall amount of iron absorbed (Bezwoda et al., 1983). Clinical examples of nutritional iron overload due to intake of large amounts of dietary iron in an unusually bioavailable form occurring in sub-Saharan Africa indicate that this control mechanism is overcome only in exceptional circumstances (see Chapter 9).

3.3. The Effect of Iron Valency and Mucosal Coating Material on Non-haem Iron Absorption

There is convincing evidence that absorption of ferrous iron is superior to ferric iron in man (Brise and Hallberg, 1962). Although not conclusive, evidence suggests that ferric iron reduction to ferrous iron is necessary for absorption to occur. Addition of the serum protein ceruloplasmin, which has oxidant properties, to the gastrointestinal lumen, significantly reduces absorption in rats (Wollenberg and Rummel, 1987). Prior washing of upper gastrointestinal tract segments significantly reduces absorption of iron suggesting that luminal fluid contains elutable factors which promote reduction. Addition of ascorbic acid to washed segments of bowel restores the ability to absorb iron from transferrin (Wollenberg and Rummel, 1987). These findings suggest that reduction of ferric iron in the rat small intestine is dependent on luminal factors which are removable by prewashing.

Mucus and the mucins coating the intestinal mucosa also play a role in non-haem iron absorption (Conrad et al., 1991; Wien and Van Campen, 1991). The previously mentioned elutable factor may be explained, in part, by the presence of mucus and the mucins it contains. The mucins bind iron at an acidic pH and maintain the iron in solution despite a rise in pH towards neutral. In this manner, iron is kept available for absorption in the alkaline milieu found in the duodenum in the absence of other chelators. Iron is bound relatively weakly and easily disassociates from the mucin. Iron ligands found in food, e.g. ascorbic acid, histidine and fructose, can donate iron to mucin. The mucins also bind other cations including lead, zinc and cobalt. The binding affinity is, however, greatest for iron (Conrad et al., 1991).

3.4. Non-haem Iron Compounds in the Diet and their Bioavailability

Non-haem iron compounds are found in foods of both plant and animal origin. Iron is present in plants in three main forms, namely as metalloproteins with the predominant example being plant ferritin (Sczekan and Joshi, 1987), as soluble iron in the sap of xylem, phloem and vacuoles, and as a non-functional form complexed either to structural components or with storage compounds predominantly in the form of phytates (Hazell, 1985). A large fraction of the iron in plant foods may be of contaminant origin as ferric oxides and hydroxides (Derman et al., 1982). Non-haem iron in animal-derived food is found in many forms including, for example, ferritin and haemosiderin in meat products, bound to the phosphoprotein, phosphovitin, in the yolk of eggs, and in milk bound to lactoferrin (±40%) and associated with fat globule membranes and low molecular weight compounds such as citrate.

Not all non-haem iron consumed enters the common non-haem iron pool equally. In this regard, non-haem iron as ferritin, haemosiderin, fortificant iron, and contaminant iron deserve special mention. Since the latter two may contribute disproportionately to food iron intake in developing regions, they may provide a false sense of nutritional security.

Once non-haem iron enters the common pool it is subject to the influence of the major dietary components namely carbohydrate, fat and protein. In addition, a number of exogenous iron ligands have been identified as promotory or inhibitory. In relation to fat and carbohydrate, the data indicate that these are relatively inert in terms of iron absorption (Monsen and Cook, 1979). The major influences that have been identified, largely in single meal studies, as affecting bioavailability are proteins and the exogenous ligands.

Based on single meal studies, a number of foods can be segregated as having low, medium and high non-haem iron bioavailability (Table 6.1). For the most part, cereals and nuts have low iron bioavailability, while bioavailability varies considerably

Table 6.1 Relative bioavailability of non-haem iron in a number of foods based largely on single meal studies (Bothwell *et al.*, 1989)

| Foods | Bioavailability | | |
	Low	Medium	High
Cereals	Maize	Cornflour	
	Oatmeal	White flour	
	Rice		
	Sorghum		
	Whole wheat flour		
Fruits	Apple	Cantaloupe	Guava
	Avocado	Mango	Lemon
	Banana	Pineapple	Orange
	Grape		Papaw
	Peach		Tomato
	Pear		
	Plum		
	Rhubarb		
	Strawberry		
Vegetables	Aubergine	Carrot	Beetroot
	Legumes	Potato	Broccoli
	Soy flour		Cabbage
	Isolated soy protein		Cauliflower
	Lupines		Pumpkin
			Turnip
Beverages	Tea	Red wine	White wine
	Coffee		
Nuts	Almond		
	Brazil		
	Coconut		
	Peanut		
	Walnut		
Animal proteins	Cheese		Fish
	Egg		Meat
	Milk		Poultry

for the individual components in the fruit and vegetable groups. These variable bioavailability measurements, determined largely on single meal studies, reflect the interplay of various proteins and inhibitory and promotory ligands. These factors will now be addressed in some detail.

3.4.1. *Enhancers of Non-haem Iron Absorption*

The main enhancers of non-haem iron absorption are first, proteins derived from animal tissues such as meat, poultry, and fish (see under Proteins in Iron Absorption, p. 164) and second, ascorbic acid. Other organic acids also have an enhancing effect as do certain spices and condiments. In addition, certain degradation products of plant proteins have also been shown to enhance non-haem iron bioavailability.

(a) *Ascorbic acid.* Bioavailability of iron in foods containing significant amounts of ascorbic acid is high (Gillooly *et al.*, 1983; Ballot *et al.*, 1987). In addition, ascorbic acid increases absorption from meals of low bioavailability containing potent inhibitors of absorption (Hallberg *et al.*, 1989; Siegenberg *et al.*, 1991) and from meals of medium availability (Hallberg *et al.*, 1987a). Addition of a fixed amount of ascorbic acid to different meals results in varied responses in absorption (Hallberg *et al.*, 1987a). A linear increase in absorption occurs with increasing content of ascorbic acid in a given meal up to a threshold molar excess. This has been demonstrated with foods containing phytates and polyphenols. Addition of 30 mg ascorbic acid to a bread meal containing 58 mg phytate doubled absorption (absorption ratio 2.08), while addition of 50 mg ascorbic acid further increased the absorption ratio to 2.97. Addition of 150 mg ascorbic acid had a minimal further enhancing effect (Siegenberg *et al.*, 1991). The nature of food preparation must, however, be borne in mind since heating ascorbic acid results in its destruction and hence reduction of its enhancing qualities.

Ascorbic acid potentiates non-haem iron absorption by two mechanisms, namely by reduction of ferric to ferrous iron in the stomach and as a chelator in the stomach and upper small bowel. These both help to maintain iron in a soluble state by preventing its polymerization and binding to other inhibitory ligands.

Based on the enhancing effects of ascorbic acid in single meal absorption studies, it would seem that long-term ingestion of foods containing adequate to raised amounts of ascorbic acid would lead to improved iron status. However, this has not been clearly demonstrated. Despite enhanced absorption from a test meal given with ascorbic acid both at the start and after several months of high dose ascorbic acid ingestion, iron status remained unchanged after 24 months of ascorbic acid supplementation (Cook *et al.*, 1984). Similarly, a study in women taking high dose ascorbic acid over an 8 week period failed to demonstrate significant changes in iron status (Malone *et al.*, 1986) and in a further study, iron status did not differ in populations taking vitamin–mineral supplements as compared with those not taking them (Looker *et al.*, 1988). The most feasible explanation for the apparent lack of an effect of ascorbic acid on iron nutrition is that the normal Western diet contains adequate amounts of ascorbic acid and meat. Taking additional ascorbic acid has no further positive effect on iron assimilation. A further explanation is that significant adaptation at the level of the mucosal cell occurs to limit absorption (Cook, 1990). A more recent study in women in whom iron deficiency was induced by repeated phlebotomy followed by eating a diet of low bioavailability during a 5½ week repletion period showed an apparent improvement in iron status in those taking high dose ascorbic acid compared with those taking a placebo. Although iron status was apparently minimally improved as judged by haemoglobin, zinc protoporphyrin and serum iron levels, serum ferritin levels did not change (Hunt *et al.*, 1990). Additional comments on this study are presented in Chapter 7. This finding suggests that ingestion of ascorbic acid on a long-term basis may have a beneficial effect on iron status only when the diet consists mainly of poorly available foods and iron deficiency is present. Further work in this area is needed to confirm or refute the role of ascorbic acid.

(b) *Organic acids*. Besides ascorbic acid, other organic acids also have enhancing effects on non-haem iron absorption. Citric acid present in citrus fruits and certain vegetables induces a significant three- to four-fold enhancing effect on non-haem iron absorption from a rice meal (Gillooly *et al.*, 1983; Ballot *et al.*, 1987). Addition of ascorbic acid to citric acid induces a further increase in absorption from this meal. Malic acid, a component of deciduous fruits, causes a significant two-fold enhancing effect on absorption from the rice meal (Gillooly *et al.*, 1983; Ballot *et al.*, 1987) and tartaric acid found in white wines displays a similar effect. Lactic acid has an enhancing effect and may be responsible for the favourable absorption from sauerkraut (Gillooly *et al.*, 1983). Lactic acid is also responsible for the enhanced absorption occurring from maize and sorghum beer in sub-Saharan Africa (Derman *et al.*, 1980). Oxalic acid, on the other hand, appears to have an inhibitory effect on absorption from cabbage (Gillooly *et al.*, 1983).

3.4.2. *Inhibitors of Non-haem Iron Absorption*

A significant portion of the diet eaten in developing countries is derived from cereals and vegetables, and the dietary fruit and animal protein content, while varying widely, is often suboptimal. This type of diet tends to contain disproportionately large quantities of factors inhibitory to non-haem iron absorption. This, along with increased demands as outlined in Chapter 7, contributes to the high incidence and prevalence of iron deficiency in these areas.

(a) *Phytate*. Bran is a major inhibitor of non-haem iron absorption and a quantitative inhibitory effect occurs with increasing bran content of a meal (Bjorn-Rasmussen, 1974). Similarly, rice has low intrinsic bioavailability (Ballot *et al.*, 1987; Hallberg *et al.*, 1977). Unpolished rice has an inhibitory effect on non-haem iron absorption which does not occur with polished rice or rice flour (Tuntawiroon *et al.*, 1990). The inhibitory effects present in beans, rice, and a number of other cereals including sorghum, oat products, and in certain vegetables are partly related to their phytate content (Gillooly *et al.*, 1983, 1984a; Rossander-Hulthen *et al.*, 1990). Small amounts of phytate in a meal reduce non-haem iron absorption (Hallberg, 1987; Siegenberg *et al.*, 1991). Removal of phytate from bran using endogenous phytase or dilute hydrochloric acid results in significantly improved absorption (Hallberg *et al.*, 1987b). The phytate content of rice may vary from region to region based on differences in soil nutrients and also on differences in milling practice (Tuntawiroon *et al.*, 1990). Wet milling of bran reduces phytate content (Siegenberg *et al.*, 1991). The inhibitory effects of phytate are significantly counter-balanced by both meat and ascorbic acid (Hallberg, 1987; Tuntawiroon *et al.*, 1990; Siegenberg *et al.*, 1991).

The exact mechanism by the inhibition of phytate is unknown. Monoferric phytate, which typically constitutes only a small portion of the phytate content of bran, does not possess significant inhibitory effects (Simpson *et al.*, 1981). The formation of diferric and tetraferric phytate complexes in the gastrointestinal tract renders the iron unavailable for absorption by the mucosal cell (Morris and Ellis, 1982).

In strict vegetarians, with a chronic intake of a high phytate diet, there is poor iron absorption from single phytate-containing meals. This finding suggests that populations eating a high phytate-containing diet are unable to improve iron assimilation from this type of diet by adaptation of the intestinal mucosal cell (Brune *et al.*, 1989a). However, the extent to which phytate consumption has a negative impact on iron nutrition has yet to be shown in population studies.

(b) *Polyphenols*. The polyphenols are common constituents of certain vegetables and beverages such as tea and coffee and have significant inhibitory effects on non-haem iron absorption. Tea has a potent inhibitory effect (Disler *et al.*, 1975; Hallberg and Rossander, 1982a; Morck *et al.*, 1983) as does coffee (Hallberg and Rossander, 1982a; Morck *et al.*, 1983). Inhibition of absorption by vegetables is not only related

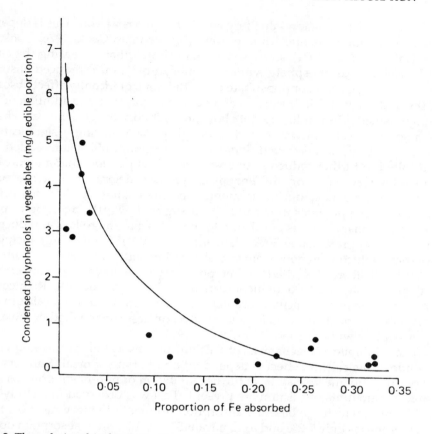

Fig. 6.2 The relationship between the condensed polyphenol content of vegetables (total-extractable polyphenols) and iron absorption from them (Gillooly *et al.*, 1983).

to their phytate content but also to their polyphenol content. The extent of inhibition is inversely related to the polyphenol content (Fig. 6.2) and specifically to the non-hydrolysable condensed polyphenols (Gillooly *et al.*, 1983). A similar inverse relationship between absorption occurs when increasing amounts of tannic acid are added to wheat rolls (Brune *et al.*, 1989b) or to dephytinized bread (Siegenberg *et al.*, 1991). Small amounts of tannic acid (5 mg) produce inhibition. The dose response curve is initially steep but maximal inhibition is achieved rapidly, with no further inhibition of iron absorption occurring beyond a tannic acid content of 50 mg (Brune *et al.*, 1989b; Siegenberg *et al.*, 1991). The inhibition of absorption is thought to be due to formation of complexes between the hydroxyl groups of the phenolic compounds and iron molecules. The ten galloyl groups present in tannic acid are the reactive sites for binding iron molecules. Other polyphenols such as chlorogenic acid, a constituent found in coffee, also have inhibitory effects on absorption but are less potent inhibitors than are gallic acid residues on an equimolar basis (Brune *et al.*, 1989b). As with the phytates, addition of ascorbic acid to foods reverses the inhibitory effect of the polyphenols (Siegenberg *et al.*, 1991; Tuntawiroon *et al.*, 1991). Most of these data have been generated in studies based on single meals. Again, the future challenge is to define the role that dietary polyphenols play in population iron nutrition.

(c) *Calcium*. Calcium has an inhibitory effect on iron absorption. This is dependent on the amount and form of calcium present (Monsen and Cook, 1976; Cook *et al.*, 1991b; Hallberg *et al.*, 1991). Early studies had shown that increasing the content of both calcium and phosphate within a semi-synthetic meal reduced absorption while addition of calcium or phosphate alone did not significantly affect absorption (Monsen and Cook, 1976). In studies of food iron absorption, the addition of 40 mg calcium to baked wheat rolls did not show an inhibitory effect, whereas when the same amount of calcium was added to dough prior to baking a significant 40% reduction in absorption occurred. Increasing the amount of calcium added to the rolls resulted in further reduction in absorption. It is possible that added calcium has an inhibitory effect on the enzymatic phytase degradation of the phytate contained in the wheat during fermentation and baking, leading to increased amounts of active phytates in the rolls (Hallberg *et al.*, 1991). Ingestion of milk or cheese with similar amounts of calcium to that added to the rolls also reduces iron absorption by approximately 50% (Hallberg *et al.*, 1991). Even an enhancing meal shows some reduction in non-haem iron absorption with addition of calcium (Cook *et al.*, 1991b; Hallberg *et al.*, 1991). When pharmaceutical doses of calcium carbonate are taken without food no reduction in iron absorption occurs. Reduced iron absorption occurs when calcium carbonate is taken with food. Both calcium citrate and calcium phosphate have an inhibitory effect on absorption whether the calcium is taken with or without food (Cook *et al.*, 1991b).

The exact inhibitory mechanism of calcium on absorption is not known. The magnitude of the calcium effect is dependent on the type of meal. Subjects eating low bioavailability meals may have further inhibition of non-haem iron absorption if significant amounts of calcium are present. This was observed in a study (Cook *et al.*, 1991b) in which the baseline absorption from an inhibitory meal containing 4.7 mg of iron was only 1.2% and a significant 55% reduction in absorption occurred with ingestion of calcium supplements. When taken with an enhancing meal, iron absorption was reduced by approximately 30% with calcium carbonate and calcium phosphate while no difference in absorption was seen with calcium citrate.

(d) *Fibre*. Although there is evidence that components of fibre bind iron *in vitro* (Reinhold *et al.*, 1981; Fernandez and Phillips, 1982), studies in humans indicate only a modest decrease in iron absorption with dietary fibre except for bran. Bran, however, contains large amounts of phytates which are associated with significant inhibition of absorption. Other components of dietary fibre appear to play less of a role. Ispagula causes a mild reduction in absorption, while pectin and cellulose do not have an inhibitory effect (Cook *et al.*, 1983; Gillooly *et al.*, 1983; Rossander, 1987).

3.4.3. Proteins in Iron Absorption

Dietary protein in western countries has traditionally been derived from animals, while in developing countries a significantly larger proportion of protein intake is derived from vegetable sources. Recently, there has been an increasing trend to replace traditional meat sources of dietary protein with proteins derived from non-animal sources. This is especially notable in commercial sources of infant foods and formulae. The source of dietary protein has an important impact on both non-haem and haem iron absorption. While protein derived from animal tissue may have enhancing properties on non-haem iron absorption, other animal derived protein constituents and most plant derived protein may not, or may even have inhibitory properties.

(a) *Iron absorption from proteins of animal origin.* High absorption rates from animal tissues occur when these are taken by themselves (Martinez-Torres and Layrisse, 1973), with absorption being in the 15–20% range. Animal tissue protein has an enhancing effect on iron absorption from the non-haem iron pool whether the iron is derived from other constituents of the meal or from the meat itself. Veal muscle induces a ten-fold increase in non-haem iron absorption from a maize meal (Layrisse *et al.*, 1973). Further studies using other animal tissue sources, show similar enhancing properties on non-haem iron absorption (Cook and Monsen, 1975; Hallberg and Rossander, 1984; Lynch *et al.*, 1989a). No significant differences in the enhancing effect of beef, pork, lamb, liver, chicken or fish have been observed (Cook and Monsen, 1976). Increasing the quantity of tissue protein in a meal results in only a modest further increase in non-haem iron absorption (Lynch *et al.*, 1989a).

While proteins derived from animal tissues have an enhancing effect on non-haem iron absorption, non-tissue proteins of animal origin do not display this effect. Early studies using intrinsically radiolabelled eggs indicated low iron absorption (Callender *et al.*, 1970). When animal products such as milk, cheese, eggs or egg albumin are substituted for beef in a standard meal, significantly reduced absorption occurs (Cook and Monsen, 1976). Absorption from a semisynthetic meal containing the same amount and constituents as a standard meal but with egg albumin instead of beef as the protein source, is significantly lower at 1.6% as compared with 8.3% from the standard meal (Cook and Monsen, 1976). When the protein fraction of the semi-synthetic meal is substituted with animal tissue proteins, absorption increases to levels comparable to those seen with the standard meal. The protein constituents of animal tissues, such as bovine albumin, may have an enhancing or inhibitory effect in different meals. A 60% enhancing effect occurs in a bread meal, while a 47% inhibition occurs with a semi-purified liquid meal containing no protein (Hurrell *et al.*, 1988).

Many attempts to isolate the potentiating 'meat factor' of animal tissue proteins have been made, since understanding the nature of this factor and its isolation could be of potential value in promoting iron absorption from less bioavailable foods. This is particularly true in the age of molecular biology since if a specific enhancing peptide could be identified the corresponding gene might be engineered into the genome of cereals and legumes in developing regions. Several candidates have been identified as contributing to the 'meat factor'. A prerequisite for promoting non-haem iron absorption is the maintenance of iron in solution during progressive alkalinization within the small intestine (Hazell, 1985). Water-soluble extracts (Bjorn-Rasmussen and Hallberg, 1979; Slatkavitz and Clydesdale, 1988) and dilute acid soluble extracts of muscle do not have significant iron solubilizing properties (Slatkavitz and Clydesdale, 1988). A number of studies have shown that free amino acids, and particularly the divalent amino acids asparagine, glycine and serine, enhance iron absorption in the rat (Christensen *et al.*, 1984). However, other proteins undergoing digestion should also liberate these amino acids. Another group has identified cysteine-containing residues as contributing to the meat effect (Martinez-Torres and Layrisse, 1970; Martinez-Torres *et al.*, 1981). It is, however, uncertain whether proteolysis is sufficiently complete early on to provide an adequate amino acid content to account for the effect, which occurs in the first part of the small intestine. To address this problem, cysteine-containing peptides obtained by simulated digestion were studied and shown to enhance non-haem iron absorption from a maize meal (Layrisse *et al.*, 1984; Taylor *et al.*, 1986). These peptides are stable in the gastrointestinal tract and their thiol groups tend to remain unoxidized. The myofibrillary proteins actin and myosin contain significant numbers of cysteine residues per molecule and it is possible that these proteins supply significant numbers of binding sites to iron in the gastrointestinal tract, thus maintaining it in solution (Hurrell *et al.*, 1988). Data contradictory to the cysteine findings have been generated by *in vitro* study of iron complex formation with amino acids and peptides. These show that complex formation involves only carboxylic groups and not thiol groups (Fitzsimmons *et al.*, 1985; Shears *et al.*, 1987). To complicate the issue further, it has been reported that soluble ferrous iron increases during *in vitro* beef digestion suggesting that the meat factor may enhance reduction (Kapsokefalou and Miller, 1991). This, however, has not been observed in other *in vitro* studies (Slatkavitz and Clydesdale, 1988). Further work is clearly required to resolve these issues.

Besides solubilization of iron by peptides, stimulation of gastric acid secretion is enhanced by meat and the time taken to reach a pH <3 is significantly less from meat than from other proteins. The relationship between the time taken from the gastric contents to reach a pH <3 and enhanced absorption from different protein sources has been noted (Zhang *et al.*, 1990) although direct measurements to confirm this are not available.

(b) *Iron absorption from vegetable proteins*. Iron absorption from vegetable protein sources tends to be lower than that from animal tissue sources. Because of their relative low cost and wide availability as a source of protein, soybean products are widely used in infant formulae, as extenders in meat products, in baked goods, and in dairy type products (Erdman and Fordyce, 1989). Non-haem iron absorption from soybean protein is significantly reduced (Cook *et al.*, 1981; Morck *et al.*, 1982; Gillooly *et al.*, 1984b; Derman *et al.*, 1987), although this is partly offset by the relatively high iron content of soy products (Hallberg and Rossander, 1982b) and the apparent enhancing effect on haem iron absorption (Lynch *et al.*, 1985). Similar to the findings of poor iron bioavailability from soybeans, other members of the legume family (Lynch *et al.*, 1984; MacFarlane *et al.*, 1988a) and nut family (MacFarlane *et al.*, 1988b) also have low iron bioavailability. Because of the extensive use and importance of soy products, vigorous attempts have been made to isolate the soybean factor responsible for the inhibitory effect on iron absorption. Baking isolated soy protein, whole soybeans and soy products of low availability was reported to result in a modest improvement in iron bioavailability (Morck *et al.*, 1982). This observation was not, however, confirmed by other workers (Derman *et al.*, 1987). The use of various soy fractions such as full fat soy flour, textured soy flour, and fermented soy products such as silken tofu, sufu, tempeh, natto and miso are associated with an improvement in bioavailability which correlates roughly with the size of the predominant polypeptides present in the given product (MacFarlane *et al.*, 1990). Indeed, extensively degraded soy protein, such as is found in the fermentation products miso (MacFarlane *et al.*, 1990) and soy sauce (Baynes *et al.*, 1990), actually act as promoters of non-haem iron absorption.

A cause, in addition to the protein composition, for the inhibitory effect of intact soy protein has not been isolated. The possible relationship of phytate content to the inhibition is controversial. Hydroponically radioiron labelled soybeans containing varying phosphate and phytate contents did not show differences in iron absorption studies in rats or man (Hallberg and Rossander, 1982b; Beard *et al.*, 1988). Absorption from phytate-free soy flour was two-fold greater than from nondephytenized soy flour but this difference was not of sufficient magnitude by itself to explain the soy effect (MacFarlane *et al.*, 1990). The soybean contains only modest amounts of polyphenols (Rao and Prabhavathi, 1982). Soy products containing high calcium contents have reduced non-haem iron absorption (MacFarlane *et al.*, 1990). Soy protein itself may affect iron absorption in *in vivo* studies (Schricker *et al.*, 1982; Berner and Miller, 1985). An additional factor in the effect of soy protein on non-haem iron absorption relates to the possibility that adequate proteolysis to yield non-inhibitory peptides might be complete only at a level in the gut beyond the point of maximal iron absorption.

While the inhibitory effect of soy protein on iron absorption is well established in single meal studies its presence in the diet has a less clearly defined impact on iron nutrition. In a study of various forms of infant formulae, a soybean based formula had no disadvantage in terms of infant nutrition (Hertrampf *et al.*, 1986). Long-term ingestion of soy protein over 6 months did not result in any changes in iron status in males (Morris *et al.*, 1987). While dietary manoeuvres are unlikely, *per se*, to modify iron sufficiency in meals (Chapter 7), the suggestion is that soybean in the mixed diet has limited adverse influence on iron nutrition.

(c) *Interactions of protein and promoting and inhibitory ligands.* Ultimately, absorption of non-haem iron in a mixed meal is dependent upon the complex interactions of the various components of that meal. Whether absorption is unaffected, enhanced or reduced reflects, in part, the outcome of these interactions. While the hydroxyl moieties of the polyphenols contained in the food strongly bind iron, they also form complexes with proteins which may interfere with iron binding to the polyphenol complex. Thus the presence of protein in a meal may lead to reduction of the inhibitory effect of polyphenols.

Improved iron absorption from phytate-containing food in the presence of meat may be due to the formation of complexes between phytate and peptides or amino acids released from meat at low pH in the stomach. These complexes are fairly insoluble below pH 3 and may therefore limit iron complexing to the phytate molecule (Lynch *et al.*, 1989a). Furthermore, the amino acids, or more likely, peptide products of protein digestion may form chelates with iron thus impeding iron complexing with phytate present (Berner and Miller, 1985). These observations indicate that, direct promotor–inhibitor interactions may be as important as iron–chelator interactions. Further investigation is required to understand these complex interactions.

3.5. Reservations about Single Meal Studies

The wealth of data collected concerning food iron bioavailability in man is derived predominantly from single meal studies. The setting used to study the single meal does not reflect the usual conditions encountered during the absorptive process, consisting as it does of a protracted overnight fast, the single meal administration, and subsequently another period of fasting. The observations already outlined, indicating a discrepancy between promotory ligand (e.g. ascorbic acid) and inhibitory factor (e.g. soy protein) activity as judged by single meals and their lack of impact on observed human nutrition, raise the possibility that single meal studies exaggerate the measurement of food iron bioavailability. This suspicion was further highlighted in a recent study (discussed more fully in Chapter 7) in which chronically labelled diets achieved a ratio of only 2.5 for a maximally promotory diet, whereas in a maximally inhibitory diet for non-haem iron bioavailability the ratio based on single meal studies was 6 (Cook *et al.*, 1991a). Since the models used to predict dietary iron bioavailability are heavily predicated on single meal data, further work is required to define more clearly the relationship between single meal and dietary bioavailability estimates.

3.6. Mechanism of Non-haem Iron Absorption

Non-haem iron absorption involves a series of overlapping steps. These mechanistically distinct, yet temporally synchronous, stages include iron binding to the brush border, uptake of bound iron into the interior of the cell, intracellular handling of the iron, transcellular transport and finally, transport from the basolateral surface of the mucosal cell into the portal circulation. Iron uptake occurs predominantly in the proximal small bowel with the duodenum being the site of maximal absorption (Becker *et al.*, 1979; Johnson *et al.* 1983; Muir and Hopfer, 1985; Conrad *et al.*, 1987). It is at this level that the regulation of absorption is most apparent.

3.6.1. *Mucosal Iron Uptake*

A number of different mechanisms of non-haem iron uptake by the mucosal cell have been described in a variety of models. Three main mechanisms of non-haem iron-binding to the brush border have been reported, namely non-specific low affinity binding, binding to a high affinity receptor and binding to an elutable factor responsible for presentation to the mechanism involved in shuttling iron into the interior of the cell. It is likely that several mechanisms co-exist, for example, a saturable high affinity iron uptake mechanism via a specific receptor along with a non-saturable low affinity mechanism with linear uptake mainly evident at higher iron concentrations (Srai *et al.*, 1988).

In terms of specific receptors, one of the first putatively identified was the transferrin receptor. This was thought to be expressed on the luminal surface and to bind diferric transferrin resulting from the combination of luminal non-haem iron with apotransferrin of biliary and intestinal origin (Huebers *et al.*, 1983). Enthusiasm for this model has waned as contrary evidence has mounted. Neither transferrin nor transferrin receptors have been detected in the apical microvillous brush borders in the proximal small bowel using immunolocalization techniques (Levine and Seligman, 1984; Parmley *et al.*, 1985; Banerjee *et al.*, 1986; Osterloh *et al.*, 1988; Levine and Woods, 1990). *In vivo* studies administering ^{59}Fe-labelled transferrin to achlorhydrics did not show enhanced iron absorption suggesting that transferrin does not play a physiological role in iron absorption in humans (Bezwoda *et al.*, 1986). The hypotransferrinaemic mouse has enhanced iron absorption despite a lack of transferrin in the bowel lumen, mucosal cells and plasma suggesting that transferrin is not important for iron uptake or transport across the mucosal cell (Simpson *et al.*, 1991). Based on these observations, transferrin and its receptor are unlikely to be the major iron transporter from the lumen into the mucosal cell (Osterloh *et al.*, 1987a).

Despite these contrary data, numerous studies have demonstrated the presence of putative transferrin and lactoferrin receptors in a number of different species (Cox *et al.*, 1979; Mazurier *et al.*, 1985; Hu *et al.*, 1988; Kawakami *et al.*, 1990; Hisayasu *et al.*, 1991). Their presence in suckling animals may have particular ontogenetic relevance and suggests that they may well be involved in binding their respective iron transport proteins in milk. Given their relatively low affinity constant, ranging from 1.03 to $4.9 \times 10^6 \, M^{-1}$ (Kawakami *et al.*, 1990; Hisayasu *et al.*, 1991), suggested shared specificities and paucity of complete characterization, further work is required before their relevance to iron absorption in these species and, more particularly, in man can be evaluated.

A new iron-binding protein has recently been isolated in microvillous membrane vesicles of the upper small intestine. This putative receptor has high affinity for ferric iron and facilitates ferric iron transport across the microvillous membrane vesicles. Uptake is temperature dependent and is inhibited by pronase pretreatment. The receptor is a glycoprotein of 160 kDa consisting of three 54 kDa monomeric peptides (Teichmann and Stremmel, 1990). The receptor protein is also present in the stomach and liver, but is not found in the oesophagus. Based on its physicochemical and immunological features, it is distinct from other iron-binding proteins. The concentration in the duodenum is increased in iron deficiency and reduced in secondary iron overload suggesting that its concentration is responsive to iron status (Stremmel *et al.*, 1991).

A variety of fatty acids present in lipid extracts of brush border membrane vesicles have iron binding capabilities. Iron binding to these fatty acids is pH dependent. Purified lipid extracts including phosphatidic acid, phosphatidyl serine, oleic acid and stearic acid have significant iron binding capabilities. It is possible that these lipid components in the duodenal brush border membrane vesicles have a role in iron binding and uptake into the mucosal cell (Simpson and Peters, 1987).

Understanding post-surface adsorption transmembrane iron transport is clearly dependent upon which binding mechanism and which valency state appear to be predominant. One candidate mechanism would be that of simple diffusion (Sheehan, 1976; Eastham *et al.*, 1977; Savin and Cook, 1978). In this regard, there are conflicting data as to whether the process is energy independent (MacDermott and Greenberger, 1969) or not (Cox and Peters, 1979). A transmembrane protein, identified as an integrin and located in microvilli, which consists of two protein chains of 150 kDa and 90 kDa, has recently been described as playing a role in transmembrane iron transport (Conrad *et al.*, 1993). Other candidate mechanisms might include facilitated diffusion, entry via a ferrous or ferric iron channel, fluid phase endocytosis, adsorptive pinocytosis, or receptor mediated endocytosis. Not only is understanding this process of relevance to iron absorption it may also provide insight to the general issue of transmembrane iron transport.

3.6.2. *Mucosal Iron Handling and Intracellular Iron Transport*

With respect to internalized iron, the mucosal cell may be viewed as two separate compartments, an iron storage compartment and an iron transfer pathway. Little is known regarding the transfer mechanism through the cell. Iron moves rapidly through this transfer pathway since most is absorbed into the body within a 2–4 hour period after ingestion (Worwood and Jacobs, 1972). Iron absorption from a meal is essentially complete within 24 hours and only trivial amounts will be absorbed into the circulation from the mucosal cell after this time. The excess iron taken up into the mucosal cell from the gastrointestinal lumen and which has not entered the transfer pathway, is diverted to the storage compartment. Only small amounts of the iron that have entered the storage compartment re-enter the transfer pathway. Estimates of this late release compartment are of the order of 10% (Wheby *et al.*, 1964).

The mechanism of transcellular iron transport is unknown. Transferrin has been implicated as playing a role. Transferrin isolated from mucosal cells is similar to serum transferrin but differences in amino acid composition have been suggested (Huebers *et al.*, 1976; Pollack and Lasky, 1976). Its original structure may be modified by proteolysis (Purves *et al.*, 1988). Significant amounts of iron are found in the transferrin fraction of mucosal cell homogenates early after radiolabelled iron administration to rats (Huebers, 1975). After instillation of radioiron into gut loops, lower levels of radioiron were bound to transferrin in animals with normal iron stores than in iron deficient rats (Huebers, 1975). Other studies in the rat indicated that the magnitude of iron absorbed into the carcass, reflecting mucosal cell transfer, correlate directly with mucosal cell transferin concentration (Savin and Cook, 1978, 1980). The mucosal cell transferrin content was observed to be inversely related to iron status thereby mimicking transferrin in the serum. While these studies suggest a possible role for transferrin in the transfer of iron across the mucosal cell, these observations have been questioned as, for example, in a rat model with induced inflammation where iron absorption was reduced despite raised mucosal transferrin concentrations (Savin, 1984). As already discussed on p. 169, atransferrinaemic mice (Simpson *et al.*, 1991), and patients, have iron overload due to enhanced absorption, while hypoxic rats with increased iron absorption do not have appreciable changes in mucosal transferrin concentration despite increases in plasma transferrin levels (Osterloh *et al.*, 1987b).

Studies in man reveal that mucosal transferrin levels are not different in iron deficient subjects and subjects with normal iron stores, and do not show a correlation with iron storage status or with non-haem or haem iron absorption from a standard meal (Whittaker *et al.*, 1989c). Furthermore, mucosal transferrin levels in patients with idiopathic haemochromatosis and increased iron absorption were decreased, rather than elevated. Mucosal transferrin levels may rise only when severe iron deficiency is present. These observations suggest that mucosal cell transferrin does not play a regulating role in iron transfer through the cell, at least in the absence of severe iron deficiency.

Perhaps the most persuasive argument against a transfer role for mucosal transferrin is the finding that transferrin mRNA is absent in rat and human gastroduodenal mucosal cells (Idzerda *et al.*, 1986; Pietrangelo *et al.*, 1992). The lack of transferrin mRNA within the mucosal cell suggests that transferrin is not produced within the mucosal cell. It is likely that mucosal transferrin is derived from entry through transferrin receptors at the basolateral surface of the cells which is the mechanism responsible for supplying iron for cellular growth and development (Banerjee *et al.*, 1986). In addition, the presence of transferrin in mucosal cell isolates may be partly due to serum contamination of mucosal cell preparations (Osterloh *et al.*, 1987a).

The newly identified iron-binding protein, mobilferrin, localized in the apical cytoplasm of proximal small bowel mucosa is capable of reversibly binding iron, one mole of protein binding one mole of iron (Conrad *et al.*, 1990, 1992). This protein has a lower affinity for iron than iron binding proteins such as transferrin. The protein is not found in other organs and is capable of binding other metals such as copper, zinc, cobalt and lead. The ability of this protein to transport iron across the cell has not been established. Its location in the apical cytoplasm, and its apparent close association with integrin (Conrad *et al.*, 1993), does suggest a possible role in iron transit. Further work is required to confirm and extend these observations.

Ferritin acts as a repository for excess iron within a cell. In the latter phases of absorption, proportionately increased amounts of iron are deposited in the ferritin fraction while iron in the transferrin fraction progressively decreases (Huebers, 1975). In iron deficient animals, reduced amounts of radioiron are incorporated into the ferritin fraction during absorption. It is possible that the ferritin content of the mucosal cells has some effect on determining the amount of iron entering the circulation from the cell although, with its major function related to sequestration of excess cellular iron, its concentration may only passively reflect the transcellular kinetics of absorbed and delivered iron. The ferritin content of the mucosal cell correlates directly with iron status, levels being low in iron deficient states and high in secondary iron overload in both animals and man (Halliday *et al.*, 1978; Savin and Cook, 1980; Whittaker *et al.*, 1989c).

Both L- and H-rich ferritin are found in the mucosal cell in man (Halliday *et al.*, 1978; Whittaker *et al.*, 1989c). The L-rich ferritin content of the mucosal cell correlates with storage iron status and bears an indirect relationship to non-haem and haem iron absorption, the relationship with non-haem iron absorption being more significant. The L-rich ferritin concentration of the duodenal mucosal cell rises with the administration of oral iron, reflecting the amount of iron entering the cell (Halliday *et al.*, 1978). While L-rich ferritin is well established as an iron storage protein, the role played by H-rich ferritin is less well understood. H-rich ferritin has been shown to incorporate and release iron more rapidly than L-rich ferritin in other cells. Whether H-rich ferritin plays a role in intracellular shuttling or short-term storage of iron is unknown: like red blood cell precursors, duodenal mucosal cells have an active internal iron circuit and their isoferritin distribution is similar, the ratio of L- to H-ferritin being approximately 1.5 in situations of normal iron status. The isoferritin ratio is equal or reversed in iron deficiency (Whittaker *et al.*, 1989c). H-rich ferritin also displays an inverse relationship with non-haem and haem iron absorption and a direct relationship with storage iron status. Patients with idiopathic haemochromatosis and a demonstrated increase in iron absorption have lower than expected mucosal ferritin concentrations relative to serum ferritin concentrations. This has suggested that dysregulation of ferritin synthesis, reduced stability or enhanced degradation may be the metabolic defect in idiopathic haemochromatosis. This conclusion may be inappropriate since disproportionate cellular ferritin content may result from dysregulated transcellular transfer or release of the absorbed iron. Support for this latter view is found in the observation that raised mucosal cell ferritin levels are induced in these patients by oral iron administration (Halliday *et al.*, 1978).

While transferrin mRNA has not been detected in mucosal cells from gastric or duodenal tissue, mRNAs for both L- and H-ferritin subunits are present. The mRNA levels for both subunits are reduced in patients with iron deficiency and are raised in patients with secondary iron overload. The mRNA levels for both are higher in duodenal cells than in gastric mucosal cells. This suggests that the ferritin mRNA level in the duodenal mucosal cell reflects, in part, the amount of iron absorbed, with the intracellular ferritin content being, in part, transcriptionally regulated by the amount of iron in the cell or passing through the cell (Pietrangelo *et al.*, 1992).

3.6.3. *Mucosal Cell Iron Transfer to Plasma*

The final step in the absorptive process is the transfer of iron across the basal surface of the mucosal cell into the portal circulation. Information regarding this mechanism is scanty. Iron may exit not only along the basal portion of the mucosal cell, but also along the sides of the cells into the lateral intercellular spaces (Parmley *et al.*, 1978). Having left the cell, the iron then has to traverse the interstitial space and the endothelial cell to enter the portal venous system. Macrophages in the villous interstitium have been implicated as providing a further late control step in determining iron absorption (Bjorn-Rasmussen, 1983; Refsum and Schreiner, 1984). The relative constancy and trivial size of the late release compartment determined ferrokinetically as well as the lack of a relationship to iron storage status argue against any significant physiological role for this.

The finding of transferrin receptors on the basolateral surface of mucosal cells initially was presumed to be the pathway for iron transfer from the mucosal cell to the portal circulation. Transferrin receptor levels increase in iron deficiency and this correlates with increased iron absorption occurring in iron deficiency. Iron overload is associated with reduced numbers of transferrin receptors. However, a number of studies have dispelled this theory. With normal iron status, receptors are found on the basolateral surfaces of mucosal cells located in the crypts and basal portions of the villi with decreased density of receptors towards the apical segments of the villi. In iron deficiency, transferrin receptors extend up to apical villous cells as well (Anderson *et al.*, 1990, 1991). However, while mucosal cell transferrin receptors increase in iron deficiency along with increased iron absorption, when iron absorption is increased by inducing haemolysis in rats, receptor density and binding affinity remain unchanged from control animals indicating no relationship between iron absorption and receptor numbers (Anderson *et al.*, 1990). Similar changes in transferrin receptor levels related to iron status occur in non-absorbing areas of the bowel such as the gastric mucosa and distal segments of the intestine (Anderson *et al.*, 1991). Transferrin receptor mRNA is found in mucosal cells of the stomach and duodenum and mRNA levels do not differ in these two bowel segments in subjects with normal iron stores (Pietrangelo *et al.*, 1992). In iron deficiency, transferrin receptor mRNA levels increase only in duodenal mucosal cells. This is thought to occur due to rapid iron transfer through the iron deficient mucosal cell contributing to perceived cellular iron deficiency relative to the rest of the intestinal mucosa. This feature is further substantiated by reduced ferritin mRNA levels in these cells in iron deficiency (Pietrangelo et al., 1992). In patients with secondary iron overload, transferrin receptor mRNA levels are reduced. Based on observations in neonatal and adult rats, transferrin receptors in the basolateral surface of mucosal cells sequester iron from portal blood, via binding of diferric transferrin, to meet the iron requirements of proliferation and cellular metabolism (Anderson et al., 1991). The available data suggest that, in part, mucosal transferrin receptor content may be transcriptionally regulated.

An in vitro model examining iron transfer from the mucosal cell, using cultured mouse duodenal enterocytes, indicates that iron release is temperature dependent. Addition of previously dialysed serum to the culture medium leads to failure of iron release from the cells to the medium, and addition of the dialysate back into the medium restores the ability to release iron to transferrin. These observations suggest that low molecular weight serum components may mediate iron transfer out of the mucosal cell (Snape and Simpson, 1991). Addition of bicarbonate, amino acids and various organic acids to dialysed serum leads to restoration of iron release from the mucosal cells (Snape and Simpson, 1991). The relevance of these observations to the in vivo situation requires further refinement given that serum does not directly bathe the basal aspect of mucosal cells. Iron appears in the portal blood within minutes of its instillation into small bowel loops in a rat model and peak levels occur in 6 to 8 minutes. Most of the iron appearing in the portal blood of rats whose iron binding capacity had been saturated with exogenous iron was in the ferrous state, irrespective of whether ferrous or ferric iron was instilled in the bowel loop: 63% of the iron in the portal blood was in the ferrous state after administration of ferric iron and 86% was in the ferrous state when ferrous iron was administered (Wollenberg et al., 1990). These findings suggest that iron is released by the mucosal cell in the ferrous state and is probably reduced from ferric iron at the basolateral membrane prior to release by unknown mechanisms (Eastham et al., 1977; Wollenberg et al., 1990). The model may be a reflection of the situation pertaining in idiopathic haemochromatosis where the presence of non-transferrin iron in circulation is well documented.

After release from the mucosal cell, iron traverses the interstitial space and has to pass through endothelial cells of the portal capillary system. It is possible that small molecular weight chelators or ligands are involved (Snape and Simpson, 1991). Ceruloplasmin may also be involved in the transfer. Iron absorption is enhanced by the intravenous injection of ceruloplasmin in copper deficient rats. This increase in absorption occurs rapidly after ceruloplasmin injection. It is assumed that the ferrous iron that diffuses to the portal capillary system, bound to low molecular weight ligand, is oxidized by ceruloplasmin upon entry into the capillary wall, thus producing a ferric moiety for binding to transferrin (Wollenberg et al., 1990).

4. REGULATION OF IRON ABSORPTION

4.1. Factors Affecting Iron Absorption

Complex interrelationships between food and its iron constituents occur in the gastro-intestinal lumen which influence the amount of iron made available to the mucosal cells for absorption. Dietary non-haem iron is significantly more affected by these factors than is haem iron. The interplay of enhancing and inhibiting ligands with the non-haem iron pool in the gastrointestinal lumen has some importance in affecting the amount of iron absorbed. The proportion of haem iron and non-haem iron contained in an individual mixed meal is probably of greater importance. While non-haem iron absorption is influenced by the total iron contained in a meal, haem iron is relatively unaffected (Bezwoda *et al.*, 1983). Populations eating a diet with a high meat content, and thus a high haem iron content, tend to have adequate amounts of available dietary iron which leads to a reduced incidence of iron deficiency (Chapter 7). This situation pertains to industrialized countries and may contribute to raised iron absorption and an increased incidence of iron overload in subjects who carry the gene for idiopathic haemochromatosis. In situations where the diet contains no meat or haem iron, iron assimilation is reduced and maintenance of a normal iron balance becomes more problematic. This is especially true when the total daily iron intake is marginal, where the diet lacks other enhancers of iron absorption, and where total iron content reflects a significant contribution from contaminant iron. The latter circumstance pertains to many developing regions. When iron demands are greatest, such as in pregnancy, growing children and menstruating women, such dietary considerations assume major importance. When demands are less, as in adult men, these considerations have less impact on iron balance (Cook, 1990).

The mucosal cell itself influences iron absorption. Transplantation of small intestine from iron deficient rats and iron overloaded rats into isogeneic iron deficient rats reveal significant differences in iron absorption. Iron uptake by the mucosal cells and iron transfer into the carcass is significantly increased from intestines transplanted from iron deficient animals compared with intestines transplanted from iron overloaded animals (Adams *et al.*, 1991). Short-term control of absorption at the level of the mucosal cell, independent of body iron storage status, has also been demonstrated in other experiments, where altering mucosal cell iron concentration with a high iron containing meal results in reduction in absorption from a test meal given subsequently (Fairweather-Tait and Wright, 1984; Fairweather-Tait *et al.*, 1985). Thus, mucosal cell iron content appears to play a role in determining the amount of iron absorbed. The iron content of the mucosal cell may be partly self-regulated to ensure a sufficient concentration for its own metabolic requirements. This may be achieved by iron entering from the gastrointestinal lumen or via the transferrin receptors at the base of the mucosal cells, or by both of these pathways. When the mucosal cell achieves sufficient iron content, transferrin receptor mRNA levels are down-regulated and, at the same time, ferritin mRNA levels are increased so that sufficient amounts of apoferritin are produced to sequester excess iron in the internal cellular environment (Pietrangelo *et al.*, 1992). While this suggests control in the mucosal cell at a transcriptional level, further work is required to establish whether post-transcriptional regulation, well-described in other cell types (Chapter 5), is also operative. This control may occur to a greater degree in younger cells at the base of the crypts and is perhaps not entirely lost in older cells which have migrated towards the apical portions of the villi.

Absent synthesis of NF-E2, a nuclear DNA-binding protein, and of its corresponding mRNA due to defective gene encoding, has been associated with the hypochromic microcytic anaemia and defective iron uptake by red blood cells and intestinal mucosal cells seen in homozygous Mk mice (Peters *et al.*, 1993). Further evaluation of the potential role of such a regulatory factor in other mammals and man will be of great interest.

A number of internal factors affect iron absorption. Major determinants include storage iron status, erythropoietic activity and hypoxia. The extent to which this latter effect is mediated through increased erythropoiesis or by a direct effect of hypoxia on the mucosal cell itself remains to be fully defined. Direct relationships between absorption and the plasma iron turnover, transferrin saturation and whole body transferrin receptor concentrations have also been described. How these various influences affect the ability of the mucosal cell to modulate iron entry into the body remains one of the major important unanswered questions in ferrobiology.

4.2. Sites at which Absorption may be Regulated

The major sites at which non-haem iron absorption is regulated are at the level of iron uptake by the mucosal cell from the intestinal lumen and at the level of iron transfer from the basal surface of the mucosal cell to the portal circulation. Both these steps are influenced by storage iron status. Uptake by the mucosal cell appears to be the main site of regulation of non-haem iron absorption (Nathanson and McLaren, 1987). Prior intake of a high iron diet or parenteral iron loading in rats diminishes iron uptake by the mucosal cell (Charlton *et al.*, 1965). This could not be attributed to increased iron content of the mucosal cell itself. The observation of a delay between systemic iron loading and a reduction in absorption is compatible with the notion that absorptive capacity is conditioned in the young crypt cell but that a delay for migration to the villous apex is required for these cells to participate maximally in absorption. Haem iron absorption is controlled largely at the site of transfer from the mucosal cell to the portal circulation although the entry of haem from the gut lumen to the mucosal cell may be increased in iron deficiency (Wheby and Spyker, 1981). This difference in sites of control of non-haem and haem iron absorption results in a greater sensitivity of non-haem iron absorption to changes in iron stores.

That these two sites are implicated in the regulation of absorption is emphasized by observations in idiopathic haemochromatosis where the defect in absorption appears to be at the level of iron transfer from the mucosal cell to the portal circulation. Abnormal control at this level is evident by loss of the inverse relationship between haem iron absorption and body iron stores (Lynch *et al.*, 1989b). Absorption of non-haem iron is also excessive in relation to iron stores but some regulation of absorption, compatible with the controlling step being that of non-haem iron entry into the mucosal cell, is retained (Powell *et al.*, 1970; Marx, 1979; Lynch *et al.*, 1989b). Increased transfer of iron from the mucosal cell into the portal circulation was also identified as the major site of abnormal absorption control in idiopathic haemochromatosis patients using a kinetic model of absorption (McLaren *et al.*, 1991). Diminished ferritin protein content occurs in reticuloendothelial cells as well as the mucosal cells in these patients. This has been implicated as the cause of the disordered internal and external iron exchange. The diminished ferritin levels in the mucosal cell are more likely, however, to be due to enhanced transfer of iron from the mucosal cell into the portal circulation. The finding of increased numbers of transferrin receptors on the basal surface of the mucosal cells in idiopathic haemochromatosis is in keeping with enhanced transfer of iron out of the mucosal cell rendering the cell relatively iron deficient. The disturbance of iron absorption in idiopathic haemochromatosis is discussed further in Chapter 8.

4.3. Effect of Iron Status

Storage iron status is one of the best known internal factors regulating absorption and a number of examples depicting this relationship exist in both animal models and humans (Cook et al., 1974; Walters et al., 1975; Magnusson et al., 1981; Baynes et al., 1987; Cook, 1990). Despite vast knowledge regarding the relationship between iron stores and absorption, the mechanism by which the duodenal mucosal cell is appraised of storage iron status is unknown. While it is conventional to plot the relationship between serum ferritin and iron absorption on a log–log basis, the arithmetic relationship between serum ferritin and absorption in humans shows two absorptive phases in relation to stores, i.e. slowly increasing absorption as iron stores decline from high to normal levels of approximately 200–300 mg and a second phase characterized by a steeper rise in absorption as iron stores decline further (Baynes et al., 1987). This suggests two phases of body iron regulation of absorption. At normal iron stores, a minor level of control is apparent which is responsible for fine adjustments in iron absorption whereas, when iron stores are depleted, a major level of control becomes operative and is responsible for significantly increased absorption rates. Similar data are evident from the relationship between serum transferrin receptor concentration and iron absorption. More specifically, a direct relationship was observed over the iron deficient range but no relationship was seen in the non-deficient range (Cook et al., 1990).

Using the regression line derived from the log of non-haem food iron absorption obtained from a number of food iron absorption studies, on the log of serum ferritin, a slope of approximately −1.0 is observed (Cook et al., 1991a). Although absolute absorption levels from different meals may vary depending on the nature of the food constituents, the slope of the regression line between log absorption and log serum ferritin tends to remain constant (Taylor et al., 1988; Cook et al., 1991a). Other measurements of iron status have been examined to establish their relationship with iron absorption, including per cent transferrin saturation, but these measurements are less satisfactory than serum ferritin (Baynes et al., 1987; Taylor et al., 1988). In vitro studies of iron transfer from cultured rat mucosal cells indicate that iron release is enhanced by the presence of unsaturated rather than saturated transferrin (Levine et al., 1972). However, in vivo models have not defined a clear association between transferrin saturation and absorption. Iron absorption still proceeds despite saturation of transferrin with iron (Wheby and Jones, 1963).

A liver transplantation model in rats has been used to establish whether the liver has a specific regulatory function in relation to iron absorption. Prior to transplantation, the livers of donor animals were iron loaded using carbonyl iron to label predominantly the hepatocytes or parenteral iron dextran to label predominantly the Kupffer cells. These livers were transplated into isogeneic rats with normal iron status. Significant differences in absorption were noted, with a 20-fold reduction in absorption where the transplanted liver had predominantly hepatocyte iron loading, as compared with a 0.5-fold reduction with predominant Kupffer cell iron loading (Adams *et al.*, 1989). The findings suggest that hepatocyte iron content may be related to a putative messenger controlling absorption. Attempts to alter absorption by infusion of various proteins including transferrin, ferritin, and extracts from rat liver and spleen, have not shown any significant effect. However, infusion of plasma from pregnant women into rats has shown enhanced iron absorption suggesting a possible hormonal regulator (Apte and Brown, 1969).

4.4. Effect of Erythropoiesis

Evidence for increased iron absorption due to enhanced erythropoiesis is based on clinical observations in patients with chronic haematological disorders associated with significant ineffective erythropoiesis as seen in thalassaemia major and sideroblastic anaemias (Bothwell *et al.*, 1979). In haemolytic disorders with effective red cell production such as hereditary spherocytosis, glucose-6-phosphate dehydrogenase deficiency and chronic autoimmune haemolytic anaemias, only modest effects on iron absorption occur and it is unusual for these patients to develop significant iron overload. Patients with ineffective erythropoiesis, however, develop iron overload due to enhanced iron absorption (Bothwell *et al.*, 1979; Pippard *et al.*, 1979). Enhanced erythropoiesis is probably responsible for the increased absorption noted in subjects who have been transported to high altitudes. However, hypoxia itself may have a direct effect on the bowel mucosa and cause enhanced iron absorption. Studies examining the role of erythropoiesis in absorption during hypoxia are not fully conclusive and the quantitative importance of enhanced erythropoiesis is unclear (Raja *et al.*, 1986). However, differential effects of hypoxia and enhanced erythropoiesis, on mucosal iron uptake and subsequent iron transfer to the body respectively were found in mice (Raja *et al.*, 1988, 1989) suggesting independent regulatory effects of these two variables at different stages of the iron absorptive process. Recent data showing that enhanced erythropoiesis is commonly associated with iron deficient erythropoiesis despite normal iron stores raises the possibility that distinction between an erythropoietic and iron status related signal may be spurious (Cazzola *et al.*, 1987).

A possible mechanism for an effect of erythropoiesis on iron absorption has been suggested by Cavill *et al.* (1975). These workers postulated that the rate of tissue iron uptake from the plasma and the size of the labile iron pool in various body tissues influences iron absorption. The bowel mucosal cell normally contains proportionally larger labile iron pools. Iron absorption is predicted to increase when outflow of iron from the plasma is increased. The outflow is determined by the total mass of transferrin receptors which are normally predominantly present on the erythroid precursors. Thus, stimulation of erythropoiesis with resultant increased transferrin receptor mass in the erythroid marrow leads to increased uptake of diferric transferrin from the circulating transferrin pool. Iron then shifts out of various intracellular labile iron pools including the gastrointestinal mucosal cell. The findings from a number of studies support this hypothesis. Increased iron absorption occurs following exchange transfusion of reticulocytes in rodents (Finch *et al.*, 1982; Raja *et al.*, 1989). The increase in absorption is not accompanied by a decrease in plasma iron or increase in unsaturated iron binding capacity suggesting that the iron delivered to the transfused reticulocytes is indirectly derived from labile iron pools in various tissues including the gastrointestinal tract. Absorption increased between 50 and 130% from baseline in the rat model (Finch *et al.*, 1982). Similarly, in iron deficiency, the number of transferrin receptors increase on iron deficient cells, especially those in the erythroid bone marrow where a similar increase in uptake of diferric transferrin occurs. The process whereby the increased consumption of iron on diferric transferrin by erythroid and other cellular elements is relayed to the cells of iron procurement so they may increase iron release remains unclear. The data suggest that it is not transferrin or 'empty site' mediated nor is it related to an 'activated' transferrin (Aron *et al.*, 1985).

The serum transferrin receptor concentration is a sensitive measurement of tissue receptor mass and levels rise in iron deficiency or enhanced erythropoiesis. In normal subjects there is a significant relationship between absorption from both food iron and inorganic iron, and transferrin receptor concentration. However, this is less clear cut than is the relationship between serum ferritin and absorption. The correlation between serum transferrin receptor and absorption is, as previously mentioned, no longer significant when subjects with depleted iron stores are excluded (Cook *et al.*, 1990). These findings are in line with the observation that the concentration of serum transferrin receptors is a better index of functional iron deficiency than of iron storage status (Skikne *et al.*, 1990).

In order to quantitate the component effects of erythropoiesis and iron deficiency on iron absorption a recent study was conducted in which recombinant human erythropoietin was administered to normal subjects. Significantly increased absorption due to the combined effect of enhanced erythropoiesis and mobilization of iron from stores occurred. Enhanced erythropoiesis accounted for a two- to three-fold increase in non-haem iron absorption over baseline after correction for the change occurring in iron stores with iron mobilization. This increase in erythropoiesis was approximately equal in magnitude to the effect of the reduced iron stores on absorption observed in the study as a consequence of redistribution (Skikne and Cook, 1991). While haem iron absorption also increased, it was significantly less impressive.

5. CONCLUSION

From the foregoing discussion it is clear that although much has been learnt about the mechanisms underlying, and the factors influencing iron absorption, there are still major gaps in our understanding. While gastrointestinal luminal factors which alter mucosal iron uptake from single meals are increasingly well described, their quantitative relationship to iron bioavailability from a diet taken over a long period requires further work. The precise molecular mechanisms underlying mucosal iron uptake, mucosal intracellular iron transport and subsequent transfer of iron to the plasma have still to be defined with certainty, as have the pathophysiological changes giving rise to the enhanced iron absorption seen in association with iron deficiency, with erythroid hyperplasia (particularly when this is ineffective erythropoiesis), and hypoxia. Definition of these mechanisms is likely to provide the key to understanding not only iron absorption, but also the normal close matching of iron supply to tissue iron demands in the processes of internal iron exchange (Chapter 2), and its dysregulation in pathological states of iron overload (Chapters 8 and 9).

ACKNOWLEDGEMENTS

Supported by NIH grant DK 39246 and AID Cooperative Agreement DAN-5115-A-00-7908-00. The authors thank Ms L. Kuharich for preparation of the manuscript.

REFERENCES

Adams, P. C., Reece, A. S., Powell, L. W. and Halliday, J. W. (1989) Hepatic iron in the control of iron absorption in a rat liver transplantation model. *Transplantation* **48**, 19–21.

Adams, P. C., Zhong, R., Haist, J., Flanagan, P. R. and Grant, D. R. (1991) Mucosal iron in the control of iron absorption in a rat intestinal transplant model. *Gastroenterology* **100**, 370–374.

Anderson, G. J., Powell, L. W. and Halliday, J. W. (1990) Transferrin receptor distribution and regulation in the rat small intestine. Effect of iron stores and erythropoiesis. *Gastroenterology* **98**, 576–585.

Anderson, G. J., Walsh, M. D., Powell, L. W. and Halliday, J. W. (1991) Intestinal transferrin receptors and iron absorption in the neonatal rat. *Br. J. Haematol.* **77**, 229–236.

Apte, S. V. and Brown, E. B. (1969) Effects of plasma from pregnant women on iron absorption by the rat. *Gastroenterology* **57**, 126–133.

Aron, J., Baynes, R., Bothwell, T. H., Lyons, G., Graham, B. and Torrance, J. D. (1985) Does plasma transferrin regulate iron absorption? *Scand. J. Haematol.* **35**, 451–454.

Ballot, D., Baynes, R. D., Bothwell, T. H. *et al.* (1987) The effects of fruit juices and fruits on the absorption of iron from a rice meal. *Br. J. Nutr.* **57**, 331–343.

Banerjee, D., Flanagan, P. R., Cluett, J. and Valberg, L. S. (1986) Transferrin receptors in the human gastrointestinal tract. Relationship to body iron stores. *Gastroenterology* **91**, 861–869.

Baynes, R. D., Bothwell, T. H., Bezwoda, W. R., MacPhail, A. P. and Derman, D. P. (1987) Relationship between absorption of inorganic and food iron in field studies. *Ann. Nutr. Metab.* **31**, 109–116.

Baynes, R. D., MacFarlane, B. J., Bothwell, T. H. *et al.* (1990) The promotive effect of soy sauce on iron absorption in human subjects. *Eur. J. Clin. Nutr.* **44**, 419–424.

Beard, J. L., Weaver, C. M., Lynch, S. R., Johnson, C. D., Dassenko, S. and Cook, J. D. (1988) The effect of soybean phosphate and phytate content on iron bioavailability. *Nutr. Res.* **8**, 345–352.

Becker, G., Korpilla-Schafer, S., Osterloh, K. and Forth, W. (1979) Capacity of the mucosal transfer system and absorption of iron after oral administration in rats. *Blut* **38**, 127–134.

Berner, L. A. and Miller, D. D. (1985) Effects of dietary proteins on iron bioavailability – a review. *Food Chem.* **18**, 47–69.

Bezwoda, W., Charlton, R., Bothwell, T., Torrance, J. and Mayet, F. (1978) The importance of gastric hydrochloric acid in the absorption of nonheme food iron. *J. Lab. Clin. Med.* **92**, 108–116.

Bezwoda, W. R., Bothwell, T. H., Charlton, R. W. *et al.* (1983) The relative dietary importance of haem and non-haem iron. *S. Afr. Med. J.* **64**, 552–556.

Bezwoda, W. R., MacPhail, A. P., Bothwell, T. H., Baynes, R. D., Derman, D. P. and Torrance, J. D. (1986) Failure of transferrin to enhance iron absorption in achlorhydric human subjects. *Br. J. Haematol.* **63**, 749–752.

Bjorn-Rasmussen, E. (1974) Iron absorption from wheat bread. Influence of various amounts of bran. *Nutr. Metab.* **16**, 101–110.

Bjorn-Rasmussen, E. (1983) Iron absorption: present knowledge and controversies. *Lancet* i, 914–916.

Bjorn-Rasmussen, E. and Hallberg, L. (1979) Effect of animal proteins on the absorption of food iron in man. *Nutr. Metab.* **23**, 192–202.

Bothwell, T. H., Charlton, R. W., Cook, J. D. and Finch, C. A. (1979) *Iron Metabolism in Man*, Blackwell Scientific, Oxford.

Bothwell, T. H., Baynes, R. D., MacFarlane, B. J. and MacPhail, A. P. (1989) Nutritional iron requirements and food iron absorption. *J. Int. Med.* **226**, 357–365.

Brise, H. and Hallberg, L. (1962) Absorbability of different iron compounds. *Acta Med. Scand. (Suppl.)* **17**, 23–37.

Brune, M., Rossander, L. and Hallberg, L. (1989a) Iron absorption: no intestinal adaptation to a high-phytate diet. *Am. J. Clin. Nutr.* **49**, 542–545.

Brune, M., Rossander, L. and Hallberg, L. (1989b) Iron absorption and phenolic compounds: Importance of different phenolic structures. *Eur. J. Clin. Nutr.* **43**, 547–558.

Callender, S. T., Marney, S. R., Jr and Warner, G. T. (1970) Eggs and iron absorption. *Br. J. Haematol.* **19**, 657–665.

Calvo, E., Hertrampf, E., de Pablo, S., Amar, M. and Stekel, A. (1989) Haemoglobin-fortified cereal: an alternative weaning food with high iron bioavailability. *Eur. J. Clin. Nutr.* **43**, 237–243.

Cavill, I., Worwood, M. and Jacobs, A. (1975) Internal regulation of iron absorption. *Nature* **256**, 328–329.

Cazzola, M., Pootrakul, P., Bergamaschi, G., Huebers, H. A., Eng, M. and Finch, C. A. (1987) Adequacy of iron supply for erythropoiesis: in vivo observations in humans. *J. Lab. Clin. Med.* **110**, 734–739.

Charlton, R. W., Jacobs, P., Torrance, J. D. and Bothwell, T. H. (1965) The role of the intestinal mucosa in iron absorption. *J. Clin. Invest.* **44**, 543–554.

Chidambaram, M. V., Reddy, M. B., Thompson, J. L. and Bates, G. W. (1989) In vitro studies of iron bioavailability: probing the concentration and oxidation–reduction reactivity of pinto bean iron with ferrous chromogens. *Biol. Trace Elem. Res.* **19**, 25–39.

Christensen, J. M., Ghannam, M. and Ayres, J. W. (1984) Effects of divalent amino acids on iron absorption. *J. Pharm. Sci.* **73**, 1245–1248.

Conrad, M. E. and Schade, S. G. (1968) Ascorbic acid chelates in iron absorption: a role for hydrochloric acid and bile. *Gastroenterology* **55**, 35–45.

Conrad, M. E., Cortell, S., Williams, H. L. and Foy, A. L. (1966) Polymerization and intraluminal factors in the absorption of hemoglobin iron. *J. Lab. Clin. Med.* **68**, 659–668.

Conrad, M. E., Parmley, R. T. and Osterloh, K. (1987) Small intestinal regulation of iron absorption in the rat. *J. Lab. Clin. Med.* **110**, 418–426.

Conrad, M. E., Umbreit, J. N., Moore, E. G., Peterson, R. D. and Jones, M. B. (1990) A newly identified iron binding protein in duodenal mucosa of rats. Purification and characterization of mobilferrin. *J. Biol. Chem.* **265**, 5273–5279.

Conrad, M. E., Umbreit, J. N. and Moore, E. G. (1991) A role for mucin in the absorption of inorganic iron and other metal cations. *Gastroenterology* **100**, 129–136.

Conrad, M. E., Umbreit, J. N., Moore, E. G. and Rodning, C. R. (1992) Newly identified iron-binding protein in human duodenal mucosa. *Blood* **79**, 244–247.

Conrad, M. E., Umbreit, J. N., Peterson, R. D. A., Moore, E. G. and Harper, K. P. (1993) Function of integrin in duodenal mucosal uptake of iron. *Blood* **81**, 517–521.

Cook, J. D. (1990) Adaptation in iron metabolism. *Am. J. Clin. Nutr.* **51**, 301–308.

Cook, J. D. and Monsen, E. R. (1975) Food iron absorption. I. Use of semisynthetic diet to study absorption of nonheme iron. *Am. J. Clin. Nutr.* **28**, 1289–1295.

Cook, J. D. and Monsen, E. R. (1976) Food iron absorption in human subjects. III. Comparison of the effect of animal proteins on nonheme iron absorption. *Am. J. Clin. Nutr.* **29**, 859–867.

Cook, J. D., Brown, G. M. and Valberg, L. S. (1964) The effect of achylia gastrica on iron absorption. *J. Clin. Invest.* **43**, 1185–1191.

Cook, J. D., Lipschitz, D. A., Miles, L. E. and Finch, C. A. (1974) Serum ferritin as a measure of iron stores in normal subjects. *Am. J. Clin. Nutr.* **27**, 681–687.

Cook, J. D., Morck, T. A. and Lynch, S. R. (1981) The inhibitory effect of soy products on nonheme iron absorption in man. *Am. J. Clin. Nutr.* **34**, 2622–2629.

Cook, J. D., Morck, T. A., Skikne, B. S. and Lynch, S. R. (1982) The importance of animal products in human iron nutrition. In: *Animal Products in Human Nutrition* (eds D. C. Beitz and R. G. Hansen), Academic Press, New York, p. 321.

Cook, J. D., Noble, N. L., Morck, T. A., Lynch, S. R. and Petersburg, S. J. (1983) Effect of fiber on nonheme iron absorption. *Gastroenterology* **85**, 1354–1358.

Cook, J. D., Watson, S. S., Simpson, K. M., Lipschitz, D. A. and Skikne, B. S. (1984) The effect of high ascorbic acid supplementation on body iron stores. *Blood* **64**, 721–726.

Cook, J. D., Dassenko, S. and Skikne, B. S. (1990) Serum transferrin receptor as an index of iron absorption. *Br. J. Haematol.* **75**, 603–609.

Cook, J. D., Dassenko, S. A. and Lynch, S. R. (1991a) Assessment of the role of nonheme-iron availability in iron balance. *Am. J. Clin. Nutr.* **54**, 717–722.

Cook, J. D., Dassenko, S. A. and Whittaker, P. (1991b) Calcium supplementation: Effect on iron absorption. *Am. J. Clin. Nutr.* **53**, 106–111.

Cox, T. M. and Peters, T. J. (1979) The kinetics of iron uptake in vitro by human duodenal mucosa: studies in normal subjects. *J. Physiol.* **289**, 469–478.

Cox, T. M., Mazurier, J., Spik, G., Montreuil, J. and Peters, T. J. (1979) Iron binding proteins and influx of iron across the duodenal brush border. Evidence for specific lactotransferrin receptors in the human intestine. *Biochim. Biophys. Acta* **588**, 120–128.

Derman, D. P., Bothwell, T. H., Torrance, J. D. *et al.* (1980) Iron absorption from maize (*Zea mays*) and sorghum (*Sorghum vulgare*) beer. *Br. J. Nutr.* **43**, 271–279.

Derman, D. P., Bothwell, T. H., Torrance, J. D. *et al.* (1982) Iron absorption from ferritin and ferric hydroxide. *Scand. J. Haematol.* **29**, 18–24.

Derman, D. P., Ballot, D., Bothwell, T. H. *et al.* (1987) Factors influencing the absorption of iron from soya-bean protein products. *Br. J. Nutr.* **57**, 345–353.

Disler, P. B., Lynch, S. R., Charlton, R. W. *et al.* (1975) The effect of tea on iron absorption. *Gut* **16**, 193–200.

Eastham, E. J., Bell, J. I. and Douglas, A. P. (1977) Iron-transport characteristics of vesicles of brush-border and basolateral plasma membrane from the rat enterocyte. *Biochem. J.* **164**, 289–294.

Erdman, J. W., Jr and Fordyce, E. J. (1989) Soy products and the human diet. *Am. J. Clin. Nutr.* **49**, 725–737.

Fairweather-Tait, S. J. and Wright, A. J. (1984) The influence of previous iron intake on the estimation of bioavailability of Fe from a test meal given to rats. *Br. J. Nutr.* **51**, 185–191.

Fairweather-Tait, S. J., Swindell, T. E. and Wright, A. J. (1985) Further studies in rats on the influence of previous iron intake on the estimation of bioavailability of Fe. *Br. J. Nutr.* **54**, 79–86.

Fernandez, R. and Phillips, S. F. (1982) Components of fiber bind iron in vitro. *Am. J. Clin. Nutr.* **35**, 100–106.

Finch, C. A., Huebers, H., Eng, M. and Miller, L. (1982) Effect of transfused reticulocytes on iron exchange. *Blood* **59**, 364–369.

Fitzsimmons, B. W., Hume, A., Larkworthy, L.-F., Turnbull, M. H. and Yavari, A. (1985) The preparation and characterisation of some complexes of iron (II) with amino acids. *Inorg. Chim. Acta* **106**, 109–114.

Fomon, S. J., Ziegler, E. E., Rogers, R. R. *et al.* (1989) Iron absorption from infant foods. *Pediatr. Res.* **26**, 250–254.

Forbes, A. L., Adams, C. E., Arnaud, M. J. *et al.* (1989) Comparison of in vitro, animal, and clinical determinations of iron bioavailability: International Nutritional Anemia Consultative Group Task Force report on iron bioavailability. *Am. J. Clin. Nutr.* **49**, 225–238.

Gabbe, E. E., Heinrich, H. C., Bruggemann, J. and Pfau, A. A. (1979) Iron absorption from hemiglobin (stable oxidation product of hemoglobin) in relation to the dose in subjects with normal and depleted iron stores. *Nutr. Metab.* **23**, 17–25.

Gillooly, M., Bothwell, T. H., Torrance, J. D. *et al.* (1983) The effects of organic acids, phytates and polyphenols on the absorption of iron from vegetables. *Br. J. Nutr.* **49**, 331–342.

Gillooly, M., Bothwell, T. H., Charlton, R. W. *et al.* (1984a) Factors affecting the absorption of iron from cereals. *Br. J. Nutr.* **51**, 37–46.

Gillooly, M., Torrance, J. D., Bothwell, T. H. *et al.* (1984b) The relative effect of ascorbic acid on iron absorption from soy-based and milk-based infant formulas. *Am. J. Clin. Nutr.* **40**, 522–527.

Grasbeck, R., Kuovonen, I., Lundberg, M. and Tenhunen, R. (1979) An intestinal receptor for heme. *Scand. J. Haematol.* **23**, 5–9.

Grasbeck, R., Majuri, R., Kuovonen, I. and Tenhunen, R. (1982) Spectral and other studies on the intestinal haem receptor of the pig. *Biochim. Biophys. Acta* **700**, 137–142.

Hallberg, L. (1980) Food iron absorption. In: *Methods in Hematology: Iron* (ed. J. D. Cook), Churchill Livingstone, New York, p. 116.

Hallberg, L. (1981) Bioavailable nutrient density: a new concept applied in the interpretation of food iron absorption data. *Am. J. Clin. Nutr.* **34**, 2242–2247.

Hallberg, L. (1987) Wheat fiber, phytates and iron absorption. *Scand. J. Gastroenterol.* (Suppl.), **129**, 73–79.

Hallberg, L. and Rossander, L. (1982a) Effect of different drinks on the absorption of non-heme iron from composite meals. *Hum. Nutr. Appl. Nutr.* **36**, 116–123.

Hallberg, L. and Rossander, L. (1982b) Effect of soy protein on nonheme iron absorption in man. *Am. J. Clin. Nutr.* **36**, 514–520.

Hallberg, L. and Rossander, L. (1984) Improvement of iron nutrition in developing countries: comparison of adding meat, soy protein, ascorbic acid, citric acid, and ferrous sulphate on iron absorption from a simple Latin American-type of meal. *Am. J. Clin. Nutr.* **39**, 577–583.

Hallberg, L., Bjorn-Rasmussen, E., Rossander, L. and Suwanik, R. (1977) Iron absorption from Southeast Asian diets. II. Role of various factors that might explain low absorption. *Am. J. Clin. Nutr.* **30**, 539–548.

Hallberg, L., Bjorn-Rasmussen, E., Howard, L. and Rossander, L. (1979) Dietary heme iron absorption. A discussion of possible mechanisms for the absorption-promoting effect of meat and for the regulation of iron absorption. *Scand. J. Gastroenterol.* **14**, 769–779.

Hallberg, L., Brune, M. and Rossander-Hulthen, L. (1987a) Is there a physiological role of vitamin C in iron absorption? *Ann. NY Acad. Sci.* **498**, 324–332.

Hallberg, L., Rossander, L. and Skanberg, A. B. (1987b) Phytates and the inhibitory effect of bran on iron absorption in man. *Am. J. Clin. Nutr.* **45**, 988–996.

Hallberg, L., Brune, M. and Rossander, L. (1989) Iron absorption in man: ascorbic acid and dose-dependent inhibition by phytate. *Am. J. Clin. Nutr.* **49**, 140–144.

Hallberg, L., Brune, M., Erlandsson, M., Sandberg, A.-S. and Rossander-Hulten, L. (1991) Calcium: Effect of different amounts on nonheme- and heme-iron absorption in humans. *Am. J. Clin. Nutr.* **53**, 112–119.

Halliday, J. W., Mack, U. and Powell, L. W. (1978) Duodenal ferritin content and structure: relationship with body iron stores in man. *Arch. Intern. Med.* **138**, 1109–1113.

Hazell, T. (1985) Minerals in foods: Dietary sources, chemical forms, interactions, bioavailability. *Wld. Rev. Nutr. Diet.* **46**, 1–123.

Hertrampf, E., Cayazzo, M., Pizarro, F. and Stekel, A. (1986) Bioavailability of iron in soy-based formula and its effect on iron nutriture in infancy. *Pediatrics* **78**, 640–645.

Hisayasu, S., Mugitani, K., Orimo, H. *et al.* (1991) The role of diferric transferrin in iron absorption and transferrin concentration in rat pancreatic juice and milk. *Int. J. Hematol.* **54**, 201–208.

Hu, W. L., Mazurier, J., Sawatzki, G., Montreuil, J. and Spik, G. (1988) Lactotransferrin receptor of mouse small-intestinal brush border. Binding characteristics of membrane-bound and Triton X-100-solubilized forms. *Biochem. J.* **249**, 435–441.

Huebers, H. (1975) Identification of iron binding intermediates in intestinal mucosal tissue of rats during absorption. In: *Proteins of Iron Storage and Transport in Biochemistry and Medicine* (ed. R. R. Crichton), North Holland, Amsterdam, p. 381.

Huebers, H., Huebers, E., Rummel, W. and Crichton, R. R. (1976) Isolation and characterization of iron-binding proteins from rat intestinal mucosa. *Eur. J. Biochem.* **66**, 447–455.

Huebers, H. A., Huebers, E., Csiba, E., Rummel, W. and Finch, C. A. (1983) The significance of transferrin for intestinal iron absorption. *Blood* **61**, 283–290.

Hungerford, D. M., Jr and Linder, M. C. (1983) Interactions of pH and ascorbate in intestinal iron absorption. *J. Nutr.* **113**, 2615–2622.

Hunt, J. R., Mullen, L. M., Lykken, G. I., Gallagher, S. K. and Nielsen, F. H. (1990) Ascorbic acid: Effect on ongoing iron absorption and status in iron-depleted young women. *Am. J. Clin. Nutr.* **51**, 649–655.

Hurrell, R. F., Lynch, S. R., Trinidad, T. P., Dassenko, S. A. and Cook, J. D. (1988) Iron absorption in humans: bovine serum albumin compared with beef muscle and egg white. *Am. J. Clin. Nutr.* **47**, 102–107.

Hurrell, R. F., Lynch, S. R., Trinidad, T. P., Dassenko, S. A. and Cook, J. D. (1989) Iron absorption in humans as influenced by bovine milk proteins. *Am. J. Clin. Nutr.* **49**, 546–552.

Idzerda, R. L., Huebers, H., Finch, C. A. and McKnight, G. S. (1986) Rat transferrin gene expression: tissue-specific regulation by iron deficiency. *Proc. Natl. Acad. Sci. USA* **83**, 3723–3727.

Jacobs, A. and Miles, P. M. (1970) The formation of iron complexes with bile and bile constituents. *Gut* **11**, 732–734.

Jacobs, A. and Owen, G. M. (1969) Effect of gastric juice on iron absorption in patients with gastric atrophy. *Gut* **10**, 488–490.

Jacobs, A., Rhodes, J. and Eakins, J. D. (1967) Gastric factors influencing iron absorption in anaemic patients. *Scand. J. Haematol.* **4**, 105–110.

Jacobs, P., Charlton, R. W. and Bothwell, T. H. (1968) The influence of gastric factors on the absorption of iron salts. *S. Afr. J. Med. Sci.* **33**, 53–57.

Johnson, G., Jacobs, P. and Purves, L. R. (1983) Iron binding proteins of iron-absorbing rat intestinal mucosa. *J. Clin. Invest.* **71**, 1467–1476.

Kapsokefalou, M. and Miller, D. D. (1991) Effects of meat and selected food components on the valence of nonheme iron during in vitro digestion. *J. Food Sci.* **56**, 352–358.

Kawakami, H., Dosako, S. and Lonnerdal, B. (1990) Iron uptake from transferrin and lactoferrin by rat intestinal brush-border membrane vesicles. *Am. J. Physiol.* **258**, G535–G541.

Layrisse, M., Cook, J. D., Martinez, D. *et al.* (1969) Food iron absorption: a comparison of vegetable and animal foods. *Blood* **33**, 430–443.

Layrisse, M., Martinez-Torres, C., Cook, J. D., Walker, R. and Finch, C. A. (1973) Iron fortification of food: its measurement by the extrinsic tag method. *Blood* **41**, 333–352.

Layrisse, M., Martinez-Torres, C., Leets, I., Taylor, P. and Ramirez, J. (1984) Effect of histidine, cysteine, glutathione or beef on iron absorption in humans. *J. Nutr.* **114**, 217–223.

Levine, D. S. and Woods, J. W. (1990) Immunolocalization of transferrin and transferrin receptor in mouse small intestinal absorptive cells. *J. Histochem. Cytochem.* **38**, 851–858.

Levine, D. S., Huebers, H. A., Rubin, C. E. and Finch, C. A. (1988) Blocking action of parenteral desferrioxamine on iron absorption in rodents and men. *Gastroenterology* **95**, 1242–1248.

Levine, J. S. and Seligman, P. A. (1984) The ultrastructural immunocytochemical localization of transferrin receptor (TFR) and transferrin in the gastrointestinal tract in man. *Gastroenterology* **86**, 1161a.

Levine, P. H., Levine, A. J. and Weintraub, L. R. (1972) The role of transferrin in the control of iron absorption: Studies on a cellular level. *J. Lab. Clin. Med.* **80**, 333–341.

Looker, A., Sempos, C. T., Johnson, C. and Yetley, E. A. (1988) Vitamin-mineral supplement use: association with dietary intake and iron status of adults. *J. Am. Diet. Assoc.* **88**, 808–814.

Lynch, S. R., Beard, J. L., Dassenko, S. A. and Cook, J. D. (1984) Iron absorption from legumes in humans. *Am. J. Clin. Nutr.* **40**, 42–47.

Lynch, S. R., Dassenko, S. A., Morck, T. A., Beard, J. L. and Cook, J. D. (1985) Soy protein products and heme iron absorption in humans. *Am. J. Clin. Nutr.* **41**, 13–20.

Lynch, S. R., Hurrell, R. F., Dassenko, S. A. and Cook, J. D. (1989a) The effect of dietary proteins on iron bioavailability in man. *Adv. Exp. Med. Biol.* **249**, 117–132.

Lynch, S. R., Skikne, B. S. and Cook, J. D. (1989b) Food iron absorption in idiopathic hemochromatosis. *Blood* **74**, 2187–2193.

MacDermott, R. P. and Greenberger, N. J. (1969) Evidence for a humoral factor influencing iron absorption. *Gastroenterology* **57**, 117–125.

MacFarlane, B. J., Baynes, R. D., Bothwell, T. H., Schmidt, U., Mayet, F. and Friedman, B. M. (1988a) Effect of lupines, a protein-rich legume, on iron absorption. *Eur. J. Clin. Nutr.* **42**, 683–687.

MacFarlane, B. J., Bezwoda, W. R., Bothwell, T. H. *et al.* (1988b) Inhibitory effect of nuts on iron absorption. *Am. J. Clin. Nutr.* **47**, 270–274.

MacFarlane, B. J., van der Riet, W. B., Bothwell, T. H. *et al.* (1990) Effect of traditional soy products on iron absorption. *Am. J. Clin. Nutr.* **51**, 873–880.

Magnusson, B., Bjorn-Rasmussen, E., Hallberg, L. and Rossander, L. (1981) Iron absorption in relation to iron status. Model proposed to express results to food iron absorption measurements. *Scand. J. Haematol.* **27**, 201–208.

Malone, H. E., Kevany, J. P., Scott, J. M., O'Broin, S. D. and O'Connor, G. (1986) Ascorbic acid supplementation: its effects on body iron stores and white blood cells. *Ir. J. Med. Sci.* **155**, 74–79.

Martinez-Torres, C. and Layrisse, M. (1970) Effect of amino acids on iron absorption from a staple vegetable food. *Blood* **35**, 669–682.

Martinez-Torres, C. and Layrisse, M. (1973) Nutritional factors in iron deficiency: Food iron absorption. *Clin. Haematol.* **2**, 339–352.

Martinez-Torres, C., Romano, E. and Layrisse, M. (1981) Effect of cysteine on iron absorption in man. *Am. J. Clin. Nutr.* **34**, 322–327.

Marx, J. J. (1979) Mucosal uptake, mucosal transfer and retention of iron, measured by whole-body counting. *Scand. J. Haematol.* **23**, 293–302.

Mazurier, J., Montreuil, J. and Spik, G. (1985) Visualization of lactotransferrin brush-border receptors by ligand-blotting. *Biochim. Biophys. Acta* **821**, 453–460.

McLaren, G. D., Nathanson, M. H., Jacobs, A., Trevett, D. and Thomson, W. (1991) Regulation of intestinal iron absorption and mucosal iron kinetics in hereditary hemochromatosis. *J. Lab. Clin. Med.* **117**, 390–401.

Miller, D. D., Schricker, B. R., Rasmussen, R. R. and Van Campen, D. (1981) An in vitro method for estimation of iron availability from meals. *Am. J. Clin. Nutr.* **34**, 2248–2256.

Monsen, E. R. and Cook, J. D. (1976) Food iron absorption in human subjects. IV. The effects of calcium and phosphate salts on the absorption of nonheme iron. *Am. J. Clin. Nutr.* **29**, 1142–1148.

Monsen, E. R. and Cook, J. D. (1979) Food iron absorption in human subjects. V. Effects of the major dietary constituents of semisynthetic meal. *Am. J. Clin. Nutr.* **32**, 804–808.

Morck, T. A., Lynch, S. R. and Cook, J. D. (1982) Reduction of the soy-induced inhibition of nonheme iron absorption. *Am. J. Clin. Nutr.* **36**, 219–228.

Morck, T. A., Lynch, S. R. and Cook, J. D. (1983) Inhibition of food iron absorption by coffee. *Am. J. Clin. Nutr.* **37**, 416–420.

Morris, E. R. and Ellis, R. (1982) Phytate, wheat bran, and bioavailability of dietary iron. In: *Nutritional Bioavailability of Iron* (ACS Symposium Series 203), (ed. C. Kies), American Chemical Society, Washington, DC, p. 121.

Morris, E. R., Bodwell, C. E., Miles, C. W., Mertz, W., Prather, E. S. and Canary, J. J. (1987) Long-term consumption of beef extended with soy protein by children, women and men: III. Iron absorption by adult men. *Plant Foods Hum. Nutr.* **37**, 377–389.

Muir, A. and Hopfer, U. (1985) Regional specificity of iron uptake by small intestinal brush-border membranes from normal and iron-deficient mice. *Am. J. Physiol.* **248**, G376–G379.

Nathanson, M. H. and McLaren, G. D. (1987) Computer simulation of iron absorption: regulation of mucosal and systemic iron kinetics in dogs. *J. Nutr.* **117**, 1067–1075.

Osterloh, K. R., Simpson, R. J. and Peters, T. J. (1987a) The role of muscosal transferrin in intestinal iron absorption [editorial]. *Br. J. Haematol.* **65**, 1–3.

Osterloh, K. R., Simpson, R. J., Snape, S. and Peters, T. J. (1987b) Intestinal iron absorption and mucosal transferrin in rats subjected to hypoxia. *Blut* **55**, 421–431.

Osterloh, K., Snape, S., Simpson, R. J., Grindley, H. and Peters, T. J. (1988) Subcellular distribution of recently absorbed iron and of transferrin in the mouse duodenal mucosa. *Biochim. Biophys. Acta* **969**, 166–175.

Parmley, R. T., Barton, J. C., Conrad, M. E. and Austin, R. L. (1978) Ultrastructural cytochemistry of iron absorption. *Am. J. Pathol.* **93**, 707–727.

Parmley, R. T., Barton, J. C., Conrad, M. E., Austin, R. L. and Holland, R. M. (1981) Ultrastructural cytochemistry and radioautography of hemoglobin–iron absorption. *Exp. Mol. Pathol.* **34**, 131–144.

Parmley, R. T., Barton, J. C. and Conrad, M. E. (1985) Ultrastructural localization of transferrin, transferrin receptor, and iron-binding sites on human placental and duodenal microvilli. *Br. J. Haematol.* **60**, 81–89.

Peters, L. L., Andrews, N. C., Eicher, E. M., Davidson, M. B., Orkin, S. H. and Lux, S. E. (1993) Mouse microcytic anaemia caused by a defect in the gene encoding the globin enhancer-binding protein NF-E$_2$. *Nature* **362**, 768–770.

Pietrangelo, A., Rocchi, E., Casalgrandi, G. *et al.* (1992) Regulation of transferrin, transferrin receptor, and ferritin genes in human duodenum. *Gastroenterology* **102**, 802–809.

Pippard, M. J., Callender, S. T., Warner, G. T. and Weatherall, D. J. (1979) Iron absorption and loading in beta-thalassaemia intermedia. *Lancet* **ii**, 819–821.

Pollack, S. and Lasky, F. D. (1976) A new iron-binding protein isolated from intestinal mucosa. *J. Lab. Clin. Med.* **87**, 670–679.

Powell, L. W., Campbell, C. B. and Wilson, E. (1970) Intestinal mucosal uptake of iron and iron retention in idiopathic haemochromatosis as evidence for a mucosal abnormality. *Gut* **11**, 727–731.

Purves, L. R., Purves, M., Linton, N., Brandt, W., Johnson, G. and Jacobs, P. (1988) Properties of the transferrin associated with rat intestinal mucosa. *Biochim. Biophys. Acta* **966**, 318–327.

Raja, K. B., Pippard, M. J., Simpson, R. J. and Peters, T. J. (1986) Relationship between erythropoiesis and the enhanced intestinal uptake of ferric iron in hypoxia in the mouse. *Br. J. Haematol.* **64**, 587–593.

Raja, K. B., Simpson, R. J., Pippard, M. J. and Peters, T. J. (1988) *In vivo* studies on the relationship between intestinal iron (Fe^{3+}) absorption, hypoxia and erythropoiesis in the mouse. *Br. J. Haematol.* **68**, 373–378.

Raja, K. B., Simpson, R. J. and Peters, T. J. (1989) Effect of exchange transfusion of reticulocytes on *in vitro* and *in vivo* intestinal iron (Fe^{3+}) absorption in mice. *Br. J. Haematol.* **73**, 254–259.

Rao, B. S. and Prabhavathi, T. (1982) Tannin content of foods commonly consumed in India and its influence on ionisable iron. *J. Sci. Food Agric.* **33**, 1–8.

Reddy, M. B. and Cook, J. D. (1991) Assessment of dietary determinants of nonheme-iron absorption in humans and rats. *Am. J. Clin. Nutr.* **54**, 723–728.

Refsum, S. B. and Schreiner, B. B. (1984) Regulation of iron balance by absorption and excretion. A critical review and a new hypothesis. *Scand. J. Gastroenterol.* **19**, 867–874.

Reinhold, J. G., Garcia, J. S. and Garzon, P. (1981) Binding of iron by fiber of wheat and maize. *Am. J. Clin. Nutr.* **34**, 1384–1391.

Rossander, L. (1987) Effect of dietary fiber on iron absorption in man. *Scand. J. Gastroenterol.* (Suppl.), **129**, 68–72.

Rossander-Hulthen, L., Gleerup, A. and Hallberg, L. (1990) Inhibitory effect of oat products on non-haem iron absorption in man. *Eur. J. Clin. Nutr.* **44**, 783–791.

Sanyal, A. J., Hirsch, J. I. and Moore, E. W. (1990) Premicellar taurocholate avidly binds ferrous (Fe + +) iron: a potential physiologic role for bile salts in iron absorption. *J. Lab. Clin. Med.* **116**, 76–86.

Savin, M. A. (1984) Duodenal mucosal transferrin as a regulation of iron absorption in the rat: Role in blood loss and lack of role in inflammation. *Blood* **64**, 41a.

Savin, M. A. and Cook, J. D. (1978) Iron transport by isolated rat intestinal mucosal cells. *Gastroenterology* **75**, 688–694.

Savin, M. A. and Cook, J. D. (1980) Mucosal iron transport by rat intestine. *Blood* **56**, 1029–1035.

Schricker, B. R., Miller, D. D., Rasmussen, R. R. and Van Campen, D. (1981) A comparison of in vivo and in vitro methods for determining availability of iron from meals. *Am. J. Clin. Nutr.* **34**, 2257–2263.

Schricker, B. R., Miller, D. D. and Van Campen, D. (1982) In vitro estimation of iron availability in meals containing soy products. *J. Nutr.* **112**, 1696–1705.

Sczekan, S. R. and Joshi, J. G. (1987) Isolation and characterization of ferritin from soybeans (*Glycine max*). *J. Biol. Chem.* **262**, 13780–13788.

Shears, G. E., Ledward, D. S. and Neale, R. J. (1987) Iron complexation to carboxyl groups in a bovine serum albumin digest. *Int. J. Food Sci. Tech.* **22**, 265–272.

Sheehan, R. G. (1976) Unidirectional uptake of iron across intestinal brush border. *Am. J. Physiol.* **231**, 1438–1444.

Siegenberg, D., Baynes, R. D., Bothwell, T. H. *et al.* (1991) Ascorbic acid prevents the dose-dependent inhibitory effects of polyphenols and phytate on nonheme iron absorption. *Am. J. Clin. Nutr.* **53**, 537–541.

Simpson, K. M., Morris, E. R. and Cook, J. D. (1981) The inhibitory effect of bran on iron absorption in man. *Am. J. Clin. Nutr.* **34**, 1469–1478.

Simpson, R. J. and Peters, T. J. (1987) Iron-binding lipids of rabbit duodenal brush-border membrane. *Biochim. Biophys. Acta* **898**, 181–186.

Simpson, R. J., Lombard, M., Raja, K. B., Thatcher, R. and Peters, T. J. (1991) Iron absorption by hypotransferrinaemic mice. *Br. J. Haematol.* **78**, 565–570.

Skikne, B. and Cook, J. (1991) Iron balance during recombinant erythropoietin administration (rHEPO) in normal subjects. *Blood* **78**, 90a.

Skikne, B. S., Lynch, S. R. and Cook, J. D. (1981) Role of gastric acid in food iron absorption. *Gastroenterology* **81**, 1068–1071.

Skikne, B. S., Lynch, S. R., Robinson, R. G., Spicer, J. A. and Cook, J. D. (1983) The effect of food consistency on iron absorption. *Am. J. Gastroenterol.* **78**, 607–610.

Skikne, B. S., Flowers, C. H. and Cook, J. D. (1990) Serum transferrin receptor: A quantitative measure of tissue iron deficiency. *Blood* **75**, 1870–1876.

Slatkavitz, C. A. and Clydesdale, F. M. (1988) Solubility of inorganic iron as affected by proteolytic digestion. *Am. J. Clin. Nutr.* **47**, 487–495.

Snape, S. and Simpson, R. J. (1991) Iron binding to, and release from, the basolateral membrane of mouse duodenal enterocytes. *Biochim. Biophys. Acta* **1074**, 159–166.

Srai, S. K., Debnam, E. S., Boss, M. and Epstein, O. (1988) Age-related changes in the kinetics of iron absorption across the guinea pig proximal intestine in vivo. *Biol. Neonate* **53**, 53–59.

Stekel, A. (1981) Fortification from the laboratory to a national program. Two Chilean experiences. In: *Proceedings of the Annual Meeting of the International Nutritional Anaemia Consultative Group. Section 7.* Nutrition Foundation, New York.

Stremmel, W., Teichmann, R., Arweiler, D. *et al.* (1991) Iron uptake by enterocytes represents a carrier mediated transport mechanism: Significance of the microvillous membrane iron binding protein in primary hemochromatosis. In: *Proceedings of the Third International Conference on Haemochromatosis,* Demeter Verlag Gmblt., Dusseldorf, p. 16.

Taylor, P. G., Martinez-Torres, C., Romano, E. L. and Layrisse, M. (1986) The effect of cysteine-containing peptides released during meat digestion on iron absorption in humans. *Am. J. Clin. Nutr.* **43**, 68–71.

Taylor, P., Martinez-Torres, C., Leets, I., Ramirez, J., Garcia-Casal, M. N. and Layrisse, M. (1988) Relationships among iron absorption, percent saturation of plasma transferrin and serum ferritin concentration in humans. *J. Nutr.* **118**, 1110–1115.

Teichmann, R. and Stremmel, W. (1990) Iron uptake by human upper small intestine microvillous membrane vesicles. Indication for a facilitated transport mechanism mediated by a membrane iron-binding protein. *J. Clin. Invest.* **86**, 2145–2153.

Tuntawiroon, M., Sritongkul, N., Rossander-Hulten, L. *et al.*(1990) Rice and iron absorption in man. *Eur. J. Clin. Nutr.* **44**, 489–497.

Tuntawiroon, M., Sritongkul, N., Brune, M. *et al.* (1991) Dose-dependent inhibitory effect of phenolic compounds in foods on nonheme-iron absorption in men. *Am. J. Clin. Nutr.* **53**, 554–557.

Walters, G. O., Jacobs, A., Worwood, M., Trevett, D. and Thomson, W. (1975) Iron absorption in normal subjects and patients with idiopathic haemochromatosis: a relationship with serum ferritin concentration. *Gut* **16**, 188–192.

Wheby, M. S. and Jones, L. G. (1963) Role of transferrin in iron absorption. *J. Clin. Invest.* **42**, 1007–1016.

Wheby, M. S. and Spyker, D. A. (1981) Hemoglobin iron absorption kinetics in the iron-deficient dog. *Am. J. Clin. Nutr.* **34**, 1686–1693.

Wheby, M. S., Jones, L. G. and Crosby, W. H. (1964) Studies on iron absorption. Intestinal regulatory mechanisms. *J. Clin. Invest.* **41**, 1433–1442.

Whittaker, P., Mahoney, A. W. and Hendricks, D. G. (1984) Effect of iron-deficiency anemia on percent blood volume in growing rats. *J. Nutr.* **114**, 1137–1142.

Whittaker, P., Fox, M. R. S. and Forbes, A. L. (1989a) In vitro prediction of iron bioavailability for food fortification. *Nutr. Rep. Int.* **39**, 1205–1215.

Whittaker, P. G., Lind, T., Williams, J. G. and Gray, A. L. (1989b) Inductively coupled plasma mass spectrometric determination of the absorption of iron in normal women. *Analyst* **114**, 675–678.

Whittaker, P., Skikne, B. S., Covell, A. M. *et al.* (1989c) Duodenal iron proteins in idiopathic hemochromatosis. *J. Clin. Invest.* **83**, 261–267.

Wien, E. M. and Van Campen, D. R. (1991) Mucus and iron absorption regulation in rats fed various levels of dietary iron. *J. Nutr.* **121**, 92–100.

Wollenberg, P. and Rummel, W. (1987) Dependence of intestinal iron absorption on the valency state of iron. *Arch. Pharmacol.* **336**, 578–582.

Wollenberg, P., Mahlberg, R. and Rummel, W. (1990) The valency state of absorbed iron appearing in the portal blood and ceruloplasmin substitution. *Biol. Met.* **3**, 1–7.

Woodhead, J. C., Drulis, J. M., Rogers, R. R. *et al.* (1988) Use of the stable isotope, ^{58}Fe, for determining availability of nonheme iron in meals. *Pediatr. Res.* **23**, 495–499.

Worwood, M. and Jacobs, A. (1972) The subcellular distribution of 59Fe in small intestinal mucosa: Studies with normal, iron deficient and iron overloaded rats. *Br. J. Haematol.* **22**, 265–272.

Zempsky, W. T., Rosenstein, B. J., Carroll, J. A. and Oski, F. A. (1989) Effect of pancreatic enzyme supplements on iron absorption. *Am. J. Dis. Child* **143**, 969–972.

Zhang, D., Carpenter, C. E. and Mahoney, A. W. (1990) A mechanistic hypothesis for meat enhancement of nonheme iron absorption: Stimulation of gastric secretions and iron chelation. *Nutr. Res.* **10**, 929–935.

7. Iron Deficiency

R. D. BAYNES

Division of Hematology, University of Kansas Medical Center, 3901 Rainbow Boulevard, Kansas City, KS 66160, USA

I. INTRODUCTION

The critical dependence of body tissues on iron (Dallman, 1986) means that elaborate mechanisms have evolved for its efficient absorption, transport, cellular uptake, storage and conservation. Perturbations of any of these components may result in iron deficiency. The clearer definition, in recent years, at both a clinical and biochemical level, of the liabilities of iron deficiency have made its eradication a medical, social and economic necessity (Scrimshaw, 1991; UN Admin. Comm., 1991). At the same time, however, it has become apparent that the notion that subjects exposed to additional dietary iron are safe from any ill-effects unless they are homozygous for the HLA-linked iron loading gene coding for idiopathic haemo-chromatosis, or are affected by an iron loading anaemia, may be excessively optimistic.

2. BODY IRON COMPARTMENTS

A detailed quantitative breakdown of the distribution of the total body iron (around 50 mg/kg in adults) is given in Chapter 2. Understanding and discussion of iron deficiency is greatly facilitated by the consideration of body iron as two major compartments, namely functional and storage iron (Bothwell *et al.*, 1979). Functional iron, accounting for 35–40 mg/kg, consists largely of erythrocyte haemoglobin. The functional compartment also includes a smaller amount in muscle myoglobin, and in a number of haem and non-haem iron-containing enzymes which are essential for cellular metabolism, growth and division (Beutler and Fairbanks, 1980; Dallman, 1986). The storage iron compartment is an intrinsically more variable compartment accounting in normal individuals for between 0 and 20 mg iron/kg body weight. The iron in this compartment is stored in association with the proteins ferritin and haemosiderin. It is located primarily in the reticuloendothelial system which consists of macrophage elements found predominantly in the bone marrow, liver and spleen, and in parenchymal cells of the liver. It serves both as a repository for dietary iron absorbed in excess of functional requirements in order that this be stored in non-toxic form and as an emergency reserve supply from which sudden deficits in functional iron are replenished. A third compartment in the form of a transport system interfacing between storage and functional compartments exists as iron bound to transferrin. Quantitatively, at any one time this compartment is insignificant. However, measurement of this transport iron provides important information in defining the stage of iron deficiency.

3. STAGES OF IRON DEFICIENCY

Employing the concept of two major compartments of body iron, it is logical to divide deficiency into three sequentially developing stages. In summary, these include depleted stores, iron deficient erythropoiesis and iron deficiency anaemia (Bothwell et al., 1979). The former stage reflects reduction of iron within the storage compartment while the latter two stages reflect deficits in the functional compartment.

3.1. Depleted Iron Stores

The condition of depleted stores exists when iron in the storage compartment is absent but without any reduction in the functional compartment (Cook and Skikne, 1989). Iron stores that are reduced but still present do not constitute iron deficiency since this state has never been documented to be associated with any liability. The gold standard for assessing adequacy of storage iron remains the evaluation of macrophage iron in an adequate bone marrow sample (Cook, 1982). Retrospective precise quantitation of stores can also be obtained by quantitative phlebotomy (Chapter 14). Clearly, however, such invasive approaches are not routinely justifiable and are obviously inappropriate for the survey of populations. The measurement of serum ferritin is of greater clinical utility since, in the concentration range of 20–200 ng/ml, it bears a semi-quantitative relationship with iron stores, with 1 ng/ml roughly equivalent to 8 mg of storage iron (Worwood, 1979; Cook, 1982). Once stores are depleted the serum ferritin concentration falls to a value $\leqslant 12$ ng/ml. Some information about iron stores can also be obtained from the serum transferrin concentration since it has been shown to bear an inverse relationship with the serum ferritin concentration (Cook et al., 1974). The predictive value of this measurement as reflecting stores is, however, limited (Bothwell et al., 1979; Cavill et al., 1986).

3.2. Iron Deficient Erythropoiesis

Data from normal subjects undergoing serial phlebotomy indicate that simultaneously with depletion of iron stores, the size of the transport compartment becomes critically reduced. Stated differently, as serum ferritin concentration reaches the 12 ng/ml level, the transferrin saturation falls below 16% (Skikne et al., 1990). The latter has been well documented to correspond to the point at which depletion of the functional compartment of iron commences (Bainton and Finch, 1964). Since the tissue requirement for iron is greatest in developing erythroid elements the resultant deficit in the functional iron compartment is associated with the development of iron deficient erythropoiesis. The measurable correlates include an increase in the concentration of the serum transferrin receptor (Skikne et al., 1990), a progressive accumulation of free protoporphyrin (FEP) in the developing erythroid elements (Labbe and Rettmer, 1989) secondary to reduced incorporation of iron to form haemoglobin, an increase in red cell heterogeneity as determined by such indicators as the red cell size distribution width (RDW) (Bessman et al., 1983) a reduction in the sideroblast count determined from a bone marrow aspirate stained for iron (Bainton and Finch, 1964) and finally, the development of microcytosis or a reduced mean cell volume (MCV) (Bothwell et al., 1979; Cook, 1982) secondary to reduced erythrocyte haemoglobinization.

3.3. Iron Deficiency Anaemia

The erythropoietic endpoint of functional iron depletion is anaemia. This corresponds to a haemoglobin concentration $< 130 \, g/l$ in men and $< 120 \, g/l$ in women (Cook and Skikne, 1989). The mechanisms of the anaemia are incompletely understood. Clearly, iron deficient erythropoiesis significantly curtails haemoglobin synthesis within individual erythroid precursors (Finch and Huebers, 1982). However, given that erythropoietin concentrations rise appropriately (Spivak et al., 1989) and that erythropoiesis appears predominantly hypoproliferative with a reduced reticulocyte production index and a reduced erythropoietic to granulopoietic ratio in the marrow (Hillman and Finch, 1985), a situation of impaired erythropoietin responsiveness must pertain. Erythroid ontogeny involves sequential passage through the interleukin-3, granulocyte macrophage colony stimulating factor and stem cell factor (kit-ligand) responsive burst forming unit (BFU-E), the erythropoietin, insulin-like growth factor 1, and insulin responsive colony forming unit (CFU-E), before sequential maturation as various morphologically distinct transferrin receptor bearing stages of normoblasts to yield mature red blood cells (Krantz, 1991) (see also Chapter 2). Study of iron deficiency in the rat by clonal culture techniques has revealed a normal number of BFU-Es, a mildly increased number of normoblasts but a markedly increased number of CFU-Es (Kimura et al., 1986). Similar data have been found in man (Misago et al., 1987). The anaemia of iron deficiency therefore appears to involve, in addition to impaired haemoglobinization of individual cells, a highly selective maturation defect between CFU-E and the early normoblast.

4. DETERMINANTS OF IRON BALANCE

The maintenance of iron balance resides with the gastrointestinal mucosal cell. Initial pioneering observations subsequently confirmed by radioisotopic data (Green et al., 1968) established that iron excretion is a limited and constant obligatory phenomenon. Obligatory losses in iron replete man are of the order of 1 mg/day. These losses are passive, reflecting iron delivery by transferrin to cells destined for exfoliation. Absorptive behaviour of the mucosal cell is far more responsive to changes in iron status (Bothwell *et al.*, 1958). More specifically, mucosal cells in iron deficiency increase absorptive performance by a factor five times that in normal iron replete subjects (Bothwell *et al.*, 1979).

Given the constancy of obligatory iron loss there are three major determinants of iron balance. First, is the iron demand reflecting basal, physiological, pathological, or therapeutic processes. Second, is the supply of iron from the diet. Third, is the process of adaptation reflecting the ability of mucosal cells to balance supply and demand. Negative iron balance is the consequence of excessive demands, impaired dietary supply, a failure of adaptation, or a combination of these (Cook, 1990).

4.1. Iron Demands

4.1.1. *Basal Iron Losses*

Iron is passively lost, incorporated in cells, either to the exterior from skin or to the lumen of the gastrointestinal and urinary tracts. Small amounts of red blood cells are also lost via the gastrointestinal tract. The total amount of iron lost in normal adult males is approximately 14 µg/kg/day (Green *et al.*, 1968). These losses are divided between gastrointestinal tract, skin and urinary tract in a proportion of approximately 6:3:1. In a 70 kg male obligatory iron loss would represent 0.98 mg/day. Extrapolating directly to a 55 kg woman this would amount to 0.77 mg/day. The coefficient of variation on these estimates is calculated to be 15% (FAO/WHO Joint Expert Consultation Report, 1988). In iron deficiency, these losses may be reduced by 50% (Cook, 1990). Sweat iron losses are negligible and can be disregarded in calculating iron losses (Green *et al.*, 1968; Brune *et al.*, 1986; Hallberg and Rossander-Hulten, 1991), despite claims to the contrary.

4.1.2. *Increased Iron Losses*

(a) *Menstruation*. Menstrual blood loss is highly variable between women but constant within any individual (Hallberg *et al.*, 1966). Data suggest that individual menstrual loss is largely genetically determined (Rybo and Hallberg, 1966). Exogenous causes of variation in menstrual losses include anovulatory medications which reduce losses by approximately 50% (Nilsson and Solvell, 1967) and intrauterine devices which double losses (Guillebaud *et al.*, 1976). A number of surveys of menstrual losses indicate similar values and that the distribution of blood lost per period is skewed (Hallberg *et al.*, 1966; Hefnawi *et al.*, 1980; Hallberg and Rossander-Hulten, 1991). A study conducted at a time when use of anovulatory agents and intrauterine devices was infrequent provides unique data (Hallberg *et al.*, 1966). The median blood loss in this sample of 476 women was 30 ml. The 75th, 90th and 95th percentile values were 52.4, 83.9 and 118.0 ml, respectively.

Allowing for the many assumptions intrinsic to converting menstrual blood to iron losses, adding these to basal losses indicate that 50% of women will require absorption of 1.36 mg/day to maintain iron balance. To achieve this balance in 95% of females, the required absorption would be up to 2.84 mg/day.

(b) *Pregnancy*. Despite protracted amenorrhoea, pregnancy places a significant stress on iron homeostasis. Most of the negative balance relates to iron which will be lost. The iron needs of pregnancy calculated over a 9-month gestation for a 55 kg woman are as follows: 230 mg for basal losses, 360 mg for the products of conception (fetus 270 mg, placenta and umbilical cord 90 mg) and around 150 mg as peripartum blood loss. Thus, pregnancy results in a 740 mg iron loss. There is an additional 450 mg of iron required for expanded red cell mass. This is, however, returned to the mother during postpartum contraction of red cell mass (Bothwell *et al.*, 1979; Hallberg, 1988). Since the greatest increase in iron requirements for fetal growth and erythropoietic expansion occur later in gestation, the major increases in absorption (up to 6 mg/day) are required in the second and third trimesters (Baynes and Bothwell, 1990). Lactation results in a further loss of 0.3–0.6 mg/day postpartum (Siimes *et al.*, 1979). This is, however, balanced to some extent by accompanying amenorrhoea.

(c) *Pathological blood loss*. Any pathological blood loss will impact negatively on iron economy, thereby increasing demand for absorbed iron. Predominant causes are to be found in the gastrointestinal tract (Bothwell *et al.*, 1979). To some degree these causes do have a geographic relationship. In developed regions, gastrointestinal blood loss results from a host of pathological entities including oesophagitis, gastritis, varices, peptic ulcers, neoplasms, diverticulosis, angiodysplasia, haemorrhagic telangiectasis, inflammatory bowel disease and haemorrhoids (Beveridge *et al.*, 1965; Skikne, 1988). In developing areas, while all of the above can occur, they are quantitatively surpassed in significance by pathological blood loss secondary to parasitic infestation, particularly by hookworm. It is estimated that in excess of 450 million people are infested worldwide and heavy parasitization with faecal egg loads in the region of 5000/g may increase daily iron requirements by as much as 3–4 mg (Layrisse and Roche, 1964). In the majority of cases, however, the level of parasitization is much lower (Layrisse and Roche, 1964). Pathological blood loss may occasionally be urinary, pulmonary, factitious or iatrogenic in origin.

(d) *Non-pathological blood loss*. A number of situations arise in which blood loss increases as a consequence of neither overt pathology nor normal physiology. These include the widespread use of aspirin for its cardio-protective and anti-inflammatory properties, blood donation and autologous blood banking prior to elective surgery, and the trained athlete. Regular ingestion of aspirin has been well-documented to enhance intestinal loss of red blood cells (Fleming *et al.*, 1987). This can be as much as ten times the basal loss. A number of other therapeutic agents including corticosteroids, non-steroidal anti-inflammatory agents and anticoagulants have similar effects. Blood donation obviously increases iron losses. One donation of 500 ml blood/year imposes an additional iron requirement of 0.5 mg/day (Finch *et al.*, 1977). Clearly such losses will be profoundly increased by the increasing practice of preoperative collection of autologous blood, sometimes with concomitant erythropoietic stimulation with erythropoietin (Goodnough *et al.*, 1989; Goodnough and Brittenham, 1990; Skikne and Cook, 1991). Increased gastrointestinal blood loss occurs frequently in endurance athletes (Newhouse and Clement, 1988;

Nickerson *et al.*, 1989). Factors which may contribute to this phenomenon include transient gut ischaemia, stress gastritis, use of anti-inflammatory agents and recurrent mechanical trauma (Newhouse and Clement, 1988).

4.1.3. *Enhanced Tissue Iron Requirements*

The high prevalence of iron deficiency in infants, children and adolescents reflects enhanced requirements for iron consequent upon growth and expansion of erythropoiesis. Iron deficiency may result from pharmacologic stimulation of erythro-poiesis with the haemopoietic growth factor erythropoietin as in the treatment of anaemia of chronic renal insufficiency and for increasing the yield of autologous blood banked for elective surgery. The increased iron absorption noted in a number of disorders with marked ineffective erythropoiesis (Chapters 6 and 9) is also associated with relative iron deficient erythropoiesis in these disorders.

(a) *Growth*. (i) Infancy: A normal term infant has a total body iron content of approximately 80 mg/kg. Of this, two-thirds is in circulating haemoglobin and one-third in storage form (Bothwell *et al.*, 1979). Rapid growth in early infancy increases requirements markedly. At this time, however, the infant is independent of nutritional iron to meet these requirements. This is because more effective tissue oxygenation *ex utero* reduces erythropoiesis transiently, resulting in a fall in haemoglobin concentration of about 60 g/l within the first six weeks, with a concomitant rise in hepatic iron stores and plasma ferritin concentration (Saarinen and Siimes, 1978; Bothwell *et al.*, 1979; Dallman, 1981). Growth and subsequent erythropoiesis exhausts these stores within six months. With these composite influences, a full-term infant has a daily iron requirement of 0.3 mg/day (Bothwell *et al.*, 1979). This situation is severely prejudiced by factors such as low birth weight and premature umbilical cord clamping such that these infants may require up to 1 mg iron/day. Neonatal iron status is relatively independent of maternal iron status reflecting the remarkable efficiency of the placenta in supplying iron to the developing fetus (Rios *et al.*, 1975; Wallenburg and van Eijk, 1984).

(ii) Childhood and Adolescence: Growth requirements in the second year of life increase iron demand to approximately 0.4 mg/day. Demands from two years to the beginning of adolescence are proportionately less than those of infancy on account of the reduced growth rate (Bothwell *et al.*, 1979). Ongoing growth, a slow rise in haemoglobin concentration and an increase in obligatory losses necessitate an increase in daily iron requirements from 0.5 to 0.8 mg during this period. Daily iron needs increase at adolescence in relation to the pubertal growth spurt and a further increase in erythropoiesis, reaching approximately 2.4 mg in females and 1.6 mg in males (Bothwell *et al.*, 1979), the higher value in adolescent females being related to the concomitant menarche.

(b) *Therapeutically enhanced erythropoiesis*. With the cloning of the erythropoietin gene and the commercial production of recombinant erythropoietin, haemopoietic growth factor therapy for enhancing erythropoiesis has become a reality for the treatment of a number of anaemias, particularly that of chronic renal insufficiency (Eschbach *et al.*, 1987) and for facilitating autologous blood banking prior to elective surgery (Goodnough *et al.*, 1989; Goodnough and Brittenham, 1990). It has rapidly become appreciated that this approach markedly enhances iron requirements, and indeed iron deficiency may become limiting to the erythropoietic response

(Eschbach *et al.*, 1989; Eschbach, 1991). Iron limited erythropoiesis may occur prior to development of depleted iron stores (Kooistra *et al.*, 1991) suggesting that relative deficiency may develop in relation to a limited ability of the transport compartment to reconcile stores with need. Quantitative aspects of the effect of recombinant erythropoietin were provided in a recent study in which it was administered to normal subjects for ten consecutive days. Calculation of redistribution from stores to erythropoietic elements indicated that requirements for functional iron increased by approximately 25 mg/day. This was associated with an increase in haemoglobin concentration of about 10 g/l (Skikne and Cook, 1991).

(c) *Endogenously enhanced erythropoiesis.* Shortened red cell survival results in anaemia with consequent stimulation of erythropoietic activity by endogenously produced haemopoietic growth factors. This results in increased erythroid demands. The erythropoiesis may be either effective, as in spherocytosis or sickle cell anaemia, or ineffective with a high rate of intramedullary cell death, as in thalassaemia. Increased iron requirements, particularly in ineffective erythropoiesis, are reflected in increased plasma iron turnover and iron absorption. Iron stores often increase secondary to the enhanced absorption and any accompanying therapeutic transfusions (Chapter 9). Despite the increased stores, increased red cell-free protoporphyrin is observed in subjects with hereditary spherocytosis who have not been splenectomized (Zanella *et al.*, 1989) and thalassaemia (Pootrakul *et al.*, 1984). Sophisticated ferrokinetic data (Cazzola *et al.*, 1987) have confirmed that erythroid hyperplasia may result in the paradox of iron deficient erythropoiesis despite seemingly adequate stores. This situation, and that occurring when anaemia of renal failure is treated with erythropoietin, suggest that the inability of the transport compartment to meet the erythroid iron requirements despite seemingly adequate stores is a not uncommon occurrence. This may have certain important physiological implications. First, relative iron deficiency may impose some limit on enhanced erythropoiesis. Second, the possibility exists that the erythropoietic signal and iron deficient signal controlling iron absorption (Bothwell *et al.*, 1958) may in fact be the same (Cazzola *et al.*, 1987).

4.2. Dietary Iron

The role of dietary iron in iron balance refers to the luminal phase of iron absorption. This encompasses two essential components, namely the absolute iron content of ingested food and the relative bioavailability of iron in ingested food. This is determined by dietary composition.

4.2.1. Food Iron Content

The typical Western diet has remarkably consistent iron content. Expressed in relation to food caloric value the diet contains approximately 6 mg/1000 kCal. Although bioavailability issues will be addressed in the next section it can be assumed that the availability of food iron in a Western diet is in the region of 14–17% (Hallberg and Rossander-Hulten, 1991). Thus, a 2000 kCal food intake could provide 1.8 mg iron/day. This is insufficient to meet the requirements of many menstruating women and all pregnant women. To obtain sufficient iron, many subjects must ingest in excess of a 2000 kCal diet. To prevent the development of iron deficient erythro-poiesis, a mean dietary intake of 3440 kCal would be required for 95% of iron depleted menstruating females in Sweden. The comparable figure for US women would be 3264 kCal (Hallberg and Rossander-Hulten, 1991). From these calculations, it is impossible to reach the recommended iron store goal (National Research Council, 1989) of 300 mg in 95% of women. The trend for women in Western countries is to ingest a calorie restricted diet and consequently many are ingesting amounts of iron well below that required to prevent iron deficiency (Barber et al., 1985). The relationship between calorie and iron ingestion has been further emphasized by data showing that obese subjects have better measures of iron nutriture than non-obese subjects (Fricker et al., 1990). The distinction between haem and non-haem iron will be made in the next section. Most non-haem iron enters a common absorption pool. Contaminant iron may, in developing regions, contribute significantly to measured dietary iron intake but is poorly absorbed (Hallberg and Bjorn-Rasmussen, 1981). Contaminant iron is insensitive to the effect of promotory ligands. Consequently, dietary iron content in developing regions may not accurately reflect bioavailable iron.

4.2.2. Food Iron Bioavailability

This topic has been extensively covered in Chapter 6. Consequently, it will be outlined only briefly here to facilitate discussion of mucosal adaptation.

There are two pathways whereby dietary iron enters the gastrointestinal mucosal cell. These reflect the major forms of dietary iron, namely non-haem and haem iron. Non-haem iron is the largest component. It enters a common pool and its absorption, as measured by single meal studies, is determined by the balance between the large number of potential promotory and inhibitory influences discussed in Chapter 6. The extremes of bioavailability are profoundly dependent on this interplay. Indeed, estimates of bioavailability indicate a 15-fold variation between the extremes (Cook, 1990).

The second pathway is that of haem iron. This is absorbed into the mucosal cell as the intact porphyrin complex via a luminal surface haem receptor (Grasbeck et al., 1982). After mucosal uptake, haem is rapidly catabolized by haem oxygenase (Raffin et al., 1974) and the released iron then enters a common cellular pool. The intact porphyrin complex is not subject to the non-haem iron promoters and inhibitors (Lynch et al., 1985). Its absorption is facilitated by digestion products of dietary protein (Lynch et al., 1985). Although haem iron accounts for only approximately 10–15% of food iron in meat-eating communities, with percentage absorption five- to ten-fold higher than from non-haem iron it accounts for fully one-third of absorbed iron (Bjorn-Rasmussen et al., 1974).

Bioavailability of non-haem iron as established by single meal studies has been utilized to try to predict nutritional impact of dietary patterns. Using the single meal studies it is possible to arrange foods in terms of relative bioavailability of the inorganic iron (Bothwell et al., 1989; Baynes et al., 1990). Using this total dietary iron content and haem iron content of the diet, models for predicting food iron absorption have been developed (Monsen et al., 1978; Monsen and Balintfy, 1982). These do not, however, reflect the role of a number of inhibitory ligands. In addition, recent data questioning single meal studies necessitate a re-evaluation of these models. In an important study, a maximally promotory single meal increased non-haem iron absorption by approximately 120% over a neutral self-selected meal, while a maximally inhibitory one caused a 62% reduction. By contrast, when the diet was chronically labelled, a maximally promotory diet caused a mere 25% increase while the maximally inhibitory one caused a 50% reduction. While inorganic iron from the facilitating single meal was absorbed six times better than from the inhibitory single meal, this difference fell to a factor of only 2.5 times for labelled diets (Cook *et al.*, 1991). The future challenge in the area of bioavailability is to document its impact on population nutrition (Cook, 1990). The reasons for these discrepant findings require elucidation. It should also be noted that these findings relate to a Western type diet. Bioavailability continues to be of greater significance in developing regions where diets are relatively or absolutely devoid of haem iron.

4.2.3. Adaptation

This refers to the process whereby the gastrointestinal mucosal cell balances the absorption of available luminal iron with body iron demands. The theories relating to the regulation of iron absorption have been extensively reviewed in Chapter 6. These will not be restated but adaptation will be addressed in relation to iron absorption and measurements of iron nutriture. More specifically the adaptation to variations in iron demand and to variations in dietary iron supply will be briefly addressed.

(a) *Adaptation to variations in iron demand.* The inverse relationship between body iron status and food iron absorption in normal subjects is well established (Cook *et al.*, 1974; Baynes *et al.*, 1987b). This adaptation is far more dramatic for non-haem than for haem iron. In normal iron-replete males absorption of haem iron is of the order of 26% while that of non-haem iron is only 2.5%. In iron deficient subjects, haem iron absorption increases modestly to 47% (1.8 times increase) whereas non-haem iron absorption increases to 22% (8.8 times increase) (Cook, 1990). These data were obtained from doubly tagged composite meals. Similar data have been obtained using single meals (Bezwoda *et al.*, 1983). Based on western diets, Cook has calculated that in iron deficiency, males could absorb 4.25 mg/day (2.75 mg from non-haem and 1.49 mg from haem sources) while women could achieve maximal absorption of 2.92 mg/day (1.89 mg from non-haem and 1.03 mg from haem sources). The picture would be dramatically different in the absence of haem iron since, in addition to losing the haem iron fraction, lack of meat-derived promotory factors means that absorption of non-haem iron would decrease by 50%. In this scenario, not unlike that in developing regions, ceiling absorption for iron deficient males would be 1.73 mg and for females 1.19 mg. Females in such circumstances could not meet their basal requirement unless calorie intake was markedly enhanced or food iron content was much higher than current Western averages (Cook, 1990). Further studies are required to define which of these latter two variables is the major determinant of iron status in this situation. This emphasizes the marked importance of meat in preventing iron deficiency. Indeed, meat is the only dietary component documented to modify measurements of iron nutrition (Worthington-Roberts *et al.*, 1988;

Snyder *et al.*, 1989; Leggett *et al.*, 1990). The relative non-suppressability of haem iron absorption also makes it a major contributor to iron overload.

(b) *Adaptation to variations in iron supply.* In the absence of excessive losses or increased demands it is inordinately difficult to induce iron deficiency by dietary means. Cook (1990) has calculated that after removing iron from the diet of an iron-replete male it would require 3–5 years to deplete iron stores. A 50% reduction could take as long as 10 years. Consequently, adaptation to iron supply must be addressed by examining the storage consequence of enhancing factors. To this end a study of long-term ingestion of high dose vitamin C failed to show any increase in iron stores (Cook *et al.*, 1984). This was true even of iron deficient subjects. This finding has been confirmed in a study in which iron status of 10 515 subjects examined in the NHANES II survey did not differ between users and non-users of vitamin-mineral supplements (Looker *et al.*, 1988). These studies demonstrate that it is inordinately difficult to induce changes in iron status by modifying dietary constituents other than meat. The reason for this is unclear, however, since in single meal studies vitamin C markedly enhances iron absorption even when subjects have been receiving high dose vitamin C for many months (Cook *et al.*, 1984).

A contrary finding was reported in women rendered iron deficient by phlebotomy combined with a diet of relatively low bioavailability, where ascorbic acid supplementation caused a short-term more favourable haemoglobin concentration, FEP content and serum iron concentration (Hunt *et al.*, 1990). The study was intrinsically flawed, however, by small groups, different iron intakes between the ascorbate and placebo groups (presumably reflecting differences in weight), a trend towards more favourable initial status in the ascorbate group in terms of serum ferritin, haemoglobin concentration and serum iron, as well as more unfavourable measures of haemoglobin, FEP and serum iron in the placebo group prior to ascorbic acid supplementation.

5. RECOMMENDED DAILY IRON INTAKE

This is a relatively controversial area and will be addressed only superficially. While daily iron requirements are relatively well established, problematic areas relate to whether dietary intake should be calculated to allow for moderate iron stores and whether dietary iron intake can be based on bioavailability models derived in large measure from single meal studies. The issue of pregnancy has been addressed in a prior section and suffice it to say that the second and third trimester requirements cannot be met by diet alone. The information presented here is based largely on the relatively recent report of the FAO/WHO Expert Consultative Group (FAO/WHO Joint Expert Consultation Report, 1988). The values employed for the various groups stratified by age and sex reflect the values estimated to apply to the 95th percentile of the population. The estimated iron requirements and recommended daily iron intakes are summarized in Table 7.1.

While these recommended intakes provide guidelines, the FAO/WHO Group recommended additional research in relation to variations in losses, bioavailability from complete diets across the spectrum of populations, the availability of

Table 7.1 Calculated daily iron requirements and recommended daily iron intake as a function of estimated dietary iron bioavailability in various categories by age and sex. Values are based on 95th percentile calculations

Group	Age (yrs)	Requirements (μg/kg/day)	Recommended intake (mg/day)		
			Low (5%)	Intermediate (10%)	High (15%)
Children	0.25–1	120	21	11	7
	1–2	56	12	6	4
	2–6	44	14	7	5
	6–12	40	23	12	8
Boys	12–16	34	36	18	12
Girls	12–16	40	40	20	13
Adult men		18	23	11	8
Adult women:					
menstruating*		43	48	24	16
post-menopausal		18	19	9	6
lactating		24	26	13	9

*Recommended intakes for Low and Intermediate bioavailability are unlikely to be achieved with conventional diet

contaminant iron and the iron content of diets (FAO/WHO Joint Expert Consultation Report, 1988).

6. CAUSES OF IRON DEFICIENCY

From Section 4 it is evident that iron deficiency may result from inadequate intake, increased iron requirements, increased blood loss or decreased absorption of iron. Inadequate dietary iron intake may result in the settings of single food diets in infancy, voluntary or involuntary calorie restriction, and developing communities in which haem iron is absent from the diet which is otherwise depleted of other promotory ligands. Increased iron requirements are observed during growth in infants, children and adolescents, during pregnancy and with either endogenously or exogenously stimulated erythropoiesis. Increased blood loss may be physiological as in menstruation, non-pathological, or pathological as outlined previously. Finally, food iron may rarely be poorly absorbed as a consequence of a primary pathological process involving the stomach or small intestine. In practical terms, however, iron deficiency is commonly a consequence of a combination of factors. For example, menstrual losses or pregnancy occurring in the setting of either voluntary caloric restriction as in Western societies or in the face of poor dietary iron intake as a consequence of a low haem iron diet as in developing communities may result in iron deficiency. Highly trained athletes often have the combined influences of enhanced gastrointestinal blood losses together with reduced dietary iron intake (Newhouse and Clement, 1988; Haymes and Spillman, 1989; Nickerson et al., 1989). An infant born prematurely in a developing community as a consequence of iron deficiency may, in addition to already impaired iron stores, be subject to poor dietary iron intake and increased blood loss secondary to hookworm

Table 7.2 Laboratory measurements commonly used in the assessment of iron deficiency along with the body iron compartment evaluated, the diagnostic range, and the stage of iron deficiency that the findings are associated with

Sequential stage of iron deficiency	Measurement	Body iron compartment	Diagnostic range
Depleted stores	Bone marrow iron	Stores	Absent
	Total iron binding capacity	Stores	$>400\ \mu g/dl$ ($71.5\ \mu mol/l$)
	Serum ferritin	Stores	$<12\ ng/ml$
Iron deficient erythropoiesis	Transferrin saturation	Transport	$<16\%$
	Free erythrocyte protoporphyrin	Functional	$>70\ \mu g/dl$ red cells
	Mean cell volume	Functional	$<80\ fl$
	Red cell distribution width	Functional	$>16\%$
	Serum transferrin receptor*	Functional	$>8.5\ mg/l$
Iron deficiency anaemia	Haemoglobin concentration	Functional	$<130\ g/l$ (σ) $<120\ g/l$ (φ)

*Kansas City monoclonal antibody ELISA

infestation. A renal dialysis patient may become iron deficient as a combined consequence of a protein restricted diet, anorexia, blood loss on dialysis, and exogenously stimulated erythropoiesis by means of erythropoietin.

7. ASSESSMENT OF IRON DEFICIENCY

7.1. Commonly Used Iron Measurements

Assessment of iron status both in individual subjects and in populations has, in recent years, undergone progressive refinement. Obtaining maximal information both in the individual subject and in populations is predicated on knowledge of the compartment addressed by a particular measurement. A number of commonly used measurements and the compartments they address are summarized in Table 7.2.

These laboratory measurements have been discussed in Section 3 as correlates of stages of iron depletion. A precise measurement of storage iron, can be obtained using quantitative phlebotomy (Chapter 14), but clearly, this approach is used only in an investigational setting. Similar information can be obtained by semi-quantitative assessment of an adequate bone marrow aspirate sample stained for iron or the quantitative non-haem iron determination on a bone marrow biopsy sample. The former analysis is performed most commonly for distinguishing iron deficiency anaemia from other anaemias and particularly that associated with chronic inflammation. It is not required for the evaluation of an uncomplicated case of iron deficiency anaemia and is obviously not used for assessing population nutrition. The value of serum ferritin as a non-invasive measure of iron stores has already been outlined. A concentration of 12 ng/ml indicates storage iron depletion, but the

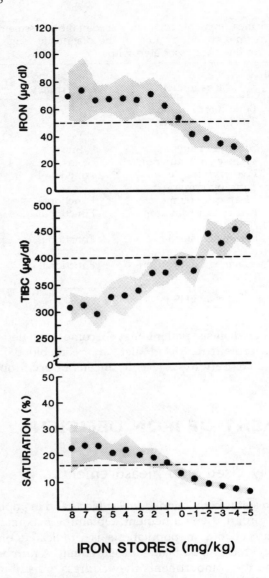

Fig. 7.1 Relationship between differences in iron nutrition and serum iron measurements (top), total iron binding capacity (middle) and per cent transferrin saturation (bottom). Iron stores were assessed by quantitative phlebotomy, a negative value indicating an additional deficit in functional iron compounds, particularly haemoglobin. Threshold value is indicated by dotted line. Mean ± 2 SE indicated. (Skikne *et al.*, 1990; used with permission of authors and the editor of *Blood*).

measurement below this threshold does not have value as an indicator of more severe stages of iron deficiency. The value of the serum ferritin concentration is therefore mainly as an indicator of iron sufficiency rather than of severity of deficiency. The measurement has diminished utility in the presence of factors known to cause a rise in its serum concentration unrelated to iron storage status. Such factors include

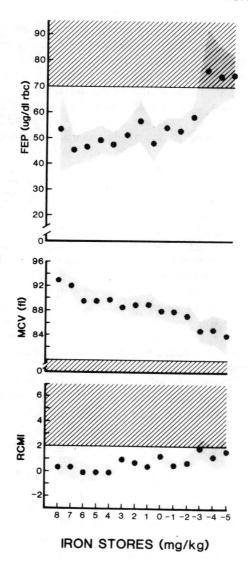

Fig. 7.2 Relationship between differences in iron nutrition as determined by quantitative phlebotomy (see legend to Fig. 7.1) and free-erythrocyte protoporphyrin (top), mean cell volume (middle) and a measure of anisocytosis (red cell mean index – RCMI) (bottom). Threshold regions are shaded. Mean ± 2 SE indicated. (Skikne *et al.*, 1990; used with permission of authors and the editor of *Blood*).

infection, neoplasia, hepatic disease and heavy alcohol consumption (Worwood, 1979; Cook, 1982; Cook *et al.*, 1992a,b).

To some extent, these variables can be controlled by the concomitant use of markers of inflammation such as C-reactive protein or erythrocyte sedimentation rate (Witte *et al.*, 1988), markers of hepatic injury such as transaminase concentrations and markers of heavy alcohol consumption such as gammaglutamyl transpeptidase

(Meyer *et al.*, 1984) or desialated transferrin. Clearly this adds to the cost and complexity of the evaluation. A guide to the use of serum ferritin concentrations in the setting of inflammation is that if the concentration is $\leqslant 12$ ng/ml the patient has depleted iron stores and if > 100 ng/ml the patient probably does not. The range of 12–100 ng/ml represents an area without diagnostic certainty (Guyatt *et al.*, 1990; Cook *et al.*, 1992a). A new measure of iron status, namely the serum transferrin receptor, may prove to be of great value in the settings outlined above.

Serum ferritin concentration is also of limited utility in subjects who, because of physiological conditions, would be expected to have limited iron stores, such as children or pregnant women. The latter situation is compounded since transferrin concentration is elevated as a hormonal consequence, per cent saturation is border-line, and red cell indices take some period of iron deficient erythropoiesis to show the appropriate changes. Even the haemoglobin concentration cannot be relied on since physiological variations occur in plasma volume and red cell mass (Carriaga *et al.*, 1991). Here again, the serum transferrin receptor concentration shows promise as an indicator of functional compartment depletion.

A recent investigation employing quantitative phlebotomy has provided very important data concerning the relationship between iron nutrition and the various measurements reflecting the transport and functional iron compartments (Skikne *et al.*, 1990). The relationship between iron stores and the measurements of serum iron, total iron binding capacity and per cent transferrin saturation is summarized in Fig. 7.1. It can be seen that reduction of the per cent saturation below the critical 16% level occurs as stores are exhausted. The picture in regard to the red cell indices is not so favourable. The relationships between iron stores and FEP, MCV and erythrocyte anisocytosis are summarized in Fig. 7.2. It can be seen that functional deficit of iron is already profound before red cell abnormalities are manifest. This is not surprising given the relatively slow red cell turnover but does emphasize that these measurements of functional depletion become abnormal relatively late in the evolution of iron deficiency.

Haemoglobin concentration or haematocrit are well established indicators because they identify a more severe level of iron deficiency. Their major limitations are that they lack sensitivity and specificity, and the definition of a threshold value is very problematic. In a study in which an arbitrary cut-off was employed, and a response to iron therapy monitored in putative anaemic and non-anaemic groupings, one-fifth of anaemic subjects were wrongly labelled normal and one-third of normal subjects were wrongly considered anaemic (Garby *et al.*, 1969). The lower end of a population can, to some extent, be segregated into a normal tail and a second anaemic population by means of probability analysis of the cumulative frequency (Cook *et al.*, 1971).

7.2. The Serum Form of the Transferrin Receptor

The last decade has seen vast progress in the understanding of how cells procure the iron so essential for their metabolic integrity and propagation from circulating transferrin by means of the transferrin receptor (Morgan, 1981; Huebers and Finch, 1987). This subject has been extensively reviewed in Chapter 3. The receptor is a transmembrane glycoprotein comprising identical 95 K monomers linked by a pair

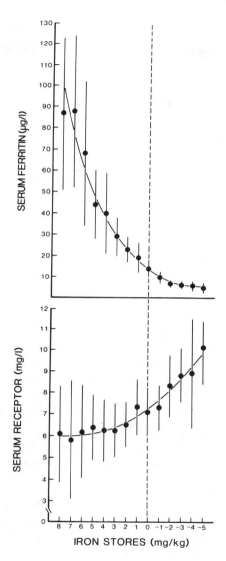

Fig. 7.3 Relationship between differences in iron nutrition as determined by quantitative phlebotomy (see legend to Fig. 7.1) and serum ferritin (top) and serum transferrin receptor (bottom) concentrations. The point of storage iron depletion is indicated by the vertical dashed line. Mean ± 2 SE indicated. (Skikne *et al.*, 1990; used with permission of authors and the editor of *Blood*).

of disulfide bridges. Each monomer consists of 760 amino acids organized into an N-terminal cytoplasmic domain of 61 amino acids, a membrane spanning region of 28 amino acids and a carboxy terminal extracellular domain of 671 amino acids (McClelland *et al.*, 1984). Immunoreactive transferrin receptor has been shown to be uniformly detected in human serum (Kohgo *et al.*, 1986, 1987a,b; Flowers *et al.*, 1989; Huebers *et al.*, 1990). This serum form of receptor was believed to be intact

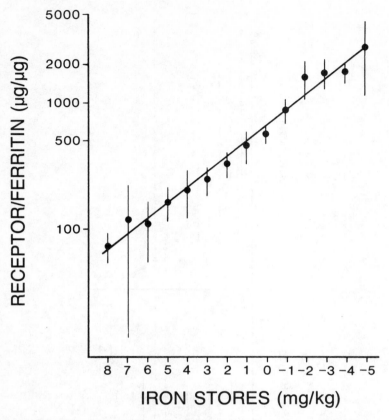

Fig. 7.4 Relationship between differences in iron nutrition as determined by quantitative phlebotomy (see legend to Fig. 7.1) and the ratio of serum transferrin receptor to serum ferritin. Mean ± 2 SE indicated. (Skikne *et al.*, 1990; used with permission of authors and the editor of *Blood*).

receptor related to the exosome (Harding *et al.*, 1983; Pan and Johnstone, 1983) released from the multivesicular endosome of transferrin receptor bearing cells (Kohgo, 1986; Kohgo *et al.*, 1986, 1987a,b; Beguin *et al.*, 1988; Huebers *et al.*, 1990; Chitambar *et al.*, 1991). More detailed evaluation of immunoaffinity purified receptor, including sequence data (Shih *et al.*, 1990; Baynes *et al.*, 1991b) indicate that this is in fact a truncated soluble receptor consisting of the extracellular domain monomer. Recent preliminary data indicate that the appropriate soluble form of the receptor can be generated by a cell membrane associated serine protease, and that this proteolysis appears to be maximal at the exosome surface while contained in an intracellular organelle (Baynes *et al.*, 1993). Since receptor is expressed on all growing cells and particularly erythroid progenitors after the CFU-E stage, and since cellular receptor concentration varies inversely with the size of the cellular iron pool, it may be reasonably anticipated that the concentration would be increased in situations of functional iron deficiency, stimulated erythropoiesis, and reduced in situations of suppressed erythropoiesis. This has been confirmed in clinical studies (Flowers *et al.*, 1989), *in vivo* with sophisticated ferrokinetic investigations (Huebers *et al.*, 1990) and *in vitro* cell culture experiments (Baynes *et al.*, 1991a).

The role of the soluble form of the transferrin receptor in the evaluation of functional iron deficiency was well characterized in a study which employed quantitative phlebotomy to establish a progressive reduction in iron status (Skikne et al., 1990). The relationship between iron stores and the serum concentrations of ferritin and soluble transferrin receptor are summarized in Fig. 7.3. From this, it can be seen that the serum ferritin concentration is most informative in the range where iron stores are greater than zero. The serum receptor concentration is most informative in the range reflecting a deficit in functional iron compounds (iron stores <0). Clearly, it becomes increased earlier in the development of functional iron depletion than any of the red cell related parameters. The combination of serum receptor and ferritin provides complete information about storage and functional compartments. This information can be made linear by plotting the ratio of receptor to ferritin against stores, as is shown in Fig. 7.4. Using this combination along with the haemoglobin concentration it is possible completely to define iron nutritional status. Experience with the serum receptor is currently limited to a few laboratories, and widespread confidence in the measurement must obviously await general availability and a well-validated, well-standardized assay.

The soluble form of the transferrin receptor has been evaluated in relation to certain of the diagnostically problematic areas already alluded to. In the situation of inflammatory disease, anaemia is common and is frequently associated with hypoferraemia, reduced transferrin saturation, reduced MCV and increased FEP (Lee, 1983). Measurements which may be helpful in distinguishing this picture from that of iron deficiency include a reduced transferrin concentration and ferritin concentration >100 ng/ml. However, the transferrin concentration lacks sensitivity and specificity and serum ferritin concentration is commonly in the 12–100 ng/ml non-diagnostic zone. The RDW was initially presented as a powerful discriminator of the two conditions (Bessman et al., 1983) but this did not stand up to further evaluation (Baynes et al., 1986, 1987a). This situation, therefore, commonly requires a bone marrow evaluation to resolve the diagnosis. A recent evaluation of the serum form of the transferrin receptor demonstrated a remarkable ability of this measurement to resolve subjects with the anaemia of chronic disease (where serum transferrin receptor concentrations were normal or only slightly increased) from those with iron deficiency anaemia (Ferguson et al., 1992). In the same study, it was demonstrated that acute and chronic liver disease, well-known causes of a spuriously raised serum ferritin concentration, had no effect on the concentration of the serum transferrin receptor. Serum transferrin receptor was also recently evaluated in pregnancy. In this situation it appears to be a useful indicator of functional iron deficiency, thereby identifying those subjects with low serum ferritin concentrations who have more significant iron deficiency (Carriaga et al., 1991). Studies are still required to evaluate the receptor as an indicator of iron deficiency in children.

7.3. Red Cell Ferritin

This is another potentially useful measurement of iron supply to the erythron. Numerous earlier studies documented the presence of ferritin in red blood cells and showed a relationship between it and disturbances of iron metabolism (Chapter 14). The test is predicated on the notion that red cell ferritin reflects the balance between supply of iron by transferrin to the erythron and incorporation into haemoglobin. Both liver (basic) and heart (acidic) ferritins in the red cell show a direct relationship to body stores as reflected by serum ferritin concentration (Cazzola *et al.*, 1983a) and percentage transferrin saturation (Cazzola *et al.*, 1983b), but in both circumstances the slope of this relationship is steeper for basic than for acidic ferritins. Consequently, the ratio of L- to H-ferritin in the erythrocyte would appear to provide most information about iron status. A more complete assessment of the relationship between this ratio, or L-ferritin alone, in red cells to precisely determined iron stores, and a comparative assessment of the duration of iron deficiency required for the measurement to become abnormal, are essential before this approach can be placed in clinical perspective. The fact that a pure red cell population is required for lysis together with subsequent removal of stroma makes the work of evaluation intensive.

7.4. Screening for Iron Deficiency

In the subsequent sections it will be seen that iron deficiency is an undesirable state on account of its many liabilities. Attempts to relieve this by untargeted fortification increase iron intake in subjects already iron replete. A second approach is targeted fortification but this is not uniformly applicable. A third approach is targeted supplementation of groups at high risk. This may take the form of supplementing the whole group or only those identified by screening. The latter is probably the ideal circumstance. Primary targets for screening include infants, preschool children, pregnant women, regular blood donors, trained athletes, vegetarians and communities with low haem iron intake (Cook *et al.*, 1992b). As will be seen, the screened supplemental approach improves compliance, therapeutic efficacy, and protects those who require no additional iron. The disadvantages include cost, labour and inconvenience. Only measurements which can be performed on a capillary sample are considered appropriate for screening (Cook *et al.*, 1992b). To limit costs, one or occasionally two measurements will be employed. The choice of these should be guided by the expected prevalence. Since the liabilities of iron deficiency have been best correlated with anaemia, an assessment of circulating red cell mass either by haemoglobin concentration or haematocrit is one of the most commonly performed investigations. Its major value is in the situation where prevalence of iron deficiency is high. As discussed previously, it has low specificity and use of an arbitrary threshold is problematic. The utility of this measurement is greatly enhanced in combination with a second indicator of iron nutrition.

As discussed previously, serum ferritin concentration is a good indicator of stores but gives little information as to the severity of iron deficiency. Its major utility is in settings where the prevalence of anaemia is low. It is of limited use when depleted iron stores are common, as in pregnancy and in infants. The combination of haemoglobin concentration and serum ferritin concentration is, however, a very useful one. If both measures are normal, iron deficiency is excluded. If both are reduced, iron deficient anaemia is present. A low serum ferritin with normal haemoglobin concentration implies that the subject is at risk for iron deficiency. A low haemoglobin concentration with normal serum ferritin dictates the need for further evaluation.

FEP is now readily determined by means of the haematofluorometer. An elevated measurement indicates either absolute or relative iron deficient erythropoiesis or lead poisoning. The latter finding limits its usefulness in the evaluation of children. In combination with haemoglobin concentration it may suggest that iron deficiency is the cause of the anaemia or if haemoglobin concentration is still normal that iron deficient erythropoiesis is occurring. In combination with serum ferritin concentration it could theoretically resolve normality, depleted iron stores and iron deficient erythropoiesis.

As mentioned, the serum transferrin receptor appears to be the earliest indicator of functional iron deficiency. Its use in screening is yet to be fully evaluated but would appear to hold great promise. In combination with the serum ferritin concentration it appears destined for a major role in defining very accurately iron nutrition within the individual. This combination, together with haemoglobin concentration, can completely define iron status.

7.5. Evaluation of Population Iron Nutrition

The accurate determination of population iron nutritional status is crucial to the identification of problematic regions, and is therefore of importance in defining national and international nutritional priorities and programmes. Once a region is identified with an unacceptable prevalence of iron deficiency and an interventional strategy implemented, further surveillance is mandatory to determine efficacy of the programme. Population analysis is also of importance in determining long-term nutritional trends. This may in future prove to be of greater significance in relation to iron overload rather than iron deficiency.

The approach to population survey has been to use increasing numbers of measurements to define iron nutritional status better. In general, this approach leads to more complete population assessment. The manner in which the data are handled statistically is as important as the data themselves. The crudest handling is to employ somewhat arbitrary threshold values. This has the major disadvantage that prevalence will be critically determined by the threshold value. As outlined, the threshold value cannot separate with certainty the normal population tail from a distinct abnormal second population. When multiple measurements are being performed the use of multiple threshold values leads, not unexpectedly, to conflicting estimates of prevalence. The advantage of the use of multiple measures in this way is to enhance the specificity of the prevalence data (Cook et al., 1976; Cook and Finch, 1979). This, however, is at the expense of sensitivity (Hallberg and Rossander-Hulten, 1991). Combinations of measurements can be used to define prevalence by category of compartment depleted (Pilch and Senti, 1984). This approach is adequate for iron deficiency but does little to define degrees of iron sufficiency.

A more sophisticated approach to the handling of population survey data has recently been developed (Cook et al., 1986). Using this, body iron status is established for each individual surveyed thus giving meaningful data over the whole range of iron status. In iron replete subjects, iron stores are quantitated from the serum ferritin concentration. In subjects with iron deficiency anaemia functional deficiency is derived from the deficit in circulating haemoglobin. In the situation between these extremes, reflecting iron depletion and iron deficient erythropoiesis, the approach employs empirical formulae based on the degree of abnormality in transferrin saturation, serum ferritin and FEP. The usefulness of this approach has been confirmed in a targeted fortification trial in South Africa (Ballot *et al.*, 1989).

Given the recent development of the serum transferrin receptor as a quantitative measure of functional iron depletion, along with the serum ferritin established as a quantitative measure of iron stores and haemoglobin concentration it should, in the future, be possible to give an even more accurate portrayal of population iron nutrition. It will, however, be important to establish the effects of folic acid deficiency and other confounding influences on serum transferrin receptor concentration.

8. PREVALENCE OF IRON DEFICIENCY

Given that many of the liabilities of iron deficiency correlate with the presence of anaemia and that much survey material has been generated with the measurement of haemoglobin concentration or haematocrit, the prevalence of anaemia will be used as the departure point and then certain extrapolations will be made. By far the most comprehensive assessment of the prevalence of anaemia can be obtained from a meta-analysis of 523 studies by DeMaeyer and Adiels-Tegman (DeMaeyer and Adiels-Tegman, 1985). Inclusion criteria for the analysis included adequate standardization data, studies published after 1960, and studies covering at least 50 subjects other than in the adolescent category. The WHO threshold criteria for haemoglobin concentration and haematocrit were employed (WHO Scientific Group, 1968) and studies not conducted at sea level were corrected for altitude. Clearly, the data have the problems intrinsic to the use of threshold values. The mean percentage prevalence data derived from this analysis are summarized in Table 7.3 by continent, by region defined as either developed or developing, and by age and sex. Based on these data, it is estimated that 30% of the world population is anaemic (1.3 billion people). A marked discrepancy exists between developing and developed regions with 36% of subjects (1.2 billion people) being anaemic in the former, compared with a mere 8% (100 million people) in the latter. Geographically, South Asia and Africa appeared worst off. Although these data give no indication of the severity of the anaemia they certainly speak to the sheer magnitude of the problem.

Clearly not all anaemia is due to iron deficiency. A crude correction to obtain the iron deficiency anaemia number involves the assumption that anaemia in adult males is not iron deficient in origin. This would then indicate the prevalence of non-iron related anaemia. Clearly, this correction factor is intrinsically unsound given that iron deficiency is well documented in males in a number of regions. However, with this correction a very conservative estimate of global iron deficient anaemia can be arrived at of between 0.5 and 0.6 billion people. Since iron deficient anaemia is merely the tip of the iceberg, with roughly two to three times that number affected by storage or functional compartment depletion (Cook *et al.*, 1976), the enormity of the problem is apparent. A number of subsequent investigations have confirmed the very low prevalence in iron deficiency anaemia in developed regions in all age groups (Looker *et al.*, 1989; Manore *et al.*, 1989; Yip, 1989; Borch-Iohnsen *et al.*, 1990; English and Bennett, 1990; Benjamin *et al.*, 1991; Greene-Finestone *et al.*, 1991; Tershakovec and Weller, 1991). Indeed, with these very low prevalence data in these regions, anaemia

Table 7.3 Mean percentage prevalence of anaemia as determined by WHO threshold criteria for various age groups by continent, region and for certain age groups by sex (adapted from data of DeMaeyer and Adiels-Tegman, 1985)

Geographic region*	0–5 years[†]	6–12 years[†]	Adolescents		Adults		
			Male	Female	Male	Female**	Elderly[†]
Africa	59	52	57	45	27	48	47
North America	8	13	8	7	4	8	12
Latin America	34	29	22	12	11	34	18
East Asia	46	24	17	19	15	14	32
South Asia	51	43	12	17	40	57	65
Europe	11	10	5	7	1	14	12
Oceania	36	35	43	45	29	41	43
Less developed	51	38	27	26	26	50	25
More developed[††]	10	12	5	7	2	13	12
World data	49	36	15	15	15	25	16

*Regions are those of the United Nations
[†]Males and females
**Includes pregnant, lactating, and all other women of childbearing age
[††]More developed regions include North America, Japan, Europe, Australia, New Zealand and the former USSR

is increasingly likely to be unrelated to iron deficiency (Yip, 1989; Tershakovec and Weller, 1991). The reasons for reduction of iron deficiency in developed regions are multifactorial and will be addressed in a subsequent section. The implication, however, is that traditional thoughts on screening in developed regions may have to be re-evaluated (Yip, 1989).

9. LIABILITIES OF IRON DEFICIENCY

As will be appreciated from the prior sections, the obvious and inevitable liability of progressive iron deficiency in a haematological sense is the development of anaemia. The clinical manifestations and consequences of anaemia *per se* are generally well known. In recent years, however, it has become well recognized that a number of non-haematological liabilities result from both iron deficiency and iron deficiency anaemia (Dallman, 1982; Finch and Huebers, 1982; Finch and Cook, 1984; Cook and Lynch, 1986; Dallman 1986). This is not unexpected given the plethora of tissue compounds which, because of their dependence on iron, may result in dysfunction in the presence of iron deficiency. Clearly, the iron required by these compounds is neither inviolate nor necessarily reduced proportionally to the degree of anaemia (Beutler and Fairbanks, 1980). Indeed, iron deficiency may affect these compounds somewhat unevenly with this being determined in part by the rate of growth of the tissue, the rate of turnover of the individual iron compound, the work load of the tissue and the developmental stage at which functional iron deficiency develops (Dallman, 1986). As a corollary, the rate at which the relative deficiency is reversed may also vary for various compounds. Although the clinically manifest liabilities of iron deficiency are now being more widely appreciated, in most instances, the biochemical and mechanistic basis of the particular liability are less well understood.

9.1. Central Nervous System Dysfunction

A number of early animal studies indicated a cause and effect relationship between a brief period of iron deficiency anaemia at a young age, reduced brain iron content and behavioural abnormalities. That dietary iron replenishment did not reverse these processes was clearly cause for concern (Dallman et al., 1975; Dallman and Spirito, 1977; Findlay et al., 1981). Human investigations then addressed this problem as, for example, in a study of Israeli children where it was noted that iron deficient infants followed for as many as 4 years had lower developmental scores and IQ test results than non-anaemic controls after such variables as maternal education, socioeconomic status and birth weight were factored out (Palti et al., 1983). Despite methodological criticism, such observations suggest that iron deficiency anaemia is associated with impaired psychomotor development which may not be fully corrected by reversing the iron deficiency anaemia.

A number of subsequent studies have evaluated iron deficiency and central nervous system function. Many have methodological deficiencies and will not be extensively reviewed. Methodological requirements for adequate data have recently been outlined (Wilson-Fairchild et al., 1989). The establishment of causality between iron deficiency anaemia and impaired psychomotor development requires that studies have internal validity, plausibility and external validity. Internal validity for a positive finding requires the absence of differentiating characteristics between the normal and iron deficient anaemia groups other than iron deficiency. Such characteristics might include maternal intelligence, socioeconomic status, paternal intelligence, and the fact that iron deficiency may enhance the absorption of toxic trace elements such as lead (Hallberg, 1989). Internal validity also requires that there be no confounders of behavioural response to iron supplementation such as the ceiling effect or a differential practice effect. In the ceiling effect, the control group already performs maximally for the particular test such that no improvement could be detectable over time, whereas the abnormal population starting at a lower level does have room for improvement. The differential practice effect refers to the concept that while merely repeating a behavioural test is known to cause score improvement, this may be greater for the group with the abnormality. Thus, response to iron supplementation may in fact be apparent rather than real. This does, however, presuppose a positive response. Other internal validity issues for a positive finding include randomization, placebo groups and true blinding. While epidemiologically valid, the ethics of protracted placebo administration to iron deficient children remain highly questionable. Internal validity for negative findings relates to test selection, correctness of the diagnosis of iron deficiency and adequacy of the sample size. In terms of the tests themselves, the commonly used Bayley Scale has, on account of its wide recognition, coefficient of reliability and reproducibility, been widely applied. Its use across age groups has been challenged as well as its ability to define specific components of abnormal behaviour. Scholastic achievement tests suffer the same deficiency. Tests with greater ability to define the abnormal component of behaviour include the attention–retention test, and the Bayley infant behaviour record. Plausibility of a study depends on the demonstration that the observed changes in behaviour correlate with differences in iron status. Epidemiologically, much is made of a dose response between iron administration and degree of response or level of iron depletion and severity of abnormality. The former is all predicated on the notion that a response will be observed to iron replenishment. As already described, much of the available evidence suggests that this does not occur. Plausibility is also enhanced by defining the metabolic basis of observed abnormalities. External validity relates to the presence or absence of effect modifiers of response to iron therapy and thus again assumes a response to the iron.

A number of investigations have addressed the question of behavioural sequelae of iron deficiency at different ages (Oski and Honig, 1978; Deinard et al., 1981; Seshadri et al., 1982; Soemantri et al., 1985; Pollitt et al., 1986, 1989). In a number of these methodological criticisms apply. Two investigations of the impact of iron deficiency on psychomotor development in infants have attempted to address the epidemiological concerns articulated.

These studies were conducted by Lozoff and coworkers in Costa Rica (Lozoff et al., 1987; Lozoff, 1989) and by Walter and colleagues in Chile (Walter et al., 1989; Walter, 1989). In both studies, infants were rigorously classified in terms of iron status by multiple tests and by response to iron therapy. Both studies employed the Bayley scale. Infants with iron deficiency anaemia had significantly lower mental and motor test scores. Reversal of iron deficiency anaemia by iron treatment for three months did not correct the behavioural abnormalities. One methodological problem with the Costa Rican data was the finding that the children with iron deficiency anaemia tended to come from less stimulating home environments and to have mothers with lower IQ tests. However, these variables appeared not to account for the observed differences in infant test scores (Lozoff et al., 1987; Lozoff, 1989). In the Chilean study, this problem of internal validity was obviated by studying a homogeneous population which had been randomized either to receive or not receive iron-fortified foods from the age of 3 months. Re-evaluation at 12 months of age identified iron deficiency almost exclusively in the non-fortified group. This was accompanied by abnormal test scores. The intrinsic differences observed in the Costa Rican study were not detected in the Chilean study. The follow-up of the children from the Costa Rican study indicated impaired cognitive function in those who had had iron deficiency anaemia as infants even after controlling for their different socioeconomic backgrounds (Lozoff et al., 1991).

Studies conducted in school children reveal that iron deficiency anaemia is accompanied by poor IQ test scores (Soemantri et al., 1985; Pollitt et al., 1989). In this age group, it also appears that correction of the iron deficiency anaemia is not accompanied by improved IQ performance.

The most convincing evidence that iron deficiency prejudices central nervous system function would be the demonstration of the metabolic basis of this finding. Data are beginning to appear demonstrating abnormalities of dopaminergic neurotransmission in animals consequent upon central nervous system depletion of iron. This results from a reduction in D_2 receptor expression which appears related to the iron deficiency (Yehuda and Youdim, 1989; Youdim et al., 1989).

At this moment, we must therefore accept that iron deficiency anaemia is associated with impaired psychomotor development and function in children. The data suggest that central nervous system dysfunction persists despite reversal of the deficiency.

9.2. Impaired Work Performance and Response to Exercise

There is unequivocal evidence that iron deficiency anaemia limits work performance. Seminal studies in Sri Lankan tea pickers and Indonesian rubber tappers indicate that reduced productivity is a direct consequence of iron deficiency anaemia (Basta et al., 1979; Edgerton et al., 1979). Indeed, the economics of this have been calculated for three countries and the conclusion reached that the benefits of eradicating iron deficiency in these areas by either a supplementation or fortification programme would outweigh the costs of such programmes by a factor of 4 and 70, respectively (Levin, 1986). There is general acceptance that iron deficient subjects tire more rapidly, experience more severe tachycardia, and have enhanced lactic acid production on exercise (Dallman, 1989). There has long been debate of whether this effect is predominantly due to anaemia or to functional tissue iron depletion. While mechanistically important, practically, the argument is spurious since iron therapy corrects both. The role of functional tissue iron depletion is better established in relation to animal studies (Perkkio et al., 1985; Willis et al., 1990). The data in humans are less clear-cut. While investigations in athletes suggest functional tissue deficiency of iron as being mechanistically important (Schoene et al., 1983) this has not been found in other studies. Phlebotomy studies of iron deficiency anaemia with subsequent correction by transfusion failed to show any effect additional to the anaemia (Celsing et al., 1986). A phlebotomy study in subjects with polycythaemia vera failed to show any clearly definable effect of chronic functional tissue iron depletion on muscle function (Rector et al., 1982). Further work is required to resolve this issue fully.

9.3. Impaired Immune Response

There is much conflicting information on the roles that iron deficiency and, conversely, iron administration play in the causation of infection (Dallman, 1987). This topic is reviewed in Chapter 11. A practical problem, however, is evidence that the malarial parasite appears to thrive in an iron-rich environment and be growth restricted in an iron-poor one (Gordeuk et al., 1992b). Clearly, the liabilities of iron deficiency are such that it should be treated and eradicated (Cook and Lynch, 1986; Dallman, 1989). The practical problem is that high prevalence is often found in endemic malaria areas. Consequently, in such regions iron deficiency eradication must go hand-in-hand with a malaria control programme and surveillance for other infections (Fleming, 1982).

9.4. Adverse Outcome of Pregnancy

Two large epidemiological surveys have reported that maternal anaemia is associated with low birth weight, prematurity and an increased perinatal mortality (Garn et al., 1981; Murphy et al., 1986). Another large study addressed the question of prematurity more directly. Again, a strong association between reduced haematocrit and premature labour was observed (Lieberman et al., 1988). Using the serum ferritin concentration other workers have reported that premature labour was four times more frequent if the concentration was less than 20 ng/ml (Goepel *et al.*, 1988). While a strong association has been found, just as with iron and neurological dysfunction, appropriate studies are now indicated definitively to establish causality between iron deficiency and an adverse outcome of pregnancy. The first prospective study attempting to address this issue has recently supported such a causal relationship (Scholl *et al.*, 1992).

9.5. Miscellaneous Liabilities

The first four liabilities have been discussed on account of their enormous economic implications, their adverse effect on human development and on account of recent pertinent data. A number of other liabilities of iron deficiency have also been described. These will be only briefly listed. The gastrointestinal tract may respond to iron deficiency in the form of glossitis, stomatitis, gastritis and the development of oesophageal webs (Cook and Lynch, 1986). A number of structural and chemical changes in the hair, nails and skin as a consequence of iron deficiency are also well described (Sato, 1991). A number of metabolic sequelae of iron deficiency have also been reported including impaired thermogenesis, thyroid metabolism and catecholamine turnover (Beard *et al.*, 1990a,b). Finally, iron deficiency enhances the absorption of other cations. In particular, enhanced lead absorption may result in severe toxicity particularly in children as may enhanced aluminium absorption in the setting of renal insufficiency.

10. TREATMENT AND PREVENTION

The liabilities of iron deficiency and the significant global prevalence necessitate that treatment and prevention receive high priority. The problem, however, is neither simple nor correctable by a single approach. Possible strategies include all of the following: treatment of individual proven cases, supplementation of groups at risk with or without prior screening, targeted fortification, global fortification, and finally, dietary modification. Treatment of the diagnosed individual is self-evident. The point, however, must be stressed that iron deficiency is *per se* not a diagnosis. Consequently, it is of importance, particularly in the low risk situation, to exclude non-physiological blood loss and to treat this appropriately. Most cases of iron deficiency can be adequately treated by oral administration of a simple iron salt (e.g. ferrous sulfate). Reasons for treatment failures include inadequate dose, a poorly available iron salt, poor compliance, ingestion with food or inhibitory beverages and significant undiagnosed blood loss. Therapeutic failure due to malabsorption is a rare phenomenon usually related to intrinsic gastrointestinal disease. This can be screened for by measuring the serum iron value before and after ingestion of two ferrous sulfate tablets. Poor compliance is often related to gastrointestinal upset. Since such upset is related to the amount of available iron in the therapeutic preparation the problem should first be addressed by giving a smaller dose of the simple iron salt, or a preparation such as ferrous gluconate which contains less elemental iron in each tablet. The recent demonstration of high bioavailability and low level of gastrointestinal side-effects of ferrous sulfate added to a gastric delivery system (GDS) holds great promise (Cook *et al.*, 1990). It is to be hoped that this gastric delivery system will be developed commercially in the near future. In the rare case of true iron malabsorption or severe gastrointestinal intolerance, iron may be administered parenterally with the appropriate precautions. Whether the goal of treatment should be repair of functional deficit or replenishment of stores is a debatable point and, to some extent, depends on the physician's practice philosophy.

The use of dietary modification can be dispensed with fairly rapidly. While the wealth of data from single meal studies make dietary modification, either by increasing promotory ligands or reducing inhibitory ones, an intellectually attractive exercise this would, at this moment, be decidedly premature. The only factor convincingly shown to modify population iron nutrition is meat intake. Increasing meat intake in regions of low socioeconomic status or where religious considerations pertain is hardly practical. Indeed, increasing meat intake may, by virtue of its lipid and protein composition, have other health ramifications. Other promoters or inhibitors have, to date, not been convincingly documented to modify population iron nutrition. Further study of this is required before the dietary modification approach can be seriously recommended.

10.1. Choice of Iron Intervention Strategy

Before considering specific intervention strategies it is important to document the iron status of the particular population and the prevalence of iron deficiency anaemia. Where prevalence of iron deficiency anaemia is low, two considerations are pertinent. First, any public health initiative aimed at improving the overall iron nutrition is inappropriate. Second, the only appropriate intervention should be screening of high risk groups such as infants, pre-school children, pregnant women, and trained athletes and supplementation of identified deficient subjects. Indeed, in the USA, levels of iron deficiency have reached such low levels in pre-school children on account of improved socioeconomic status, infant food fortification, improved infant feeding practices and public health programmes, that it is questionable whether screening of this group is required any longer (Yip, 1989).

If the population has a medium prevalence of iron deficiency then two strategies are appropriate (International Nutritional Anemia Consultative Group, 1977), either a pilot fortification trial or a prophylactic supplementation trial. If successful, these should then be extended to regional or national programmes. In regions of high prevalence, a pilot therapeutic supplementation trial should be undertaken and, if successful, translated into a regional or national programme.

Initial evaluations for a supplementation strategy include establishing the source of supply, adequate budgetary provision, the size of the supply, storage, quality control of the supplements, the level of supplementation, the infrastructure for delivery, the training of health professionals, methods for ensuring and monitoring compliance, methods and infrastructure for monitoring response and, if applicable, methods and infrastructure for screening at-risk groups (UN Admin. Comm., 1991). Clearly, the population coverage is based on individuals, the time to achieve a response is usually short (months), the initial costs are very high, the continuing costs are high, public participation has to be active, personnel requirements are high and compliance is a problem (International Nutritional Anemia Consultative Group, 1977). The advantages are that iron exposure is fairly brief and, if accompanied by screening, is focused to avoid exposure of normal subjects to increased iron intake.

By contrast, fortification requires very intensive initial research to establish the optimal centrally processed vehicle, the optimal fortificant, acceptable bioavailability, stability, and acceptability of vehicle and fortificant in food. Close collaboration is required with food processing industries. Population coverage by fortification is broad and unscreened. It may be targeted, as with infant cereal fortification, or global. The time required for response is longer, being of the order of a few years. The initial costs are moderate and the continuing costs are low. Public participation is not required and the personnel requirements are minimal. The degree of expertise required is high. A major advantage is that compliance is high. The major disadvantage is that increased iron intake is protracted and unfocused as many normal people will be ingesting greater than normal amounts of iron (International Nutritional Anemia Consultative Group, 1977). It is also important to ensure that the fortificant has no untoward side-effects on population health such as, for example, the depletion of other divalent cations when FeEDTA is used as the fortificant. Several strategies have been employed in pilot fortification trials including the use of NaFeEDTA as the fortificant and a variety of staples, such as sugar, and condiments such as fish sauce, fish paste and curry powder, as vehicles (Layrisse and Martinez-Torres, 1977; Viteri et al., 1978; Lamparelli et al., 1987; Ballot et al., 1989). A rather novel approach has been the use of animal haemoglobin as the fortificant baked into cookies as part of a school lunch programme (Stekel, 1981; Walter et al., 1993). At a national level, many Western countries employ moderate to high levels of fortification. The low prevalence of iron deficiency in these areas has already been outlined. The extent to which this reflects success of the programme, additional supplemental programmes, or other socioeconomic or dietary factors is as yet not fully resolved (Yip, 1989).

Clearly, in many regions addressing the question of suboptimal iron nutrition is merely one component of a public health issue of enormous proportions. In many developing areas, the iron problem co-exists with other nutritional deficiencies such as vitamin A or iodine, and with major infection-related problems including intestinal parasitism, malaria, and epidemic and endemic infectious processes. In these circumstances, iron fortification or supplementation is but one component of the public health initiative. Supplementation of other deficient micronutrients, treatment of intestinal parasitism, control of malaria and eradication of other infectious diseases need to proceed *pari passu*. Indeed, an indirect benefit of vitamin A supplementation appears to be an increase in iron status, and when combined with iron supplementation, results in better iron nutrition than either modality applied on its own (Mejia and Chew, 1988). Since hookworm infestation contributes directly to iron deficiency and iron replacement may exacerbate malarial infection, eradication programmes for each of these should accompany a strategy aimed at improving iron nutrition.

10.2. Concerns about Broad-based Fortification or Supplementation

It is obvious that fortification and unscreened supplementation indiscriminately supply increased iron to subjects who need it and those that do not. The danger has been considered acceptable in that the only people thought to be at risk are those with the HLA-linked iron loading disease, idiopathic haemochromatosis, and those with iron loading anaemias (Bothwell and Charlton, 1982). However, in recent years disturbing information has begun to appear suggesting that excess iron intake may not be as innocuous as was once believed. As discussed in detail in Chapters 8 and 11, epidemiological studies indicating that subjects who develop malignancy, even several years later, tend to have had higher iron stores have generated much controversy, as have reports of an increased risk of ischaemic heart disease in subjects with higher levels of iron stores, albeit still within the normal range (Chapter 8). In addition, the suggestion that idiopathic haemochromatosis homozygotes are the only group other than subjects with iron-loading anaemias at risk from fortification or supplementation needs to be re-evaluated. Recent data from Zimbabwe suggest that there may be hereditary iron-loading conditions other than for the HLA-linked condition (Gordeuk et al., 1992a). Finally, longitudinal survey data in the USA give additional cause for concern. When the NHANES II study (1976–1980), the HHANES study (1982–1984) and the pilot data from the NHANES III survey (1987–1988) are compared in all age group categories and both sexes, there appears to be a progressive increase in serum ferritin concentrations (Looker et al., 1991). While interpretation of these data is complex, taken together there would appear to be reason for conservatism in relation to fortification and unscreened supplementation, particularly in more iron-replete regions. In addition, the urgent need for more comprehensive research evaluation of the various issues raised is obvious.

ACKNOWLEDGEMENTS

Supported by NIH grant DK 39246 and AID Cooperative Agreement DAN-5115-A-00-7908-00. The author thanks Ms L. Kuharich for preparation of the manuscript and Dr B. S. Skikne for helpful comments during preparation.

REFERENCES

Bainton, D. F. and Finch, C. A. (1964) The diagnosis of iron deficiency anemia. Am. J. Med. **37**, 62–70.
Ballot, D. E., MacPhail, A. P., Bothwell, T. H., Gillooly, M. and Mayet, F. G. (1989) Fortification of curry powder with NaFe(III)EDTA in an iron-deficient population: report of a controlled iron-fortification trial. Am. J. Clin. Nutr. **49**, 162–169.
Barber, S. A., Bull, N. L. and Buss, D. H. (1985) Low iron intakes among young women in Britain. Br. Med. J. **290**, 743–744.
Basta, S. S., Soekirman, M. S., Karyadi, D. and Scrimshaw, N. S. (1979) Iron deficiency anemia and the productivity of adult males in Indonesia. Am. J. Clin. Nutr. **32**, 916–925.
Baynes, R. D. and Bothwell, T. H. (1990) Iron deficiency. Annu. Rev. Nutr. **10**, 133–148.
Baynes, R. D., Flax, H., Bothwell, T. H., Bezwoda, W. R., Atkinson, P. and Mendelow, B. (1986) Red blood cell distribution width in the anemia secondary to tuberculosis. Am. J. Clin. Pathol. **85**, 226–229.
Baynes, R. D., Bothwell, T. H., Bezwoda, W. R., Gear, A. J. and Atkinson, P. (1987a) Hematologic and iron-related measurements in rheumatoid arthritis. Am. J. Clin. Pathol. **87**, 196–200.

Baynes, R. D., Bothwell, T. H., Bezwoda, W. R., MacPhail, A. P. and Derman, D. P. (1987b) Relationship between absorption of inorganic and food iron in field studies. *Ann. Nutr. Metab.* **31**, 109–116.

Baynes, R. D., MacFarlane, B. J., Bothwell, T. H. *et al.* (1990) The promotive effect of soy sauce on iron absorption in human subjects. *Eur. J. Clin. Nutr.* **44**, 419–424.

Baynes, R. D., Shih, Y. J. and Cook, J. D. (1991a) Production of soluble transferrin receptor by K562 erythroleukemia cells. *Br. J. Haematol.* **78**, 450–455.

Baynes, R. D., Shih, Y. J., Hudson, B. G. and Cook, J. D. (1991b) Characterization of transferrin receptor released by K562 erythroleukemia cells. *Proc. Soc. Exp. Biol. Med.* **197**, 416–423.

Baynes, R. D., Shih, Y. J. and Cook, J. D. (1993) Mechanism of production of the serum transferrin receptor. 11th International Conference on Iron and Iron Proteins, Jerusalem, 1993.

Beard, J. L., Borel, M. J. and Derr, J. (1990a) Impaired thermoregulation and thyroid function in iron-deficiency anemia. *Am. J. Clin. Nutr.* **52**, 813–819.

Beard, J. L., Tobin, B. W. and Smith, S. M. (1990b) Effects of iron repletion and correction of anemia on norepinephrine turnover and thyroid metabolism in iron deficiency. *Proc. Soc. Exp. Biol. Med.* **193**, 306–312.

Beguin, Y., Huebers, H. A., Josephson, B. and Finch, C. A. (1988) Transferrin receptors in rat plasma. *Proc. Natl. Acad. Sci. USA* **85**, 637–640.

Benjamin, J. T., Dickens, M. D., Ford, R. F. *et al.* (1991) Normative data of hemoglobin concentration and free erythrocyte protoporphyrin in a private pediatric practice: A 1990 update. *Clin. Pediatr.* **30**, 74–76.

Bessman, J. D., Gilmer, P. R. and Gardner, F. H. (1983) Improved classification of anemias by MCV and RDW. *Am. J. Clin. Pathol.* **80**, 322–326.

Beutler, E. and Fairbanks, V. F. (1980) The effects of iron deficiency. In: *Iron in Biochemistry and Medicine* 2nd edn, (eds A. Jacobs and M. Worwood), Academic Press, London, p. 393.

Beveridge, B. R., Bannerman, R. M., Evanson, J. M. and Witts, L. J. (1965) Hypochromic anaemia. A retrospective study and follow-up of 378 in-patients. *Q. J. Med.* **34**, 145–161.

Bezwoda, W. R., Bothwell, T. H., Charlton, R. W. *et al.* (1983) The relative dietary importance of haem and non-haem iron. *S. Afr. Med. J.* **64**, 552–556.

Bjorn-Rasmussen, E., Hallberg, L., Isaksson, B. and Arvidsson, B. (1974) Food iron absorption in man. Applications of the two-pool extrinsic tag method to measure heme and nonheme iron absorption from the whole diet. *J. Clin. Invest.* **53**, 247–255.

Borch-Iohnsen, B., Meltzer, H. M., Stenberg, V. and Reinskou, T. (1990) Iron status in a group of Norwegian menstruating women. *Eur. J. Clin. Nutr.* **44**, 23–28.

Bothwell, T. H. and Charlton, R. W. (1982) A general approach to the problems of iron deficiency and iron overload in the population at large. *Semin. Hematol.* **19**, 54–67.

Bothwell, T. H., Pirzio-Biroli, G. and Finch, C. A. (1958) Iron absorption I. Factors influencing absorption. *J. Lab. Clin. Med.* **51**, 24–36.

Bothwell, T. H., Charlton, R. W., Cook, J. D. and Finch, C. A. (1979) *Iron Metabolism in Man*, Blackwell Scientific, Oxford.

Bothwell, T. H., Baynes, R. D., MacFarlane, B. J. and MacPhail, A. P. (1989) Nutritional iron requirements and food iron absorption. *J. Intern. Med.* **226**, 357–365.

Brune, M., Magnusson, B., Persson, H. and Hallberg, L. (1986) Iron losses in sweat. *Am. J. Clin. Nutr.* **43**, 438–443.

Carriaga, M. T., Skikne, B. S., Finley, B., Cutler, B. and Cook, J. D. (1991) Serum transferrin receptor for the detection of iron deficiency in pregnancy. *Am. J. Clin. Nutr.* **54**, 1077–1081.

Cavill, I., Jacobs, A. and Worwood, M. (1986) Diagnostic methods for iron status. *Ann. Clin. Biochem.* **23**, 168–171.

Cazzola, M., Arosio, P., Barosi, G., Bergamaschi, G., Dezza, L. and Ascari, E. (1983a) Ferritin in the red cells of normal subjects and patients with iron deficiency and iron overload. *Br. J. Haematol.* **53**, 659–665.

Cazzola, M., Dezza, L., Bergamaschi, G. *et al.* (1983b) Biologic and clinical significance of red cell ferritin. *Blood* **62**, 1078–1087.

Cazzola, M., Pootrakul, P., Bergamaschi, G., Huebers, H. A., Eng, M. and Finch, C. A. (1987) Adequacy of iron supply for erythropoiesis: in vivo observations in humans. *J. Lab. Clin. Med.* **110**, 734–739.

Celsing, F., Blomstrand, E., Werner, B., Pihlstedt, P. and Ekblom, B. (1986) Effects of iron deficiency on endurance and muscle enzyme activity in man. *Med. Sci. Sports Exerc.* **18**, 156–161.

Chitambar, C. R., Loebel, A. L. and Noble, N. A. (1991) Shedding of transferrin receptor from rat reticulocytes during maturation in vitro: Soluble receptor is derived from receptor shed in vesicles. *Blood* **78**, 2444–2450.

Cook, J. D. (1982) Clinical evaluation of iron deficiency. *Semin. Hematol.* **19**, 6–18.

Cook, J. D. (1990) Adaptation in iron metabolism. *Am. J. Clin. Nutr.* **51**, 301–308.

Cook, J. D. and Finch, C. A. (1979) Assessing iron status of a population. *Am. J. Clin. Nutr.* **32**, 2115–2119.

Cook, J. D. and Lynch, S. R. (1986) The liabilities of iron deficiency. *Blood* **68**, 803–809.

Cook, J. D. and Skikne, B. S. (1989) Iron deficiency: Definition and diagnosis. *J. Intern. Med.* **226**, 349–355.

Cook, J. D., Alvarado, J., Gutniskey, A. *et al.* (1971) Nutritional deficiency and anemia in Latin America: a collaborative study. *Blood* **38**, 591–603.

Cook, J. D., Lipschitz, D. A., Miles, L. E. and Finch, C. A. (1974) Serum ferritin as a measure of iron stores in normal subjects. *Am. J. Clin. Nutr.* **27**, 681–687.

Cook, J. D., Finch, C. A. and Smith, N. J. (1976) Evaluation of the iron status of a population. *Blood* **48**, 449–455.

Cook, J. D., Watson, S. S., Simpson, K. M., Lipschitz, D. A. and Skikne, B. S. (1984) The effect of high ascorbic acid supplementation on body iron stores. *Blood* **64**, 721–726.

Cook, J. D., Skikne, B. S., Lynch, S. R. and Reusser, M. E. (1986) Estimates of iron sufficiency in the US population. *Blood* **68**, 726–731.

Cook, J. D., Carriaga, M., Kahn, S. G., Schalch, W. and Skikne, B. S. (1990) Gastric delivery system for iron supplementation. *Lancet* **335**, 1136–1139.

Cook, J. D., Dassenko, S. A. and Lynch, S. R. (1991) Assessment of the role of nonheme-iron availability in iron balance. *Am. J. Clin. Nutr.* **54**, 717–722.

Cook, J. D., Baynes, R. D. and Skikne, B. S. (1992a) Iron deficiency and the assessment of iron status. *Nutr. Res. Rev.*, **5**, 189–202.

Cook, J. D., Skikne, B. S. and Baynes, R. D. (1992b) Screening strategies for nutritional iron deficiency. In: *Nutritional Anemias* (eds S. Fomon and S. Zlotkin), Nestlé Nutrition Workshop Series, Vol. 30, pp. 159–168. Nestec and Raven Press, New York.

Dallman, P. R. (1981) Anemia of prematurity. *Annu. Rev. Med.* **32**, 136–160.

Dallman, P. R. (1982) Manifestations of iron deficiency. *Semin. Hematol.* **19**, 19–30.

Dallman, P. R. (1986) Biochemical basis for the manifestations of iron deficiency. *Annu. Rev. Nutr.* **6**, 13–40.

Dallman, P. R. (1987) Iron deficiency and the immune response. *Am. J. Clin. Nutr.* **46**, 329–334.

Dallman, P. R. (1989) Iron deficiency: does it matter? *J. Intern. Med.* **226**, 367–372.

Dallman, P. R. and Spirito, R. A. (1977) Brain iron in the rat: extremely slow turnover in normal rats may explain long-lasting effects of early iron deficiency. *J. Nutr.* **107**, 1075–1081.

Dallman, P. R., Siimes, M. A. and Manies, E. C. (1975) Brain iron: persistent deficiency following short-term iron deprivation in the young rat. *Br. J. Haematol.* **31**, 209–215.

Deinard, A., Gilbert, A., Dodds, M. and Egeland, B. (1981) Iron deficiency and behavioral deficits. *Pediatrics* **68**, 828–833.

DeMaeyer, E. and Adiels-Tegman, M. (1985) The prevalence of anaemia in the world. *Wld. Hlth. Statist. Quart.* **38**, 302–316.

Edgerton, V. R., Gardner, G. W., Ohira, Y., Gunawardena, K. A. and Senewiratne, B. (1979) Iron-deficiency anaemia and its effect on worker productivity and activity patterns. *Br. Med. J.* **2**, 1546–1549.

English, R. M. and Bennett, S. A. (1990) Iron status of Australian children. *Med. J. Aust.* **152**, 582–586.

Eschbach, J. W. (1991) Recombinant human erythropoietin (epoetin alpha) in patients on hemodialysis: United States. In: *Erythropoietin Molecular, Cellular and Clinical Biology* (eds A. J. Ersler, J. W. Adamson, J. W. Eschbach and C. G. Winearls), Johns Hopkins University Press, Baltimore, p. 211.

Eschbach, J. W., Egrie, J. C., Downing, M. R., Browne, J. K. and Adamson, J. W. (1987) Correction of the anemia of end-stage renal disease with recombinant human erythropoietin. Results of a combined phase I and II clinical trial. *N. Engl. J. Med.* **316**, 73–78.

Eschbach, J. W., Abdulhadi, M. H., Browne, J. K. *et al.* (1989) Recombinant human erythropoietin in anemic patients with end-stage renal disease. Results of a phase II multicenter clinical trial. *Ann. Intern. Med.* **111**, 992–1000.

FAO/WHO Joint Expert Consultation Report (1988) Requirements of Vitamin A, Iron, Folate and Vitamin B12. FAO Food and Nutrition Series 23, Food and Agriculture Organization, Rome.

Ferguson, B. J., Skikne, B. S., Simpson, K. M., Baynes, R. D. and Cook, J. D. (1992) Serum transferrin receptor distinguishes the anemia of chronic disease from iron deficiency anemia. *J. Lab. Clin. Med.* **119**, 385–390.

Finch, C. A. and Cook, J. D. (1984) Iron deficiency. *Am. J. Clin. Nutr.* **39**, 471–477.

Finch, C. A. and Huebers, H. (1982) Perspectives in iron metabolism. *N. Engl. J. Med.* **306**, 1520–1528.

Finch, C. A., Cook, J. D., Labbe, R. F. and Culala, M. (1977) Effect of blood donation on iron stores as evaluated by serum ferritin. *Blood* **50**, 441–447.

Findlay, E., Ng, K. T., Reid, R. L. and Armstrong, S. M. (1981) The effect of iron deficiency during development on passive avoidance learning in the adult rat. *Physiol. Behav.* **27**, 1089–1096.

Fleming, A. F. (1982) Iron deficiency in the tropics. *Clin. Haematol.* **11**, 365–388.

Fleming, J. L., Ahlquist, D. A., McGill, D. B., Zinsmeister, A. R., Ellefson, R. D. and Schwartz, S. (1987) Influence of aspirin and ethanol on fecal blood levels as determined by using the HemoQuant assay. *Mayo Clin. Proc.* **62**, 159–163.

Flowers, C. H., Skikne, B. S., Covell, A. M. and Cook, J. D. (1989) The clinical measurement of serum transferrin receptor. *J. Lab. Clin. Med.* **114**, 368–377.

Fricker, J., LeMoel, G. and Appelbaum, M. (1990) Obesity and iron status in menstruating women. *Am. J. Clin. Nutr.* **52**, 863–866.

Garby, L., Irnell, L. and Werner, I. (1969) Iron deficiency in women of fertile age in a Swedish community. III. Estimation of prevalence based on response to iron supplementation. *Acta Med. Scand.* **185**, 113–117.

Garn, S. M., Ridella, S. A., Tetzold, A. S. and Falkner, F. (1981) Maternal haematological levels and pregnancy outcomes. *Semin. Perinatol.* **5**, 155–162.

Goepel, E., Ulmer, R. D. and Neth, R. D. (1988) Premature labor contractions and the value of serum ferritin during pregnancy. *Gynecol. Obstet. Invest.* **26**, 265–273.

Goodnough, L. T. and Brittenham, G. M. (1990) Limitations of the erythropoietic response to serial phlebotomy: implications for autologous blood donor programs. *J. Lab. Clin. Med.* **115**, 28–35.

Goodnough, L. T., Rudnick, S., Price, T. H. *et al.* (1989) Increased preoperative collection of autologous blood with recombinant human erythropoietin therapy. *N. Engl. J. Med.* **321**, 1163–1168.

Gordeuk, V., Mukiibi, J., Hasstedt, S. J. *et al.* (1992a) Iron overload in Africa. Interaction between a gene and dietary iron intake. *N. Engl. J. Med.* **326**, 95–100.

Gordeuk, V. R., Thuma, P. E., Brittenham, G. M. *et al.* (1992b) Iron chelation with desferroxamine B in adults with asymptomatic plasmodium falciparum parasitemia. *Blood* **79**, 308–312.

Grasbeck, R., Majuri, R., Kouvonen, I. and Tenhunen, R. (1982) Spectral and other studies on the intestinal haem receptor of the pig. *Biochim. Biophys. Acta* **700**, 137–142.

Green, R., Charlton, R., Seftel, H. *et al.* (1968) Body iron excretion in man. A collaborative study. *Am. J. Med.* **45**, 336–353.

Greene-Finestone, L., Feldman, W., Heick, H. and Luke, B. (1991) Prevalence and risk factors of iron depletion and iron deficiency anemia among infants in Ottawa-Carleton. *J. Can. Diet. Assoc.* **52**, 20–23.

Guillebaud, J., Bonnar, J., Morehead, J. and Matthews, A. (1976) Menstrual blood loss with intrauterine devices. *Lancet* **i**, 387–390.

Guyatt, G. H., Patterson, C., Ali, M. *et al.* (1990) Diagnosis of iron-deficiency anemia in the elderly. *Am. J. Med.* **88**, 205–209.

Hallberg, L. (1988) Iron balance in pregnancy. In: *Vitamins and Minerals in Pregnancy and Lactation* (ed. H. Berger), Nestlé Ltd/Raven, Vevey/New York, p. 115.

Hallberg, L. (1989) Search for nutritional confounding factors in the relationship between iron deficiency and brain function. *Am. J. Clin. Nutr.* **50**, 598–606.

Hallberg, L. and Bjorn-Rasmussen, E. (1981) Measurement of iron absorption from meals contaminated with iron. *Am. J. Clin. Nutr.* **34**, 2808–2815.

Hallberg, L. and Rossander-Hulten, L. (1991) Iron requirements in menstruating women. *Am. J. Clin. Nutr.* **54**, 1047–1058.

Hallberg, L., Hogdahl, A.-M., Nilsson, L. and Rybo, G. (1966) Menstrual blood loss – a population study. Variation at different ages and attempts to define normality. *Acta Obstet. Gynaecol. Scand.* **45**, 320–351.

Harding, C., Heuser, J. and Stahl, P. (1983) Receptor-mediated endocytosis of transferrin and recycling of the transferrin receptor in rat reticulocytes. *J. Cell Biol.* **97**, 329–339.

Haymes, E. M. and Spillman, D. M. (1989) Iron status of women distance runners, sprinters, and control women. *Int. J. Sports Med.* **10**, 430–433.

Hefnawi, F., El Zayat, A. F. and Yacout, M. M. (1980) Physiologic studies of menstrual blood loss. I. Range and consistency of menstrual blood loss in and iron requirements of menstruating Egyptian women. *Int. J. Gynaecol. Obstet.* **17**, 343–348.

Hillman, R. S. and Finch, C. A. (1985) *Red Cell Manual*, 5th edn, F. A. Davis Co., Philadelphia.

Huebers, H. A. and Finch, C. A. (1987) The physiology of transferrin and transferrin receptors. *Physiol. Rev.* **67**, 520–582.

Huebers, H. A., Beguin, Y., Pootrakul, P., Einspahr, D. and Finch, C. A. (1990) Intact transferrin receptors in human plasma and their relation to erythropoiesis. *Blood* **75**, 102–107.

Hunt, J. R., Mullen, L. M., Lykken, G. I., Gallagher, S. K. and Nielsen, F. H. (1990) Ascorbic acid: Effect on ongoing iron absorption and status in iron-depleted young women. *Am. J. Clin. Nutr.* **51**, 649–655.

International Nutritional Anemia Consultative Group (1977) *Guidelines for the Eradication of Iron Deficiency Anemia*, The Nutrition Foundation, Washington, D.C., pp. 1–29.

Kimura, H., Finch, C. A. and Adamson, J. W. (1986) Hematopoiesis in the rat: quantitation of hematopoietic progenitors and the response to iron deficiency anemia. *J. Cell. Physiol.* **126**, 298–306.

Kohgo, Y. (1986) Structure of transferrin and transferrin receptor. *Acta Haematol. Jpn.* **49**, 1627–1634.

Kohgo, Y., Nishisato, T., Kondo, H., Tsushima, N., Niitsu, Y. and Urushizaki, I. (1986) Circulating transferrin receptor in human serum. *Br. J. Haematol.* **64**, 277–281.

Kohgo, Y., Niitsu, Y., Kondo, H. *et al.* (1987a) Serum transferrin receptor as a new index of erythropoiesis. *Blood* **70**, 1955–1958.

Kohgo, Y., Niitsu, Y., Nishisato, T. *et al.* (1987b) Externalization of transferrin receptor in established human cell lines. *Cell Biol. Int. Rep.* **11**, 871–879.

Kooistra, M. P., Van As, A., Struyvenberg, A. and Marx, J. J. (1991) Iron metabolism in patients with the anaemia of end stage renal disease during treatment with recombinant human erythropoietin. *Br. J. Haematol.* **79**, 634–639.

Krantz, S. B. (1991) Erythropoietin. *Blood* **77**, 419–434.

Labbe, R. F. and Rettmer, R. L. (1989) Zinc protoporphyrin: A product of iron-deficient erythropoiesis. *Semin. Hematol.* **26**, 40–46.

Lamparelli, R. D., MacPhail, A. P., Bothwell, T. H. *et al.* (1987) Curry powder as a vehicle for iron fortification: effects on iron absorption. *Am. J. Clin. Nutr.* **46**, 335–340.

Layrisse, M. and Martinez-Torres, C. (1977) Fe(III)-EDTA complex as iron fortification. *Am. J. Clin. Nutr.* **30**, 1166–1174.

Layrisse, M. and Roche, M. (1964) The relationship between anemia and hookworm infection. *Am. J. Hyg.* **79**, 279–301.

Lee, G. R. (1983) The anemia of chronic disease. *Semin. Hematol.* **20**, 61–80.

Leggett, B. A., Brown, N. N., Bryant, S. J., Duplock, L., Powell, L. W. and Halliday, J. W. (1990) Factors affecting the concentrations of ferritin in serum in a healthy Australian population. *Clin. Chem.* **36**, 1350–1355.

Levin, H. M. (1986) A benefit–cost analysis of nutritional programs for anaemia reduction. *Res. Observ.* **1**, 219–245.

Lieberman, E., Ryan, K. J., Monson, R. R. and Schoenbaum, S. C. (1988) Association of maternal hematocrit with premature labor. *Am. J. Obstet. Gynecol.* **159**, 107–114.

Looker, A., Sempos, C. T., Johnson, C. and Yetley, E. A. (1988) Vitamin-mineral supplement use: association with dietary intake and iron status of adults. *J. Am. Diet. Assoc.* **88**, 808–814.

Looker, A. C., Johnson, C. L., McDowell, M. A. and Yetley, E. A. (1989) Iron status: prevalence of impairment of three Hispanic groups in the United States. *Am. J. Clin. Nutr.* **49**, 553–558.

Looker, A. C., Gunter, E. W., Cook, J. D., Green, R. and Harris, J. W. (1991) Comparing serum ferritin values from different population studies. National Center for Health Statistics. *Vital Health Stat.* **2**(III), 1–18.

Lozoff, B. (1989) Methodologic issues in studying behavioral effects of infant iron-deficiency anemia. *Am. J. Clin. Nutr.* **50**, 641–654.

Lozoff, B., Brittenham, G. M., Wolf, A. W. *et al.* (1987) Iron deficiency anemia and iron therapy: Effects on infant developmental test performance. *Pediatrics* **79**, 981–995.

Lozoff, B., Jimenez, E. and Wolf, A. W. (1991) Long-term developmental outcome of infants with iron deficiency. *N. Engl. J. Med.* **325**, 687–694.

Lynch, S. R., Dassenko, S. A., Morck, T. A., Beard, J. L. and Cook, J. D. (1985) Soy protein products and heme iron absorption in humans. *Am. J. Clin. Nutr.* **41**, 13–20.

Manore, M. M., Vaughan, L. A. and Carroll, S. S. (1989) Iron status in free living, low income elderly. *Nutr. Rep. Int.* **39**, 1–11.

McClelland, A., Kuhn, L. C. and Ruddle, F. H. (1984) The human transferrin receptor gene: genomic organization and the complete primary structure of the receptor deduced from a cDNA sequence. *Cell* **39**, 267–274.

Mejia, L. A. and Chew, F. (1988) Hematological effect of supplementing anemic children with vitamin A alone and in combination with iron. *Am. J. Clin. Nutr.* **48**, 595–600.

Meyer, T. E., Kassianides, C., Bothwell, T. H. and Green, A. (1984) Effects of heavy alcohol consumption on serum ferritin concentrations. *S. Afr. Med. J.* **66**, 573–575.

Misago, M., Chiba, S., Kikuchi, M., Tsukada, J. and Eto, S. (1987) Population size of erythroid progenitor cells (CFU-E) and erythropoiesis in iron deficiency anemia. *Acta Haematol. Jpn.* **50**, 1126–1133.

Monsen, E. R. and Balintfy, J. L. (1982) Calculating dietary iron bioavailability: refinement and computerization. *J. Am. Diet. Assoc.* **80**, 307–311.

Monsen, E. R., Hallberg, L., Layrisse, M. *et al.* (1978) Estimation of available dietary iron. *Am. J. Clin. Nutr.* **31**, 134–141.

Morgan, E. H. (1981) Transferrin, biochemistry, physiology and clinical significance. *Mol. Aspects Med.* **4**, 1–123.

Murphy, J. F., O'Riordan, J., Newcombe, R. G., Coles, E. C. and Pearson, J. F. (1986) Relation of haemoglobin levels in first and second trimesters to outcome of pregnancy. *Lancet* **i**, 992–994.

National Research Council (1989) *Recommended Daily Allowances*, 10th edn, National Academy Press, Washington DC.

Newhouse, I. J. and Clement, D. B. (1988) Iron status in athletes. An update. *Sports Med.* **5**, 337–352.

Nickerson, H. J., Holubets, M. C., Weiler, B. R., Haas, R. G., Schwartz, S. and Ellefson, M. E. (1989) Causes of iron deficiency in adolescent athletes. *J. Pediatr.* **114**, 657–663.

Nilsson, L. and Solvell, L. (1967) Clinical studies on oral contraceptives – a randomized, double blind, crossover study of four different preparations. *Acta Obstet. Gynaecol. Scand. (Suppl)* **46**, 1–31.

Oski, F. A. and Honig, A. S. (1978) The effects of therapy on the developmental scores of iron-deficient infants. *J. Pediatr.* **92**, 21–25.

Palti, H., Peusner, B. and Adler, B. (1983) Does anemia in infancy affect achievement on developmental and intelligence tests? *Hum. Biol.* **55**, 189–194.

Pan, B. T. and Johnstone, R. M. (1983) Fate of the transferrin receptor during maturation of sheep reticulocytes in vitro: selective externalization of the receptor. *Cell* **33**, 967–978.

Perkkio, M. V., Jansson, L. T., Brooks, G. A., Refino, C. J. and Dallman, P. R. (1985) Work performance in iron deficiency of increasing severity. *J. Appl. Physiol.* **58**, 1477–1480.

Pilch, S. M. and Senti, F. R. (eds) (1984) *Assessment of the Iron Nutritional Status of the U.S. Population Based on Data Collected in the Second National Health and Nutrition Examination Survey, 1976–1980.* Life Sciences Research Office, FASEB, Bethesda, MD.

Pollitt, E., Saco-Pollitt, C., Leibel, R. L. and Viteri, F. E. (1986) Iron deficiency and behavioral development in infants and preschool children. *Am. J. Clin. Nutr.* **43**, 555–565.

Pollitt, E., Hathirat, P., Kotchabhakdi, N. J., Missell, L. and Valyasevi, A. (1989) Iron deficiency and educational achievement in Thailand. *Am. J. Clin. Nutr.* **50**, 687–697.

Pootrakul, P., Wattanasaree, J., Anuwatanakulchai, M. and Wasi, P. (1984) Increased red blood cell protoporphyrin in thalassemia: a result of relative iron deficiency. *Am. J. Clin. Pathol.* **82**, 289–293.

Raffin, S. B., Woo, C. H., Roost, K. T., Price, D. C. and Schmid, R. (1974) Intestinal absorption of hemoglobin iron-heme cleavage by mucosal heme oxygenase. *J. Clin. Invest.* **54**, 1344–1352.

Rector, W. G., Jr, Fortuin, N. J. and Conley, C. L. (1982) Non-hematologic effects of chronic iron deficiency. A study of patients with polycythemia vera treated solely with venesections. *Medicine* **61**, 382–389.

Rios, E., Lipschitz, D. A., Cook, J. D. and Smith, N. J. (1975) Relationship of maternal and infant iron stores as assessed by determination of plasma ferritin. *Pediatrics* **55**, 694–699.

Rybo, G. and Hallberg, L. (1966) Influence of heredity and environment on normal menstrual blood loss. *Acta Obstet. Gynaecol. Scand.* **45**, 389–410.

Saarinen, U. M. and Siimes, M. A. (1978) Developmental changes in red blood cell counts and indices of infants after exclusion of iron deficiency by laboratory criteria and continuous iron supplementation. *J. Pediatr.* **92**, 412–416.

Sato, S. (1991) Iron deficiency: Structural and microchemical changes in hair, nails and skin. *Semin. Dermatol.* **10**, 313–319.

Schoene, R. B., Escourrou, P., Robertson, H. T., Nilson, K. L., Parsons, J. R. and Smith, N. J. (1983) Iron repletion decreases maximal exercise lactate concentrations in female athletes with minimal iron-deficiency anemia. *J. Lab. Clin. Med.* **102**, 306–312.

Scholl, T. O., Hediger, M. L., Fisher, R. L. and Shearer, J. W. (1992) Anemia vs iron deficiency increased risk of pre-term delivery in a prospective study. *Am. J. Clin. Nutr.* **55**, 985–988.

Scrimshaw, N. S. (1991) Iron deficiency. *Scient. Am.* **265**, 46–52.

Seshadri, S., Hirode, K., Naik, P. and Malhotra, S. (1982) Behavioural responses of young anaemic Indian children to iron-folic acid supplements. *Br. J. Nutr.* **48**, 233–240.

Shih, Y. J., Baynes, R. D., Hudson, B. G., Flowers, C. H., Skikne, B. S. and Cook, J. D. (1990) Serum transferrin is a truncated form of tissue receptor. *J. Biol. Chem.* **265**, 19077–19081.

Siimes, M. A., Vuori, E. and Kuitunen, P. (1979) Breast milk iron – a declining concentration during the course of lactation. *Acta Paediatr. Scand.* **68**, 29–31.

Skikne, B. S. (1988) Current concepts in iron deficiency anemia. *Food Rev. Int.* **4**, 137–173.

Skikne, B. and Cook, J. (1991) Iron balance during recombinant erythropoietin administration (rHEPO) in normal subjects. *Blood* **78**, 90a.

Skikne, B. S., Flowers, C. H. and Cook, J. D. (1990) Serum transferrin receptor: A quantitative measure of tissue iron deficiency. *Blood* **75**, 1870–1876.

Snyder, A. C., Dvorak, L. L. and Roepke, J. B. (1989) Influence of dietary iron source on measures of iron status among female runners. *Med. Sci. Sports Exerc.* **21**, 7–10.

Soemantri, A. G., Pollitt, E. and Kim, I. (1985) Iron deficiency anemia and educational achievement. *Am. J. Clin. Nutr.* **42**, 1221–1228.

Spivak, J. L., Barnes, D. C., Fuchs, E. and Quinn, T. C. (1989) Serum immunoreactive erythropoietin in HIV infected patients. *JAMA* **261**, 3104–3107.

Stekel, A. (1981) Fortification from the laboratory to a national program. Two Chilean experiences. In: Proceedings of the Annual Meeting of the International Nutritional Anemia Consultative Group. Section 7. Nutrition Foundation, New York.

Tershakovec, A. M. and Weller, S. C. (1991) Iron status of inner-city elementary school children: lack of correlation between anemia and iron deficiency. *Am. J. Clin. Nutr.* **54**, 1071–1076.

United Nations Administrative Committee on Coordination/Subcommittee on Nutrition. (1991) Controlling Iron Deficiency. Nutrition Policy Discussion Paper No. 9.

Viteri, F. E., Garcia-Ibanez, R. and Torun, B. (1978) Sodium iron NaFeEDTA as an iron fortification compound in Central America. Absorption studies. *Am. J. Clin. Nutr.* **31**, 961–971.

Wallenburg, H. C. and van Eijk, H. G. (1984) Effect of oral iron supplementation during pregnancy on maternal and fetal iron status. *J. Perinat. Med.* **12**, 7–12.

Walter, T. (1989) Infancy: mental and motor development. *Am. J. Clin. Nutr.* **50**, 655–666.

Walter, T., De Andraca, I., Chadud, P. and Perales, C. G. (1989) Iron deficiency anemia: Adverse effects on infant psychomotor development. *Pediatrics* **84**, 7–17.

Walter, T., Hertranpf, E., Pizarro, F. *et al.* (1993) Effect of bovine-hemoglobin-fortified cookies on iron status of school children: A nationwide program in Chile. *Am. J. Clin. Nutr.* **57**, 190–194.

WHO Scientific Group (1968) Nutritional Anaemias, WHO Technical Report Series No. 405, WHO, New York.

Willis, W. T., Gohil, K., Brooks, G. A. and Dallman, P. R. (1990) Iron deficiency: improved exercise performance within 15 hours of iron treatment in rats. *J. Nutr.* **120**, 909–916.

Wilson-Fairchild, M., Haas, J. D. and Habicht, J. P. (1989) Iron deficiency and behavior criteria for testing causality. *Am. J. Clin. Nutr.* **50**, 566–574.

Witte, D. L., Angstadt, D. S., Davis, S. H. and Schrantz, R. D. (1988) Predicting bone marrow iron stores in anemic patients in a community hospital using ferritin and erythrocyte sedimentation rate. *Am. J. Clin. Pathol.* **90**, 85–87.

Worthington-Roberts, B. S., Breskin, M. W. and Monsen, E. R. (1988) Iron status of premenopausal women in a university community and its relationship to habitual dietary sources of protein. *Am. J. Clin. Nutr.* **47**, 275–279.

Worwood, M. (1979) Serum ferritin. *CRC Crit. Rev. Clin. Lab. Sci.* **10**, 171–204.

Yehuda, S. and Youdim, M. B. (1989) Brain iron: a lesson from animal models. *Am. J. Clin. Nutr.* **50**, 618–629.

Yip, R. (1989) The changing characteristics of childhood iron nutritional status in the United States. In: *Dietary Iron: Birth to Two Years* (ed. L. J. Filer), Raven Press, New York, p. 37.

Youdim, M. B., Ben Shachar, D. and Yehuda, S. (1989) Putative biological mechanisms of the effect of iron deficiency on brain biochemistry and behavior. *Am. J. Clin. Nutr.* **50**, 607–617.

Zanella, A., Barosi, G., Berzuini, A. *et al.* (1989) Relative iron deficiency in hereditary spherocytosis. *Am. J. Hematol.* **31**, 81–86.

8. Primary Iron Overload

L. W. POWELL, E. JAZWINSKA AND J. W. HALLIDAY

Queensland Institute of Medical Research, Liver Unit, The Bancroft Center, 300 Herson Road, Brisbane 4029 QLD, Australia

I. INTRODUCTION AND TERMINOLOGY

The association of cirrhosis with heavy hepatic deposits of iron-containing pigment was first recognized about 100 years ago with the term 'haemosiderin' being given to the iron-containing compound, and 'haemochromatosis' (HC) to the condition (Troisier, 1871; Hanot, 1888; von Recklinghausen, 1889). The disease (variously described as genetic haemochromatosis, hereditary haemochromatosis or idiopathic haemochromatosis) is now known to result from an inborn error of iron metabolism leading to inappropriately increased iron absorption from the diet. Although the basic defect is still not elucidated much is now known about the genetics, the sequence of events leading to symptomatic disease and rational, effective therapy is available.

It is now considered likely that most, if not all, primary iron overload in Caucasoid populations (i.e. iron overload not associated with thalassaemia major, sideroblastic anaemia or multiple blood transfusions) is due to homozygosity for HC, the genetic locus for which is known to be closely linked to the HLA-A locus on chromosome 6. Furthermore, a recent study has suggested that iron overload in South African blacks who ingest large quantities of iron from alcoholic beverages brewed in iron drums, is caused by an interaction between the increased dietary iron and an iron-loading gene, although this appears not to be HLA-linked (Gordeuk et al., 1992).

There is an increasing tendency to confine the term haemochromatosis (HC) to the inherited form or forms of parenchymal iron overload and refer to the other disorders as iron overload secondary to the specific cause (see classification of iron overload in Chapter 9). This also avoids the need for the use of the somewhat confusing term 'haemosiderosis'.

2. GENETICS OF HLA-LINKED HAEMOCHROMATOSIS

2.1. Prevalence and Mode of Inheritance

HLA-linked HC is inherited as an autosomal recessive trait. It is the most common inherited liver disease in caucasoids, affecting approximately 1 in 300 in populations of Northern European origin with a carrier rate of 1 in 20. This high prevalence makes HC one of the most common autosomal recessive disease traits (Table 8.1).

A recent survey of over 5000 male blood donors in Utah revealed a frequency of nearly 1 in 200 (Edwards et al., 1988) and the prevalence in an unselected group of asymptomatic Australians was estimated to be approximately 1 in 300 (Leggett et al., 1990). Indeed the high prevalence of HC can give rise to homozygote/heterozygote matings and a pseudo-dominant mode of inheritance (Fig. 8.1).

2.2. Rate of Expression

Expression of the disorder is influenced by dietary iron intake, thus in countries where there are sufficient quantities of absorbable iron in the diet the majority of people homozygous for the defect will eventually develop full clinical and biochemical expression of the disease. In a recent study by Powell et al. (1990), 47 of 50 putative homozygous relatives expressed the disease, either at first assessment or during a follow-up period of up to 8 years. In contrast, heterozygotes may demonstrate minor biochemical abnormalities of iron status, but do not develop a progressive increase in body iron stores of the order seen in homozygotes (Bassett et al., 1981, 1986) unless there is an additional disease present (Section 6.3).

2.3. Location of the Gene and Role of HLA Studies

The responsible gene has not yet been identified but it is known to be located on the short arm of chromosome 6 (6p) very close to the HLA class I complex, HLA-A

Table 8.1 Approximate prevalence of autosomal recessive diseases

Disease	Homozygote frequency (q^2)	Mutant gene frequency (q)	Heterozygote frequency $(2pq)^*$
Haemochromatosis	1:400	1:20	1:10
A1 AT** deficiency	1:1600	1:40	1:20
Cystic fibrosis	1:2500	1:50	1:25
Phenylketonuria	1:10 000	1:100	1:50
Wilson disease***	1:100 000	1:300	1:150

* Hardy-Weinberg Equilibrium
** Alpha-1 antitrypsin deficiency
*** Current momenclature no longer includes 's in disease name

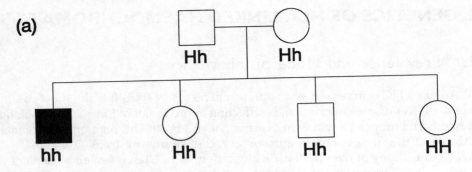

(a)

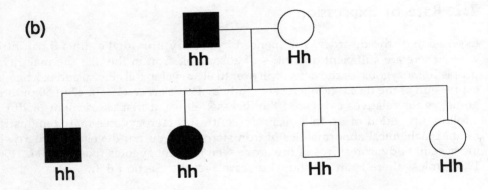

(b)

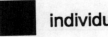

H = normal allele
h = haemochromatosis allele

individuals with haemochromatosis

Fig. 8.1 Pattern of inheritance of haemochromatosis. (a) Mendelian autosomal recessive mode of inheritance. (b) Apparent dominant mode of inheritance. Reproduced from *Medicine International*, **84**, 3496, by courtesy of The Medicine Group (Journals) Ltd.

in particular. The HLA linkage was first noted by Simon and co-workers (1976) who reported an increased frequency of HLA-A3-B14 and HLA-A3-B7 in this disease. Studies in Salt Lake City (Edwards *et al.*, 1977) and Australia (Doran *et al.*, 1981; Summers *et al.*, 1989) showed a stronger association of HC with HLA-A3-B7 than with HLA-A3-B14. This reflects the strong linkage disequilibrium between HLA-A3 and B7 in these populations. HLA linkage cannot be used to screen for HC in the

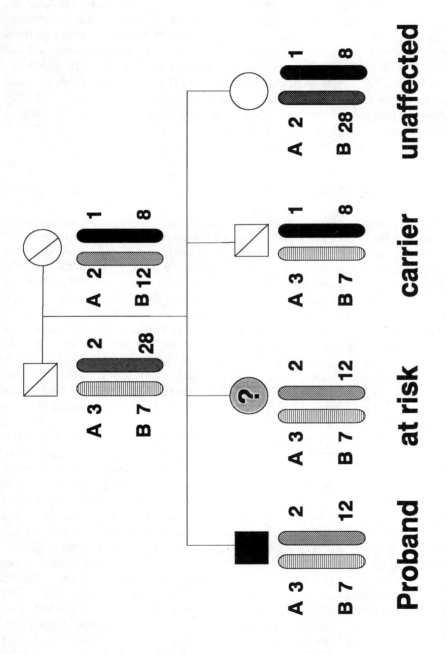

Fig. 8.2 HLA linkage for gene tracking in pedigrees with haemochromatosis. In this pedigree the haemochromatosis allele is carried on the HLA haplotypes A3 B7 and A2 B12; thus the sibling with an HLA type identical with the proband is also at risk of developing the disorder. The sibling sharing only one HLA haplotype with the proband is a putative carrier □. Reproduced from *Today's Life Science* 5(1), 34–36, 1933, with permission.

general population as the genetic locus for HC is sufficiently separate from the HLA loci for genetic recombination to have occurred with time, such that different HLA-A alleles – not only HLA-A3 – may be found in association with HC in different kindreds. In Australia, A2 and A11 are the next most common alleles encountered with the disease (Summers *et al.*, 1990). Furthermore all of these HLA alleles (A3, A2 and A11) occur with a high frequency in asymptomatic caucasians. HLA linkage has, however, been used very successfully for many years to track the gene in affected pedigrees. Affected siblings of the proband usually have two haplotypes identical to those of the proband, whereas unaffected siblings have one or neither haplotype identical to the proband (Fig. 8.2). In sibships resulting from a homozygous–heterozygous mating, affected individuals share the affected HLA haplotype from the heterozygous parent but may inherit either haplotype from the affected (homozygous) parent (Fig. 8.2).

2.4. Identification of the Gene

The biochemical abnormality underlying HC is unknown, and the gene is thus a candidate for positional cloning, i.e. cloning on the basis of chromosomal location. The first stage in positional cloning has been completed; recombination mapping has been used in order to define more closely the region of chromosome 6p which contains the gene. Recombination mapping involves saturating 6p with highly polymorphic markers and then recording the pattern of their inheritance in association with inheritance of the disorder (Boretto *et al.*, 1992). Recombination mapping using the highly polymorphic markers known as microsatellites has confirmed that the gene for HC is indeed very closely linked to HLA-A (Gruen *et al.*, 1992; Gasparini *et al.*, 1993; Jazwinska *et al.*, 1993) and this region of the chromosome is now being analysed for the presence of cDNAs which may encode the HC gene (El Kahloun *et al.*, 1993). Identification of the gene and a knowledge of the gene product will be a significant advance in diagnosis and management of the disorder.

Several theories have been proposed to account for the origin and prevalence of the gene for HC. One hypothesis, proposed by Simon *et al.* (1980), is that HC is basically a disease of Celtic peoples (because of the similarity in geographic distribution of case reports and the current settlements of Celtic peoples), and that the HC mutation arose on a chromosome carrying HLA-A3 and -B7, and spread among European populations by migration. This conclusion is supported by the pattern of HLA association in North America (Edwards *et al.*, 1977) and Australia (Summers *et al.*, 1989). A study of HLA haplotypes associated with HC among South Africans of Afrikaner origin (Meyer *et al.*, 1987, 1988) found multiple HLA haplotypes to be involved and suggested that the abnormal gene was prevalent among European populations before settlement of that colony in 1652. The gene was then presumably introduced into the colony with different haplotypes as opposed to a 'founder' effect with a single haplotype. The high prevalence of the gene in European populations may have resulted from a selective advantage conferred by it, for example protection against iron deficiency, or from a selective advantage for the HLA-A3 allele or another closely linked gene.

3. NATURE OF GENETIC DEFECT AND METABOLIC ABNORMALITY

The basic defect leading to an inappropriately high iron absorption in HC is still unknown. Theoretically, it could be a defect in the intestinal mucosal cell of the upper small intestine, or a more widespread disorder affecting the liver and/or the reticuloendothelial system: a defect in the iron-proteins transferrin or ferritin or their receptors potentially could be involved (Powell, 1992b). It is also tempting to speculate that the HC gene involves an iron transport abnormality analogous to that recently demonstrated in the copper-loading disorder, Menkes disease, in which the gene product is a member of a cation transporting P-type ATPase family (Davies, 1993).

3.1. The Intestinal Mucosal Cell

Several observations have suggested that the intestinal mucosal cell functions abnormally in HC and contains less ferritin than normal. Thus, the intestinal mucosal cell is behaving as if the body is iron deficient (Bothwell *et al.*, 1979; Klausner, 1988).

3.1.1. Intestinal Cell Iron-binding Proteins

Peters (1989) investigated the association of increased iron absorption with increased erythropoiesis in mice with experimentally altered erythropoietic activity. He showed enhanced iron uptake *in vitro* in response to hypoxia. *In vivo*, the transfer of iron to the carcass was markedly reduced in animals with obliterated bone marrow. Nevertheless, such animals did respond to an induced reticulocytosis although not to erythropoietin. Although his findings suggested regulation both at the point of uptake and the point of transfer to the body, the mechanism by which increased erythropoiesis results in a rapid increase in iron absorption was not elucidated by these experiments.

Several membrane iron-binding proteins have been described recently, one by Teichmann and Stremmel (1990) and others, mucosal in origin, by Conrad and colleagues (Conrad *et al.*, 1990; Conrad and Umbreit, 1993). The former is a 160 kDa iron-binding protein (a trimer of 54 kDa monomers) prepared from solubilized human microvillous membrane proteins. It was localized to brushborder membranes and was present in human intestinal mucosa, liver and heart but not in the oesophagus. An antibody against this protein inhibited Fe^{3+} uptake by more than 50%. These data indicate that the transport of Fe^{3+} across human microvillous membranes represents a facilitated transport mechanism which is mediated, at least in part, by this membrane iron-binding protein (Teichman *et al.*, 1991). Recently reported studies from this group have indicated that the protein is upregulated in HC and remains so after phlebotomy therapy (Stremmel *et al.*, 1991a). The mucosal iron-binding proteins include mucin (Conrad *et al.*, 1991), integrin (Conrad *et al.*, 1993) and mobilferrin (Conrad *et al.*, 1990). Their identification and characterization have led Conrad and his co-workers to describe a pathway of absorption of iron across the duodenal mucosal cell as follows: (i) mucin binds iron at acid pH to solubilize it for absorption in the alkaline pH of the duodenum; (ii) integrin (90/150 kD) as a transmembrane protein, facilitates iron transfer through the microvilli; and (iii) mobilferrin (56 kD), a cytosolic protein, may serve to maintain iron in an appropriate redox state. Thus, they propose that the absorptive process is driven by a cascade of differences in the binding constants of these proteins, so that iron moves from luminal mucin to mucosal mobilferrin to plasma transferrin.

These iron-binding proteins and their potential biological significance in iron metabolism are also considered in Chapter 6.

3.1.2. *The Role of Low Molecular Weight Iron Carriers in Mucosal Cells*

Because of the technical difficulties in studying low molecular weight iron carriers there are few data available on this aspect of HC and the results to date have been inconclusive. Iron chelates such as citrate and ascorbate may act on IRE-binding proteins to result in upregulation of intracellular ferritin synthesis in response to increased cellular iron content, but this remains speculative.

3.1.3. *Serosal Transfer of Iron*

In vivo studies of iron absorption in patients with HC have suggested that both net mucosal iron uptake and transfer of mucosal iron to the plasma are increased (Boender and Verloop, 1969; Powell *et al.*, 1970; Marx, 1979). However, at least two *in vivo* studies have provided data which indicate that the defective control of iron absorption in this disease is mediated at the level of intestinal cell transfer to the plasma (i.e. serosal transfer as opposed to mucosal uptake). The first of these studies (Powell *et al.*, 1970) used a double-labelled radio isotope technique to distinguish between mucosal uptake of iron from the lumen and body iron retention. In the second study (McLaren *et al.*, 1991) mucosal iron kinetics were analysed using a compartmental model of intestinal iron absorption and systemic ferrokinetics. In subjects with HC, transfer of mucosal iron to the plasma, although inappropriately high, was inversely related to body iron stores as in normal subjects, and this increase in mucosal iron transfer rate was the major determinant of increased iron absorption.

3.2. Transferrin and the Transferrin Receptor

Numerous studies have concluded that both transferrin and its receptor function normally in HC (Banerjee *et al.*, 1986; Pietrangelo *et al.*, 1992). Moreover, the genes for each of these proteins are on chromosome 3 rather than chromosome 6. Recent work supports the hypothesis that the transferrin receptor is concerned more with the transport of iron from the plasma to the mucosal cell presumably for use within the cell especially during cell growth (Anderson *et al.*, 1990, 1991).

It has been suggested that HC relates to a failure to 'switch' from neonatal to adult control of iron absorption (Srai *et al.*, 1984, 1987), but there are few studies to support this concept. Anderson *et al.* (1991) showed that the intestine of the pre-term rat demonstrated a high level of duodenal transferrin receptor (TfR) along the full length of the crypt–villous axis but soon after birth it reduced towards the villous tip.

The crypt receptor density remained high at all ages. There was no correlation between iron absorption and transferrin receptor expression in either neonates or adult animals.

3.3. Non-transferrin-bound Iron and Hepatocyte Membrane Transport

Hepatic transferrin receptors are reduced in HC (Sciot *et al.*, 1987) suggesting that hepatic iron overload is not due to increased clearance of transferrin-bound iron from the plasma. In contrast, recent attention has focused on the low molecular weight iron complexes referred to collectively as 'non-transferrin-bound' iron (NTBI). Although the NTBI accounts normally for less than 1% of the total serum iron, it may account for up to 35% of serum iron in subjects with HC (Batey *et al.*, 1978). Hepatic clearance of this form of iron is remarkably efficient and not reduced by hepatic iron loading (Wright *et al.*, 1986). Thus, NTBI may be quantitatively much more important than transferrin-bound iron in hepatic iron accumulation in HC. Using the isolated perfused liver model, Wright and colleagues (1988) provided evidence that the hepatic uptake of NTBI is mediated by a membrane carrier and occurs by an electrogenic mechanism in which there is a net movement of positive charge into the cell. Further, uptake of NTBI did not appear to depend on the presence of transmembrane gradients for sodium, chloride or bicarbonate. These authors concluded that since there is evidence that copper, zinc and manganese share a common carrier with iron (Wright *et al.*, 1986), hepatic uptake and accumulation of these metal ions may be driven by similar transmembrane gradients.

Sheldon (1935) and MacDonald (1964) reported that the concentration of other metal ions, specifically calcium, copper, lead and sulfur (but not zinc or manganese) is also increased in the liver and other organs affected in HC. Thus, other transition metal ions may compete with NTBI for incorporation into a cytosolic binding site (Wright *et al.*, 1986; Wright and Lake, 1990). Against this background, the recent demonstration of a membrane transport protein for copper that is defective in Menkes disease (Davies, 1993; Mercer *et al.*, 1993) is of particular interest.

3.4. Regulation of Ferritin Synthesis and Transferrin Receptor Expression

Despite the recent advances in the elucidation of the coordinate regulation of ferritin synthesis and transferrin receptor expression (Hentze *et al.*, 1988, 1989a,b; Kuhn, 1991) (Chapter 5) no new evidence for a defect of this coordinate regulation in HC has come to light. In subjects with HC, intestinal mucosal H- and L-ferritin as well as immunohistochemical ferritin fail to rise in parallel with the serum ferritin levels (Fracanzani *et al.*, 1989; Whittaker *et al.*, 1989) and it has also been shown that the steady-state messenger RNA (mRNA) for both H and L is inappropriately low, while the mRNA for transferrin receptor (TfR) is inappropriately increased (Pietrangelo *et al.*, 1992). The activity of the recently described IRE-binding protein which coordinately regulates translation of the mRNAs for ferritin and transferrin receptor (Chapter 5) is also normal in HC patients (Pietrangelo *et al.*, 1993).

These results could be interpreted as indicating a primary defect in ferritin transcription or pretranslational control of ferritin gene expression in the intestinal mucosal cells. However, they can also be interpreted as indicating that the coordinate regulation of the genes for TfR and for ferritin in the gut is still intact and that the demonstrated abnormality in intestinal ferritin in HC is secondary to a primary abnormality elsewhere. The latter could involve the mucosal cell, a more remote defect (e.g. in the liver or the monocyte/macrophage system), or a more generalized cellular or membrane defect, perhaps involving the recently reported 160 kilodalton iron-binding glycoprotein (Teichman and Stremmel, 1990) described in detail elsewhere (Chapter 6). Since this protein may be up-regulated in HC (Stremmel *et al.*, 1991a), it is possible that if such a membrane iron transport protein or proteins were present on parenchymal cells of a number of organs, defects in its function could lead to iron accumulation in those tissues. Alternatively, if confined to the intestine and monocyte/macrophage system (e.g. Kupffer cells of the liver), such a protein could be responsible for the rapid removal of iron from these cells: they may then respond to an apparent iron deficient state with reduced ferritin synthesis and a concomitant increase in TfR expression, accompanied by a sustained and inappropriately increased iron absorption.

Positional cloning has not yet provided additional clues. The gene for the IRE-binding protein is located on chromosome 9 (Hentze *et al.*, 1989b) and recent mapping and linkage studies (Summers *et al.*, 1991) have placed at least one of the H-ferritin pseudogenes on chromosome 6 centromeric to the HC locus which makes this unlikely to be a candidate gene for the disease.

Thus, the available evidence suggests that ferritin synthesis and function in the gut and liver are normal in HC. It is possible that the ferritin receptor (Mack *et al.*, 1983; Adams *et al.*, 1988) is involved in the pathobiology of HC but evidence for this must await elucidation of its structure and physiological role. The available molecular data indicate that there is a deficit in 'sensing' by the mucosal cytoplasmic regulatory system which fails to 'see' and/or trap incoming iron into the storage compartment of the enterocyte (Pietrangelo *et al.*, 1993).

3.5. The Liver

In HC in contrast to iron overload in other circumstances, the abnormal iron accumulation occurs in the hepatocytes and it is only late in the disease that Kupffer cells, macrophages and biliary epithelial cells of the liver become involved. In addition, the high percentage iron saturation of circulating transferrin is observed long before the accumulation of large amounts of iron. The deposition of iron in hepatocytes and parenchymal cells of other organs could occur as a passive consequence of the saturated transferrin (Cook *et al.*, 1973). Once the circulating transferrin is fully saturated, iron is also delivered to hepatocytes by non-transferrin-bound iron. The nature of this iron is ill-defined but could include ferritin (Batey *et al.*, 1978) (see above). Thus, a primary role for hepatocytes in the control of iron accumulation seems unlikely.

The results of studies of iron absorption after cross-transplantation of liver or gut from iron-loaded and normal rats (Adams *et al.*, 1989, 1991) would be consistent with a role for the intestinal mucosal cell in regulating iron uptake and body absorption according to its iron content. However, a further role for a humoral factor in down-regulating iron transfer across the intestinal cell is possible, particularly where hepatocytes (rather than Kupffer cells) are iron loaded, and a primary defect of such regulation cannot be excluded in HC.

Human liver transplantation has also provided some insight into this problem. The available data to June 1992, which included some 22 subjects with HC successfully transplanted for end-stage liver disease and a further four instances where a liver from an HC subject was inadvertently transplanted into a non-HC recipient, have recently been reviewed by Powell (1992b) who concluded that the combined data could best be explained by both a hepatic and an extrahepatic defect being necessary before the disease is fully expressed.

3.6. The RE System

The observation that Kupffer cells and intestinal macrophages contain little iron in subjects with HC has led to the suggestion that a primary defect in iron metabolism may lie in reticuloendothelial cells leading to reduced iron storage within these cells and the delivery of increased amounts of iron via the plasma to hepatocytes and other parenchymal cells. Kinetic studies involving reticuloendothelial function in HC lend support to this concept. A defect in storing iron, which is common to the two cells types, is certainly compatible with a number of observations in HC including the paucity of iron present in these cells, the increased iron absorption, and an early rise in transferrin saturation.

To date studies have failed to reveal any defect in the ferritin synthetic capabilities of these cells or in their ability to take up iron. However, increased release of iron as ferritin has been observed in mononuclear cells of patients with HC, whether treated or not. Fillet *et al.* (1989) showed that the early release phase of iron from RE cells was considerably enhanced in patients with HC. The mechanism by which this enhanced release occurs has not been elucidated but may be related to the basic defect in HC.

3.7. A Widespread Parenchymal Cell Defect?

As discussed above there is increasing evidence that HC results from a generalized membrane transport or other defect in multiple organs, such as occurs in cystic fibrosis and Menkes disease. This evidence comes from studies of the membrane iron carrier protein described by Stremmel and co-workers (discussed above), also from our analysis of the global experience of liver transplants in HC (see above), and from the recent demonstration that the abnormal gene for the copper loading disorder, Menkes disease, results in a defective membrane copper transport protein (Davies, 1993).

However, the elucidation of the basic metabolic defect must presumably await the cloning and sequencing of the HLA-A linked gene on the short arm of chromosome 6. The fact that the major iron-loading gene so far documented is tightly linked to the HLA loci and displays linkage disequilibrium with HLA-A suggests that abnormalities of a key protein coded at a single locus result in overt haemochromatosis. A number of genes have been considered potential candidates for the HC gene on the basis of the function of their gene product (e.g. transferrin, transferrin receptor, ferritin, etc.). Modern genetic techniques such as genetic linkage analysis, *in situ* hybridization, and somatic cell hybrid deletion mapping panel analysis, have demonstrated that most of these can be excluded on the basis of incorrect chromosome location. However, the development of techniques to analyse di- and tri-nucleotide repeats (microsatellites) should lead eventually to identification of the HC gene (Jazwinska *et al.*, 1993).

4. ROLE OF ENVIRONMENTAL FACTORS IN PRIMARY IRON OVERLOAD

4.1. Dietary Iron

The phenotypic expression of iron overload in subjects homozygous for the HC disease trait is clearly influenced by the amount of iron in the diet and its bioavailability (Chapter 6), and by physiological and pathological blood loss.

Haem iron is readily absorbed whatever the dietary composition, and meat-containing diets also promote the absorption of non-haem iron. In contrast, non-haem iron is of low bioavailability and is influenced by other dietary ingredients. Thus, non-haem iron absorption is inhibited by phytates in bran, tannates in tea and polyphenols in vegetables but it is promoted by ascorbic acid (Bothwell *et al.*, 1979). It is not surprising therefore that in Australia, a country with a comparatively high meat consumption, almost all homozygous subjects for HC express the disease (Powell *et al.*, 1990). The higher oral iron intake in men than women, coupled with physiological demands for iron in women, adequately accounts for the greater iron load and earlier expression of the disease in males. However, a recent study has shown strong concordance of expression of HC between siblings irrespective of environmental factors, emphasizing that genetic factors are the predominant factor in determining the degree of iron overload in all subjects (Crawford *et al.*, 1993).

4.2. Physiological and Pathological Blood Loss

Regular blood donation, heavy menstrual blood loss, multiple pregnancies and pathological blood loss (e.g. from peptic ulceration or hookworm infestation) will all delay the expression of the disease in homozygotes. Failure to express the disease in putative homozygotes (see below) or failure to reaccumulate iron after a course of venesection therapy should lead to suspicion of occult blood loss, especially in males.

4.3. Alcohol Ingestion and Iron Overload

The role of alcohol ingestion in the development of iron overload has been a subject of considerable controversy and confusion. However, recent studies particularly of the genetic aspects of HC have greatly clarified the picture. An important and consistent observation in numerous reports has been that a high proportion (approximately 20–30%) of cases of fully developed HC have consumed alcohol in excess of 50 g per day. This observation was primarily responsible for the former view that HC was not a genetic disorder, but merely a form of alcoholic or nutritional cirrhosis in subjects whose dietary intake of iron was high. It is now established however, that

1. Caucasian subjects with heavy alcohol consumption and iron overload of the degree seen in symptomatic HC are homozygous for haemochromatosis (Powell, 1965, 1970, 1975; Powell and Kerr, 1975; Le Sage et al., 1983).
2. Subjects heterozygous for HC do not develop significant iron overload if they consume alcohol to excess (Powell, 1975).
3. Those subjects with mild siderosis do not have an increased frequency of the HLA antigens associated with HC (Simon et al., 1977b).
4. In alcoholic subjects with mild hepatic haemosiderosis but without evidence of HC the hepatic iron concentration is not significantly elevated and the hepatic iron index (see below) is under 2.0, in contrast to subjects homozygous for HC (Bassett et al., 1986; Summers et al., 1990). In these alcoholic subjects the stainable iron is found in macrophages and Kupffer cells and probably represents iron released from damaged hepatocytes.
5. For practical purposes the only situation encountered in which heavy alcohol consumption leads to significant iron overload is in the South African blacks who ingest large amounts of iron from home-made beer brewed in iron drums or pots. However, even in this situation recent evidence suggests that the additional presence of an iron-loading gene is necessary if significant iron overload is to develop (Gordeuk et al., 1992).

Despite this recent evidence that alcohol itself seldom, if ever, leads to severe iron overload in Caucasian subjects, there is no doubting the association between an increased alcohol intake and the development of the clinical manifestations of HC. Alcohol may contribute to the organ damage associated with iron overload, and therefore accelerate the onset of the clinical phase of the condition. Alcoholic subjects with HC have the clinical features of HC but, in addition, manifest signs and symptoms of superimposed alcoholic liver disease (Powell, 1975). Their liver histopathology also shows features of alcoholic liver disease superimposed on HC (Powell and Kerr, 1975). Moreover, venesection therapy is less effective in these subjects (Powell, 1970; Grace and Powell, 1974; Grace, 1978).

One is left with the conclusion that prolonged heavy alcohol consumption may accelerate the symptomatic stage of homozygous HC and in addition such patients may have superimposed symptoms and signs of alcoholism and alcoholic liver disease. Clinically, the distinction between HC in an alcoholic subject and mild hepatic haemosiderosis associated with alcoholism can be made in most instances by hepatic biopsy and measurement of hepatic iron concentration and the hepatic iron index (see below). The distinction between HC and alcoholic liver disease associated with haemosiderosis or increased histochemical staining of iron is reviewed in specific detail by Powell *et al.* (1994).

Alcohol ingestion and modest degrees of iron overload are also associated with porphyria cutanea tarda. This disorder, and the possible role of the gene for HC in the iron overload, are discussed in Chapter 9.

5. PATHOLOGY

The major pathological findings in HC relate to the massive amounts of iron found in the parenchymal cells of most organs, particularly liver, pancreas, heart and endocrine glands. The liver is enlarged and nodular and along with the pancreas presents a striking reddish-brown colour. On histological examination iron is found in large amounts in the parenchymal cells and, in the late stage, in Kupffer cells, macrophages and biliary epithelial cells. This iron deposition is associated with dense fibrosis in the liver and pancreas, and in the liver the fibrosis leads eventually to a mixed macro-micronodular cirrhosis. Cell necrosis and inflammation are usually absent and the parenchymal cells otherwise usually appear normal. Of particular interest (and possible relevance to the pathobiology of the disease) is the pattern of iron distribution in the liver. It is seen first within the periportal hepatocytes and in a peri-canalicular distribution within lysosomes. With increasing iron loading, hepatocytes in zones 2 and 3 become iron loaded, followed by fibrosis in the portal areas eventually linking up to form a 'holly-leaf' pattern but with a large area of preserved parenchyma (Powell and Kerr, 1975; Searle *et al.*, 1993).

Microscopic examination of the pancreas usually shows heavy deposits of haemosiderin in the acinar cells. Haemosiderin is also found in the heart muscle fibres in nearly all cases of well-established HC but fibrosis is rare. Haemosiderin is also deposited in the conducting fibres of the atrioventricular node and is presumably responsible for the cardiac arrhythmias which occur in this disease. The pituitary, adrenal, thyroid and parathyroid glands frequently contain extensive haemosiderin deposits, although evidence of functional impairment is usually confined to the pituitary. The epidermis of the skin is atrophic with increased melanin in the cells of the basal layer. The characteristic metallic grey hue results from increased melanin (with or without iron) in the dermis in association with the atrophic epidermis. Increased iron deposition in the skin is very variable and tends to occur around the sweat glands.

6. CLINICAL FEATURES

6.1. Symptomatic Stage

The clinical features of HC are easily recognizable in patients with advanced disease but they are not pathognomonic for this disorder. Such patients usually present with one or more of the following symptoms: skin pigmentation, loss of libido, joint pain or symptoms related to the onset of diabetes (Bothwell et al., 1979). Skin pigmentation, hepatomegaly, testicular atrophy, loss of body hair and arthropathy are the most prominent physical signs. In young patients with symptomatic disease, endocrine and cardiac manifestations are frequently prominent.

Since the positive iron balance is limited to a few milligrams per day, the accumulation of 20–40 g surplus iron takes many years. Most subjects are, therefore, aged between 40 to 60 years at the time of diagnosis, although a number of younger patients have been described, including some in early adulthood and even children (Perkins et al., 1965). The symptomatic stage of the disease is encountered approximately ten times more frequently in males than in females and at an earlier age of onset. This is because of physiological blood loss in women in the reproductive age group and also because of a higher iron intake in men (dietary iron being linked to meat and carbohydrate intake). In many affected females there is a history of scanty menstruation for several years preceding the onset of symptoms.

It should be emphasized, however, that in keeping with the autosomal recessive mode of inheritance, homozygosity for HC is as common in women as in men and population studies reveal equal sex distribution (Leggett et al., 1990) (see below). Moreover, the genetic effect in HC is such that homozygous siblings of the same sex have comparable iron stores irrespective of environmental influences, and female siblings of males with heavy iron overload have significantly larger iron stores than unrelated female homozygotes (Crawford et al., 1993) (Fig. 8.3).

6.1.1. Skin

Excessive pigmentation is present in the majority of symptomatic patients, but is absent in the early stages of iron accumulation. As noted above the characteristic metallic grey or bronze hue is largely due to melanin deposition in the dermis. Pigmentation usually is generalized, but frequently is deeper on the face, neck, extensor aspects of the lower forearms, dorsa of the hands, lower legs and genital region and in old scars. There is generalized atrophy of both epidermis and dermis. Pigmentation of the hard palate and retina has also been described.

6.1.2. Liver

The liver is usually the first organ to be affected, and hepatomegaly is present in more than 95% of symptomatic patients. This is a result principally of the increase in iron content. Hepatic enlargement usually precedes the development of symptoms or abnormal liver function tests. Signs of chronic liver disease such as palmar erythema, spider angiomata, loss of body hair and gynaecomastia are seen but less often than in other forms of cirrhosis (Powell et al., 1971). Manifestations of portal hypertension may also occur but are less common than in alcoholic cirrhosis. Hepatocellular carcinoma develops in some 25–30% of patients who present with symptoms of HC, particularly in males with established cirrhosis (see later). Hepatic function is usually well preserved and liver function tests may be quite normal despite substantial hepatic iron content and fibrosis.

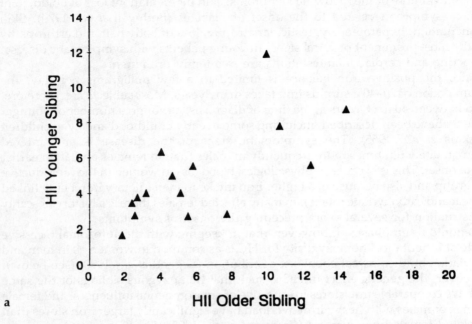

a

Fig. 8.3a The correlation of the hepatic iron index between siblings of the same sex (r=0.70, P=0.004).

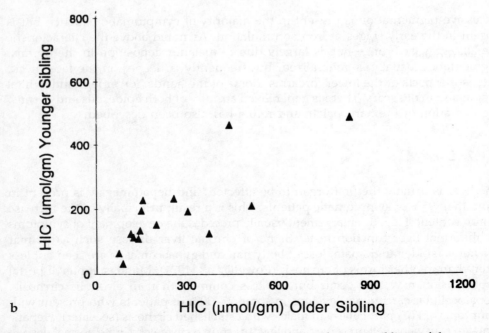

b

Fig. 8.3b The correlation of the hepatic iron concentration between siblings of the same sex (r=0.81, P=0.0003). Reproduced from Hepatology 17(5), 833–837, 1993, with permission.

6.1.3. *The Endocrine System*

Diabetes mellitus develops in 30% to 60% of patients with advanced disease. However, in a more recent study from Australia (Phelps *et al.*, 1989) a higher figure was found, which would justify screening patients attending diabetic clinics for HC. The inheritance of the gene for type I diabetes mellitus, cirrhosis and direct damage to the pancreas by deposition of iron probably all contribute to the frequency of diabetes in HC subjects. The high occurrence rate of diabetes in first- and second-degree relatives of patients with HC suggests that diabetes is not simply due to islet cell damage from deposition of iron.

Insulin resistance develops in cirrhotic patients but in addition it has been described in non-cirrhotic patients and attributed to iron-loading of hepatocytes. Diabetic complications such as retinopathy, nephropathy and peripheral neuropathy may be observed. However, retinopathy of the proliferative type is comparatively rare.

Loss of libido and testicular atrophy are common in HC and may antedate other clinical manifestations of the disease especially in young subjects and in both sexes. Hypogonadal symptoms may occur also before liver function is abnormal. The cause of hypogonadism in HC is debated, although most evidence favours hypothalamic or pituitary failure with selective impairment of gonadotropin or gonadotrophin releasing hormone secretion (Strohmeyer *et al.*, 1989). Yet, normal or even elevated gonadotropin concentrations have been found in some patients with testicular atrophy, suggesting primary testicular failure. The results of studies employing clomiphene stimulation of the hypothalamic–pituitary axis have suggested that there is a defect in normal feedback between the testes and the hypothalamic–pituitary axis rather than in the anterior pituitary itself. A decreased prolactin reserve has also been demonstrated. Other additional aetiological factors, such as liver damage and in some cases the direct effect of alcohol on gonadal function, may also be important. Gynaecomastia is uncommon compared with patients with alcoholic liver disease (Powell *et al.*, 1971).

Deposition of iron is frequently seen in other endocrine glands in addition to the pituitary. However, diseases such as Addison's disease, hypothyroidism and hypoparathyroidism, although documented, are rare in patients with HC.

6.1.4. *The Joints*

Arthropathy associated with HC has been reported in from 20 to 70% of symptomatic patients with HC, and may be the presenting feature. HC should be suspected if joint symptoms of osteoarthritis occur under 40 years of age. The association was first studied in detail in 1964 by Schumacher (1964). The arthropathy is unrelated to either the extent or duration of iron overload and may arise or progress after the removal of the excess iron stores. The arthropathy is identical to that of degenerative osteoarthritis except for the common finding of calcium pyrophosphate deposition (chondrocalcinosis) (see below). Acute attacks of synovitis (pseudogout) may occur and require appropriate treatment including the use of non-steroidal anti-inflammatory agents.

Chondrocalcinosis, due to the deposition of calcium pyrophosphate dihydrate crystals, can be demonstrated radiologically in one or more joints, most often the knees and the wrists. The incidence and severity increase with age and irrespective of removal of the iron by venesection therapy. Similar findings in other forms of iron overload suggest that the iron is in some way responsible; it has been reported to inhibit pyrophosphatase activity and thus to interfere with the hydrolysis of pyrophosphate to soluble orthophosphate. Iron is present in the chondrocytes, but there is no constant relationship with the pyrophosphate crystals. The synovial lining cells are heavily laden with haemosiderin.

Arthritis with loss of joint space, cysts and destruction of articular surfaces also occur, especially of the hands in the second and third metacarpophalangeal joints. These features distinguish haemochromatotic chondrocalcinosis from the idiopathic variety. Clinically there is bony swelling, deformity and limitation of movement, usually without serious disablement.

Although these associated joint lesions may progress despite venesection therapy, destructive arthropathy of the type seen in rheumatoid arthritis rarely occurs and symptoms can usually be controlled with non-steroidal anti-inflammatory agents. However, hip replacement is commonly indicated for this condition and can be expected to restore normal mobility.

6.1.5. *The Heart*

Cardiac involvement is the presenting manifestation in 5 to 15% of patients although ECG abnormalities are seen in about 30% (Strohmeyer *et al.*, 1993). The most common cardiac complications are congestive heart failure and cardiac arrhythmias. These are usually observed in long-standing iron overload, but they also occur in young adults, sometimes being precipitated by moderate to large doses of ascorbic acid. Cardiac manifestations are common presenting features of HC in young subjects. Symptoms of congestive cardiac failure may develop suddenly and the disorder may be misdiagnosed if other overt manifestations of HC are absent.

Clinically the picture is usually that of a congestive cardiomyopathy with bilateral ventricular dilatation. On radiographic investigation the cardiac profile is globular with a decrease in the amplitude of the cardiac pulsations. However, restrictive features have also been described.

Arrhythmias are also common. Ventricular ectopic beats are the most common manifestation, but supraventricular and ventricular tachycardias, ventricular fibrillation and varying degrees of heart block may also occur (Bothwell *et al.*, 1979). The presence of supraventricular arrhythmias correlates with the extent of iron deposition in the atrium and sinoatrial nodes. Cardiac manifestations are usually improved by phlebotomy if instituted early. Even with severe cardiac impairment, if the cardiac state can be managed by appropriate therapy and iron removal is undertaken simultaneously, including by the use of desferrioxamine if phlebotomy is contraindicated (see below), a good result may ensue.

6.1.6. *Neoplasia*

Malignant hepatoma (primary hepatocellular carcinoma or HCC) develops in about 30% of patients with cirrhosis and it is now the most common cause of death in treated patients. Indeed, the relative risk of HCC in patients with HC and cirrhosis is

200-fold (Bradbear *et al.*, 1985, Niederau *et al.*, 1986). Although rare cases of HCC have been described in non-cirrhotic patients, fibrosis has usually been observed (Deugnier *et al.*, 1993) for practical purposes cirrhosis is virtually always present. This is important since regular screening with ultrasound examination and estimation of α-fetoprotein is not cost-effective in non-cirrhotic patients (Colombo *et al.*, 1991). Indeed more suitable screening tests are needed urgently for cirrhotic patients since early diagnosis gives the only hope of prolonging life in such subjects.

Aetiological factors that seem relevant to the development of HCC include the presence of cirrhosis, male gender and longevity (Bradbear *et al.*, 1985; Niederau *et al.*, 1986). A recent large collaborative study (Deugnier *et al.*, 1993) has shown that chronic alcoholism and tobacco smoking are further risk factors for HCC in HC patients and that iron-free foci are probable precursors, particularly when proliferative and dysplastic.

Malignant change is suggested by the onset of unexplained weight loss, fever, nodular enlargement of the liver, ascites, jaundice, abdominal pain, anaemia or insulin insensitivity or more rarely by the occurrence of metabolic abnormalities associated with HCC, for example hypercalcaemia and hypoglycaemia.

There has been much interest in the frequency of extrahepatic malignancy in HCC, especially following early reports of an increased incidence of colo-rectal and lung cancer in patients with HC (Bomford and Williams, 1976) (Chapter 11). However, the two large controlled studies cited above failed to demonstrate an increase in incidence of malignancy other than primary HCC.

6.1.7. Rarer Clinical Manifestations

Other less common manifestations of HC include: acute severe upper abdominal pain of unknown cause, endocrine and neurological manifestations. Porphyria cutanea tarda (PCT) tends to be associated with iron overload, and may occur with haemo-chromatosis, but probably this occurrence is coincidental (Adams and Powell, 1987).

The acute onset of severe pain, often associated with shock, is a rare but well documented manifestation of HC, and *Yersinia enterocolitica* has been particularly incriminated in some instances. Unlike most micro-organisms, this bacterium does not possess a high affinity iron chelating system and seldom causes systemic infections because it is unable to obtain sufficient iron from the internal environment of the body. However, it is able to proliferate in HC and other iron-overload states. Despite much interest and research on the subject, there is no convincing evidence of increased susceptibility to infection in HC and no properly controlled study has been performed (Chapter 11).

6.2. Presymptomatic Stage

Since HC is inherited as an autosomal recessive trait the HC genotype occurs with equal frequency in both sexes. However, clinical symptoms and signs occur more frequently in men. Increased iron absorption occurs throughout the lifetime of patients with HC with iron accumulating silently in the early stages. Gradually, iron stores reach toxic levels and tissue damage is initiated. Only after sufficient tissue damage has occurred (usually with >10 g of storage iron) do symptoms develop. Most patients present with insidiously developing non-specific symptoms such as lethargy, apathy, lack of interest, or weight loss. Lethargy is almost universally present in the early stages of the disease, and is often recognized retrospectively after the patient has been diagnosed and treated.

With the widespread use of biochemical screening tests (often included with a standard physical examination, e.g. for insurance purposes), HC is being recognized earlier in the natural history of the disease and before symptoms or physical signs develop. Since neither the gene causing iron loading nor its protein product have been identified, phenotypic tests for iron overload are used for diagnosis. Once HC is suspected, the diagnosis is reasonably straightforward in otherwise uncomplicated patients (Sections 7.2 and 7.3 below).

6.3. Expression in the Heterozygote

Although the mutant gene for HC has not been identified, the tight linkage of the disease to the HLA-A locus on chromosome 6p can be used to follow HC alleles within families (Fig. 8.2) and thereby designate family members as putative homozygotes (hh) for the abnormal gene, putative heterozygotes (Hh) and homozygote normals (HH). The practical importance of this lies in the fact that the disease is inherited as a Mendelian recessive trait and full expression occurs only in hh subjects. Approximately 25% of Hh subjects manifest minor phenotypic expression, usually as slight to moderate increase in serum levels of serum ferritin or transferrin saturation (Simon et al., 1980; Bassett et al., 1981; Dadone et al., 1982; Borwein et al., 1983; Milman, 1991). However, significant iron loading does not occur unless there is another disorder such as hereditary spherocytosis (Edwards et al., 1982; Fargion et al., 1986; Mohler and Wheby, 1986) beta-thalassaemia minor (Edwards et al., 1981), idiopathic refractory sideroblastic anaemia (Cartwright et al., 1980; Barron et al., 1989), or sporadic porphyria cutanea tarda (Edwards et al., 1989). As stated earlier (Section 4.3) Hh subjects do not develop significant iron overload with alcohol abuse and heavy drinkers with increased iron stores are usually homozygous for HC (Powell, 1975).

7. DIAGNOSIS AND DIFFERENTIAL DIAGNOSIS

7.1. In Symptomatic Patients

Diagnosis of HC involves not only a high index of clinical suspicion, but screening of high risk individuals, and careful clinicopathological correlation, i.e. the demonstration of excess stainable iron in parenchymal cells in the liver, elevated hepatic iron content and a clinical history that excludes other causes of liver iron overload such as thalassaemia. Most causes of secondary iron overload (Chapter 9) can be identified by a careful history and appropriate laboratory investigations.

Thus, the diagnosis of HC is usually made on the basis of the classic clinical features described elsewhere together with laboratory investigations indicative of excessive iron stores and tissue damage. The diagnosis should be considered in any patient with unexplained hepatomegaly, abnormal skin pigmentation, idiopathic cardiomyopathy, diabetes, arthritis, or loss of libido. Particular attention in the history should focus on the amount of alcohol ingested as well as previous oral and parenteral iron administration, excessive menstrual blood loss, multiple pregnancies, blood donations and other causes of blood loss. A haematologic examination should be performed for evidence of anaemia and abnormal erythropoiesis to exclude iron loading secondary to a haematologic disorder, such as thalassaemia major or sideroblastic anaemia. Biochemical tests may indicate the presence of liver damage, although results of these 'liver function tests' are frequently normal, even in the presence of gross hepatic iron overload. Evidence of pancreatic, cardiac and joint disease should be obtained by physical examination, roentgenological examination and routine function tests of these organs.

7.1.1. Laboratory Investigations

Laboratory findings in patients with fully developed HC usually include: (1) an elevated serum iron concentration (greater than 30 μmol/litre or 170 μg/100 ml); (2) increased transferrin saturation (greater than 60% in men and 50% in women); (3) increased serum ferritin levels. Infrequently untreated symptomatic patients may have one or more of these within the normal range on some occasions (Edwards et al., 1988; Powell et al., 1990), particularly if they are tested early in life (Chapter 14). For a firm diagnosis of HC with iron overload, excessive parenchymal deposits of iron must be identifiable on liver biopsy sections, together with an increased level of tissue iron. Histological examination is important in defining the extent of tissue damage (fibrosis or cirrhosis) as well as iron deposition. However, chemical analysis of hepatic iron obtained by biopsy or at necropsy is usually necessary to distinguish HC from other disorders leading to stainable hepatic iron (see later). Because of an age-related rise in liver iron concentration in homozygous HC subjects and to a considerably lesser extent in heterozygotes and normal subjects, calculation of a hepatic iron index (hepatic iron concentration ÷ age) has proved useful in diagnosing pre-symptomatic homozygotes (see below).

As emphasized above, the degree of total body iron overload is influenced by many factors, including age, sex and blood loss, and these may result in a delay in diagnosis in some patients. Nevertheless increased body iron stores with primarily parenchymal cell deposition of iron has been the hallmark of HC for diagnostic and therapeutic purposes. This is clearly strengthened by a family history of HC and evidence of HLA-linked iron-overload disease, e.g. HLA identity in an affected sibling.

7.1.2. Methods of Assessing Body Iron Stores

(a) Transferrin saturation. Serum iron and saturation of transferrin are elevated early in the course of disease. However, the specificity of these tests is reduced by the relatively high frequency of false-positive and false-negative values, especially in relatives of patients with the disease. In a study of 242 members of 43 families, the serum iron concentration was elevated in only 76% of relatives with increased iron stores and in 10% of relatives with normal iron stores. The percentage saturation of transferrin was elevated in all relatives with increased iron stores and in 33% of relatives with normal iron stores. The transferrin saturation is increased in some 25% of heterozygous subjects (Bassett *et al.*, 1984). An increased serum iron concentration may be present in patients with alcoholic liver disease without excess iron stores. In this situation, however, the percentage saturation of the transferrin is often still normal. With very severe alcoholic liver disease and impaired protein synthesis, serum transferrin level may be decreased and thus percentage saturation increased.

(b) *Serum ferritin.* The serum ferritin levels rise slightly with age in normal subjects but steadily in homozygous HC subjects in direct proportion to the increasing iron stores (Summers *et al.*, 1990). In untreated patients with endstage HC the serum ferritin level is greatly increased (as much as ten times normal or greater) and correlates well with the magnitude of body iron stores. The serum ferritin test is thus very useful as a non-invasive screening test for HC. Levels of serum ferritin in some young HC patients, especially females, may be low and some heterozygotes have raised serum ferritin levels. Therefore, regular monitoring of serum ferritin levels in individuals at risk for HC is necessary, with a diagnostic liver biopsy performed when there is evidence of a progressive rise in serum ferritin concentration. Serum ferritin levels may be elevated out of proportion to total body iron stores in patients with infection, malignancy (especially leukaemia) and hepatocellular necrosis. The serum ferritin concentration may be raised in patients with alcoholic liver disease with a raised AST but when the AST returns to the normal range the serum ferritin falls to a level proportional to the body iron stores.

Representative values for the above iron indices in HC are given in Fig. 8.4.

(c) *Chelation tests.* Chelation tests using desferrioxamine-induced urinary iron excretion can be used where liver biopsy is contra-indicated. The test most widely used involves measurement of the 24 h urinary iron excretion after an IM injection of 0.5 g desferrioxamine (Harker *et al.*, 1968) although a rapid four hour test has been advocated (Bonkovsky *et al.*, 1990a). An excretion of more than 2 mg iron in 24 h is indicative of excess parenchymal iron deposits. In patients with untreated HC the amount will often exceed 10 mg in 24 h. The test requires meticulous urine collection and for this reason, but also because of frequent contamination by exogenous iron, it has now been largely replaced by liver biopsy with quantitative assessment of iron concentration.

(d) *Liver biopsy.* This is the definitive test for the diagnosis of HC and should be performed if any of the above test results is abnormal or equivocal. Liver biopsy permits histochemical estimation of tissue iron assessment of the extent of fibrosis and cirrhosis, and chemical measurement of hepatic iron concentration. Part of the specimen should be fixed in formalin for histological examination, and the remainder carefully washed to remove extraneous blood, wrapped in clean aluminium foil, and dried to constant weight, for determination of hepatic iron concentration.

Stainable haemosiderin iron is assessed using Perls' Prussian blue stain. This test should be performed routinely on all liver biopsy specimens, whether HC is suspected or not. In HC, haemosiderin deposits characteristically appear first in the hepatocytes in the periportal area. Later, they are distributed widely throughout

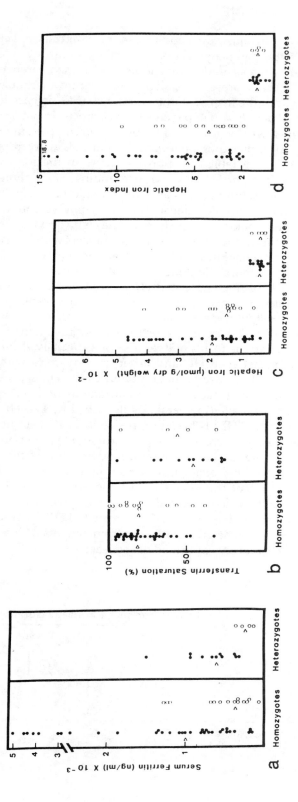

Fig. 8.4 Iron indices in haemochromatosis homozygotes and heterozygotes. Arrowheads indicate mean values; solid circles = men; open circles = women. (a) Serum ferritin. (b) Transferrin saturation. (c) Hepatic iron concentration. (d) Hepatic iron index. Reproduced from *Hepatology* **12(1)**, 20–25, 1990, with permission.

the lobules, as well as in biliary duct epithelium, Kupffer cells and connective tissue. The degree of stainable parenchymal iron is usually arbitrarily graded 0 to 4. Grades 0 and 1 are normal, whereas grades 2 to 4 indicate increased parenchymal iron stores (Scheuer et al., 1962). The presence of slight to moderate amounts of stainable iron in parenchymal cells of the liver without a demonstrable increase in total body iron may occur in normal people and in patients with cirrhosis. In patients with advanced HC, stainable iron is usually grade 4, although in young patients it may be lower.

The histologic appearance of the liver may be normal, apart from increased iron. Before cirrhosis is fully established, fibrosis occurs in the form of narrow septa radiating from expanded portal tracts and surrounding intact lobules. The liver cells may contain fat vacuoles but necrosis and inflammation are usually absent. As the liver slowly becomes cirrhotic, dense fibrous septa surround large areas of comparatively normal looking parenchyma. The deposition of iron precedes the development of fibrosis in the disease. Thus, in subjects with early precirrhotic HC, if the extent of iron deposition is only moderate (grades 2 or 3), cirrhosis would be uncommon; if more than a slight increase in fibrosis is present with lower grades of iron, the diagnosis of uncomplicated HC should be seriously questioned. It is in this situation that the measurement of liver iron concentration and the hepatic iron index are very useful (Searle et al., 1993).

(e) *Chemical estimation of liver iron concentration.* Because hepatic iron deposition may be increased in various forms of liver disease especially alcoholic liver disease (ALD) discrimination between HC and other liver diseases with secondary iron overload is important. This discrimination requires the chemical determination of hepatic iron content and is facilitated by calculation of the hepatic iron index [(μmoles Fe/gm dry wt) ÷ age (in years)] as described by Bassett et al. (1986). Use of the hepatic iron index (HII) is based on the concept that, in homozygotes with HC, there is a progressive increase in hepatic iron deposition with increasing age, whereas, in heterozygotes and in patients with other forms of chronic liver disease, there is minimal increase in hepatic iron concentration with age. Thus in alcoholic subjects, in the absence of the gene for HC, the upper limit of the hepatic iron concentration generally does not exceed 80 μmol/g dry weight, i.e. twice the upper limit of normal, and the HII is less than 2. An elevated HII (>2) separates patients with homozygous HC from heterozygotes and from patients with alcoholic siderosis. This concept has now been confirmed in at least four studies, summarized in Table 8.2.

Table 8.2 Studies of hepatic iron index in haemochromatosis

Study	Normal	ALD	Hh	hh
Bassett et al. (1986)	<1.0	<1.4	<1.8	>2.0
Summers et al. (1990)	—	—	<1.5	>1.9
Olynyk et al. (1990)	<1.1	<1.6	—	>2.1
Bonkovsky et al. (1990b)	<0.7	<1.1	<1.8	>2.0*
Sallie et al. (1991)	—	<1.6	—	>2.0

ALD = Alcoholic liver disease.
Hh = Haemochromatosis, heterozygote.
hh = Haemochromatosis, homozygote.
*Two patients (of 14) thought to have HC had HII<2.0.

Measurement of iron concentration in other tissues, such as bone marrow and skin, is of little use in the diagnosis of HC.

Quantitative Phlebotomy. An accurate, though retrospective, assessment of body iron stores may be made by careful quantitative phlebotomy, provided a few simple guidelines are adopted (Chapter 14). Weekly or twice weekly phlebotomy (each of 500 ml or approximately 250 mg iron) is continued until the haemoglobin concentration falls below 11 g/dl and fails to rise on the cessation of phlebotomy; individuals with normal iron stores become iron deficient after removal of approximately 1.5–2.0 g of iron.

Computed Tomography. Severe iron overload can increase the density of the liver on a plain film of the abdomen. This finding can be demonstrated more precisely with computed tomography (Chapman *et al.*, 1980). Severe iron overload is probable if the tomographic density of the liver exceeds 36 CT units (72 Hounsfield units) (Howard *et al.*, 1983). However, density values less than 36 CT units do not exclude milder degrees of iron overload. Thus CT scanning lacks sensitivity and falsely low values occur when iron overload and fatty liver co-exist (Guyader *et al.*, 1989). Dual energy CT overcomes this, as well as interference from fibrosis and cirrhosis, but it is technically more difficult and is not widely available.

Magnetic Resonance Imaging (MRI). MRI is another noninvasive method for measuring hepatic iron content that is currently under evaluation (Kaltwasser *et al.*, 1990; Anderson *et al.*, 1991; Siegelman *et al.*, 1991). Use of relaxation rates (1/T1 and especially 1/T2) and optimized spin-echo sequence can provide an accurate assessment of iron content at high iron concentrations but the cost and relatively poor sensitivity at lower iron concentrations greatly limit its value. Indeed, some studies have shown a poor correlation between MRI determination of hepatic iron and biochemical measurements (Guyader *et al.*, 1992). It is hoped that technical refinements in pulse sequence, time intervals and spin-echo methods will lead to better correlation between T2 calculations and hepatic iron content.

Magnetic Susceptibility Measurement of Human Iron Stores. The paramagnetic properties of ferritin and haemosiderin have also been exploited as a way to measure hepatic iron stores using a superconducting quantum-interference-device (SQUID) susceptometer, which is available in only a few specialized referral centres (Cleveland, Hamburg). Comparison of measurements of hepatic iron content by magnetic susceptibility with biochemically determined iron content in patients showed close agreement over a range extending from normal to 30 times normal (Brittenham *et al.*, 1982). While this technique appears much more accurate and reliable than either CT or MRI, its lack of availability seriously hinders its usefulness.

Thus, each of these non-invasive techniques has significant limitations for the diagnosis of iron overload, especially early in the disease, and the most definitive method for diagnosing HC remains the liver biopsy with measurement of iron content and HII. It should also be emphasized that liver biopsy provides precise information as to the histologic state of the liver, in particular the presence of fibrosis of cirrhosis, information that is of great importance to the clinician in predicting prognosis (Bradbear *et al.*, 1985) and determining the follow-up schedule and programme (Niederau *et al.*, 1986).

7.2. Detection of Disease in Asymptomatic Relatives

Among patients who present with symptomatic HC, approximately 50–70% have cirrhosis, 20% fibrosis and no cirrhosis, and 10–20% have no cirrhosis or fibrosis (Powell *et al.*, 1971; Strohmeyer *et al.*, 1993). In contrast, subjects diagnosed in family studies following detection of the index case usually show lesser degrees of iron overload and are often asymptomatic.

Once an index case or proband has been diagnosed all first-degree, and probably second-degree, relatives should be investigated. Although the optimum age to begin screening has not been addressed systematically in family studies, it seems justifiable to delay investigation until the age of 10 years because established disease is very rare before then, and because rises in serum ferritin and hepatic iron concentration are age related.

The serum iron concentration, percentage saturation of transferrin and serum ferritin concentration should be determined and if any one test is abnormal (particularly on more than one occasion) liver biopsy should be performed and stainable iron and hepatic iron concentration assessed. Chelation studies may be used to give some idea of the extent of iron overload if liver biopsy is contraindicated or refused.

It is important to emphasize that the presence of normal iron and ferritin studies does not preclude the development of iron overload at a later date. Thus, serial testing may be required. The frequency of these tests will depend on the likelihood of homozygosity or heterozygosity for the disease as determined by HLA typing. As a general rule putative homozygotes (those sharing both HLA haplotype with the proband) should be checked annually for evidence of increasing iron stores, while putative heterozygotes (those sharing only one haplotype with the proband) need be checked less frequently, e.g. every 5 years. The alternative approach of recommending that putative homozygotes become blood donors has been proposed (Edwards and Kushner, 1993), but we consider it less satisfactory because it prevents precise diagnosis both in individuals and in families (see below). A suggested protocol for the management of first degree relatives of patients with HC is given in Fig. 8.5.

Until recently, the diagnosis of HC was rarely made in patients under the age of 30 years. However, with the advent of screening of relatives for latent HC, the diagnosis is now frequently made in the second and third decades. Such subjects are usually asymptomatic and physical findings are few; hepatomegaly may be mild and the percentage saturation of transferrin may be moderately elevated. The serum ferritin concentration is usually elevated (Bassett *et al.*, 1984, 1986). Liver biopsy may show excess stainable iron, but usually no evidence of fibrosis or cirrhosis, and hepatic iron concentration is often less than 100 μmol/g dry weight of tissue, although the hepatic iron index is usually greater than 1.9. However, the rate of iron accumulation in young homozygotes is very variable. The reason is not understood but it is presumably related to differences in iron intake and physiological blood loss.

7.3. Detection in the Normal Population

Population studies in several countries have confirmed a prevalence rate for homozygous HC of between 1:250 and 1:400 (Simon *et al.*, 1980; Valberg *et al.*, 1980;

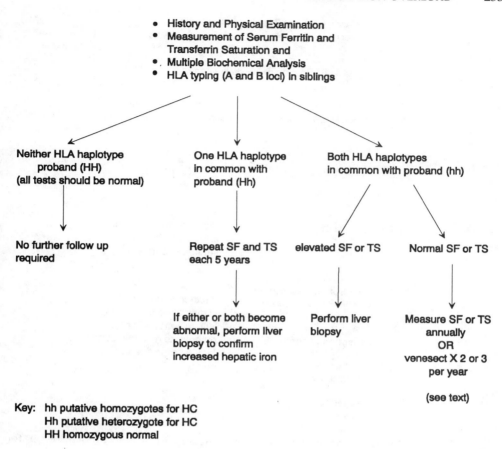

- History and Physical Examination
- Measurement of Serum Ferritin and Transferrin Saturation and
- Multiple Biochemical Analysis
- HLA typing (A and B loci) in siblings

Neither HLA haplotype proband (HH) (all tests should be normal)

One HLA haplotype in common with proband (Hh)

Both HLA haplotypes in common with proband (hh)

No further follow up required

Repeat SF and TS each 5 years

elevated SF or TS

Normal SF or TS

If either or both become abnormal, perform liver biopsy to confirm increased hepatic iron

Perform liver biopsy

Measure SF or TS annually OR venesect X 2 or 3 per year

(see text)

Key: hh putative homozygotes for HC
Hh putative heterozygote for HC
HH homozygous normal

Fig. 8.5 Protocol for the management of relatives of patients with haemochromatosis.

Dadone et al., 1982; Borwein et al., 1983; Leggett et al., 1990; Wiggers et al., 1991). Since early detection and treatment can prevent virtually every complication of the disease, a strong case can be made for population-based screening (Edwards and Kushner, 1993). However, of the available biochemical tests to detect iron overload, only the serum iron concentration is suitable for inclusion on automated multiple biochemical analysis, and this is an imprecise test with numerous false positives.

Thus, at the present time, it seems appropriate to confine screening to subjects who have a family history of HC or who are undergoing a health-check, e.g. for medical insurance purposes. In such circumstances the most cost-effective test is the serum transferrin saturation, preferably on a fasting morning specimen. If the result is greater than 60% in men or 50% in women then serum ferritin should also be performed. A suggested protocol for haemochromatosis screening and treatment is given in Fig. 8.6.

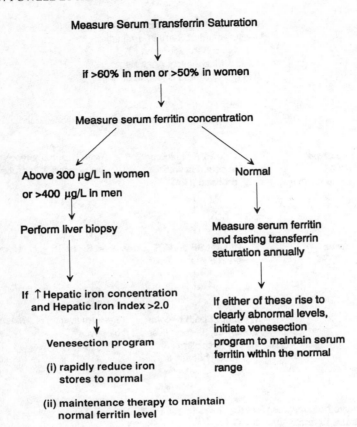

Measure Serum Transferrin Saturation

if >60% in men or >50% in women

Measure serum ferritin concentration

Above 300 µg/L in women
or >400 µg/L in men

Normal

Perform liver biopsy

Measure serum ferritin
and fasting transferrin
saturation annually

If ↑ Hepatic iron concentration
and Hepatic Iron Index >2.0

If either of these rise to
clearly abnormal levels,
initiate venesection
program to maintain serum
ferritin within the normal
range

Venesection program

(i) rapidly reduce iron
    stores to normal

(ii) maintenance therapy to maintain
     normal ferritin level

Fig. 8.6 Protocol for the screening for and management of haemochromatosis in the population.

8. IRON AS A RISK FACTOR FOR OTHER DISEASES

In addition to the direct complications of tissue iron excess that occur as manifestations or complications of HC (discussed in Section 6 above), increased body iron stores have been implicated or possibly implicated in the pathogenesis of several other disease states. Of particular interest has been the possibility that even within normal subjects with no excess of body iron as assessed by conventional reference ranges for tests of iron status, greater iron stores may be related to an increased risk of diseases including neoplasia, cardiovascular disease and infection. It has also been suggested that sudden infant death syndrome may bear some relationship to increased iron stores (Moore and Worwood, 1989), but so far the evidence is unconvicing.

8.1. Porphyria Cutanea Tarda

There is good evidence for a pathogenetic role of iron in PCT and most patients respond to phlebotomy therapy. This disorder is considered in greater detail in Chapter 9.

8.2. Extra-hepatic Malignancy

As discussed above (Section 6.1.6), early reports suggested an increased incidence of colo-rectal and lung cancer in patients with HC. However, two large controlled studies have failed to demonstrate an increase in incidence of malignancy other than HCC in symptomatic patients with HC (Bradbear *et al.*, 1985; Niederau *et al.*, 1986). Nevertheless, epidemiological studies have raised the possibility that subjects with an elevated serum ferritin concentration (with or without decreased serum transferrin level) may be predisposed to the subsequent development of intestinal malignancy. The role of iron as a potential carcinogen thus remains controversial and this subject is discussed in detail in Chapter 11.

8.3. Ischaemic Heart Disease

Much recent interest has centred on a suggestion that increased body iron stores may predispose to ischaemic heart disease and that this may occur at stored iron levels far lower than those encountered in HC (Sullivan, 1981, 1989; Lauffer, 1990; Salonen *et al.*, 1992a,b).

Sullivan (1981) hypothesized that the difference in the observed rates of heart disease between men and women could be explained by their different levels of stored iron. Premenopausal women in affluent societies enjoy relative protection from heart disease, compared with men, however this relative protection ends with the menopause (Kannel *et al.*, 1976). Although usually ascribed to the effect of oestrogens, Sullivan instead suggested that the greater incidence of heart disease in men and post-menopausal women is related to the higher levels of stored iron in these two groups. Iron stores as assessed by serum ferritin concentration, rise steadily in males after adolescence (Cook *et al.*, 1976) although levels may plateau after the age of 40–50 years (Leggett *et al.*, 1990). In contrast, serum ferritin concentrations remain low in premenopausal women before rising after the age of 45 years. These changes parallel the incidence of ischaemic heart disease seen in the Western world. In addition Sullivan postulated that the low rates of heart disease in developing countries may be related to the presence of endemic iron deficiency in these populations.

Epidemiological support for the role of iron stores as a possible explanation for the global variation in incidence of ischaemic heart diseases was provided by Lauffer (1990). In an analysis of previously published data from several different countries, he found that the correlation between the reported median value of hepatic storage iron and the ischaemic heart disease mortality rate was moderate ($r=0.55$, $P<0.025$). The correlation was stronger if the liver iron–serum cholesterol product was used ($r=0.74$, $P<0.005$). He concluded that it may be possible to identify individuals at risk of ischaemic heart disease and reduce this risk by venesection.

The debate has intensified following the recent report of Salonen *et al.* (1992b) that identified modestly elevated serum ferritin levels as a risk factor for acute myocardial infarction. In a prospective study of Eastern Finnish men, followed for an average of three years, subjects with a serum level ferritin $>200\,\mu g/l$ had a 2.2-fold relative risk (95% confidence interval 1.2–4.0, $P<0.01$) for acute myocardial infarction compared with men with a serum ferritin level $<200\,\mu g/l$. The risk was highest in those who had both a serum ferritin above 200 µg/l and a serum low density lipoprotein of greater than 5.0 mmol/l. Measurements of hepatic iron concentration were not available, but the assumption was made that the elevated ferritin levels reflected elevated tissue iron stores. Although elevated serum ferritin levels may also be related to an inflammatory response, meat intake or alcohol consumption (Leggett et al., 1990), these factors did not appear to be sufficient to explain either the differences in ferritin levels or rates of myocardial infarction. As yet no other group has confirmed these results (Riemersma et al., 1991).

A proposed mechanism implicating iron in the pathogenesis of ischaemic heart disease involves post-secretory modifications of low-density lipoprotein that appear to increase its atherogenic potential (Steinberg et al., 1989). Oxidatively modified low-density lipoprotein demonstrates chemotactic activity for circulating monocytes, enhanced uptake by macrophages via 'scavenger receptors' resulting in foam cell formation, and may be cytotoxic to endothelial cells. The oxidative modification of low-density lipoprotein by cells of the arterial subendothelium is dependent on the concentration of iron and copper (Heinecke et al., 1984) and can be inhibited in vitro by metal chelators (Steinbrecher et al., 1984). The modification of low-density lipoprotein renders it immunogenic: antibodies are detectable in human serum and can recognize material in atherosclerotic vessel walls but not in normal arteries (Palinski et al., 1989). Antibodies to oxidized low-density lipoprotein have been detected in the serum of some patients with ischaemic heart disease, and some elderly patients but not in healthy young adults (Parums et al., 1990). In addition the titre of autoantibodies to malondialdehyde-lysine (a prominent epitope of oxidatively modified low-density lipoprotein) has been proposed as an independent predictor of the progress of carotid atherosclerosis (Salonen et al., 1992a), and Probucol, a lipid lowering agent with antioxidant properties, can inhibit the development of atherosclerosis in hypercholesterolaemic rabbits independently of its cholesterol lowering effect (Carew et al., 1987). Trials in humans are awaited.

There is also experimental evidence implicating iron in the genesis of the myocardial ischaemic or reperfusion injury. This has shown that iron may be utilized in the production of free radicals that mediate tissue injury (Halliwell and Gutteridge, 1990) and treatment with desferrioxamine can reduce the degree of myocardial injury (Williams et al., 1991). Conversely iron loading increases the susceptibility of the rat heart to reperfusion damage (Van der Kraaij et al., 1988). Although this may be important after an ischaemic event, it does not relate to the pathogenesis or incidence of coronary artery atherosclerosis.

If iron plays a significant role in the pathogenesis of atherosclerosis and ischaemic heart disease, one would expect that subjects homozygous or heterozygous for genetic haemochromatosis might have a high incidence of ischaemic heart disease. We have performed a retrospective analysis of the causes of death in a cohort of 425 subjects with haemochromatosis–only 19 of 161 deaths were attributed to ischaemic heart disease. As 25 deaths were predicted, the relative risk of death from ischaemic heart disease was 0.77 in the cohort (Bradbear et al., unpublished). These findings support the clinical experience where there is no disproportionate incidence of ischaemic cardiac events in haemochromatosis patients. A minority of heterozygotes have mildly increased iron stores but an increased incidence of ischaemic heart disease does not appear to occur in this group either.

Thus the possible role of iron in the pathogenesis of ischaemic heart disease remains interesting but unproven. It raises questions about the optimal levels of body iron stores, optimal dietary requirements and potential risks of population-based food iron fortification programmes (Chapter 7). The control of iron availability and factors preventing tissue toxicity are largely unknown but critical to the understanding of diseases that may be iron related.

8.4. Infection

There is an on-going and unresolved debate over the interaction of iron and infections. The subject has been well reviewed recently (Peto and Hershko, 1989), and is discussed in detail in Chapter 11. Although increased susceptibility to infections has not been unequivocally demonstrated in subjects with HC (either homozygotes or heterozygotes) some situations of iron overload are associated with infections. However, a cause-and-effect relationship has not been established. *Yersinia enterocolitis* has been described in HC and thalassaemia in uncontrolled studies (Francois *et al.*, 1987). Iron therapy has been associated with acute exacerbations of infection, in particular malaria, and in the neonate parenteral iron has been associated with serious *E. coli* sepsis. However, Harvey *et al.* (1989), in a study of prepubescent children in Papua New Guinea, where malaria is endemic, showed that oral iron therapy could be carried out for iron deficiency without adverse consequences.

A possible pathophysiological basis for a predisposition of iron overload to infection has been provided by a number of studies which have demonstrated immuno-modulatory effects of iron on T-cell function (Good *et al.*, 1988; Brock, 1989) (see also Chapter 11). In addition, both desferrioxamine and the new, potent, orally effective iron chelator desferrithiocin, have been shown reversibly to inhibit T-cell proliferation (Bierer and Nathan, 1990).

Clearly, well-controlled, prospective studies are required both for malaria and other infectious diseases before iron can be implicated with certainty in pathogenesis and rational therapy instituted. The possible role of iron chelation in anti-malarial therapy (Yinnon *et al.*, 1989) is reviewed in detail in Chapter 13.

9. TREATMENT OF HAEMOCHROMATOSIS

In symptomatic patients treatment involves the removal of excess iron as quickly as possible and the treatment of complications, such as diabetes mellitus, hepatic failure and cardiac failure. Iron is best removed from the body by weekly or twice-weekly phlebotomy of 500 ml. Although the haemoglobin concentration initially undergoes modest decline to about 11 g/dl (haematocrit to about 35%) this stabilizes after several weeks. The serum iron and serum ferritin concentrations remain increased until the available iron stores are depleted. Since 500 ml of blood contains approximately 250 mg of iron and 20 g or more of storage iron may be present, 2 to 3 years of weekly phlebotomy are usually required for its removal. In younger patients with lesser iron stores, only 6 to 12 months of weekly phlebotomy may be required to reduce stores to normal.

A transient rise in serum ferritin level may follow commencement of phlebotomy and, at this stage, serum ferritin levels may not accurately reflect body iron stores. For practical purposes, estimation of the red cell haemoglobin concentration is adequate; venesection should continue at weekly intervals until the haemoglobin concentration falls below 11 g/dl. At this stage, the patient is usually marginally iron deficient and the serum ferritin concentration is less than 10 μg/l. As a guide to long-term maintenance therapy, the serum transferrin saturation and serum ferritin level should be maintained in the low normal range. One phlebotomy every 3 months usually suffices. A repeat liver biopsy at this stage usually reveals absence of stainable iron in hepatocytes and Kupffer cells. Phlebotomy leads to a marked increase in iron absorption. If the treatment is stopped, the serum iron level and percentage saturation of transferrin promptly increase followed by increase in serum ferritin concentration as iron stores progressively reaccumulate. Thus, lifelong phlebotomy therapy is required, preferably on a regular rather than intermittent basis. Chelating agents such as desferrioxamine (DFO) remove only 10–20 mg of iron per day. For patients with HC, phlebotomy is not only more effective but is also less expensive, more convenient, and safer. Chelating agents may be used as a substitute method for iron removal when anaemia, hypoproteinaemia, or cardiac disease is severe enough to preclude phlebotomy, but a negative iron balance is difficult to achieve by this means.

10. PROGNOSIS

Although no controlled prospective trials of phlebotomy therapy in HC have been published, two retrospective evaluations have been completed (Powell, 1970; Bomford and Williams, 1976). Bomford and Williams (1976) compared 85 patients receiving phlebotomy with 26 untreated patients. The mean survival in the phlebotomy group was greater than the survival of patients in the untreated group. The 5-year survival rate with therapy was increased from 33% to 89%. With removal of iron by repeated phlebotomy, patients lose their lethargy, the liver and spleen decrease in size, biochemical liver tests return to normal, skin pigmentation decreases, and cardiac failure may be reversed. Carbohydrate tolerance improves in 30% to 40% of patients, resulting in a reduction in insulin requirements or drug therapy.

Removal of excess iron has little or no effect on hypogonadism, arthropathy, or portal hypertension. Hepatic fibrosis may decrease but cirrhosis is irreversible. Apparent reversal of cirrhosis on needle biopsy is due to the development of macronodular cirrhosis. Hepatocellular carcinoma occurs as a late sequela in about 25 to 30% of patients with cirrhosis despite adequate iron removal. Although the cause of this complication is unclear, factors that are related include male sex, longevity and the degree of iron loading before therapy was commenced. Hence, the importance of family screening and early treatment of affected individuals cannot be emphasized too strongly.

Management of the hepatic failure, cardiac failure and diabetes differs little from conventional management of these conditions. Loss of libido and change in secondary sex characteristics may be partially relieved by testosterone or gonadotropin therapy.

REFERENCES

Adams, P. C. and Powell, L. W. (1987) Porphyria cutanea tarda and HLA-linked hemochromatosis – All in the family? *Gastroenterology* **92**(6), 2033–2035.

Adams, P. C., Powell, L. W. and Halliday, J. W. (1988) Isolation of a human hepatic ferritin receptor. *Hepatology* **9**, 719–721.

Adams, P. C., Reece, A. S., Powell, L. W. and Halliday, J. W. (1989) Hepatic iron in the control of iron absorption in a rat liver transplantation model. *Transplantation* **48**, 19–21.

Adams, P. C., Zhong, R., Haist, J., Flanagan, P. R. and Grant, D. R. (1991) Mucosal iron in the control of iron absorption in a rat transplantation model. *Gastroenterology* **100**, 370–374.

Aisen, P. (1980) The transferrins. In: *Iron in Biochemistry and Medicine*. II (eds A. Jacobs and M. Worwood), London: Academic Press, pp. 87–129.

Aisen, P., Liebman, A., Hu, H-YY. and Skoultchi, A. I. (1977) Studies on transferrin receptors of erythroid cells. In: *Proteins of Iron Metabolism* (eds E. B. Brown, P. Aisen, J. Fielding and R. R. Crichton), New York: Grune and Stratton, pp. 281–289.

Ames, B. N. (1983) Dietary carcinogens and anticarcinogens. *Science* **221**, 1256–1264.

Anderson, G. J., Powell, L. W. and Halliday, J. W. (1990) Transferrin receptor distribution and regulation in the rat small intestine: Effect of iron stores and erythropoiesis. *Gastroenterology* **98**, 576–585.

Anderson, G. J., Walsh, M. D., Powell, L. W. and Halliday, J. W. (1991a) Intestinal transferrin receptors and iron absorption in the neonatal rat. *Br. J. Haematol.* **77**, 229–236.

Anderson, P. B., Birgegard, G., Nyman, R. and Hemingsson, A. (1991b) Magnetic resonance imaging in idiopathic hemochromatosis. *Eur. J. Haematol.* **47**, 174–178.

Arnold, R. R., Russell, J. E., Champion, W. J. and Gauthier, J. J. (1981) Bactericidal activity of human lactoferrin: influence of physical conditions and metabolic state of the target microorganism. *Infect. Immun.* **32**, 655–660.

Arstila, A. U., Smith, M. A. and Trump, B. R. (1972) Microsomal lipid peroxidation: morphological characterization. *Science* **175**, 530–533.

Askari, A. D., Muir, W. A., Rosner, I. A. *et al.* (1983) Arthritis of hemochromatosis. Clinical spectrum, relation to histocompatibility antigens, and effectiveness of early phlebotomy. *Ann. Intern. Med.* **75**, 957–965.

Bacon, B. R. and Britton, R. S. (1990) The pathology of hepatic iron overload: A free radical-mediated process? *Hepatology* **11**(1), 127–136.

Bacon, B. R., Tavill, A. S., Recknagel, R. O. and Brittenham, C. M. (1981) Evidence for subcellular localization of lipid peroxidation in experimental chronic iron overload. *Hepatology* **1**, 493.

Bacon, B. R., Tavill, A. S., Brittenham, G. M., Park, C. H. and Recknagel, R. O. (1983) Hepatic lipid peroxidation in vivo in rats with chronic iron overload. *J. Clin. Invest.* **71**, 429–439.

Baker, E. and Morgan, E. H. (1967) The role of iron in the reaction between rabbit transferrin and reticulocytes. *Biochemistry* **8**, 2954–2958.

Baker, E. and Morgan, E. H. (1969) The kinetics of the interaction between rabbit transferrin and reticulocytes. *Biochemistry* **8**, 1133–1140.

Banerjee, D., Flanagan, P. R., Cluett, J. and Valberg, L. S. (1986) Transferrin receptors in the human gastrointestinal tract. *Gastroenterology* **91**, 861–869.

Barron, R., Grace, N. D., Sherwood, G. and Powell, L. W. (1988) Iron overload complicating sideroblastic anemia – Is the gene for hemochromatosis responsible? *Gastroenterology* **96**, 1204–1206.

Bassett, M. L., Halliday, J. W. and Powell, L. W. (1979) Early detection of idiopathic hemochromatosis, relative value of serum-ferritin and HLA typing. *Lancet* **ii**, 4–7.

Bassett, M. L., Halliday, J. W. and Powell, L. W. (1981) HLA typing in idiopathic hemochromatosis: distinction between homozygotes and heterozygotes with biochemical expression. *Hepatology* **1**, 120–126.

Bassett, M. L., Doran, T. J., Halliday, J. W., Bashir, H. V. and Powell, L. W. (1982) Idiopathic hemochromatosis: demonstration of homozygous–heterozygous mating by HLA typing of families. *Hum. Genet.* **60**, 352–357.

Bassett, M. L., Halliday, J. W. and Powell, L. W. (1984a) Genetic hemochromatosis. *Sem. Liver Disease* **4**(3), 217–227.

Bassett, M. L., Halliday, J. W., Ferris, R. A. and Powell, L. W. (1984b) Diagnosis of hemochromatosis in young subjects: predictive accuracy of serum iron, transferrin saturation and serum ferritin. *Gastroenterology* **87**, 628.

Bassett, M. L., Halliday, J. W. and Powell, L. W. (1986) Value of hepatic iron measurements in early hemochromatosis and determination of the critical iron level associated with fibrosis. *Hepatology* **6**(1), 24–29.

Batey, R. G., Pettit, J. E., Nicholas, A. W., Sherlock, S. and Hoffbrand, A. V. (1978) Hepatic iron clearance from serum in treated hemochromatosis. *Gastroenterology* **75**, 856–859.

Beasley, R. P., Lin, C. C., Hwang, L. Y. *et al.* (1981) Hepatocellular carcinoma and hepatitis B virus. *Lancet* **ii**, 1129–1133.

Beaumont, C., Simon, M., Fauchet, R. *et al.* (1979) Serum ferritin as a possible marker of the hemochromatosis allele. *N. Eng. J. Med.* **301**, 169–174.

Bierer, B. E. and Nathan, D. G. (1990) The effect of desferrithiocin, an oral iron chelator, on T-cell function. *Blood* **76**(10), 2052–2059.

Bjorn-Rasmussen, E. (1974) Food iron absorption in man. Applications of the twopool extrinsic tag method to measure heme and nonheme iron absorption from the whole diet. *J. Clin. Invest.* **53**, 247–255.

Blumberg, B. S., Lustbader, E. D. and Whitford, P. L. (1981) Changes in serum iron levels due to infection and hepatitis B virus. *Proc. Natl. Acad. Sci. USA* **78**, 3222–3224.

Boender, C. A. and Verloop, M. C. (1969) Iron absorption, iron loss and iron retention in man: studies after oral administration of a tracer dose of Fe59SO4. *Br. J. Haematol.* **17**, 45–48.

Bomford, A. and Williams, R. (1976) Long term results of venesection therapy in idiopathic hemochromatosis. *Quart. J. Med.* **45**, 611–623.

Bomford, A., Eddleston, A. L. W. F., Kennedy, L. A., Batchelor, J. R. and Williams, R. (1977) Histocompatibility antigens as marker of abdominal iron metabolism in patients with idiopathic hemochromatosis and their relatives. *Lancet* **i**, 327–329.

Bonkovsky, H. L., Weber, R. W. and Aaron, L. (1990a) Four hour measurement of urinary iron excretion after deferoxine treatment: a rapid simple method of study of iron excretion. *Am. J. Gastroenterol.* **15**, 554–557.

Bonkovsky, H. L., Slater, D. P., Bills, E. B. and Wolf, D. C. (1990b) Usefulness and limitations of laboratory and hepatic imaging studies in iron storage disease. *Gastroenterology* **99**, 1079–1091.

Boretto, J., Jouanolle, A. M., Yaouang, J. *et al.* (1992) Anonymous markers located on chromosome 6 in the HLA-A class I region: allelic distribution in genetic haemochromatosis. *Hum. Genet.* **89**, 33–36.

Borwein, S. T., Ghent, C. N., Flanagan, P. R., Chamberlain, M. J. and Valberg, L. S. (1983) Genetic and phenotype expression of haemochromatosis in Canadians. *Clin. Invest. Med.* **6**, 171–179.

Bothwell, T. H. (1968) The control of iron absorption. *Br. J. Haematol.* **14**, 453–456.

Bothwell, T. H., Charlton, R. W., Cook, J. D. and Finch, C. A. (1979) *Iron Metabolism in Man*. Blackwell Scientific Publications, Oxford, pp. 576.

Bradbear, R. A., Bain, C., Siskind, V., *et al.* (1985) Cohort study of internal malignancy in genetic hemochromatosis and other nonalcoholic liver diseases. *J.C.N.I.* **74**, 81.

Brittenham, G. M., Farrell, D. E., Harris, J. W. *et al.* (1982) Magneticsusceptibility measurement of human iron stores. *N. Eng. J. Med.* **307**(27), 1671–1675.

Brittin, G. M. and Raval, D. (1970) Duodenal ferritin synthesis during iron absorption in the iron-deficient rat. *J. Lab. Clin. Med.* **75**, 811–817.

Brittin, G. M. and Raval, D. (1971) Duodenal ferritin synthesis in iron-replete and iron-deficient rats: Response to small doses of iron. *J. Lab. Clin. Med.* **77**, 54–58.

Britton, R. S., O'Neill, R. and Bacon, B. R. (1990) Hepatic mitochondrial malondialdehyde metabolism in rats with chronic iron overload. *Hepatology* **11**(1), 93–97.

Brock, J. H. (1989) Iron and cells of the immune system. In: *Iron in Immunity, Cancer and Inflammation* (eds M. de Sousa and J. H. Brock), J. Wiley & Sons, New York.

Broxmeyer, H. E., Ralph, P., Bognacki, J., Kincade, P. W. and DeSousa, M. (1980a) A subpopulation of human polymorphonuclear neutrophils contains an active form of lactoferrin capable of binding to human monocytes and inhibiting production of granulocytemacrophage colony stimulatory activities. *J. Immunol.* **125**, 903–909.

Broxmeyer, H. E., DeSousa, M., Smithyman, A. *et al.* (1980b) Specificity and modulation of the action of lactoferrin, a negative feedback regulator of myelopoiesis. *Blood* **55**, 324–333.

Buja, L. M. and Roberts, W. C. (1971) Iron in the heart. *Am. J. Med.* **51**, 209–221.

Carew, T. E., Schwenke, D. C. and Steinberg, D. (1987) Antiatherogenic effect on probucol unrelated to its hypocholesterolemic effect: evidence that antioxidants in vivo can selectively inhibit low density lipoprotein degradation in macrophage-rich fatty streaks and slow the progression of atherosclerosis in the Watanabe heritable hyperlipidemic rabbit. *Proc. Natl. Acad. Sci. USA* **84**, 7725–7729.

Cartwright, G. E., Edwards, C. Q. and Skolnick, M. (1979) Letter to editors: Genetics of hemochromatosis. *N. Engl. J. Med.* **301**, 1291–1292.

Cartwright, G. E., Edwards, C. Q., Kravitz, K. *et al.* (1979) Hereditary hemochromatosis: phenotypic expression of the disease. *N. Engl. J. Med.* **301**, 175–179.

Cartwright, G. E., Edwards, C. Q., Skolnick, M. H. and Amos, D. B. (1980) Association of HLA-linked hemochromatosis with idiopathic refractory sideroblastic anemia. *J. Clin. Invest.* **65**, 989–992.

Casey, J. L., Di Jeso, B., Rao, K., Rouault, T. A., Klausner, R. D. and Harford, J. B. (1988a) Deletional analysis of the promoter region of the human transferrin receptor gene. *Nucl. Acid Res.* **16**, 629–646.

Casey, J. L., Di Jeso, B., Rao, K., Klausner, R. D. and Harford, J. B. (1988b) Two genetic loci participate in the regulation by iron of the gene for the human transferrin receptor. *Proc. Natl. Acad. Sci. USA* **85**, 1787–1791.

Casey, J. L., Hentze, M. W., Koeller, D. M. *et al.* (1988c) Iron-responsive elements: regulatory DNA sequences that control mRNA levels and translation. *Science* **240**, 924–928.

Caughman, S. W., Hentze, M. W., Rouault, T. A., Harford, J. B. and Klausner, R. D. (1988) The iron-responsive element is the single element responsible for iron-dependent translational regulation of ferritin biosynthesis. *J. Biol. Chem.* **263**, 19048–19052.

Cavill, I., Worwood, M. and Jacobs, A. (1975) Internal regulation of iron absorption. *Nature* **256**, 328.

Celada, A., Rudolf, H. and Donath, A. (1978) Effect of a single ingestion of alcohol on iron absorption. *Am. J. Hematol.* **5**, 225–227.

Celada, A., Rudolf, H. and Donath, A. (1979) Effect of experimental chronic alcohol ingestion and folic acid deficiency on iron absorption. *Blood* **54**, 906–915.

Chapman, R. W. G., Williams, G., Bydder, G., Dick, R., Sherlock, S. and Kreel, L. (1980) Computed tomography for determining liver iron content in primary hemochromatosis. *Br. Med. J.* **1**, 440–442.

Colombo, M., De Franchis, R., Del Ninno, E. *et al.* (1991) Hepatocellular carcinoma in Italian patients with cirrhosis. *N. Engl. J. Med.* **325**(1), 675.

Conrad, M. E. and Umbreit, J. N. (1993) A concise review: iron absorption – the mucin–mobilferrin–integrin pathway. A competitive pathway for metal absorption. *Am. J. Hematol.* **42**, 67–73.

Conrad, M. E., Umbreit, J. N., Moore, E. G., Peterson, R. D. A. and Jones, M. B. A. (1990) A newly identified iron binding protein in duodenal mucosa of rats. *J. Biol. Chem.* **265**, 5273–5279.

Conrad, M. E., Umbreit, J. N. and Moore, E. G. (1991) A role for mucin in the absorption of inorganic iron and other metal cations. A study in rats. *Gastroenterology* **100**, 129–136.

Cook, J. D., Barry, W. E. and Hershko, C. (1973) Iron kinetics with emphasis on iron overload. *Am. J. Pathol.* **72**(2), 337–343.

Cook, J. D., Finch, C. A. and Smith, N. J. (1976) Evaluation of the iron status of a population. *Blood* **48**, 449–455.

Cox, T. M. and Peters, T. (1978) Uptake of iron by duodenal biopsy specimens from patients with iron deficiency anaemia and primary haemochromatosis. *Lancet* i, 123–124.

Cox, T. M. and Peters, T. (1979) The kinetics of iron uptake in vitro by human duodenal mucosa: studies in normal subjects. *J. Physiol.* **289**, 469–478.

Cox, T. M. and Peters, T. H. (1980a) Cellular mechanisms in the regulation of iron absorption by human intestine: studies in patients with iron deficiency before and after treatment. *Br. J. Haematol.* **44**, 75–86.

Cox, T. M. and Peters, T. H. (1980b) In vitro studies of duodenal iron uptake in patients with primary and secondary iron storage disease. *Quart. J. Med.* **49**, 249–257.

Cox, T. M. and O'Donnell, M. W. (1981) Studies on the binding of iron by rabbit intestinal microvillus micromembranes. *Biochem. J.* **194**, 753–759.

Crawford, D. H. G., Halliday, J. W., Summers, K. M., Burke, M. and Powell, L. W. (1993) Concordance of iron storage in siblings with genetic haemochromatosis: Evidence for a predominantly genetic effect on iron storage. *Hepatology* (in press).

Dadone, M. M., Kushner, J. P., Edwards, C. Q., Bishop, D. T. and Skolnick, M. H. (1982) Hereditary hemochromatosis. Analysis of laboratory expression of the disease by genotype in 18 pedigrees. *Am. J. Clin. Path.* **78**, 196–207.

Davies, K. (1993) Cloning the Menkes disease gene. *Nature* **361**, 98.

de Alarcon, P. A., Donovan, M. E., Forbes, G. B., Landaw, S. and Stockman, J. A. (1979) Iron absorption in the thalassemia syndromes and its inhibition by tea. *N. Engl. J. Med.* **300**, 5–8.

Deugnier, Y. M., Guyader, D., Crantock, L. *et al.* (1993) Primary liver cancer in genetic hemochromatosis: A clinical, pathological, and pathogenetic study of 54 cases. *Gastroenterology* **104**, 228–234.

Disler, P. B., Lynch, S. R., Charlton, R. W. *et al.* (1975) The effect of tea on iron absorption. *Gut* **16**, 193–200.

Doran, T., Bashir, H. V., Trejaut, J., Bassett, M. L., Halliday, J. W. and Powell, L. W. (1981) Idiopathic hemochromatosis in the Australian population: HLA linkage and recessivity. *Human Immunol.* **2**, 191–200.

Dymock, I. W., Hamilton, E. B. D., Laws, J. W. and Williams, R. (1970) Arthropathy of hemochromatosis. Clinical and radiological analysis of 63 patients with iron overload. *Ann. Rheum. Dis.* **29**(5), 469–476.

Eason, R. J., Adams, P. C., Aston, C. E. and Searle, J. (1990) Familial iron overload with possible autosomal dominant inheritance. *Aust. N.Z. J. Med.* **20**, 226–230.

Edwards, C. Q. and Kushner, J. P. (1993) Screening for hemochromatosis. *N. Eng. J. Med.* **328**, 1616–1620.

Edwards, C. Q., Griffin, L. M., Goldgar, D. E., Skolnick, M. H. and Kushner, J. P. (1989) HLA-linked hemochromatosis alleles in sporadic prophyria cutanea tarda. *Gastroenterology* **97**, 972–981.

Edwards, C. Q., Carroll, M., Bray, P. and Cartwright, G. E. (1977) Hereditary hemochromatosis. *N. Engl. J. Med.* **297**, 7–13.

Edwards, C. Q., Skolnick, M. H. and Kushner, J. P. (1981) Coincidental nontransfusional iron overload and thalassemia minor: association with HLA-linked hemochromatosis. *Blood* **58**, 844–848.

Edwards, C. Q., Dadone, M. M., Skolnick, M. H. and Kushner, J. P. (1982) Hereditary hemochromatosis. *Clin. Haematol.* **11**, 411–435.

Edwards, C. Q., Griffin, L. M., Goldgar, D., Drummond, C., Skolnick, M. H. and Kushner, J. P. (1988) Prevalence of hemochromatosis among 11 065 presumably healthy blood donors. *N. Engl. J. Med.* **318**(1), 1355–1362.

El Kalhoun, A., Chauvel, B., Mauvieux, N. *et al.* (1993) Localization of seven new genes around the HLA-A locus. *Hum. Mol. Genet.* **2**, 55–60.

Erickson, R. P. (1978) Haemochromatosis and superoxide metabolism; free radical influence iron storage? *Lancet* ii, 743.

Fargion, S., Capellini, M. D., Piperno, A., Panajotopoulos, N., Ronchi, G., and Fiorelli, G. (1986) Association of hereditary spherocytosis and idiopathic hemochromatosis: a synergistic effect in determining iron overload. *Am. J. Clin. Pathol.* **86**, 645–649.

Fauchet, R., Simon, M., Genetet, B. *et al.* (1977) HLA-A, B, C, D and lymphocytes B antigens typing in idiopathic haemochromatosis with the study of 5 families. *Tissue Antigens* **10**, 206.

Fauchet, R., Genetet, N., Genetet, B., Simon, M. and Bourel, M. (1979) HLA determinants in idiopathic hemochromatosis. *Tissue Antigens* **14**, 10–14.

Feely, J. and Counihan, T. B. (1977) Haemochromatosis presenting as angina and responding to venesection. *Br. Med. J.* **2**, 681–682.

Fillet, G. and Marsaglia, G. (1976) Idiopathic hemochromatosis. Abnormality in RBC transport of iron by the reticuloendothelial system. (Abstract No. 19.) *Blood* **46**, 1007.

Fillet, G., Beguin, Y. and Baldelli, L. (1989) Model of reticuloendothelial iron metabolism in humans: Abnormal behaviour in idiopathic hemochromatosis and in inflammation. *Blood* **74**(2), 844–851.

Finch, S. C. and Finch, C. A. (1955) Idiopathic hemochromatosis and iron storage disease. A. Iron metabolism in hemochromatosis. *Medicine (Baltimore)* **34**, 381–430.

Finch, C. A. and Hueberg, H. (1982) Perspectives in iron metabolism. *N. Engl. J. Med.* **306**, 1520–1528.

Finch, C. A., Hueberg, H., Eng, M. and Miller, L. (1982) The effect of transferred reticulocytes on iron exchange. *Blood* **59**, 364–369.

Flanagan, P. R., Lam, D., Banerjee, D. and Valberg, L. S. (1989) Ferritin release by mononuclear cells in hereditary hemochromatosis. *J. Lab. Clin. Med.* **113**, 145–150.

Fletcher, L. M., Roberts, F. D., Irving, M. G., Powell, L. W. and Halliday, J. W. (1989) Effects of iron loading on free radical scavenging enzymes and lipidperoxidation in rat liver. *Gastroenterology* **97**, 1011–1018.

Fracanzani, A. L., Fargion, S., Romeno, R., Piperno, A., Arosio, P. and Fiorelli, G. (1989) Immunohistochemical evidence for a lack of ferritin in duodenal absorptive epithelial cells in idiopathic hemochromatosis. *Gastroenterology* **96**, 1071–1078.

Francois, P., Bachelot, C., Andrini, P. and Bost, M. (1987) Roles of iron overload and chelating treatment in *Yersinia* infections complicated by major thalassemia. *Presse Med.* **16**(32), 1574–1576.

Gasparini, P., Borgato, L., Piperno, A. *et al.* (1993) Linkage analysis of 6p21 polymorphic markers and the hereditary hemochromatosis: localization of the gene centromeric to HLA-F. *Hum. Mol. Genet.* **2**, 571–576.

Good, M. F., Powell, L. W. and Halliday, J. W. (1988) Iron status and cellular immune competence. *Blood Reviews* **2**, 43–49.

Gordeuk, V., Mukiibi, J., Hasstedt, S. J. *et al.* (1992) Iron overload in Africa: Interaction between a gene and dietary iron content. *N. Eng. J. Med.* **326**, 95–100.

Grace, N. D. (1978) Evidence of hepatic toxicity of iron. In: *Metals and the Liver* (ed. L. W. Powell), New York: Marcel Dekker, pp. 133–144.

Grace, N. D. and Greenberg, M. S. (1971) Phlebotomy in the treatment of iron overload. A controlled trial (preliminary report), *Gastroenterology* **60**, 744.

Grace, N. D. and Powell, L. W. (1974) Iron storage disorders of the liver. *Gastroenterology* **64**, 1257–1283.

Greenberger, N. J., Ruppert, R. D. and Cuppage, F. E. (1967) Inhibition of intestinal iron transport induced by tetracycline. *Gastroenterology* **53**, 590–599.

Grohlich, D., Morley, C. G. D. and Bezkorovainy, A. (1979) Some aspects of iron uptake by rat hepatocytes in suspension. *Int. J. Biochem.* **10**, 797–802.

Gruen, J. R., Goel, V. L., Summers, K. M. *et al.* (1992) Physical and genetic mapping of the telomeric major histocompatibility complex region in man and relevance to the primary hemochromatosis gene (HFE). *Genomics* **14**, 232–240.

Guyader, D., Gandon, Y., Deugnier, Y. *et al.* (1989) Evaluation of computed tomography in the assessment of liver iron overload. A study of 46 cases of idiopathic haemochromatosis. *Gastroenterology* **97**, 737–743.

Guyader, D., Gandon, Y., Robert, J. Y. *et al.* (1992) Magnetic resonance imaging and assessment of liver iron content in genetic hemochromatosis. *J. Hepatology* **75**, 304–308.

Halliday, J. W. and Powell, L. W. (1982) Iron overload. *Semin. Hematol.* **29**, 42–53.

Halliday, J. W., Cowlishaw, J. C., Russo, A. M. and Powell, L. W. (1977) Serum ferritin in the diagnosis of hemochromatosis. *Lancet* **i**, 621–624.

Halliday, J. W., Mack, U. and Powell, L. W. (1978) Duodenal ferritin content and structure. Relationship with body iron stores in man. *Arch. Int. Med.* **138**, 1109–1113.

Halliwell, B. and Gutteridge, J. M. C. (1990) Role of free radicals and catalytic metal ions in human disease: an overview. *Methods Enzymol* **186**, 1–85.

Hamilton, E. (1971) Joint disease in haemochromatosis. In: *Modern Trends in Rheumatology 2* (ed. A. G. S. Hill), Butterworths, London, pp. 338–347.

Hanot, V. and Schachmann, M. (1886) *Archives de Physiologies Normale et Pathologique* 7, 50.

Harker, L. A., Funk, D. D. and Finch, C. A. (1968) Evaluation of storage iron by chelates. *Am. J. Med.* 45, 105–115.

Harvey, P. W., Heywood, P. F., Nesheim, M. C. *et al.* (1989) The effect of iron therapy on malarial infection in Papua New Guinean schoolchildren. *Am. J. Trop. Med. Hyg.* 40(1), 12–18.

Haskins, D., Stevens, P. R., Jr, Finch, S. C. and Finch, C. A. (1952) Iron metabolism: iron stores in man as measured by phlebotomy. *J. Clin. Invest.* 31, 543–547.

Heinecke, J. W., Rosen, H. and Chait, A. (1984) Iron and copper promote modification of low density lipoprotein by human arterial smooth muscle cells in culture. *J. Clin. Invest.* 74, 1890–1894.

Hemmaplardh, D. and Morgan, E. H. (1974) Transferrin uptake and release by reticulocytes treated with proteolytic enzymes and neuraminidase. *Biochim. Biophys. Acta* 373, 84–99.

Hennigar, G. R., Greene, W. B., Walker, E. M. and deSaussure C. (1979) Hemochromatosis caused by excessive vitamin iron intake. *Am. J. Pathol.* 96, 611–624.

Hentze, M. W., Caughman, S. W., Casey, J. W. *et al.* (1988) A model for the structure and functions of iron-responsive elements. *Gene* 72, 201–208.

Hentze, M. W., Seuanez, H. N., O'Brien, S. J., Harford, J. B. and Klausner, R. D. (1989a) Chromosomal localization of nucleic acid-binding proteins by affinity mapping: assignment of the IRE-binding protein gene to human chromosome 9. *Nucleic Acids Res.* 17, 6103–6108.

Hentze, M. W., Rouault, T. A., Harford, J. B. and Klausner, R. D. (1989b) Oxidation–reduction and the molecular mechanism of a regulatory RNA–protein interaction. *Science* 244, 357–359.

Howard, J. M., Ghent, C. N., Carey, L. S., Flanagan, P. R. and Valberg, L. S. (1983) Diagnostic efficacy of hepatic computed tomography in the detection of body iron overload. *Gastroenterology* 84, 209–215.

Huebers, H., Huebers, E., Csiba, E. and Finch, C. A. (1978) Iron uptake from rat plasma transferrin by rat reticulocytes. *J. Clin. Invest.* 62, 944–951.

Huebers, H., Finch, C. A., Eng, M. and Miller, L. (1981a) Uptake and release of iron from human transferrin. *Proc. Natl. Acad. Sci. USA* 78, 2572–2576.

Huebers, H., Csiba, E., Josephson, B., Huebers, E. and Finch, C. (1981b) Interaction of human diferric transferrin with reticulocytes. *Proc. Natl. Acad. Sci. USA* 78, 621–625.

Iancu, T. C., Neustein, H. B. and Landing, B. H. (1977) The liver in thalassaemia major: Ultrastructural observations. In: *Iron Metabolism*, Ciba Foundation Symposium 51, Amsterdam: Elsevier, pp. 293–316.

Jacobs, A. and Miles, P. M. (1968) The ironbinding properties of gastric juice. *Clin. Chim. Acta* 24, 87–92.

Jazwinska, E. C., Lee, S. C., Webb, S. I., Halliday, J. W. and Powell, L. W. (1993) Localization of the hemochromatosis gene close to DG5105. *Am. J. Hum. Genet.* in press.

Jensen, P. S. (1976) Hemochromatosis: a disease often silent but not invisible. *Am. J. Roentgenol.* 126, 343–351.

Kaltwasser, J. P., Gottschalk, R., Schalk, K. P. and Hartl, W. (1990) Non-invasive quantitation of liver iron-overload by magnetic resonance imaging. *Br. J. Haematol.* 74, 360–363.

Kannel, W. B., Hjortland, M. C., McNamara, P. M. and Gordon, T. (1976) Menopause and risk of cardiovascular disease. The Framingham study. *Ann. Intern. Med.* 85, 447–452.

Kent, G. and Popper, H. (1960) Secondary hemochromatosis: its association with anemia. *Arch. Pathol.* 70, 623–642.

Klausner, R. D. (1988) From receptors to genes – insights from molecular iron metabolism. *Clin. Res.* 36(5), 494–500.

Kuhn, L. C. (1991) mRNA–protein interactions regulate critical pathways in cellular iron metabolism. *Br. J. Haematol.* 79, 1–5.

Kuhn, I. N., Layrisse, M., Roche, M., Martinez, C. and Walker, R. B. (1968) Observations on the mechanism of iron absorption. *Am. J. Clin. Nutr.* 21, 1184–1188.

Lauffer, R. B. (1990) Iron stores and the international variation in mortality from coronary artery disease. *Medical Hypotheses* 35, 96–102.

Le Sage, G. D., Baldus, W. P., Fairbanks, V. F. *et al.* (1983) Hemochromatosis: Genetic or alcohol induced? *Gastroenterology* 84, 1471–1477.

Leggett, B. A., Brown, N. N., Bryant, S. J., Duplock, L., Powell, L. W. and Halliday, J. W. (1990a) Factors affecting the concentration of serum ferritin in a healthy Australian population. *Clin. Chem.* **36**, 1350–1355.

Leggett, B. A., Halliday, J. W., Brown, N. N., Bryant, S. and Powell, L. W. (1990b) Prevalence of hemochromatosis amongst asymptomatic Australians. *Br. J. Haematol.* **74**, 525–530.

Leibman, A. and Aisen, P. (1977) Transferrin receptors of the rabbit reticulocyte. *Biochemistry* **16**, 1268–1272.

Leibold, F. A. and Munro, H. N. (1988) Cytoplasmic protein binds in vitro to a highly conserved sequence in the 5′ untranslated region of ferritin heavy and light subunit mRNA's. *Proc. Natl. Acad. Sci. USA* **85**, 2171–2175.

Leon, M. B., Borer, J. S., Bacharach, S. L. *et al.* (1979) Detection of early cardiac dysfunction in patients with severe β-thalassemia and chronic iron overload. *N. Engl. J. Med.* **301**(2), 1143–1148.

Lipschitz, D. A., Simon, M. O., Lynch, S. R., Dugard, J., Bothwell, T. H. and Charlton, R. W. (1971) Some factors affecting the release of iron from reticuloendothelial cells. *Br. J. Haematol.* **21**, 289–303.

Lundvall, O., Weinfeld, A. and Lundin, P. (1970) Iron storage in porphyria cutania tarda. *Acta Med. Scand.* **188**, 37–53.

Lynch, S. R. and Cook, J. D. (1980) Interaction of vitamin C and iron. *Proc. NY Acad. Sci.* **355**, 32–44.

MacDonald, R. A. (1964) *Hemochromatosis and Hemosiderosis*, Charles C. Thomas, Illinois.

MacSween, R. N. M. and Scott, A. R. (1973) Hepatic cirrhosis: a clinicopathological review of 520 cases. *J. Clin. Pathol.* **26**, 936.

Mack, U., Powell, L. W. and Halliday, J. W. (1983) Detection and isolation of a hepatic membrane receptor for ferritin. *J. Biol. Chem.* **258**, 4672–4675.

Marx, J. J. M. (1979) Mucosal uptake, mucosal transfer and retention of iron, measured by whole-body counting. *Scand. J. Haematol.* **23**, 293–302.

Mazur, A., Baez, P. and Shorr, E. (1955) The mechanism of iron release from ferritin as related to its biological properties. *J. Biol. Chem.* **213**, 147–160.

McLaren, G., Sachs, S. D., Muir, W. A. and Kellermeyer, R. W. (1976) Canine hemochromatosis: a model for the study of reticuloendothelial cell function. (Abstract) *Clin. Res.* **24**, 315A.

McLaren, C., Bett, J. H. N., Nye, J. A. and Halliday, J. W. (1982) Congestive cardiomyopathy and haemochromatosis – Rapid progression possibly accelerated by excessive ingestion of ascorbic acid. *Aust. NZ J. Med.* **12**, 187–188.

McLaren, G. D., Nathanson, M. H., Jacobs, A., Trevett, D. and Thomson, W. (1991) Regulation of intestinal iron absorption and mucosal iron kinetics in hereditary hemochromatosis. *J. Lab. Clin. Med.* **117**(5), 390–401.

Mercer, J. F. B., Livingston, J., Hall, B. *et al.* (1993) Isolation of a partial candidate gene for Menkes disease by positional cloning. *Nature Genetics* **3**, 20–25.

Meyer, T. E., Ballot, D., Bothwell, T. H. *et al.* (1987) The HLA linked iron loading gene in an Afrikaner population. *J. Med. Gen.* **24**, 348–356.

Meyer, T. E., Baynes, R. D., Bothwell, T. H. *et al.* (1988) Phenotypic expression of the HLA-linked iron-loading gene in the Afrikaner population of the Western Cape. *S.A. Med. J.* **73**, 269–274.

Milder, M. S., Cook, J. D., Stray, S. and Finch, C. A. (1980) Idiopathic hemochromatosis: an interim report. *Medicine* **59**, 34–49.

Milman, N. (1991) Hereditary haemochromatosis in Denmark 1950–1985: clinical, biochemical and histological features in 179 patients and 13 preclinical cases. *Dan. Med. Bull.* **38**, 385–393.

Mohler, D. N. and Wheby, M. S. (1986) Hemochromatosis heterozygotes may have significant iron overload when they also have hereditary spherocytosis. *Am. J. Med. Sci.* **292**, 320–324.

Moore, A. and Worwood, M. (1989) Iron and sudden infant death syndrome. *Br. Med. J.* **298**, 1248.

Motulsky, A. G. (1970) Genetics of hemochromatosis. *N. Engl. J. Med.* **301**(23), 1291.

Murphy, M., Nicholl, J. and O'Cathain, A. (1989) Iron and the sudden infant death syndrome. *Br. Med. J.* **298**, 1643.

Niederau, C., Fisher, R., Sonnenberg, A., Stremmel, W., Trammpisch, H. J. and Strohmeyer, G. (1986) Survival and causes of death in cirrhotic and non-cirrhotic patients with primary hemochromatosis. *N. Engl. J. Med.* **313**, 1256–1262.

Nienhuis, A. W. (1981) Vitamin C and iron. *N. Engl. J. Med.* **304**, 170–171.

Olynyk, J., Hall, P., Sallie, R., Reed, W., Shilkin, K. and MacKinnon, M. (1990) Computerised measurement of iron in liver biopsies: A comparison with biochemical iron measurement. *Hepatology* **12**, 26–30.

Oppenheimer, S. J. (1989) Iron and infection: the clinical evidence. *Acta Paediatr. Scand. Suppl.* **361**, 53–62.

Osterloh, K. R. S., Simpson, R. J., Snape, S. and Peters, T. J. (1987) Intestinal iron absorption and mucosal transferrin in rats subjected to hypoxia. *Blut* **55**, 421–431.

Palinski, W., Rosenfeld, M. E., Ylä-Herttuala, S. *et al.* (1989) Low density lipoprotein undergoes oxidative modification in vivo. *Proc. Natl. Acad. Sci. USA* **86**, 1372–1376.

Parums, D. V., Brown, D. L. and Mitchinson, M. J. (1990) Serum antibodies to oxidized low-density lipoprotein and ceroid in chronic periaortitis. *Arch. Pathol. Lab. Med.* **114**, 383–387.

Perkins, K. W., McInnes, I. W. S., Blackburn, C. R. B. and Beal, R. W. (1965) Idiopathic hemochromatosis in children. *Am. J. Med.* **39**, 118–126.

Peters, T. J. (1989) Mechanisms of Cellular Iron Uptake and Release. Proceedings of the Second International Haemochromatosis Conference, Gold Coast, Australia, p. 35.

Peters, T. J., Selden, C. and Seymour, C. A. (1977) Lysomal disruption in the pathogenesis of hepatic damage in primary and secondary haemochromatosis. In: *Iron Metabolism*. Ciba Foundation Symposium 51. Amsterdam: Elsevier, pp. 317–329.

Peto, T. E. and Hershko, C. (1989) Iron and infection. *Baillières Clin. Haematol.* **2**, 435–458.

Phelps, G., Chapman, I., Hall, P., Braund, W. and Mackinnon, M. (1989) Prevalence of genetic haemochromatosis among diabetic patients. *Lancet* **ii**, 233–234.

Phillips, S. F. and Fernandez, R. (1980) Components of dietary fibre reduce iron absorption. *Gut* **21**, A904–A905.

Pietrangelo, A., Rocchi, E., Rigo, G. *et al.* (1992) Regulation of transferrin, transferrin receptor and ferritin gene expression in the duodenum of normal anemic and siderotic subjects. *Gastroenterology* **102**, 802–809.

Pietrangelo, A., Gualdi, R., Casalguandi, G. *et al.* (1993) Molecular defects in the control of duodenal iron metabolism in genetic hemochromatosis. *Gastroenterology* **104**, A-272.

Pirzio-Biroli, G. and Finch, C. A. (1960) Iron absorption. III. The influence of the iron stores on iron absorption in the normal subject. *J. Lab. Clin. Med.* **55**, 216–220.

Powell, L. W. (1965) Iron storage in relatives of patients with hemochromatosis and in relatives of patients with alcoholic cirrhosis and hemosiderosis. A comparative study of 27 families. *Quart. J. Med.* **34**, 427–442.

Powell, L. W. (1970) Changing concepts in hemochromatosis. *Postgrad. Med. J.* **46**, 200–209.

Powell, L. W. (1975) The role of alcoholism in hepatic iron storage disease. *Ann. NY Acad. Sci.* **252**, 124–134.

Powell, L. W. and Halliday, J. W. (1981) Iron absorption and iron overload. *Clin. Gastroenterol.* **10**, 707–735.

Powell, L. W. and Kerr, J. F. R. (1975) The pathology of the liver in hemochromatosis. In: *Pathology Annual* (ed. J. Joachim), New York: Appleton-Century-Crofts, pp. 317.

Powell, L. W., Campbell, C. B. and Wilson, E. (1970) Intestinal mucosal uptake of iron and iron retention in idiopathic hemochromatosis as evidence of a mucosal abnormality. *Gut* **11**, 727–731.

Powell, L. W., Mortimer, R. and Harris, O. D. (1971) Hepatic cirrhosis. A comparison of the four major aetiological groups. *Med. J. Aust.* **1**, 941–950.

Powell, L. W., Ferluga, J., Halliday, J. W., Bassett, M. L., Kohonen-Corish, M. K. and Serjeantson, S. (1987) Genetic hemochromatosis and HLA linkage. *Hum. Genet.* **77**, 55–56.

Powell, L. W. (1992a) Haemochromatosis and related iron storage diseases. In: *Wright's Hepatobiliary Diseases*, Vol. 2, W. B. Saunders & Co. Ltd., London, pp. 976–994.

Powell, L. W. (1992b) Does transplantation of the liver cure genetic haemochromatosis? *J. Hepatol.* **16**, 259–261.

Powell, L. W., Summers, K. M., Board, P. G., Axelson, E., Webb, S. and Halliday, J. W. (1990) Expression of hemochromatosis in homozygous subjects. Implications for early diagnosis and prevention. *Gastroenterology* **98**, 1625–1632.

Powell, L. W., Fletcher, L. M. and Halliday, J. W. (1994) The distinction between haemochromatosis and alcoholic siderosis. In: *Alcoholic Liver Disease* (ed. P. Hall), in press.

Raja, K. B., Simpson, R. J., Pippard, M. J. and Peters, T. J. (1988) In vivo studies on the relationship between intestinal iron (Fe3+) absorption, hypoxia and erythropoiesis in the mouse. *Br. J. Haematol.* **68**, 373–378.

Riemersma, R. A., Wood, D. A., MacIntyre, C. C. A., Elton, R. A., Gey, K. F. and Oliver, M. F. (1991a) Risk of angina pectoris and plasma concentrations of vitamin A, C, and E and carotene. *Lancet* **337**, 1–5.

Riemersma, R. A., Wood, D. A., MacIntyre, C. C. A., Elton, R. A., Gey, K. F. and Oliver, M. S. (1991b) Anti-oxidants and pro-oxidants in coronary heart disease (letter). *Lancet* **337**, 677.

Roeser, H. P. (1983) The role of ascorbic acid in the turnover of storage iron. *Semin. Hematol.* **20**, 91–100.

Rouault, T. A., Stout, C. D., Kaptain, S., Harford, J. B. and Klausner R. D. (1991) Structural relationship between an iron-regulated RNA-binding protein (IRE-BP) and aconitase: Functional implications. *Cell* **64**, 881–883.

Sabesin, S. M. and Thomas, C. B. (1964) Parenchymal siderosis in patients with pre-existing portal cirrhosis: a pathologic entity simulating idiopathic and transfusional hemochromatosis. *Gastroenterology* **46**, 477–485.

Sallie, R. W., Reed, W. D. and Shilkin, K. B. (1991) Confirmation of the efficacy and hepatic tissue iron index in differentiating genetic hemochromatosis from alcoholic liver disease complicated by alcoholic haemosiderosis. *Gut* **32**, 207–210.

Salonen, J. T., Ylä-Herttuala, S., Yamamoto, R. et al. (1992a) Autoantibody against oxidised LDL and progression of carotid atherosclerosis. *Lancet* **339**, 883–887.

Salonen, J. T., Nyyssnen, K., Korpela, H., Tuomilehto, J. Seppnen, R. and Salonen, R. (1992b) High stored iron levels are associated with excess risk of myocardial infarction in Eastern Finnish men. *Circulation* **86**, 803–811.

Scheuer, P. J., Williams, R. and Muir, A. R. (1962) Hepatic pathology in relatives of patients with haemochromatosis. *J. Path. Bact.* **84**, 53–64.

Schumacher, H. R. (1964) Hemochromatosis and arthritis. *Arthritis Rheum.* **7**, 41–50.

Sciot, R., Paterson, A. C., Van Den Oord, J. J. and Desmet, V. J. (1987) Lack of hepatic transferrin receptor expression in hemochromatosis. *Hepatol.* **7**, 831–837.

Searle, J., Kerr, J. F. R., Halliday, J. W. and Powell, L. W. (1993) Iron storage disease. In: *Pathology of the Liver*, 3rd edn (eds R. McSween, P. P. Anthony, P. J. Scheuer, B. C. Portmann and A. D. Burt), Churchill Livingstone, London (in press).

Sheldon, J. H. (1927) The iron content of the tissues in hemochromatosis, with special reference to the brain. *Quart. J. Med.* **21**, 123–137.

Sheldon, J. H. (1935) *Haemochromatosis*, Oxford University Press, London.

Short, E. M., Winkle, R. A. and Billingham, M. E. (1981) Myocardial involvement in haemochromatosis. Morphologic and clinical improvement following venesection. *Am. J. Med.* **70**, 1275–1279.

Siegelman, E. S., Mitchell, D. G., Rubin, R. et al. (1991) Parenchymal versus reticuloendothelial iron overload in the liver: distinction with MR imaging. *Radiology* **179**, 361–366.

Simon, M. and Bourel, M. (1978) Hérédité de l'hemochromatose idiopathique demonstration de la transmission recessive et mise en evidence du gene responsable porte par le chromosome 6. *Gastroenterol. Clin. Biol.* **2**, 573–577.

Simon, M. and Brissot, P. (1988) The genetics of hemochromatosis. *Hepatol.* **6**(1), 116–124.

Simon, M., Bourel, M., Fauchet, R. and Genetet, B. (1976) Association of HLA A3 and HLA B14 antigens with idiopathic hemochromatosis. *Gut* **17**, 332–334.

Simon, M., Alexandre, J. L., Bourel, M., LeMarec, B. and Scordia, C. (1977a) Heredity of idiopathic hemochromatosis: a study of 106 families. *Clin. Genet.* **11**, 327–341.

Simon, M., Bourel, M., Genetet, B., Fauchet, R., Edan, C. and Brissot P. (1977b) Idiopathic hemochromatosis and iron overload in alcoholic liver disease: differentiation by HLA phenotype. *Gastroenterology* **73**, 655–658.

Simon, M., Bourel, M., Genetet, B. and Fauchet, R. (1977) Idiopathic hemochromatosis: demonstration of recessive transmission and early detection by family HLA typing. *N. Engl. J. Med.* **297**, 1017–1021.

Simon, M., Alexandre, J. L., Fauchet, R., Genetet, B. and Bourel, M. (1980) The genetics of haemochromatosis. *Prog. Med. Genet.* **4**, 135–168.

Simon, M., Fauchet, R., Hespel, J. P. *et al.* (1980) Idiopathic hemochromatosis: a study of biochemical expression in 247 heterozygous members of 63 families: evidence for a single major HLA-linked gene. *Gastroenterology* **78**, 703–708.

Simon, M., Le Mignon, L., Fauchet, R. *et al.* (1987) A study of 609 haplotypes marking for the hemochromatosis gene: (1) mapping of the gene near the HLA-A locus and characters required to define a heterozygous population and (2) hypothesis concerning the underlying cause of hemochromatosis-HLA association. *Am. J. Hum. Genet.* **41**, 89–105.

Simpson, R. J., Moore, R. and Peters, T. J. (1988) Significance of non-esterified fatty acids in iron uptake by intestinal brush-border membrane vesicles. *Biochim. Biophys. Acta* **941**, 39–47.

Sinclair, W. P. and Afrooz, N. (1977) Idiopathic hemochromatosis: case report of a patient presenting with neurologic symptoms. *J. Am. Geriatr. Soc.* **25**, 324–327.

Smith, C. H. and Bidlack, W. R. (1980) The effect of a scorbutic diet on ferritinhemosiderin iron stores in the liver and spleen of female guinea pigs. *Biochem. Med.* **24**, 43–48.

Srai, S. K. S., Epstein, O., Denham, E. S. and McIntyre, N. (1984) The ontogeny of iron absorption and its possible relationship to pathogenesis of haemochromatosis. *Hepatol.* **4**(5), 1033.

Srai, S. K. S., Denham, E. and Epstein, O. (1987) Development changes in the villous uptake of iron and enterocyte iron binding proteins in the guinea pig duodenum, *Gut* **28**, A1333.

Stewart, S., Fawcett, J. and Jacobson, W. (1985) Interstitial haemosiderin in the lungs of sudden infant syndrome: a histological hallmark of near-miss episodes? *J. Pathol.* **145**(1), 53–58.

Steinberg, D., Parthasarathy, S., Carew, T. K., Khoo, J. C. and Witztum, J. L. (1989) Beyond cholesterol. Modifications of low-density lipoprotein that increase its atherogenicity. *N. Engl. J. Med.* **320**, 915–924.

Steinbrecher, U. P., Parthasarathy, S., Leake, D. S., Witztum, J. L. and Steinberg, D. (1984) Modification of low density lipoprotein by endothelial cells involves lipid peroxidation and degradation of low density lipoprotein phospholipids. *Proc. Natl. Acad. Sci. USA* **81**, 3883–3887.

Stremmel, W., Arvailer, D., Vierbuchep, M., Teichmann, R., Diede, H. E. and Strohmeyer, G. (1991a) The membrane iron binding protein is enriched in the liver of patients with primary hemochromatosis. *Hepatology* **14**, 142A.

Stremmel, W., Teichmann, R. and Strohmeyer, G. (1991b) Carrier mediated cellular uptake of non-transferrin bound iron: significance and regulation of a membrane iron binding protein. *Hepatology* **13**, 574.

Strohmeyer, G., Niederau, C. and Stremmel, W. (1989) Endocrine abnormalities in HC. Proceedings of the 3rd International Conference for Hemochromatosis, Gold Coast.

Strohmeyer, G., Niederau, C. and Stremmel, W. (1993) Epidemiological clinical spectrum and prognosis of hemochromatosis. Proceedings of the 4th International Conference on Hemochromatosis, Jerusalem, p. 23.

Sullivan, J. L. (1989) The iron paradigm of ischaemic heart disease. *Am. Heart J.* **117**, 1177–1188.

Summers, K. M., Tam, K. S., Halliday, J. W. and Powell, L. W. (1989) HLA determinants in an Australian population of hemochromatosis patients and their families. *Am. J. Hum. Genet.* **45**, 41–48.

Summers, K. M., Halliday, J. W. and Powell, L. W. (1990) Identification of homozygous hemochromatosis subjects by measurement of hepatic iron index. *Hepatology* **12**, 20–25.

Summers, K. M., Tam, K. S., Bartley, P. B. *et al.* (1991) Fine mapping of a chromosome 6 ferritin heavy chain gene: Relevance to haemochromatosis. *Hum. Genet.* **88**, 175–178.

Tavill, A. S. and Morton, A. G. (1978) Transferrin metabolism and the liver. In: *Metal in the Liver* (ed. L. W. Powell), New York: Marcel Decker, pp. 93–130.

Teichmann, R. and Stremmel, W. (1990) Iron uptake by human upper small intestine microvillous membrane vesicles. Indication for a facilitated transport mechanism mediated by a membrane iron-binding protein. *J. Clin. Invest.* **86**, 2145.

Teichmann, R., Strohmeyer, G. and Stremmel, W. (1991) Iron absorption involves a membrane carrier protein. *Gastroenterology* **98**, A670.

Theil, E. C. (1990) Regulation of ferritin and transferrin receptor mRNAs. *J. Biol. Chem.* **265**, 4771–4774.

Thomas, F. B., Salsburey, M. and Greenberger, N. J. (1972) Inhibition of iron absorption by cholestyramine. Demonstration of diminished iron stores following prolonged administration. *Dig. Dis.* **17**, 263–269.

Thomson, G. and Bodmer, W. (1977) *The genetic analysis of HLA and disease associations* (eds J. Dausset and A. Svejgaard), Williams and Wilkins, Baltimore, p. 84.

Troisier, M. (1871) Diabete sucre. *Bulletin de la Société d'Anatomie Paris*, 44, 231–235.

Trump, B. F., Valigorsky, J. M., Arstila, A. U., Mergner, W. J. and Kinney, T. D. (1973) The relationship of intracellular pathways of iron metabolism to cellular iron overload and the iron storage diseases. *Am. J. Pathol.* **72**, 295–336.

Trump, B. F., Valigorsky, J. M., Arstila, A. J. and Barrett, L. A. (1975) Subcellular aspects of ferritin metabolism. In: *Iron Metabolism and its Disorders* (ed. H. Kief), Amsterdam: Excerpta Medica, pp. 97–109.

Valberg, L. S., Lloyd, D. A., Ghent, C. N. *et al.* (1980) Clinical and biochemical expression of the genetic abnormality in idiopathic hemochromatosis. *Gastroenterology* **79**, 884–892.

van Bockxmeer, F. M. and Morgan, E. H. (1979) Transferrin receptors during rabbit reticulocyte maturation. *Biochim. Biophys. Acta* **584**, 76–83.

van Bockxmeer, F., Hemmaplardh, D. and Morgan, E. H. (1975) Studies on the binding of transferrin to cell membrane receptors. In: *Proteins of Iron Storage and Transport in Biochemistry and Medicine* (ed. R. R. Crichton), (Proceedings of EMBO Workshop Conference), New York: American Elsevier Publishing Co., pp. 111–119.

Van der Heul Kroos, M. J. and Van Eijk, H. G. (1978) Binding sites of iron transferrin on rat reticulocytes. Inhibition by specific antibodies. *Biochim. Biophys. Acta* **511**, 430–441.

Van der Kraaij, A. M. M., Mostert, L. J., van Eijk, H. G. and Koster, J. F. (1988) Iron-load increases the susceptibility of rat hearts to oxygen reperfusion damage. Protection by the antioxidant (+)-cyanidanol-3 and deferoxamine. *Circulation* **78**, 443–449.

Van Thiel, D. H., Gavaler, J. S., Lester, R. and Goodman, M. D. (1975) Alcohol induced testicular atrophy. *Gastroenterology* **69**, 326–332.

Vartsky, D., Wielopolski, L., Ellis, K. J. and Kohn, S. H. (1982) The use of nuclear resonant scattering of gamma rays for in vitro measurement of iron. *Nucl. Instr. Methods* **193**, 359–364.

Velati, C., Piperno, A., Fargion, S., Colombo, S. and Fiorelli, G. (1990) Prevalence of idiopathic hemochromatosis in Italy: study of 1301 blood donors. *Haematologica* **75**, 309–312.

von Recklinghausen, F. D. (1889) Taggeblat der (62) Versammling Deutsch Naturforscher und Arzte in Heidelberg, pp. 324–325 (in German).

Walker, R. J. and Williams, R. (1974) Hemochromatosis and iron overload. In: *Iron in Biochemistry and Medicine* (eds A. Jacobs and M. Worwood), London: Academic Press, pp. 589–612.

Wapnick, A. A., Bothwell, T. H. and Seftel, H. (1970) The relationship between serum iron levels and ascorbic acid stores in siderotic Bantu. *Br. J. Haematol.* **29**, 271–276.

Wardle, E. N. and Patton, J. T. (1969) Bone and joint changes in hemochromatosis. *Ann. Rheum. Dis.* **28**, 1523.

Webb, J., Corrigan, A. B. and Robinson, R. G. (1972) Hemochromatosis and 'pseudogout'. *Med. J. Aust.* **2**, 24–29.

Whittaker, P., Skikne, B. S., Covell, A. M., Flowers, C., Cooke, A. and Lynch, S. L. (1989) Duodenal iron proteins in idiopathic hemochromatosis. *J. Clin. Invest.* **83**, 261–267.

Wiggers, P., Dalhoj, K., Kiaer, H. *et al.* (1991) Screening for haemochromatosis: prevalence among Danish blood donors. *J. Intern. Med.* **230**, 265–270.

Williams, R., Scheuer, P. T. and Sherlock, S. (1962) The inheritance of idiopathic hemochromatosis. A clinical and liver biopsy study of 16 families. *Quart. J. Med.* **31**, 249–265.

Williams, R., Smith, P. M. and Spicer, E. J. F. *et al.* (1969) Venesection therapy in idiopathic hemochromatosis. *Quart. J. Med.* **38**, 1.

Williams, R. E., Zweier, J. L. and Flahery, J. T. (1991) Treatment with deferoxamine during ischemia improves functional and metabolic recovery and reduces reperfusion-induced oxygen radical generation in rabbit hearts. *Circulation* **83**, 1006–1014.

Wright, T. L. and Lake, J. R. (1990) Mechanisms of transport of nontransferrin-bound iron in basolateral and canalicular rat liver plasma membrane vesicles. *Hepatology* **12**(3), 498–504.

Wright, T. L., Brissot, P., Ma, W.-I. and Weisiger, R. A. (1986) Characterization of non-transferrin-bound iron clearance by rat liver. *J. Biol. Chem.* **261**(23), 10909–10914.

Wright, T. L., Fitz, J. G. and Weisiger, R. A. (1988) Non-transferrin-bound iron uptake by rat liver. *J. Biol. Chem.* **263**(4), 1842–1847.

Yinnon, A. M., Theanach, E. N., Grady, R. W., Spira, D. T. and Hershko, C. (1989) Antimalarial effect on HBED and other phenolic and catecholic iron chelators. *Blood* **74**(6), 2166–2171.

Young, S. P. and Aisen, P. (1982) Transferrin receptors and the uptake and release of iron by isolated hepatocytes. *Hepatology* **1**(2), 114–119.

Zimmerman, H. J., Chomet, B., Kulesch, M. H. and McWhorter, C. A. (1961) Hepatic hemosiderin deposits. Incidence in 558 biopsies from patients with and without intrinsic hepatic disease. *Arch. Int. Med.* **107**, 494–503.

9. Secondary Iron Overload

M. J. PIPPARD

Department of Haematology, Ninewells Hospital and Medical School, University of Dundee, DD1 9SY, Scotland, UK

I. INTRODUCTION

Secondary iron overload may be defined as a quantitative increase in total body iron which is not the result of the genetically determined increase in iron absorption seen in primary (hereditary) haemochromatosis (Chapter 8). However, the boundaries of the distinction between primary and secondary iron overload are blurred. Even in HLA-related primary haemochromatosis, environmental factors play a significant role in determining the rate of iron loading. Conversely, it is possible that some of the causes of secondary iron overload shown in Table 9.1 may result from an interaction of the secondary disease or dietary factor with a genetically determined disturbance of iron metabolism. There has, for example, been much interest in the possible role of such interactions involving inheritance of a single HLA-related gene for haemochromatosis (heterozygous state) and this will be discussed later in this chapter. Furthermore, it has recently been suggested that the dietary iron overload long recognized in sub-Saharan Africa may have a non-HLA-related genetic component contributing to the risk of development of iron overload (Gordeuk et al., 1992). By contrast, it is unlikely that the iron overload associated with severe congenital or acquired anaemias (iron-loading anaemias) has any additional contribution from an 'iron-loading' genetic component. The pathogenesis of the secondary iron overload, its clinical consequences, and the approach to management, particularly the use of iron chelating therapy in iron-loading anaemias, are the major issues discussed in this chapter.

1.1. Terminology

There remains some confusion in the terminology used to describe body iron excess and underlying genetic disorders of iron metabolism. The general term 'iron overload'

Table 9.1 Causes of iron overload. Conditions in the upper part of the table may potentially give rise to severe iron overload (>5 g excess in adults) and a consequent risk of tissue damage. In those conditions below the line any increase in total iron burden is small: redistribution of body iron may play a major role, and a localized increase in tissue iron may then have more specific clinical effects than those of generalized iron overload.

Condition	Mechanism of iron overload	Prevalence of iron overload
Primary iron overload		
Hereditary (idiopathic) haemochromatosis	Increased iron absorption in homozygotes for the HLA-related gene	Common in those of North-European origin (Chapter 8)
Secondary iron overload Iron-loading anaemias		
•Massive ineffective erythropoiesis (severe β-thalassaemia syndromes, sideroblastic anaemias, congenital dyserythro-poietic anaemias)	Increased iron absorption and/or blood transfusion	Common, as a result of thalassaemia, in those of Mediterranean, Middle-Eastern, and Asian origin. Other causes rare
•Refractory hypoplastic anaemias (e.g. chronic renal failure, pure red cell aplasia, aplastic and mye-lodysplastic syndromes)	Blood transfusion	Relatively common where adequate transfusion services available
•Severe chronic haemolytic anaemias (e.g. pyruvate kinase deficiency, congenital spherocytosis, sickle cell disease)	Blood transfusion (increased iron absorption in some cases?)	Rare as causes of severe iron overload
Sub-Saharan dietary iron overload	Increase in both dietary iron and iron absorption	Common in sub-Saharan Africa
Other causes of iron overload		
•Perinatal (neonatal) haemochromatosis	Not known	Rare
•Juvenile haemochromatosis	Increased iron absorption	Rare
•Autosomal dominant familial haemochromatosis	Increased iron absorption	Single report of large kindred (Solomon Islands)
•Congenital atransferrin-aemia	Increased iron absorption	Very rare
Causes of modest iron overload		
•Chronic liver disease (alcoholic cirrhosis, portocaval anastamosis)	Increased iron absorption	Common
•Porphyria cutanea tarda	Increased iron absorption	Relatively uncommon
Local iron overload		
•Lung (idiopathic pulmonary haemosiderosis)	Pulmonary haemorrhage	Rare
•Renal (e.g. paroxysmal nocturnal haemoglobinuria, sickle cell disease)	Haemoglobinuria with renal tubular haemosiderosis	Rare

is now preferred to that of 'haemosiderosis', which is the visual, histological, counterpart of any increase in tissue iron, whether in parenchymal or reticulo-endothelial tissues (Bothwell *et al.*, 1979). Iron stores may normally extend to a maximum of 2 g, and an excess total body iron of more than 5 g in adults will arbitrarily be used in this chapter to identify significant, or severe, iron overload.

The term 'haemochromatosis' has been used to describe massive iron overload (whether primary or secondary) associated with iron-induced tissue damage (including cirrhosis of the liver and impaired heart and endocrine function): such damage is unusual unless iron stores exceed 10 g. However, with the identification of the auto-somal recessive inheritance of most primary iron overload (HLA-related hereditary haemochromatosis), as well as the realization that there are rarer causes of severe iron overload which may have a primary, genetically-determined disturbance of iron metabolism, it may now be reasonable to restrict the term haemochromatosis to these genetic disorders. This approach would have the advantage of freeing the term for use in describing the underlying genetic abnormality even if this is not yet expressed as iron overload (e.g. in young people who are homozygous for the HLA-related gene for haemochromatosis, but have not yet had time to develop the phenotype of iron overload). In discussing the iron overload which results from an underlying disease or particular environmental factor, this chapter will therefore use the term secondary iron overload, qualified as severe or modest. Severe iron overload carries the potential risk of inducing tissue damage (Chapter 10). This is not true of modest iron overload, but there may still be specific clinical effects (e.g. potentiation of the clinical expression of porphyria cutanea tarda) (Table 9.1).

1.2. Spectrum of Iron-overload Disorders

Severe iron overload (greater than 5 g excess iron–see above) is confined to the genetically determined causes of iron overload, HLA- or non-HLA-related haemo-chromatosis, together with the iron-loading anaemias (particularly the severe thalassaemia disorders and sideroblastic anaemias), and sub-Saharan dietary iron overload. As discussed in Chapter 8, chronic liver disease may be accompanied by modest increases in tissue iron, but can be clearly distinguished from the severe iron overload of primary HLA-related haemochromatosis by the hepatic iron index. Focal tissue iron overload in pulmonary haemosiderosis or chronic haemoglobinuria may eventually give rise to local tissue damage, but is not accompanied by systemic iron overload.

1.3. General Mechanisms in Secondary Iron Overload

Excess iron originates either from parenteral iron administration (usually as blood transfusions) or from increased absorption of iron from the gastrointestinal tract.

1.3.1. *Parenteral Iron Overload*

Regular blood transfusions provide approximately 200 mg iron in each unit of blood, and since iron excretion in humans is limited, even when iron stores are markedly increased (Green *et al.*, 1968), this results in a marked increase in body iron content. In congenital anaemias such as β-thalassaemia major, transfusion from early life means that an excess of as much as 100 g iron may be reached by the end of the second decade of life, by which time most such patients will have died from the effects of iron-induced tissue damage (Engle *et al.*, 1964; Modell, 1979). Regular injections of parenteral iron dextran (Imferon) led to significant iron overload in patients with chronic renal failure who were receiving treatment with haemodialysis in the 1970s, until these consequences were realized (Gokal *et al.*, 1979). This must now be an extremely rare cause of parenteral iron loading.

1.3.2. *Increased Gastrointestinal Absorption of Iron*

Increased oral intake of medicinal or dietary iron does not usually result in significant iron overload unless there is some additional factor, e.g. unusually high availability of the iron (in sub-Saharan iron overload) and/or an underlying genetic defect of iron metabolism giving rise to enhanced iron absorption. Since excessive iron absorption may occur even when the iron content of the diet is normal in patients with iron-loading anaemias associated with dyserythropoietic erythroid expansion (see below), it seems reasonable to believe that a combination of increased available iron in the diet and an intrinsic enhancement of iron absorption will increase the rate of development of iron overload in such individuals. Where treatment with blood transfusion is insufficient to suppress the erythroid hyperplasia, iron loading will result from contributions from both parenteral and oral routes.

1.3.3. *Tissue Distribution of Iron Overload*

Excess body iron may be distributed within the mononuclear macrophages of the reticuloendothelial system or in parenchymal tissues. This is an important distinction since it is iron within parenchymal tissues which gives rise to organ damage and clinical disease. Parenteral iron, whether derived from the haemoglobin of transfused red cells at the end of their life span or from iron-dextran injections, is initially cleared by the macrophages of the reticuloendothelial system. Iron absorbed from the gut, particularly any non-transferrin-bound iron in excess of the iron-binding capacity of transferrin, may be taken up directly by hepatocytes (Wheby and Umpierre, 1964). In addition, iron initially deposited in macrophages may redistribute to parenchymal cells. The factors controlling this redistribution are not fully understood. They include the rate of plasma iron turnover (with an increased rate of redistribution in patients with erythroid hyperplasia), the presence of ascorbic acid deficiency (which tends to restrict iron mobilization from macrophages (Roeser, 1983)), and the presence of coexisting inflammatory disease (e.g. as a result of sickle cell disease, where transfusional iron overload may remain in macrophages, and relatively non-toxic, for longer periods than in thalassaemia syndromes (Pippard, 1987)). A similar retention of excess iron by macrophages in chronic renal disease may also limit toxicity as well as availability of iron for erythropoiesis during treatment with recombinant human erythropoietin (Eschbach *et al.*, 1987; Hughes *et al.*, 1992). These aspects of the internal distribution of iron are clearly important considerations when considering potential toxicity of iron overload and the need for, and response to, iron chelation therapy.

2. IRON-LOADING ANAEMIAS

2.1. General Considerations

2.1.1. *Definitions*

Redistribution of body iron from its usual major component (haemoglobin) to iron stores is an inevitable accompaniment of any anaemia except that due to blood loss or iron deficiency (Chapter 14). However, increases in total body iron are characteristic of certain types of anaemia. Severe anaemias requiring regular blood transfusions have an obvious and inevitable steady input of excess iron as the transfused red blood cells reach the end of their lifespan and are degraded within the phagocytic cells of the reticuloendothelial system. However less severe anaemias may be associated with a progressive iron loading even in the absence of regular blood transfusions (Fig. 9.1), through enhanced iron absorption. It is this latter group

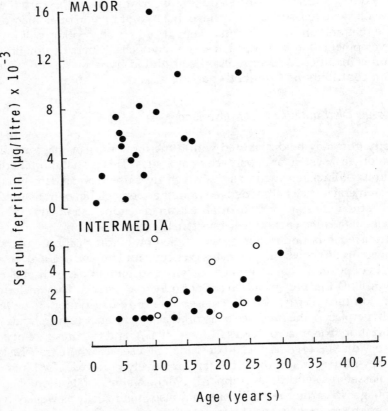

Fig. 9.1 Relationship between serum ferritin and age in patients with transfusion-dependent β-thalassaemia major (upper) or transfusion-independent β-thalassaemia intermedia (lower): some of the intermedia patients (○) had required blood transfusion in the past, a requirement which in several cases had been abolished after splenectomy. (From Pippard *et al.*, 1982b, with permission.)

which not only presents a challenge to understanding of the pathophysiological mechanisms involved, but also may cause occasional problems in identification of the risk that severe iron overload may be present in an individual patient.

In general, anaemias may result from inherited or acquired abnormalities of red cell or haemoglobin production, or from an abnormally shortened survival of red cells in circulation (haemolysis). Reduced haemoglobin production may arise from defective globin synthesis, e.g. in the thalassaemia disorders, where there is a reduced rate of production of one of the normal α- and β-globin chains which make up adult haemoglobin (HbA, $\alpha_2\beta_2$). Alternatively it may result from defective haem synthesis, e.g. in the sideroblastic anaemias. Defects of red cell production other than those related to haematinic deficiency may be the result of intrinsic marrow disease (e.g. congenital or acquired aplastic anaemias, and acquired clonal abnormalities of haemopoiesis, including myelodysplastic and myeloproliferative disorders). Alternatively in chronic renal disease there may be a defective production by the kidneys of erythropoietin, the hormone which normally regulates red cell production in response to tissue hypoxia (Pippard et al., 1992), so that there is an inadequate proliferation of developing erythroblasts within the bone marrow. Resulting abnormalities in erythropoiesis are either predominantly hypoplastic (e.g. in congenital red cell aplasia and chronic renal disease) or hyperplastic: the latter may be mainly ineffective (dyserythropoietic) (e.g. in thalassaemia syndromes and sideroblastic anaemias, where there is usually gross expansion of the erythroid marrow under the stimulus of increased erythropoietin production, as the homeostatic mechanisms attempt unsuccessfully to correct the anaemic tissue hypoxia), or effective (e.g. in haemolytic anaemias where marrow red cell production is greatly increased to compensate for shortened red cell survival). It is the dyserythropoietic anaemias with massive erythroid marrow expansion which are the main concern in relation to the risk of secondary iron overload as a result of excessive absorption of iron from the gut.

2.1.2. Iron Absorption in Iron-loading Anaemias

Increased iron absorption in thalassaemia syndromes (Section 2.2. below) was suspected after early studies showed widespread increases in tissue iron, and evidence of tissue (endocrine) damage in patients with severe β-thalassaemia syndromes, who despite anaemia and erythroid hyperplasia were able to survive with only minimal blood transfusion (Erlandson et al., 1964; Bannerman et al., 1967). Measurement of non-haem iron absorption, using test oral doses of radiolabelled iron, confirmed a marked increase in uptake in poorly-transfused patients with β-thalassaemia major (Erlandson et al., 1962), and in those who were transfusion-independent (i.e. who had β-thalassaemia intermedia) this reached a level which was more appropriate to iron deficiency than to the existing iron overload (Pippard et al., 1979). Indeed in β-thalassaemia intermedia, there was a striking direct relationship between the amount of iron absorption and plasma transferrin saturation (Pippard et al., 1982b) and measures of iron overload (Pootrakul et al., 1988), in contrast to the normal down-regulation of iron absorption in response to increasing iron stores (Chapter 6). Similar increases in iron absorption are seen in patients with sideroblastic anaemias (Pippard and Weatherall, 1984), but not in haemolytic anaemias such as hereditary spherocytosis (Erlandson et al., 1962). Iron absorption is reduced after blood transfusion in thalassaemia (Erlandson *et al.*, 1962; Heinrich *et al.*, 1973; de Alarcon *et al.*, 1979), and since blood transfusion has the effect of reducing the erythropoietin drive to erythroid proliferation, a causal relationship between increased iron absorption and expansion of the erythroid bone marrow, particularly when this is dyserythropoietic, has long been suspected.

Studies in animals have shown a variable increase in plasma iron turnover and in iron uptake from the gut in response to reticulocyte infusions (Finch *et al.*, 1982; Raja *et al.*, 1989), while experiments after marrow ablation (Raja *et al.*, 1988) also suggested an effect of the level of erythroid activity in regulating iron absorption, particularly at the stage of serosal transfer to the plasma. In human studies iron absorption was found to be directly related to plasma iron turnover, used as a measure of erythroid expansion (Chapter 2) (Pootrakul *et al.*, 1988). However, a striking finding in this study was that patients with haemolysis due to a red cell membrane defect (hereditary spherocytosis) showed a much less marked increase in iron absorption than those with thalassaemia syndromes (Fig. 9.2). This was despite the inclusion among the latter group of patients with an α-thalassaemia disorder (HbH disease) which gives rise to a predominantly haemolytic anaemia, in contrast to the dyserythropoietic anaemia seen in the other thalassaemic patients studied, who were doubly heterozygous for a structural β-globin chain defect (HbE) and β-thalassaemia (HbE/β-thalassaemia). These findings suggested that in addition to a quantitative increase in erythropoiesis, some other factor related to the disturbed erythropoiesis in thalassaemia syndromes was related to the observed increase in iron absorption, and that this factor could not be solely a function of differences between dyserythropoiesis and haemolysis. Since hypoxia is known to increase mucosal iron uptake (Raja *et al.*, 1986), differences in the degree of anaemic tissue hypoxia might lead to variation in the amount of iron available within mucosal cells for transfer to the plasma in response to increased demands by the erythron. HbF and HbH, found in HbE/β-thalassaemia and HbH disease respectively, have a much higher oxygen affinity than HbA and even with similar haemoglobin concentrations, a greater degree of tissue hypoxia might therefore be expected in the thalassaemia

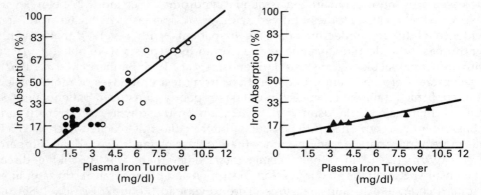

Fig. 9.2 Relationship between plasma iron turnover and iron absorption, measured using total body counting after a test oral dose of 5 mg iron as ^{59}FeSO$_4$, in Thai patients with thalassaemia intermedia syndromes (left) or hereditary spherocytosis (right): ○, β-thalassaemia/HbE double heterozygotes; ●, HbH disease; and, ▲ hereditary spherocytosis. (From Pootrakul *et al.*, 1988, with permission.)

disorders than in hereditary spherocytosis. Another possibility could involve differences in the extent to which iron is diverted away from the normal red cell circuit of macrophage recycling of iron from senescent red cells (Chapter 2). Reticuloendothelial clearance of red cells predominates in hereditary spherocytosis, but in the thalassaemia disorders, any intravascular release of haemoglobin might be expected to lead either to a shunt of haemoglobin iron, bound to plasma haptoglobin or haemopexin, to the liver, where it may be less readily available for recycling, or even to loss of iron in the form of haemoglobinuria, as may occur in HbH disease. It has been suggested that the availability of iron in the tissues which normally donate iron to the plasma (reticuloendothelial, hepatic and gastrointesinal) determines the relative contributions from each site (Cavill et al., 1975): any demand for iron by the expanded erythroid marrow that could not be met from recycled haemoglobin iron or sufficiently rapid mobilization of iron stores might then be met from increased uptake from the gastrointestinal tract. How this up-regulation of serosal transfer of iron to the plasma is mediated, particularly in the presence of increased iron saturation of the plasma transferrin, and the presence of non-transferrin-bound iron (Wang et al., 1986) remains unclear.

The availability of recombinant human erythropoietin means that it is now possible to examine the effect of changes in erythropoiesis on iron absorption in experimental studies in humans (see also Chapter 6). In normal people injections of erythropoietin lead to an enhancement of both non-haem and haem iron absorption which cannot entirely be explained by the reduction in iron stores which occurs as iron is mobilized for new haemoglobin synthesis (Skikne and Cook, 1992). In iron-loaded renal patients, erythropoietin injections had no effect on either mucosal uptake or serosal transfer of non-haem iron. However, after reduction of iron stores by regular phlebotomy in these patients, interruption of erythropoietin treatment led to a marked drop in iron absorption, due mainly to reduced serosal transfer of mucosal iron to the plasma (Hughes et al., 1992). These results suggest a regulatory role for erythropoiesis in iron absorption which is normally subordinate to that exerted by the level of iron stores. How this role may become more dominant in the thalassaemia and sideroblastic disorders may depend upon other determinants of the availability of body iron stores in different sites but, as discussed above, the exact mechanisms remain unknown.

A role for coincidental inheritance of the HLA-related gene for haemochromatosis has been postulated in the iron overload which accompanies sideroblastic and some haemolytic anaemias. This will be discussed in Section 6 below.

2.1.3. *Assessment of Iron Overload*

The clinical and laboratory assessment of iron overload secondary to anaemia follows the same pattern as in primary iron overload (Chapter 8). In transfusion-dependent anaemias the best guide to the amount of excess iron, and the current rate of iron loading, is provided by the past and present blood transfusion history respectively: where the transfusion has been adequate to suppress erythropoiesis and prevent the bony malformations typical of poorly transfused β-thalassaemia major, the contribution to the iron overload from excessive gastrointestinal absorption will be insignificant. In those iron-loading anaemias which are not transfusion-dependent, the saturation of the plasma transferrin saturation is the best guide to the current risk of excess parenchymal iron loading, while the serum ferritin provides a guide to existing iron load. As with primary iron overload, the serum ferritin may occasionally be misleadingly low in the early stages of iron loading, or where there is ascorbic acid deficiency (Cohen et al., 1981), while in the more heavily iron-loaded transfusion-dependent patients, values above 4000 μg/l, though clearly greatly raised, show a poor quantitative relationship with the size of the increased iron stores. Serum concentrations of glycosylated ferritin, measured in an attempt to distinguish secreted ferritin rather than that released as a result of iron-induced tissue damage, appeared to reach a maximum with increasing blood transfusion iron loads, to which they were even less closely related (Worwood et al., 1980). Nevertheless, serum ferritin estimations are of great value in monitoring the effects of iron chelation therapy with desferrioxamine in iron-loading anaemias. A rapid fall in serum concentrations during the first few weeks of therapy is related to reduction of hepatic tissue damage (Hoffbrand et al., 1979). Thereafter careful monitoring of serum ferritin, and adjustment of the dose of desferrioxamine, is important if on the one hand tissue iron toxicity, and on the other desferrioxamine toxicity (Chapter 12), are to be avoided (Porter et al., 1989).

Clinical investigation is directed towards assessment of the toxic effects of parenchymal iron overload in the heart, endocrine glands and liver, and to skeletal malformations in those with persistent erythroid hyperplasia. Radionuclide cardiac scanning with MUGA scans is currently the most reliable method to assess cardiac dysfunction, but may miss important early abnormalities that could respond to intensification of iron chelation therapy (Aldouri et al., 1990). This is discussed further in Section 2.5.2.

2.2. Thalassaemia Syndromes

The thalassaemia syndromes are among the commonest single gene disorders and are found in high frequency particularly in parts of the world with past or present exposure to falciparum malaria. Heterozygotes for β-thalassaemia have one remaining normally functioning β-globin gene on the unaffected chromosome 11 and have a very mild anaemia associated with slight ineffective erythropoiesis. They do not usually develop iron overload (Hussein et al., 1976; Pippard and Wainscoat, 1987). Where severe iron overload in β-thalassaemia trait has been described, it has probably been due to coincidental HLA-related haemochromatosis (Bowdler and Huehns, 1963; Edwards et al., 1981), though this may not always be the case (Parfrey et al., 1981). The possible significance of an association of heterozygous β-thalassaemia with a single HLA-related haemochromatosis allele is discussed in Section 6, below.

As with β-thalassaemia trait, subjects with a defect of only one or two of the four α-globin genes normally present (two genes on each chromosome 16) are not symptomatically anaemic and are not normally at risk of iron overload. In patients, with three of the four α-globin genes defective, the developing red cells have a marked excess of β-globin chains which form tetramers of HbH(β_4). Such patients have HbH disease, a haemolytic anaemia of variable severity, and are not normally at risk of severe iron overload (Sonakul et al., 1978) unless they become transfusion-dependent.

Patients with homozygous β-thalassaemia are most commonly transfusion-dependent from early life, and are described as having thalassaemia major. A minority have the phenotype of thalassaemia intermedia, with moderate anaemia, independence from regular blood transfusions, and persistent marked dyserythropoietic erythroid expansion (Weatherall and Clegg, 1981). This picture is also characteristic of double heterozygotes for β-thalassaemia and HbE; the latter is a structural haemoglobin variant, but the defective gene behaves as a thalassaemia gene with subnormal amounts of $β^E$ production. The defective β-globin production in the β-thalassaemia syndromes leads to an excess of α-globin chains which precipitate in developing erythroblasts, damaging cell membranes and resulting in death of the cells within the bone marrow. Erythrokinetic studies have delineated the resulting predominantly ineffective erythroid hyperplasia which is reduced after blood transfusion (Sturgeon and Finch, 1957; Cavill et al., 1978; Cazzola et al., 1987). Patients with β-thalassaemia major and intermedia are both at risk of severe iron overload (Fig. 9.1), though the clinical effects are delayed by an average of around 10 years in the intermedia group (Pippard et al., 1982a). Because the thalassaemia disorders are so numerically dominant among the iron-loading anaemias they may be taken as the prototype of these disorders. Much of the work on the pathology of iron-loading anaemias, and studies of management using iron chelation therapy (see below) have been in the thalassaemia disorders.

2.2.1. Clinical and Pathological Features

Children with untreated homozygous β-thalassaemia present during the first year of life with failure to thrive, severe anaemia and marked hepatosplenomegaly, combined with skeletal abnormalities due to expansion of erythroid tissue throughout the marrow cavity. Hypersplenism typically develops if transfusion is restricted to a minimum, bony deformities progress, and many children die from intercurrent infection: those that survive die from heart failure or cirrhosis during their second decade of life (Engle et al., 1964; Weatherall and Clegg, 1981). With adequate blood transfusions, growth and development are normal until the age of about 10 years (Wolman, 1964), but there is then failure of pubertal growth with an increasing frequency of cardiac disease (left ventricular hypertrophy, arrhythmias and failure), diabetes and cirrhosis in the second decade (Modell, 1979; Ehlers et al., 1980). Few patients survive beyond the age of 20 without intensive iron chelation therapy (see Section 2.5.2. below). Very high concentrations of iron, associated with progressive fibrosis, may be reached in the liver in the absence of iron chelation therapy (Barry et al., 1974). There has been a suggestion that cardiac iron loading may be relatively less in patients loading with iron from the gastrointestinal tract than those receiving regular blood transfusions (Sonakul et al., 1978), perhaps because of first-pass iron removal by the liver.

2.2.2. Treatment of Thalassaemic Iron Overload

Where hypersplenism has developed the blood transfusion requirement, and rate of iron loading, may be markedly increased, and splenectomy can help to reduce this (Modell, 1977) – in exceptional cases the phenotype of thalassaemia intermedia may be revealed, and regular blood transfusions no longer required (Fig. 9.1). It should be noted that there are some concerns about the effect of splenectomy on the internal distribution of iron. An increase in serum iron concentration has been noted after splenectomy in patients with HbH disease and those with HbE/β-thalassaemia (Pootrakul et al., 1980), and this does not seem to be entirely explained by an inherently greater severity of the disease in those requiring splenectomy. These results have raised the possibility that in addition to the known hazards of increased risk of infection, splenectomy may have implications for a potentially toxic redistribution of iron to parenchymal tissues.

More recently the use of bone marrow transplantation from HLA-matched sibling donors has provided the opportunity of cure for the bone marrow disease of severe β-thalassaemia. Successful extension of the procedure to older children with more significant iron overload and iron-induced tissue damage has been reported (Lucarelli, 1991). The decline in iron stores following transplantation is relatively slow and there is a need to consider intensive iron chelation therapy for this group of patients (Angelucci et al., 1992).

In some patients with milder forms of β-thalassaemia intermedia it may rarely be possible to consider cautious phlebotomy therapy as a contribution to iron removal. However, iron chelation therapy is the mainstay of the conventional approach to management of the iron overload, and this, together with the current evidence for its effects on modifying the clinical course in thalassaemia disorders, is considered in greater detail after discussion of the remaining iron-loading anaemias.

2.3. Sideroblastic Anaemias

The sideroblastic anaemias are a heterogeneous group of inherited or acquired disorders which are characterized by defective haemoglobin synthesis within erythroblasts resulting in a population of hypochromic–microcytic red cells in the peripheral blood, together with a variable accumulation of iron within the mitochondria of developing erythroblasts. Since the mitochondria are arranged in a perinuclear ring, on staining for iron the erythroblasts are seen as 'ring sideroblasts', the diagnostic feature of this form of anaemia (Bottomley, 1982). Erythrokinetic studies are consistent with ineffective erythropoiesis with a normal or only modestly reduced red cell survival (Cazzola et al., 1983a; Peto et al., 1983). Common to all the sideroblastic anaemias is a defect in the haem synthetic pathway which results in a failure to utilize the iron delivered to the mitochondria for incorporation into protoporphyrin by the enzyme ferrochelatase. This defect may be secondary to a variety of agents, including inhibitors of pyridoxine, a co-enzyme required in the first step in the synthesis of the haem prophyrin ring, i.e. synthesis of delta-aminolaevulinic acid (ALA) by the enzyme ALA synthase. These agents include antituberculous drugs and alcohol, while lead poisoning and chloramphenicol are also known to disturb haem synthesis or mitochondrial function and can give rise to a reversible sideroblastic failure of erythropoiesis. However, in the context of secondary iron overload only the inherited sideroblastic anaemias, and the sideroblastic anaemias occurring as part of the spectrum of acquired myelodysplastic disorders are of importance.

2.3.1. Inherited Sideroblastic Anaemia

These are rare forms of sideroblastic anaemia usually presenting in males in childhood or adolescence. Inheritance has followed an X-linked pattern in most reported families (Rundles and Falls, 1946; Losowsky and Hall, 1965; Weatherall and Pembrey, 1970). Female relatives may show partial expression usually with only mild or no anaemia, though families have been described in which females are more severely affected (Lee et al., 1968; Weatherall and Pembrey, 1970; Peto et al., 1983). It is possible that this may depend on variation in the severity of the defect as well as the degree of Lyonization of the affected X-chromosome. Some support for the latter hypothesis is obtained from the presence of a true dual population of microcytic and normocytic red cells in affected females, rather than simply the widening of the red cell size distribution which is seen in affected males (Peto et al., 1983). Despite these reports, many cases present sporadically in infancy or childhood with no family involvement. A proportion of patients is responsive to pharmacological doses of pyridoxine or the active form of the coenzyme, pyridoxal phosphate (Harris et al., 1956). The clinical features are dependent upon the severity of the anaemia, but it is important to realize that iron overload and its pathology may complicate long-standing disease. In patients who are not transfusion-dependent, the degree of anaemia correlates poorly with the severity of iron loading from excessive gastrointestinal iron absorption (Solomon et al., 1981; Cazzola et al., 1983a; Peto et al., 1983), the risk being much more closely related to the degree of erythroid expansion, as in other dyserythro-poietic anaemias. Indeed the anaemia may be so mild as to be asymptomatic, coming to light only after the patient presents with severe iron overload and tissue damage. This emphasizes the need for vigilance in screening for potential life-threatening iron overload, even where the disorder appears clinically benign.

2.3.2. Acquired Sideroblastic Anaemia

Primary acquired (or idiopathic refractory) sideroblastic anaemia is rather more common than the inherited disease, occurs usually in older patients, and is classified with the haemopoietic stem cell disorders which give rise to myelodysplastic syndromes (Bennett et al., 1982). In many cases the disorder is associated initially with erythroid hyperplasia and ineffective erythropoiesis, but this may progress in a minority to marrow failure with or without leukaemic transformation (Cazzola et al., 1988). Marrow failure and risk of leukaemia is particularly likely in those with multi-lineage blood cell defects (Cazzola et al., 1988; Gattermann et al., 1990). Though modest iron overload may occur in the absence of blood transfusions (Solomon et al., 1981; Cazzola et al., 1983a), life-threatening clinical manifestations of iron overload have been seen only in those who required regular blood transfusions: some of these transfusion-dependent patients will have a prolonged clinical course, and long-term iron chelation therapy may need to be considered sooner rather than later, since iron-induced tissue damage may appear relatively early in the course of transfusional iron overload, even in adults (Schafer et al., 1981).

2.3.3. Pathogenesis of Sideroblastic Anaemia

The mitochondria are the site both for the initial synthesis of δ-aminolaevulinic acid and for the final step in haem synthesis, the incorporation of iron into protoporphyrin. Failure to utilize the iron appears to underlie the mitochondrial iron accumulation. Impaired mitochondrial function, whether as the cause or result of the sideroblastic change, is likely to contribute to a defect in erythroblast maturation, premature death of the erythroblasts within the bone marrow, and consequent ineffective erythropoiesis. In many cases the exact pathogenesis of the disorder is at best only partially understood.

Reduced levels of ALA synthase are found in all types of sideroblastic anaemias (Bottomley, 1982; Fitzsimmons *et al.*, 1988). In X-linked sideroblastic anaemia, low levels of mRNA for erythroid specific ALA synthase have been reported in some patients: these were associated with increased total ALA synthase enzyme activity in bone marrow cells, perhaps representing a response of 'housekeeping' ALA synthase to low levels of cellular haem, but possibly resulting from enhanced translation of the erythroid-specific ALA synthase in response to cellular iron excess (Chapter 2) (Bottomley *et al.*, 1992). ALA synthase requires pyridoxal phosphate as a co-enzyme, and protection of a labile ALA synthase from proteolytic degradation (Aoki *et al.*, 1979), or a low affinity of the enzyme for pyridoxal phosphate (Konopka and Hoffbrand, 1979) could explain the response to pharmacological doses of pyridoxine in some cases of inherited sideroblastic anaemia. Indeed, some patients have low levels of enzyme activity which were restored by pyridoxine or pyridoxal phosphate, suggesting a structural defect of the enzyme (Murakami *et al.*, 1991; Bottomley *et al.*, 1992). In one case of pyridoxine-responsive X-linked sideroblastic anaemia a single base mutation in the gene for erythroid-specific ALA synthase (mapped to Xp11.2) led to the production of an enzyme requiring higher concentrations of pyridoxal phosphate to achieve a maximum activity (Cotter *et al.*, 1992a).

Other haem enzymes may also be affected, and a variable reduction of ferrochelatase activity has been found in both inherited and primary acquired sideroblastic anaemias. A decreased activity of ferrochelatase could explain the high levels of free erythrocyte protoporphyrin found in most patients with the primary acquired disorder, and contrasts with the reduced free erythrocyte protoporphyrin more usual in patients with inherited forms of the disorder. Rarely the abnormality may be associated with increased urinary and stool porphyrin excretion and skin photosensitivity (Lim *et al.*, 1992). In many cases the defects of haem synthetic enzymes may be secondary to general disturbances of mitochondrial protein synthesis (Aoki, 1980). This could be the result of an underlying disease process, for example an acquired clonal abnormality of haemopoiesis, or secondary to the iron accumulation itself. A genetic linkage of acquired sideroblastic anaemia to Xq13 suggests involvement of genes other than erythroid specific ALA synthase (Cotter *et al.*, 1992b).

Inherited sideroblastic anaemia has also been associated with multisystem diseases, including Pearson's syndrome of refractory sideroblastic anaemia and abnormal exocrine pancreatic function (Rotig *et al.*, 1990) and Keans-Sayre syndrome of neuromuscular dysfunction with pigmentory retinopathy (McShane *et al.*, 1991). These disorders are known to be associated with deletion of mitochondrial DNA, and such a mitochondrial DNA defect should be suspected in patients with multisystem disease, and families where there is no sex predominance (Nusbaum, 1991).

2..3.4. *Treatment of Sideroblastic Anaemia*

In many cases the anaemia may remain stable for years, but others show a progressive fall in haemoglobin concentration, or being more severe from the start require more active treatment. A trial of oral pyridoxine is rarely effective except in some kindreds with a pyridoxine-responsive inherited sideroblastic anaemia. Blood transfusions may be necessary, and will inevitably lead to secondary iron overload for which iron chelation therapy will need to be considered (see below). However, since life-threatening iron overload may develop in the absence of the need for blood transfusion due to excessive iron absorption from the gut (Peto et al., 1983), careful monitoring for a persistent rise in the saturation of the plasma total iron-binding capacity, as well as the serum ferritin concentration is needed, in the same manner as in the follow-up for patients with pre-symptomatic homozygous HLA-related haemochromatosis (Chapter 8). The aim is to anticipate and prevent the development of severe iron overload. Where the anaemia is mild, treatment with regular phlebotomy either instead of, or as an adjunct to chelation therapy, may be possible. It is of considerable interest that improvement of the anaemia in isolated cases of primary acquired sideroblastic anaemia has been reported after phlebotomy (Weintraub et al., 1966) or treatment with desferrioxamine (Haines and Wainscoat, 1991): these reports suggest that the iron damage to the mitochondria may contribute to the pathology, rather than being simply its result.

2.4. Other Iron-loading Anaemias

2.4.1. Congenital Dyserythropoietic Anaemias

The congenital dyserythropoietic anaemias (CDAs) are uncommon disorders in which the biochemical nature of the defect is not known. They are characterized by marked erythroid hyperplasia combined with reticulocytopenia (i.e. ineffective erythropoiesis). CDA type I (Heimpel, 1976; Wickramasinghe and Pippard, 1986) may present in adult life with symptoms and signs of iron overload and tissue damage, associated with a mild and asymptomatic anaemia. The anaemia in CDA type II (also known as HEMPAS – hereditary erythroblast multinuclearity associated with a positive acidified serum test) is more likely to be associated with a need for blood transfusions and hence overt iron loading by this route (Verwilghen, 1976), though occasional patients may not be diagnosed until they develop iron overload in later life (Greiner et al., 1992). Iron chelation therapy is required if the iron overload is to be prevented or reversed, though additional cautious phlebotomy is also possible in some patients.

2.4.2. Refractory Hypoplastic Anaemias

(a) Congenital red cell aplasia. Although a large proportion of patients with congenital red cell aplasia (Blackfan-Diamond syndrome) will respond to alternative therapies (e.g. steroids), others are transfusion-dependent and develop severe iron overload by the second decade of life. The same pattern of organ damage with failure of growth and sexual development, abnormal liver function and cardiac failure is seen as in other causes of severe iron overload. Iron absorption is not increased, despite very high concentrations of serum erythropoietin, ruling out a direct mediating effect of this hormone in the dysregulation of iron absorption seen in the iron-loading anaemias.

(b) *Adult hypoplastic anaemias*. Cardiac abnormalities, glucose intolerance and focal portal fibrosis have been reported in adults receiving blood transfusions for a variety of refractory, mainly hypoplastic anaemias (Schafer *et al.*, 1981). The changes were present within a transfusion period of less than four years, and liver biopsy revealed iron in both hepatocytes and Kupffer cells, confirming that the absence of erythroid hyperplasia is not a barrier to redistribution of iron to parenchymal cells. This has implications for decisions about whether and when to start iron chelation therapy in older patients with acquired refractory iron-loading anaemias. This can be a difficult decision, since the prognosis of the underlying condition is often uncertain, and effective chelation therapy is a considerable undertaking for the patient.

(c) *Renal anaemia*. In the past, patients with chronic renal failure and anaemia due to failure of erythropoietin production became iron loaded as a result of over-enthusiastic use of parenteral iron (Gokal *et al.*, 1979) or through the use of multiple blood transfusions. The latter may now be avoided since treatment with recombinant human erythropoietin is effective in reversing the anaemia of chronic renal failure (Eschbach *et al.*, 1987; Pippard *et al.*, 1992). However, the use of recombinant erythropoietin has exposed a problem in a number of patients of difficulty with mobilizing iron stores, so that patients may develop functionally iron deficient erythropoiesis in the presence of normal or increased storage iron. The latter is believed to be only slowly mobilized from reticuloendothelial stores, a situation of reduced availability similar to that seen in the anaemia of chronic diseases (Chapter 11). Several studies have indicated that iron absorption is appropriately regulated in relation to iron stores in chronic renal failure (Eschbach *et al.*, 1977; Gokal *et al.*, 1979), and this is therefore unlikely to be a significant route for iron loading. The availability of recombinant human erythropoietin also raises the possibility of treatment for excessive iron stores by regular phlebotomy combined with increased doses of erythropoietin, and this has been successfully achieved in some instances (McCarthy *et al.*, 1989; Hughes *et al.*, 1992).

2.4.3. *Haemolytic Anaemias*

In most haemolytic anaemias there is no suggestion of secondary iron overload, but this may result when the anaemia is severe enough to warrant frequent blood transfusions. Patients who are homozygous for the β-globin structural variant HbS (i.e. patients with sickle cell disease) have a haemolytic anaemia, and are not infrequently iron deficient as a result of urinary iron loss. However, they may require blood transfusions, not because of symptomatic anaemia but to suppress sickle red cell production and interrupt recurring sickle cell crises. This may give rise to transfusional iron overload and a need to consider regular iron chelation therapy (Cohen and Schwartz, 1979; Pippard, 1987). Other causes of chronic haemolysis, including hereditary spherocytosis (Barry *et al.*, 1968; Blacklock and Meerkin, 1981) and congenital non-spherocytic haemolytic anaemias such as pyruvate kinase deficiency, are occasionally associated with severe iron overload, even in the absence of blood transfusions.

Hereditary spherocytosis is the most common hereditary haemolytic anaemia in those of North European origin (prevalence approximately 1 in 5000). It is hetero-geneous in terms of inheritance, molecular basis of the red cell membrane defect, and clinical severity. Most cases have an autosomal dominant pattern of inheritance with a partial deficiency of membrane spectrin. The degree of spectrin deficiency correlates with the severity of the anaemia (Agre *et al.*, 1986), and in some cases may be secondary to reduced amounts of the membrane skeleton protein ankyrin (Coetzer *et al.*, 1988; Costa *et al.*, 1990). In the majority of patients with hereditary spherocytosis, serum ferritin concentrations are not raised, even in patients who have not had a splenectomy and therefore have a continuing chronic haemolysis (Blacklock and Meerkin, 1981). Hereditary spherocytosis is among the group of disorders in which the possibility of coincidental inheritance of an HLA-related haemochromatosis allele has attracted much comment, and the possible role of such coinheritance in the exceptional cases with severe iron overload is discussed in Section 6 below.

Pyruvate kinase deficiency is transmitted as an autosomal recessive trait, and though the anaemia may be severe and require regular blood transfusions, especially in infancy and early childhood, severe iron overload may be seen even when transfusions have been minimal (Dacie, 1985). In some cases inappropriate treatment with oral iron therapy may have contributed to the iron overload, but increased iron absorption is likely to have played an important role.

2.5. Iron Chelation Therapy

In the absence of any significant physiological iron excretion in humans, attempts to interrupt the cycle of iron overload and iron-induced tissue damage have centred on the use of iron chelating drugs. Of these only desferrioxamine (DF) is in widespread clinical use, though there has been much work over the last decade in trying to identify new, orally active iron chelating agents. The pharmacology of DF, which has to be given by parenteral injection, since it is not absorbed when given by mouth, is discussed in Chapter 12, together with the spectrum of the drug's adverse effects: it should be noted, however, that DF has been remarkably non-toxic considering the wide range of iron-dependent metabolic reactions in the body and the large doses that must be used over many years in the treatment of iron-loading anaemias. Discussion in this chapter will be confined to the clinical use of DF, and the effects of long-term treatment.

2.5.1. Clinical Use of Desferrioxamine

Because of the short life of DF in plasma the drug has to be given by continuous infusion, either subcutaneously or intravenously, to achieve sufficient iron excretion to keep pace with the rate of transfusional iron loading and to make inroads into any already established iron overload (Hussain *et al.*, 1976; Propper *et al.*, 1976). Although bolus injections of DF were able to halt the progression of liver fibrosis in a controlled trial in transfusion-dependent thalassaemic children (Barry *et al.*, 1974), very high liver iron concentrations remained. Overnight subcutaneous infusions of DF on at least five nights each week are, by contrast, able to promote sufficient iron excretion even in young children to maintain low total body burdens of iron (Pippard *et al.*, 1978a). This is important since electron microscopic studies of liver biopsies of young thalassaemic children suggest that fibrosis begins within the first year or so of life (Iancu *et al.*, 1977), and if tissue damage is to be prevented such intensive

Table 9.2 Factors influencing DF-induced iron excretion in humans (From Pippard, 1989)

Factor	Urine iron	Faecal (bile) iron
Dose of DF	Plateau with increasing dose	Linear increase with dose
Iron load	Increased	Increased
Erythron		
Expanded	Increased	Decreased
Suppressed	Decreased	Increased
Ascorbic acid	Increased	No effect
Obstructed bile flow	Increased	Decreased

iron chelation therefore needs to be started in early childhood. A number of factors influence DF-induced iron excretion in addition to the age of the patient (Table 9.2) and these will now be discussed.

(a) *Factors influencing DF-induced iron excretion.* Chelated iron (ferrioxamine) is excreted in both bile (derived directly from hepatocytes) and urine (see Chapter 12 for a review of the potential sources of this chelated iron). However, the proportion of the total excreted by each route is not fixed. An important variable is the stage of the transfusion cycle, at least in subjects with erythroid hyperplasia. Studies using a differential ferrioxamine excretion test for assessing chelatable body iron (Karabus and Fielding, 1967) first raised the suspicion that the latter might be increased in haemolytic and dyserythropoietic anaemias, while increased urinary iron excretion was seen in response to DF after prior induction of haemolysis with phenylhydrazine in patients with primary haemochromatosis (Cumming *et al.*, 1967). After the introduction of subcutaneous DF therapy, urinary iron excretion was noted to fall immediately after blood transfusion in patients with thalassaemia, but not those with red cell aplasia, while in patients with primary HLA-related haemo-chromatosis phlebotomy led to an increase in DF-induced urinary iron excretion (Pippard *et al.*, 1982b). These results suggested that mobilization of storage iron to satisfy the demands for iron by stimulated erythropoiesis might enhance the availability of iron for chelation to the urine. Iron balance studies confirmed that faecal (biliary) iron excretion changed reciprocally with the urine iron as erythroid activity altered, and the overall iron excretion was therefore much less affected than the urinary measurements alone would have suggested. As a result it is not necessary to adjust the timing of chelation therapy in relation to the transfusion cycle.

With increasing doses of DF, urine iron excretion reaches a plateau, usually at around a dose of 50 mg/kg, but higher in more heavily iron-loaded patients. However, faecal iron excretion shows no such plateau, and this provides a rationale for the use of larger doses of DF by intravenous infusion, whether occasionally at the time of blood trans-fusion when an intravenous catheter is already in place, or more intensively, as has been suggested for heavily iron-loaded patients who already have evidence of iron-induced organ damage (Cohen *et al.*, 1989). Furthermore, as iron stores are reduced during intensive iron chelation therapy, urine iron declines more steeply than faecal iron excretion, and in subjects with normal iron stores the faecal route predominates (Pippard, 1993). This may help in explaining the apparent paradox that in well chelated patients with iron-loading anaemias, the amount of urinary iron excretion sometimes appears barely adequate to keep pace with continuing transfusion requirements, yet iron stores are maintained at a low level.

Increased catabolism of ascorbic acid as a result of iron overload may result in ascorbate deficiency, as first noted in sub-Saharan iron overload (see below). Repletion of the ascorbate increases DF-induced urinary iron excretion (Wapnick *et al.*, 1969; Pippard *et al.*, 1978b), but has no consistent effect on faecal iron excretion (Nienhuis *et al.*, 1976; Pippard, 1993). A reduced rate of mobilization of macrophage iron stores (Lipschitz *et al.*, 1971; Cohen *et al.*, 1981; Roeser, 1983) and a consequent reduction in iron available for redistribution to hepatocytes, as well as for chelation, may contribute to this effect. The increased mobilization of urinary iron with ascorbate supplements led to incorporation of small doses of vitamin C (50–200 mg/day) in DF treatment programmes. Initial worries that larger doses of vitamin C might increase iron toxicity (Nienhuis *et al.*, 1979; Nienhuis, 1981) have not been borne out in clinical practice using smaller doses. However, vitamin C should be given only in parallel with DF infusions, in order that any additional iron mobilized may be chelated and excreted immediately.

(b) *Planning and monitoring of DF therapy.* Therapy with regular infusions of DF is expensive, and inconvenient. It should not be undertaken without weighing these immediate disadvantages against prospective benefits, a calculation which is especially relevant where the prognosis of the underlying disorder is uncertain. The benefits in patients with transfusion-dependent anaemia from infancy are now clear in terms of protection of organ function and survival (see below). Such patients should start iron chelation by their third birthday – a dose of around 40–50 mg DF/kg given five or six nights each week from that age is usually appropriate for the prevention of serious iron loading, while avoiding the potential toxic effect of impaired growth velocity in very young children (Chapter 12). In older patients with established iron overload, larger doses should be carefully tailored by means of individual urinary iron excretion/DF dose response curves (Pippard *et al.*, 1978a), in order to achieve maximum safe iron chelation: regular doses that exceed those required to reach the plateau in urinary iron excretion should be avoided. In patients with less severe anaemia who do not require blood transfusions, and in whom the iron overload is less easily assessed, the degree of erythroid expansion is probably the best guide to the severity of the risk of excessive iron absorption (Pippard and Weatherall, 1984), and where iron overload is suspected in adult life a confirmatory liver biopsy is usually justified before embarking on prolonged chelation therapy. In some patients the threat from undoubted iron overload may be less clear-cut than in the thalassaemia disorders. For example, the reticuloendothelial distribution of the iron in some patients with sickle cell disease may mean that parenchymal tissues are at less risk. Here a measurement of urinary iron excretion in response to a test dose of DF may be useful in assessing both the need for and likely long-term response to chelation therapy. In some cases a liver biopsy may be a further guide to the need for therapy, by allowing the distribution between macrophage and parenchymal iron to be determined, as well as the extent of any associated tissue damage.

Practical guidelines for the administration of DF infusions, including selection of dose and frequency of administration, have recently been reviewed (Pippard *et al.*, 1989). In well chelated patients with thalassaemia major the serum ferritin may be expected to be in the range 1000–2000 μg/litre. Adjustment of the dose to minimize the risks of toxicity may be on the basis of serum ferritin assay (Porter *et al.*, 1989) or by reassessment of the DF dose/urinary iron response relationship (see above). Regular ophthalmological screening and audiometry should also be carried out in order to detect early signs of neurotoxicity, which appears to be most likely in patients with relatively low levels of storage iron receiving large doses of DF (Porter and Huehns, 1989) (See also Chapter 12).

2.5.2. *Efficacy of Long-term Chelating Therapy*

The ability of DF iron chelating therapy to prevent or reverse the complications of chronic iron overload has never been proven by prospective randomized studies. In the absence of such studies, assessment of the effects of chelating therapy is limited to the comparison of morbidity and mortality figures in DF-treated patients with similar data in non-compliant patients or in historical controls. Such comparisons, however, are fraught with difficulty, as historical controls differ from patients receiving DF treatment by present-day technology in other respects. For example, chronic anaemia is an important factor contributing to the early onset and severity of congestive heart failure, hampering comparison of patients maintained by infrequent blood transfusion in the past with present-day well transfused and chelated thalassaemics. It can also be difficult to compare the results of DF therapy reported from various centres, as the manner of DF administration and methods of documenting response vary from group to group.

In spite of these difficulties there is little doubt that survival in thalassaemic patients in recent years has improved. In thalassaemic patients treated at the Cornell Medical Center with a hypertransfusion programme combined with regular subcutaneous DF chelation, median survival has increased to 31 years compared with 18 years in patients treated formerly by a low transfusion regimen and no chelation (Giardina et al., 1990; Ehlers et al., 1991). A similar improvement with respect to historical controls has been seen in the UK (Fig. 9.3). However, the most extensive and detailed information on survival in thalassaemia comes from Italy, where over 5000 patients with thalassaemia major are treated and monitored by a well coordinated national study. There, treatment with subcutaneous DF has been used systematically since 1978 (Gabutti, 1990), with a steady improvement in survival for cohorts born in 1960–1964, 1965–1969 and 1970–1974 (Borgna-Pignatti et al., 1989). The total mortality was 15.7%, but survival from birth for patients born in 1970–1974, and therefore given iron chelation therapy from an early age, was 97% at 10 years and 94% at 15 years (Zurlo et al., 1989). This marked improvement in the life expectancy of well chelated Italian thalassaemic patients is largely attributable to a decline in mortality from cardiac complications (12.3, 10.0 and 2.4% at the age of 15 years in the respective cohorts). It is difficult to be entirely certain how much of this impressive improvement over recent years may be attributed to iron chelating therapy, rather than to hypertransfusion programmes which avoid the additional strain of chronic anaemia and ineffective erythropoiesis, or to better management of infection. However, the introduction of a more effective blood transfusion programme did not alone have any significant effect on the frequency of cardiac disease or overall survival in the period 1964–1977, just before the start of the widespread use of intensive iron chelation therapy (Ehlers et al., 1980). Additional clues as to the relative importance of these factors may be gained from a comparison of patients who comply with the demands of regular subcutaneous DF therapy with those who are non-compliant.

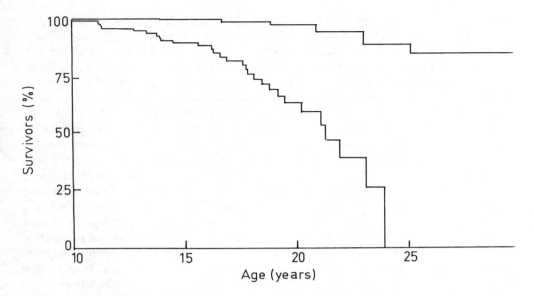

Fig. 9.3 Survival in transfusion-dependent β-thalassaemia major. The lower curve represents the survival of patients in the UK before the introduction of long-term treatment with subcutaneous desferrioxamine (Weatherall and Clegg, 1981). The upper curve describes the actuarial survival of patients among whom desferrioxamine therapy was introduced in the years 1977–78 (Hoffbrand and Wonke, 1989).

   The survival of non-compliant, unchelated thalassaemic patients continues to be poor. Thus in one study all six unchelated patients who had received 40–100 g iron by transfusion died, compared with none of seven patients with identical transfusional iron overload who were treated with a combination of long-term subcutaneous DF and intermittent high dose intravenous DF (Hyman et al., 1985). Similarly, only one of 17 compliant thalassaemic patients developed cardiac disease and died, compared with 12 of 19 non-compliant patients who developed heart failure and of whom seven have died (Wolfe et al., 1985). It should be noted, however, that the age of starting regular chelating treatment is critical if late complications are to be prevented. For instance, in patients in whom DF therapy was introduced before the age of 10 years, 90% had normal sexual development as compared with only 38% where DF treatment was started after the age of 10 (Bronspiegel-Weintrob et al., 1990). Similarly, cardiac disease-free survival among patients started on DF treatment prior to age 10 years was 92% compared with 52% where it was begun after the age of 10 years (Olivieri et al., 1991).
   Of all the consequences of iron overload, myocardial disease is undoubtedly the most severe and life-limiting. Examination of the effects of long-term iron chelating therapy on heart disease may, therefore, provide the most relevant information on the specific protective effects of DF in iron overload. The most convincing evidence supporting the beneficial effect of DF on iron-induced heart disease is the reversal of established cardiomyopathy in some far-advanced cases. Earlier experience in hereditary haemochromatosis has shown that the cardiomyopathy of iron overload is potentially curable by effective iron mobilization through phlebotomy (Short

et al., 1981). However, in transfusional iron overload, the course of established myocardial disease was uniformly fatal and, until recently, has been considered to be non-responsive to iron chelating therapy (Weatherall and Clegg, 1981). Several more recent reports indicate that such patients may still respond to aggressive chelating treatment. Reversal of established symptomatic myocardial disease was first described in three of five patients given continuous high dose (85–200 mg/kg/d) intravenous DF, albeit at the cost of severe reversible retinal toxicity (Marcus *et al.*, 1984). No such toxicity has been described in three patients on high dose subcutaneous and intravenous DF treatment who survive 2, 7 and 8 years after the onset of congestive heart failure (Hyman *et al.*, 1985). Similarly, two patients with severe cardiomyopathy recovered after receiving intensive intravenous DF therapy, with a follow-up of over two years (Cohen *et al.*, 1989, 1990), and another who developed heart failure at age 17 remains well after 11 years on iron chelating treatment (Hoffbrand and Wonke, 1989). Continuous 24-hour ambulatory intravenous infusion of DF through central venous port, using a portable infusion pump, provides a most suitable technique for the rapid reversal of established iron-induced heart disease. In addition, it is an excellent tool for improving patient compliance allowing uninterrupted delivery of 6–12 g DF per day and the effective depletion of very large iron stores (Cohen *et al.*, 1989, 1990; Berriman *et al.*, 1991).

Recognition of early cardiomyopathy is now possible using exercise radionuclide angiography. Ventricular response during exercise may be improved in about one-third of asymptomatic thalassaemic patients after one year of high dose subcutaneous DF therapy (Freeman *et al.*, 1983). More recently, using the same techniques, severe impairment of left ventricular function has been shown to improve significantly after several months of improved compliance or more intensive DF therapy, including intravenous therapy by indwelling catheter in some patients (Aldouri *et al.*, 1990).

With improved survival of patients with inherited iron-loading anaemias, in particular the modification of the cardiac effects of iron overload, it is not known whether additional later complications of chronic iron overload will eventually occur, e.g. the primary liver cell cancer which is increasingly common in HLA-related haemochromatosis (Chapter 8). However, prevention of iron-induced liver cirrhosis by regular iron chelation therapy is likely to minimize this risk.

2.5.3. *Clinical Use of Other Chelating Agents*

Alternative iron chelating agents have been used occasionally when patients have developed an allergic sensitization to DF or other DF-related toxic effects. DTPA (diethylene triamine penta-acetic acid) was introduced at the same time as DF (Fahey *et al.*, 1961), but was abandoned because it was painful when given by intramuscular injection, and caused various adverse effects related to zinc depletion. However, subcutaneous infusions of DF, given with oral zinc supplements, were painless and gave urinary excretion comparable to that of DF (Pippard *et al.*, 1986). Such treatment has been used as an alternative to DF in a small number of transfusion-dependent patients with DF-related auditory toxicity (Wonke *et al.*, 1989): serum ferritin concentrations did not increase during the several months of therapy, while the auditory toxicity improved, suggesting that this approach may be used to maintain patients, at least for short periods, when DF has to be reduced or stopped.

The search for an orally active iron chelating agent that could be much more widely available and which could overcome the major problems in compliance seen with subcutaneous DF therapy, is reviewed in detail in Chapter 12. A substantial number of patients have received oral 1,2-dimethyl-3-hydroxypyridin-4-one (also known as L1 or CP20) in studies in several countries. Although there has been some doubt about whether serum ferritin values are affected by this treatment, despite considerable though variable amounts of urinary iron excretion, recent studies have suggested both a fall in serum ferritin (Al-Refaie et al., 1992) and the potential to reduce tissue iron concentrations (Olivieri et al., 1992). A considerable pressure for further clinical studies has understandably developed (Brittenham, 1992; Hershko, 1993), but the pharmaceutical company involved has felt it necessary to withdraw from further development of this particular agent because of predictable adverse effects in animals, including bone marrow toxicity and teratogenicity (Berdoukas et al., 1993), the former problem having been seen earlier in occasional patients. Despite this disappointment, the studies with L1 have for the first time demonstrated the feasibility of oral iron chelation, and alternative drugs, including other hydroxypyridinones, may yet prove more suitable for widespread use.

3. SUB-SAHARAN DIETARY IRON OVERLOAD

3.1. Prevalence and Aetiology

A high prevalence of iron overload in black South Africans was first described in 1929, and it was later found to have a wide distribution through African countries south of the Sahara (Bothwell et al., 1979; Gordeuk, 1992). In these countries excess dietary iron is common among groups drinking traditional beer that is home-brewed in steel drums from locally-grown crops. The iron is in a particularly bioavailable ionized form (Bothwell et al., 1964; Gordeuk et al., 1986) and in rural populations drinking large amounts of the beer, iron overload is common. In the most recent study, the mean value for the total iron concentration in the traditional beer was 15.1 mg/dl of which about one-third was ferrous iron: this represented 750 times the mean value for the concentration of iron in American commercially produced beer. Although more affluent urban populations show a decreasing prevalence of the iron overload (MacPhail et al., 1979), among poor, rural populations, iron overload persists at a high frequency – in a recent survey of rural Zimbabweans, 21% of men who consumed traditional beer were found to have high serum ferritin and a transferrin saturation >70% (Gordeuk et al., 1986) indicating a risk of iron-induced parenchymal tissue damage. Liver biopsies have confirmed a moderate to severe hepatic iron overload, while previous autopsy studies showed that as many as 20% of males had severe liver iron overload with iron concentrations greater than 360 μmol/g dry weight (Bothwell and Isaacson, 1962): these high values distinguish the condition from the much milder iron excess which may be seen in alcoholic liver disease (see Section 5.1 below and Chapter 8). The hepatic iron concentration increased with age, and iron overload was less prevalent in women.

Recent studies have challenged the belief that the sub-Saharan African form of iron overload is solely due to the dietary increase in bioavailable iron. The observation that only a minority of drinkers of traditional beer developed evidence of iron overload (Gordeuk *et al.*, 1986) led to an investigation of the relatives of index subjects with iron overload. Among the family members with increased dietary iron intake from traditional beer, the serum transferrin saturation was distributed bimodally, being either normal or raised, and the serum ferritin concentration was significantly higher in the subjects with a raised transferrin saturation. Among subjects who did not have an increased dietary iron the distribution of the transferrin saturation was unimodal around a normal mean value. No linkage to HLA of the propensity to develop iron overload was detected in these pedigrees. The results were interpreted as suggesting that iron loading occurred in people heterozygous for an 'iron loading gene' but only when their iron intake was excessive (Gordeuk *et al.*, 1992).

3.2. Clinical and Pathological Features

Iron overload in sub-Saharan Africa usually presents with hepatic fibrosis and cirrhosis (Isaacson *et al.*, 1961). The hepatic iron deposition differs from that seen in patients with HLA-related haemochromatosis in that iron deposition in reticuloendothelial tissues is more prominent (Brink *et al.*, 1976), and there is a lack of a gradient in parenchymal cell iron from periportal hepatocytes decreasing towards the hepatic venule (Gordeuk *et al.*, 1992). The distribution of iron in both hepatic Kupffer and parenchymal cells (Bothwell and Bradlow, 1960) is a pattern similar to that seen in iron-loading anaemias. The spectrum of iron overload ranges from mild to severe but above a liver iron concentration of 180 μmol iron/dry weight there is an increased prevalence of portal fibrosis, and cirrhosis becomes a risk at concentrations greater than 360 μmol iron/dry weight. Other clinical effects include scurvy and osteoporosis which are thought to be caused by iron-accelerated oxidative metabolism of ascorbic acid leading to impaired formation of collagen and new bone in the presence of vitamin C deficiency (Seftel *et al.*, 1966). The dietary iron overload has also been implicated in the presentation with diabetes mellitus (Seftel *et al.*, 1961), heart failure and oesophageal carcinoma (MacPhail *et al.*, 1979).

Diagnosis of dietary iron overload is suspected on clinical grounds of a history of traditional beer drinking, hepatomegaly and hyperpigmentation. In those subjects with severe iron overload but no cirrhosis, symptoms are usually related to secondary ascorbic acid deficiency including scurvy and vertebral collapse related to osteoporosis. On laboratory testing the serum iron, transferrin saturation and serum ferritin are usually raised and the diagnosis is confirmed by liver biopsy as in primary iron overload. Treatment of the iron overload by phlebotomy is capable of removing the excess iron (Speight and Cliff, 1974) but has not been widely reported.

4. OTHER CAUSES OF SEVERE IRON OVERLOAD

4.1. Perinatal and Juvenile Haemochromatosis

Both perinatal and juvenile-onset forms of haemochromatosis are recognized (Editorial, 1984; Halliday, 1989), but the relationship, if any, with HLA-related adult haemochromatosis is unknown.

Perinatal haemochromatosis presents a picture of generally fatal neonatal liver disease with heavy stainable iron in parenchymal rather than reticuloendothelial tissues. Such an iron excess is not a feature of infants dying of known causes of severe liver disease, suggesting that the iron overload may define a specific disease entity though this is of unknown aetiology. However, it remains possible that neonatal haemochromatosis is in some way the end result of non-specific intrauterine liver damage (Witzleben and Uri, 1970). Studies of cultured skin fibroblasts from infants with neonatal haemochromatosis show no difference from normal in respect of transferrin receptor and ferritin synthesis, or their regulation by iron, a finding which is similar to that obtained in HLA-related adult haemochromatosis (Knisely et al., 1989). No family associations between adult and perinatal haemochromatosis have been established (Dalhoj et al., 1990).

Juvenile haemochromatosis presents a pattern of parenchymal organ damage which is indistinguishable from adult haemochromatosis except that cardiac damage (Charlton et al., 1967) and hypogonadotrophic hypogonadism (Cazzola et al., 1983b) are more prominent as presenting features in younger patients than liver disease. This may point to the rate of iron loading being a particularly important determinant for cardiac damage, since the latter is also an early complication in thalassaemic children dying from iron overload in the second decade of life (see above). Reported cases of juvenile haemochromatosis appear to affect males and females equally (unlike adult HLA-related haemochromatosis) (Lamon et al., 1979). Studies of possible HLA linkage in juvenile haemochromatosis are limited, and it remains uncertain whether there is a different defect in the younger patients or whether the juvenile disease is a more severe form of the adult disease.

4.2. Autosomal Dominant Haemochromatosis

A large Melanesian kindred has been described with 31 cases of iron overload and an appearance on liver biopsy similar to that of primary HLA-linked (autosomal recessive) haemochromatosis. Family studies suggested an autosomal dominant pattern of inheritance over four generations, with equal gender distribution, and no evidence of HLA linkage (Eason et al., 1990). The nature of the defect is currently unknown.

4.3. Congenital Atransferrinaemia

This is an exceedingly rare disorder in which the absence of transferrin in the plasma leads to a low serum iron concentration, inadequate delivery of iron to the erythroid bone marrow, and a microcytic hypochromic anaemia. Iron in the plasma, presumably non-transferrin-bound, is cleared rapidly by the liver and there is marked iron overload restricted to parenchymal rather than reticuloendothelial tissues (Heilmeyer et al., 1961; Goya et al., 1972). Excessive amounts of iron are absorbed from the gut, a feature which is also seen in hypo-transferrinaemic mice (Buys et al., 1991) (see Chapter 10): the mechanism for increased iron absorption is unknown, but the observation is important since it indicates that free transferrin iron-binding capacity is not an essential component of iron transfer from mucosal cell to plasma.

5. CHRONIC LIVER DISEASE

5.1. Alcohol and Alcoholic Cirrhosis

The relationship between alcohol intake and the development of iron overload and alcoholic liver disease has been discussed in Chapter 8. Synergism between iron and alcohol in promoting lipid peroxidation and collagen biosynthesis may explain early onset of fibrosis and cirrhosis in patients with iron overload who have an excessive alcohol intake (Irving *et al.*, 1988). It is doubtful whether in the absence of homozygosity for the HLA-related gene for haemochromatosis alcohol is ever responsible for more than mild liver iron excess except as a contributing factor in sub-Saharan iron overload (see above). Heavy alcohol intake does not lead to expression of haemochromatosis in subjects heterozygous for the HLA-related allele (Powell *et al.*, 1988). Nevertheless, there are a number of potential mechanisms by which alcohol and cirrhosis might favour increased iron absorption and an abnormal distribution of body iron. Alcohol increases the availability of ferric iron probably by stimulating gastric acid secretion (Charlton *et al.*, 1964), though it is unlikely that this has any major pathogenic significance in alcoholic subjects, who tend to have reduced gastric acid secretion associated with gastritis. A redistribution of body iron might be favoured by alcoholic damage to the circulating plasma transferrin resulting in its desialylation and subsequent clearance by the liver (Kapur *et al.*, 1989; Stibler, 1991; Mihas and Tavassoli, 1991), together with any bound iron. Additional potential causes of redistribution of body iron include alcohol-induced disturbances of erythropoiesis (Grace and Powell, 1974), whether by interference with folate metabolism or by induction of sideroblastic erythropoiesis, and macrophage ingestion of damaged hepatocytes.

5.2. Porphyria Cutanea Tarda

Porphyria cutanea tarda (PCT) is the most frequently recognized of the disorders of porphyrin metabolism, and results from a deficiency of hepatic uroporphyrinogen decarboxylase (URO-D), the fifth enzyme of the haem biosynthetic pathway. Clinical effects include a photosensitive bullous dermatitis with scarring and hirsutism, associated with increased hepatic accumulation and urinary excretion of uroporphyrin I and heptacarboxylporphyrins, together with increased faecal isocoproporphyrin. There are two forms of PCT, familial and sporadic (De Verneuil *et al.*, 1978). Familial PCT is due to mutations at the URO-D locus on chromosome 1 (McLellan *et al.*, 1985; Garey *et al.*, 1989), resulting in decreased URO-D activity in both liver and erythrocytes: it is inherited as an autosomal dominant trait (Kushner *et al.*, 1976), but in only a minority inheriting the trait is the disease clinically apparent. Sporadic PCT is more common than familial PCT, from which it differs by the URO-D deficiency being confined to the liver (Elder *et al.*, 1985): most cases show no identifiable inherited determinants, but in some there is evidence for inheritance as an autosomal recessive trait (Roberts *et al.*, 1988).

The majority of patients with PCT give a history of prolonged consumption of excessive quantities of alcohol, and measures of iron status show an increased transferrin saturation and mild to moderate iron excess on liver biopsy (Lundvall,

1971; Turnbull *et al.*, 1973; Edwards *et al.*, 1988). There is evidence that the hepatic iron excess plays a part in the production of the clinical manifestations, since clinical and biochemical remission follows the removal of the iron either via phlebotomy (Epstein and Redeker, 1968; Ramsay *et al.*, 1974) or by slow subcutaneous infusions of desferrioxamine (Rocchi *et al.*, 1986) (see also Chapter 12). Furthermore, treatment with iron leads to relapse of the PCT in patients in whom a remission has previously been induced by phlebotomy (Lundvall, 1971), and in both a mouse model of PCT and in patients a morphological correlation was found between the presence of uroporphyrin crystals and ferritin iron within the same hepatocyte (Siersema *et al.*, 1992). The beneficial effects of removing iron in PCT are not surprising, since ferrous iron has been shown to inhibit URO-D by direct competitive inhibition and by the generation of free radicals (Kushner *et al.*, 1975; Mukerji *et al.*, 1984). Furthermore, oxidation of uroporphyrinogen to uroporphyrin may be potentiated by iron-enhanced lipid peroxidation.

In most cases of PCT amounts of excess iron are in the range of 1.5–4.0 times normal (Lundvall, 1971; Turnbull *et al.*, 1973), though rarely the loading is more severe. The cause of the mild hepatic iron deposition in PCT is unknown. On the basis of studies of HLA haplotypes and iron status in probands with PCT and their relatives, it has been suggested that heterozygosity for an HLA-related haemochromatosis gene may be involved in the sporadic form of the disease (Kushner *et al.*, 1985; Edwards *et al.*, 1989). However, another study found no difference in frequency of HLA-A3 in patients with sporadic PCT, familial PCT and normal controls (Beaumont *et al.*, 1987). Since HLA-3 is known to be in linkage disequilibrium with the gene for primary haemochromatosis (see Chapter 8 and Section 6 below), it was concluded that there was no demonstrable relationship between the modest iron overload in PCT and inheritance of a gene for HLA-related haemochromatosis. The discrepancy between these studies is unresolved (Adams and Powell, 1987). More severe iron overload in PCT may be the result of homozygous HLA-related haemochromatosis (Edwards *et al.*, 1989; Seymour *et al.*, 1990). However, the absence of biochemical evidence of porphyria in most patients with primary haemochromatosis means that iron overload alone, without an intrinsic abnormality of URO-D, does not cause PCT. It therefore seems likely that the role of iron in PCT is to accentuate a genetically-determined enzyme deficiency.

The association of PCT with alcoholism may be a direct one or may merely reflect an association between iron overload and the consumption of alcohol (Section 5.1). A high frequency of infection by hepatitis C virus has also been reported in sporadic PCT and may be a triggering factor (Fargion *et al.*, 1992). In general it may be concluded that for expression of PCT, both an inherited enzyme deficiency and some other factor seem to be essential, and that the latter is frequently iron overload, with or without alcohol.

6. SECONDARY IRON OVERLOAD AND THE HLA-RELATED HAEMOCHROMATOSIS GENE

It is not only in PCT (see previous section) that the possibility of coincidental inheritance of an HLA-related haemochromatosis gene has been considered as a potential contributing factor in secondary iron overload. Although the heterozygous state for HLA-related haemochromatosis does not alone give rise to iron overload, a minority of carriers may show mild elevations in transferrin saturation and serum ferritin (Cartwright *et al.*, 1979; Simon *et al.*, 1981; Bassett *et al.*, 1981). The close association of the primary haemochromatosis allele with the A locus of the HLA system, and particularly HLA-A3 (Simon *et al.*, 1977b) (Chapter 8), has enabled population studies of HLA-A3 frequency in the various conditions associated with secondary iron overload, as well as family studies in which attempts have been made to identify the independent inheritance of the disease and an iron-loading trait. These two approaches, and the potential pitfalls in interpretation, were reviewed by Simon (1985). In particular HLA-A3 has a relatively high frequency in North European populations, while not all idiopathic haemochromatosis is associated with HLA-A3 – the latter is therefore a marker for the condition but not identical with it.

The presence or absence of an HLA-related haemochromatosis allele has no obvious relevance to iron loading as a result of blood transfusions. Initial suggestions that patients with chronic renal failure and one of the HLA types which have been associated with the haemochromatosis allele might have a higher frequency of iron overload and myopathy (Bregman *et al.*, 1980; Taccone-Gallucci *et al.*, 1987), have not been borne out when the effect of blood transfusion is considered (Gomez *et al.*, 1984; Simon, 1985; Carrera *et al.*, 1988).

Patients with alcoholic liver disease and mild iron overload have no HLA association, and there is no evidence that either a homozygous or heterozygous stage for the HLA-related haemochromatosis allele is involved in this form of modest iron overload (Simon *et al.*, 1977a). As discussed in Section 3 above, no HLA linkage has been detected in sub-Saharan dietary iron overload, though another 'iron-loading gene' may be involved (Gordeuk *et al.*, 1992). The conflicting evidence for HLA-related haemochromatosis in porphyria cutanea tarda has been reviewed in Section 5.2 above.

Among the iron-loading anaemias with excessive iron absorption, the close relationship between the degree of erythroid hyperplasia and iron loading in β-thalassaemia intermedia and congenital sideroblastic anaemias makes a contribution from an HLA-linked haemochromatosis allele, with a population frequency no greater than around 1:10 in populations of North European origin, most improbable. Although a limited number of family studies in idiopathic acquired sideroblastic anaemia have suggested the presence of an HLA-related haemochromatosis allele in both iron-loaded proband and family members without sideroblastic anaemia (Cartwright *et al.*, 1980; Barron *et al.*, 1989), the prevalence of HLA-A3 in such patients (0.23) was no higher than in controls (0.29) and significantly less than that seen in homozygous (0.73) and heterozygous (0.57) haemochromatosis (Simon *et al.*, 1985). Furthermore, biochemical markers of iron overload showed no differences in patients with sideroblastic anaemia whether they possessed HLA-A3 or not. A small number of patients with congenital sideroblastic anaemia and iron overload showed no association with HLA-A3 (Peto *et al.*, 1983). It seems unlikely that the presence of a haemochromatosis allele has any general role in the development of this form of secondary iron overload.

A more convincing case for a contribution from a coincidental HLA-linked haemochromatosis allele might be made in conditions where severe secondary iron overload is the exception rather than the rule. For example severe iron overload is uncommon in hereditary spherocytosis and family studies suggest that where present it may be associated with HLA-linked haemochromatosis (Blacklock and Meerkin, 1981; Edwards *et al.*, 1982; Fargion *et al.*, 1986; Mohler and Wheby, 1986). Homozygous HLA-related haemochromatosis seemed to be required for iron loading in the study by Edwards *et al.* (1982), but that of Mohler and Wheby (1986) suggested that while neither heterozygous haemochromatosis nor an autosomal dominant gene for hereditary spherocytosis alone gave rise to an abnormal iron status, the combination was associated with significant iron overload.

Heterozygous β-thalassaemia is only rarely associated with severe iron overload when there may be coincidental homozygous HLA-related haemochromatosis (Edwards *et al.*, 1981). In addition, however, a study of HLA antigens and iron status among Italian subjects suggested that in combination with β-thalassaemia trait a single coincidental haemochromatosis allele might promote modest iron overload (Fargion *et al.*, 1985). This study has been challenged since it implied an unexpectedly high frequency of the haemochromatosis allele in the general population, throwing doubt on whether HLA-A3 was truly marking this allele (Simon, 1985).

Increased iron absorption and hepatic iron have been described in some but not all members of three generations of a family with a high-oxygen-affinity haemoglobin variant, Hb Olympia. These findings could be interpreted as being the result of a coincidental inheritance of the heterozygous state for an HLA-related haemochromatosis gene (Weaver *et al.*, 1984).

It appears that while family studies have provided some evidence for heterozygous HLA-related haemochromatosis contributing to secondary iron overload, particularly where this is not usually seen with the underlying disorder, evidence of involvement from studies of the prevalence of HLA-A3 in most of the iron-loading anaemias, has not been consistent or convincing. Thus even when the HLA-related haemochromatosis gene is eventually identified, it seems probable that prediction of the likelihood of developing iron overload in the latter conditions will continue to require careful assessment of erythropoiesis, and regular monitoring of the rate of accumulation of iron stores, rather than determination of the presence or absence of an additional iron-loading gene.

7. LOCAL IRON OVERLOAD

7.1. Idiopathic Pulmonary Haemosiderosis

In this rare disease recurrent haemorrhages into the alveoli of the lung are followed by phagocytosis of the extravasculated erythrocytes by pulmonary macrophages. These macrophages retain the iron from metabolized haemoglobin as haemosiderin, and an iron deficiency anaemia develops (Apt *et al.*, 1957). The lack of recirculation of the iron by the lung macrophages may be related to their position away from the circulating plasma transferrin. The aetiology of the pulmonary haemosiderosis is uncertain, but similar haemorrhages are seen in Goodpasture's syndrome where haemorrhage into alveoli is associated with glomerulonephritis and antibodies to glomerular basement membrane, and may antedate the onset of renal disease.

7.2. Renal Haemosiderosis

With chronic intravascular haemolysis, release of haemoglobin within the circulation may exceed the binding capacity of the plasma scavenger proteins, haptoglobin and haemopexin. Haemoglobin is then filtered through the glomeruli and reabsorbed by proximal renal tubules, which thus become iron-laden. Haemosiderin in renal tubular cells, and free haemosiderin, appear in the urine sediment and as much as 15 mg of iron may be lost daily (Sears *et al.*, 1966). This may lead to iron deficiency anaemia in association with renal tubular iron overload: the latter may occasionally give rise to renal tubular dysfunction and acidosis (Riley *et al.*, 1977).

8. CONCLUSIONS

Secondary iron overload presents a number of unsolved problems. Foremost is the nature of the link between erythroid hyperplasia, particularly dyserythropoietic hyperplasia, and enhanced iron absorption. The possible role of heterozygous inheritance of the HLA-related haemochromatosis gene as a contributing factor in some forms of second iron overload also remains uncertain. It is unlikely to be important in the majority of iron-loading anaemias though it may account for occasional cases of severe iron overload in those haemolytic anaemias which are not usually associated with severe iron overload (e.g. hereditary spherocytosis). Severe secondary iron overload may be treated by iron chelation therapy and/or in some patients by phlebotomy, but in the acquired iron-loading anaemias careful consideration of the prognosis of the underlying disease is essential before embarking on an arduous and time-consuming programme of regular subcutaneous desferrioxamine infusions. The development of an inexpensive oral iron chelator could lead to a less conservative attitude to iron chelation treatment in the acquired iron-loading anaemias, as well as a wider access to iron chelation therapy in those parts of the world in which the iron-loading thalassaemia disorders are most common.

REFERENCES

Adams, P. C. and Powell, L. W. (1987) Porphyria cutanea tarda and HLA-linked hemo-chromatosis – all in the family? *Gastroenterol.* **92**, 2033–2035.

Agre, P., Asimos, A., Casella, J. F. and McMillan, C. (1986) Inheritance pattern and clinical response to splenectomy as a reflection of erythrocyte spectrin deficiency in hereditary spherocytosis. *N. Engl. J. Med.* **315**, 1579–1583.

Al-Refaie, F. N., Wonke, B., Hoffbrand, A. V., Wickens, D. G., Nortey, P. and Kontoghiorghes, G. J. (1992) Efficacy and possible adverse effects of the oral iron chelator 1,2-dimethyl-3-hydroxypyrid-4-one (L1) in thalassemia major. *Blood* **80**, 593–599.

Aldouri, M. A., Wonke, B., Hoffbrand, A. V. *et al.* (1990) High incidence of cardiomyopathy in beta-thalassaemia patients receiving regular transfusion and iron chelation: reversal by intensified chelation. *Acta Haematol.* **84**, 113–117.

Angelucci, E., Baronciani, D., Giardini, C. *et al.* (1992) Iron removal in ex-thalassaemic after bone marrow transplantation: the phlebotomy program. 2nd International Symposium on Bone Marrow Transplantation in Thalassemia, Pesaro, Abstract 48.

Aoki, Y. (1980) Multiple enzymatic defects in mitochondria in hematological cells of patients with primary sideroblastic anemia. *J. Clin. Invest.* **66**, 43–49.

Aoki, Y., Muranaka, S., Nakabayashi, K. U. and Veda, Y. (1979) δ-aminolevulinic acid synthase in erythroblasts of patients with pyridoxine-responsive anemia. Hypercatabolism caused by the increased susceptibility to the controlling protease. *J. Clin. Invest.* **64**, 1196–1203.

Apt, L., Pollycove, M., Ross, J. F., Pratt, M., Sullivan, J. and Donovan, J. (1957) Idiopathic pulmonary hemosiderosis. A study of the anemia and iron distribution using radioiron and radiochromium. *J. Clin. Invest.* **36**, 1150–1159.

Bannerman, R. M., Keusch, G., Kreimer-Birnbaum, M., Vance, V. K. and Vaughan, S. (1967) Thalassemia intermedia, with iron overload, cardiac failure, diabetes mellitus, hypopituitarism and porphyrinuria. *Am. J. Med.* **42**, 476–486.

Barron, R., Grace, N. D., Sherwood, G. and Powell, L. W. (1989) Iron overload complicating sideroblastic anemia – is the gene for hemochromatosis responsible? *Gastroenterol.* **96**, 204–206.

Barry, M., Scheuer, P. J., Sherlock, S., Ross, C. F. and Williams, R. (1968) Hereditary spherocytosis with secondary haemochromatosis. *Lancet* **ii**, 481–485.

Barry, M., Flynn, D. M., Letsky, E. A. and Risdon, R. A. (1974) Long-term chelation therapy in thalassaemia major: effect on liver iron concentration, liver histology, and clinical progress. *Br. Med. J.* **2**, 16–20.

Bassett, M. L., Halliday, J. W. and Powell, L. W. (1981) HLA typing in idiopathic hemochromatosis: distinction between homozygotes and heterozygotes with biochemical expression. *Hepatology* **1**, 120–126.

Beaumont, C., Fauchet, R., Phung, L. N., De Verneuil, H., Gueguen, M. and Nordmann, Y. (1987) Porphyria cutanea tarda and HLA-linked hemochromatosis. *Gastroenterol.* **92**, 1833–1838.

Bennett, J. M., Catovsky, D., Daniel, M. T. *et al.* (1982) Proposals for the classification of the myelodysplastic syndromes. *Br. J. Haematol.* **51**, 189–199.

Berdoukas, V., Bentley, P., Frost, H. and Schnebli, H. P. (1993) Toxicity of oral iron chelator L1. *Lancet* **341**, 1088.

Berriman, A. M., Tyler, B., Davis, S., Francombe, W. H., Liu, P. P. and Olivieri, N. F. (1991) Continuous intravenous deferoxamine in adults with severe iron overload. *Blood* **78**, 197a.

Blacklock, H. A. and Meerkin, M. (1981) Serum ferritin in patients with hereditary spherocytosis. *Br. J. Haematol.* **49**, 117–122.

Borgna-Pignatti, C., Zurlo, M. G., Destefano, P. *et al.* (1989) Survival in thalassemia with conventional treatment. In: *Advances and Controversies in Thalassemia Therapy: Bone Marrow Transplantation and Other Approaches* (eds C. D. Buckner, R. P. Gale, and G. Lucarelli), Alan R. Liss Inc., New York, pp. 27–33.

Bothwell, T. H. and Bradlow, B. A. (1960) Siderosis in the Bantu. A combined histopathological and chemical study. *Arch. Pathol.* **70**, 279–292.

Bothwell, T. H. and Isaacson, C. (1962) Siderosis in the Bantu. A comparison of the incidence in males and females. *Br. Med. J.* **i**, 522–524.

Bothwell, T. H., Seftel, H., Jacobs, P., Torrance, T. D. and Baumslag, N. (1964) Iron overload in Bantu subjects. Studies on availability of iron in Bantu beer. *Am. J. Clin. Nutr.* **14**, 47–51.

Bothwell, T. H., Charlton, R. W., Cook, J. D. and Finch, C. A. (1979) *Iron Metabolism in Man*, Blackwell Scientific Publications, Oxford.

Bottomley, S. S. (1982) Sideroblastic anaemia. *Clin. Haematol.* **11**, 389–409.

Bottomley, S. S., Healy, H. M., Brandenburg, M. A. and May, B. K. (1992) 5-aminolevulinate synthase in sideroblastic anemias: mRNA and enzyme activity levels in bone marrow cells. *Am. J. Hematol.* **41**, 76–83.

Bowdler, A. J. and Huehns, E. R. (1963) Thalassaemia minor complicated by excessive iron storage. *Br. J. Haematol.* **9**, 13–26.

Bregman, H., Gelfand, M. C., Winchester, J. F., Knepshield, J. H., Manz, H. J. and Schreiner, G. E. (1980) Iron-overload-associated myopathy in patients on maintenance haemodialysis: A histocompatibility-linked disorder. *Lancet* **ii**, 882–885.

Brink, B., Disler, P., Lynch, S., Jacobs, P., Charlton, R. and Bothwell, T. (1976) Patterns of iron storage in dietary iron overload and idiopathic hemochromatosis. *J. Lab. Clin. Med.* **88**, 725–731.

Brittenham, G. M. (1992) Development of iron-chelating agents for clinical use. *Blood* **80**, 569–574.

Bronspiegel-Weintrob, N., Olivieri, N. F., Tyler, B., Andrews, D. F., Freedman, M. H. and Holland, F. J. (1990) Effect of age at the start of iron chelation therapy on gonadal function in β-thalassemia major. *N. Engl. J. Med.* **323**, 713–719.

Buys, S. S., Martin, C. B., Eldridge, M., Kushner, J. P. and Kaplan, J. (1991) Iron absorption in hypotransferrinemic mice. *Blood* **78**, 3288–3290.

Carrera, F., Andrade, J. C., Silva, F. J. and Simoes, J. (1988) Serum ferritin and hemochromatosis alleles in chronic hemodialysis patients. *Nephron* **50**, 196–198.

Cartwright, G. E., Edwards, C. Q., Kravitz, K. *et al.* (1979) Hereditary hemochromatosis. Phenotypic expression of the disease. *N. Engl. J. Med.* **301**, 175–179.

Cartwright, G. E., Edwards, C. Q., Skolnick, M. H. and Amos, A. B. (1980) Association of HLA-linked hemochromatosis with idiopathic refractory sideroblastic anemia. *J. Clin. Invest.* **65**, 989–992.

Cavill, I., Worwood, M. and Jacobs, A. (1975) Internal regulation of iron absorption. *Nature* **256**, 328–329.

Cavill, I., Ricketts, C., Jacobs, A. and Letsky, E. (1978) Erythropoiesis and the effect of transfusion in homozygous β-thalassemia. *N. Engl. J. Med.* **298**, 776–778.

Cazzola, M., Barosi, G., Bergamaschi, G. *et al.* (1983a) Iron loading in congenital dyserythropoietic anaemias and congenital sideroblastic anaemias. *Br. J. Haematol.* **54**, 649–654.

Cazzola, M., Ascari, E., Barosi, G *et al.* (1983b) Juvenile idiopathic haemochromatosis: a life-threatening disorder presenting as hypogonadotropic hypogonadism. *Hum. Genet.* **65**, 149–154.

Cazzola, M., Pootrakul, P., Huebers, H. A., Eng, M., Eschbach, J. and Finch, C. A. (1987) Erythroid marrow function in anemic patients. *Blood* **69**, 296–301.

Cazzola, M., Barosi, G., Gobbi, P. G., Invernizzi, R., Riccardi, A. and Ascari E. (1988) Natural history of idiopathic refractory sideroblastic anemia. *Blood* **71**, 305–312.

Charlton, R. W., Jacobs, P., Seftel, H. and Bothwell, T. H. (1964) Effect of alcohol on iron absorption. *Br. Med. J.* **2**, 1427–1429.

Charlton, R. W., Abrahams, C. and Bothwell, T. H. (1967) Idiopathic hemochromatosis in young subjects. *Arch. Pathol.* **83**, 132–140.

Coetzer, T. L., Lawler, J., Liu, S. C. *et al.* (1988) Partial ankyrin and spectrin deficiency in severe, atypical hereditary spherocytosis. *N. Engl. J. Med.* **318**, 230–234.

Cohen. A. and Schwartz, E. (1979) Iron chelation therapy in sickle cell anemia. *Am. J. Hematol.* **7**, 69–76.

Cohen, A., Cohen, I. J. and Schwartz, E. (1981) Scurvy and altered iron stores in thalassemia major. *N. Engl. J. Med.* **304**, 158–160.

Cohen, A. R., Mizanin, J. and Schwartz, E. (1989) Rapid removal of excessive iron with daily high dose intravenous chelation therapy. *J. Pediatr.* **115**, 151–155.

Cohen, A. R., Martin, M. and Schwartz, E. (1990) Current treatment of Cooley's anemia. *Ann. NY Acad. Sci.* **612**, 397–404.

Costa, F. F., Agre, P., Watkins. P. C. *et al.* (1990) Linkage of dominant hereditary spherocytosis to the gene for the erythrocyte membrane-skeleton protein ankyrin. *N. Engl. J. Med.* **323**, 1046–1050.

Cotter, P. D., Baumann, M. and Bishop, D. F. (1992a) Enzymatic defect in 'X-linked' sideroblastic anemia: molecular evidence for erythroid delta-aminolevulinate synthase deficiency. *Proc. Natl. Acad. Sci. USA* **89**, 4028–4032.

Cotter, P. D., Willard, H. F., Gorski, J. L. and Bishop, D. F. (1992b) Assignment of human erythroid delta-aminolevulinate synthase (ALAS2) to a distal subregion of band Xp11.21 by PCR analysis of somatic cell hybrids containing X; autosome translocations. *Genomics* **13**, 211–212.

Cumming, R. L. C., Goldberg, A., Morrow, J. and Smith, J. A. (1967) Effects of phenylhydrazine-induced haemolysis on the urinary excretion of iron after desferrioxamine. *Lancet* **i**, 71–74.

Dacie, J. (1985) *The Haemolytic Anaemias. Vol. I The Hereditary Haemolytic Anaemias Part I.* Churchill Livingstone, Edinburgh, pp. 282–320.

Dalhoj, J., Kiaer, J., Wiggers, P., Grady, R. W., Jones, R. L. and Knisely, A. S. (1990) Iron storage disease in parents and sibs of infants with neonatal hemochromatosis: 30 year follow-up. *Am. J. Genet.* **37**, 342–345.

de Alarcon, P. A., Donovan, M. E., Forbes, G. B., Landaw, S. A. and Stockman, J. A. (1979) Iron absorption in the thalassemia syndromes and its inhibition by tea. *N. Engl. J. Med.* **300**, 5–8.

De Verneuil, H., Aitken, G. and Nordmann, Y. (1978) Familial and sporadic porphyria cutanea: two different diseases. *Hum. Genet.* **44**, 145–151.

Eason, E. J., Adams, P. C., Aston, C. E. and Searle, J. (1990) Familial iron overload with possible autosomal dominant inheritance. *Aust. NZ. J. Med.* **20**, 226–230.

Editorial (1984) Idiopathic haemochromatosis in the young. *Lancet* **ii** 145.

Edwards, C. Q., Skolnick, M. H. and Kushner, J. P. (1981) Coincidental nontransfusional iron overload and thalassemia minor: association with HLA-linked hemochromatosis. *Blood* **58**, 844–848.

Edwards, C. Q., Skolnick, M. H., Dadone, M. M. and Kushner, J. P. (1982) Iron overload in hereditary spherocytosis: association with HLA-linked hemochromatosis. *Am. J. Hematol.* **13**, 101–109.

Edwards, C. Q., Griffen, L. M. and Kushner, J. P. (1988) Increased frequency of HLA-A3 in subjects with sporadic porphyria cutanea tarda. *Tissue Antigens* **31**, 250–253.

Edwards, C. Q., Griffen, L. M., Goldgar, D. E., Skolnick, M. H. and Kushner, J. P. (1989) HLA-linked hemochromatosis alleles in sporadic porphyria cutanea tarda. *Gastroenterol.* **97**, 972–981.

Ehlers, K. H., Levin, A. R., Markenson, A. L. *et al.* (1980) Longitudinal study of cardiac function in thalassemia major. *Ann. NY Acad. Sci.* **344**, 397–404.

Ehlers, K. H., Giardina, P. J., Lesser, M. L., Engle, M. A. and Hilgartner, M. W. (1991) Prolonged survival in patients with beta-thalassemia treated with deferoxamine. *J. Pediatr.* **118**, 540–545.

Elder, G. H., Urquhart, A. J., de Salamanca, R. E., Munoz, J. J. and Bonkovsky, H. L. (1985) Immunoreactive uroporphyrinogen decarboxylase in the liver in porphyria cutanea tarda. *Lancet* **i**, 229–232.

Engle, M. A., Erlandson, M. and Smith, C. H. (1964) Late cardiac complications of chronic, severe, refractory anemia with hemochromatosis. *Circulation* **30**, 698–705.

Epstein, J. H. and Redeker, A. G. (1968) Porphyria cutanea tarda: a study of the effect of phlebotomy. *N. Engl. J. Med.* **279**, 1301–1304.

Erlandson, M. E., Walden, B., Stern, G., Hilgartner, M. W., Wehman, J. and Smith, C. H. (1962) Studies on congenital hemolytic syndromes. IV. Gastrointestinal absorption of iron. *Blood* **19**, 359–378.

Erlandson, M. E., Brilliant, R. and Smith, C. H. (1964) Comparison of sixty-six patients with thalassemia major and thirteen patients with thalassemia intermedia: including evaluations of growth, development, maturation and prognosis. *Ann. NY Acad. Sci.* **119**, 727–735.

Eschbach, J. W., Cook, J. D., Scribner, B. H. and Finch, C. A. (1977) Iron balance in hemodialysis patients. *Ann. Intern. Med.* **87**, 710–713.

Eschbach, J. W., Egrie, J. C., Downing, M. R., Browne, J. K. and Adamson, J. W. (1987) Correction of the anemia of end-stage renal disease with recombinant human erythropoietin: results of a combined Phase I and II clinical trial. *N. Engl. J. Med.* **316**, 73–78.

Fahey, J. L., Rath, C. E., Princiotto, J. V., Brick, I. B. and Rubin, M. (1961) Evaluation of trisodium calcium diethylenetriaminepentaacetate in iron storage disease. *J. Lab. Clin. Med.* **57**, 436–448.

Fargion, S., Piperno, A., Panaiotopoulos, N., Taddei, M. T. and Fiorelli, G. (1985) Iron overload in subjects with beta-thalassemia trait: role of idiopathic haemochromatosis gene. *Br. J. Haematol.* **61**, 487–490.

Fargion, S., Cappellini, M. D., Piperno, A., Panaiotopoulos, N., Ronchi, G. and Fiorelli, G. (1986) Association of hereditary spherocytosis and idiopathic hemochromatosis. *Am. J. Clin. Pathol.* **86**, 645–649.

Fargion, S., Piperno, A., Cappellini, M. D. *et al.* (1992) Hepatitis C virus and porphyria cutanea tarda: evidence of a strong association. *Hepatology* **16**, 1322–1326.

Finch, C. A., Huebers, H., Eng, M. and Miller, L. (1982) Effect of transfused reticulocytes on iron exchange. *Blood* **59**, 364–369.

Fitzsimons, E. J., May, A., Elder, G. H. and Jacobs, A. (1988) 5-Aminolaevulinic acid synthase activity in developing human erythroblasts. *Br. J. Haematol.* **69**, 281–285.

Freeman, A. P., Giles, R. W., Berdoukas, V. A., Walsh, W. F., Choy, D. and Murray, P. C. (1983) Early left ventricular dysfunction and chelation therapy in thalassemia major. *Ann. Intern. Med.* **99**, 450–454.

Gabutti, V. (1990) Current therapy for thalassemia in Italy. *Ann. NY Acad. Sci.* **612**, 268–274.

Garey, J. R., Hansen, J. L. and Kushner, J. P. (1989) A point mutation in the coding region of uroporphyrinogen decarboxylase associated with familial porphyria cutanea tarda. *Blood* **73**, 892–895.

Gattermann, N., Aul, C. and Schneider, W. (1990) Two types of acquired idiopathic sidero-blastic anaemia (AISA). *Br. J. Haematol.* **74**, 45–52.

Giardina, P. J., Grady, R. W., Ehlers, K. H. *et al.* (1990) Current therapy of Cooley's anemia. A decade of experience with subcutaneous desferrioxamine. *Ann. NY Acad. Sci.* **612**, 275–285.

Gokal, R., Millard, P. R., Weatherall, D. J., Callender, S. T. E., Ledingham, J. G. G. and Oliver, D. O. (1979) Iron metabolism in haemodialysis patients. *Q. J. Med.* **48**, 369–391.

Gomez, E., Ortega, F., Peces, R., Marin, R. and Alvarez-Grande, J. (1984) Serum ferritin in haemodialysis patients: role of blood transfusions and 'haemochromatosis alleles' HLA A3, B7 and B14. *Nephron* **36**, 106–110.

Gordeuk, V. R. (1992) Hereditary and nutritional iron overload. *Baillière's Clin. Haematol.* **5**, 169–186.

Gordeuk, V. R., Boyd, R. D. and Brittenham, G. M. (1986) Dietary iron overload persists in rural sub-saharan Africa. *Lancet* 1310–1313.

Gordeuk, V., Mukiibi, J., Med, M. *et al.* (1992) Iron overload in Africa. Interaction between a gene and dietary iron content. *N. Engl. J. Med.* **326**, 95–100.

Goya, N., Miyazaki, S., Kodate, S. and Oshio, B. (1972) A family of congenital atransferrinemia. *Blood* **40**, 239–245.

Grace, N. D. and Powell, L. W. (1974) Iron storage diseases of the liver. *Gastroenterol.* **64**, 1257–1283.

Green, R., Charlton, R., Seftel, H. *et al.* (1968) Body iron excretion in man. *Am. J. Med.* **45**, 336–353.

Greiner, T. C., Burns, C. P., Dick, F. R., Henry, K. M. and Mahmood, I. (1992) Congenital dyserythropoietic anemia type II diagnosed in a 69-year-old patient with iron overload. *Am. J. Clin. Pathol.* **98**, 522–525.

Haines, M. E. and Wainscoat, J. S. (1991) Relapsing sideroblastic anaemia. *Br. J. Haematol.* **78**, 285–286.

Halliday, J. W. (1989) Inherited iron overload. *Acta Paediatr. Scand.* **361**, 86–95.

Harris, J. W., Whittington, R. M., Weisman, R., Jr and Horrigan, D. L. (1956) Pyridoxine responsive anemia in the human adult. *Proc. Soc. Exp. Biol. Med.* **91**, 427–432.

Heilmeyer, L., Keller, W., Vivell, O. *et al.* (1961) Congenital transferrin-deficiency in a seven-year old girl. *German Medical Monthly* **vi**, 385–389.

Heimpel, H. (1976) Congenital dyserythropoietic anaemia type I: clinical and experimental aspects. In: *Congenital Disorders of Erythropoiesis*, Ciba Foundation Symposium **37**, Elsevier, Amsterdam, pp. 135–149.

Heinrich, H. C., Gabbe, E. E., Oppitz, K. H. *et al.* (1973) Absorption of inorganic and food iron in children with heterozygous and homozygous B-thalassemia. *Z. Kinderheilk.* **115**, 1–22.

Hershko, C. (1993) Development of oral iron chelator L1. *Lancet* **341**, 1088–1089.

Hoffbrand, A. V. and Wonke, B. (1989) Results of long-term subcutaneous desferrioxamine therapy. *Baillière's Clin. Haematol.* **2**, 345–362.

Hoffbrand, A. V., Gorman, A., Laulicht, M. *et al.* (1979) Improvement in iron status and liver function in patients with transfusional iron overload with long-term subcutaneous desferrioxamine. *Lancet* **i**, 947–949.

Hughes, R. T., Smith, T., Hesp, R. *et al.* (1992) Regulation of iron aborption in iron loaded subjects with end stage renal disease: effects of treatment with recombinant human erythropoietin and reduction of iron stores. *Br. J. Haematol.* **82**, 445–454.

Hussain, M. A. M., Flynn, D. M., Green, N., Hussein, S. and Hoffbrand, A. V. (1976) Subcutaneous infusion and intramuscular injection of desferrioxamine in patients with transfusional iron overload. *Lancet* **ii**, 1278–1280.

Hussein, S., Hoffbrand, A. V. and Laulicht, M. (1976) Serum ferritin levels in beta-thalassaemia trait. *Br. Med. J.* **ii**, 920.

Hyman, C. B., Agness, C. L., Rodriguez-Funes, R. and Zednikova, M. (1985) Combined subcutaneous and high-dose intravenous deferoxamine therapy of thalassemia. *Ann. NY Acad. Sci.* **445**, 293–303.

Iancu, T. C., Neustein, H. B. and Landing, B. H. (1977) The liver in thalassaemia major: ultrastructural observation. In: *Iron Metabolism*, Ciba Foundation Symposium **51**, Elsevier, North Holland, pp. 293–309.

Irving, M. G., Halliday, J. W. and Powell, L. W. (1988) Association between alcoholism and increased hepatic iron stores. *Alcoholism* **12**, 7–13.

Isaacson, C., Seftel, H. C., Keeley, K. J. and Bothwell, T. H. (1961) Siderosis in the Bantu: The relationship between iron overload and cirrhosis. *J. Lab. Clin. Med.* **58**, 845–852.

Kapur, A., Wild, G., Milford-Ward, A. and Triger, D. R. (1989) Carbohydrate deficient transferrin: a marker for alcohol abuse. *Br. Med. J.* **299**, 427–431.

Karabus, C. D. and Fielding, J. (1967) Desferrioxamine chelatable iron in haemolytic, megaloblastic and sideroblastic anaemias. *Br. J. Haematol.* **13**, 924–933.

Knisely, A. S., Harford, J. B., Klausner, R. D. and Taylor, S. R. (1989) Neonatal hemochromatosis. The regulation of transferrin-receptor and ferritin synthesis by iron in cultured fibroblastic-line cells. *Am. J. Pathol.* **134**, 439–445.

Konopka, L. and Hoffbrand, A. V. (1979) Haem synthesis in sideroblastic anaemia. *Br. J. Haematol.* **42**, 73–83.

Kushner, J. P., Steinmuller, D. P. and Lee, G. R. (1975) The role of iron in the pathogenesis of porphyria cutanea tarda. II. Inhibition of uroporphyrinogen decarboxylase. *J. Clin. Invest.* **56**, 661–667.

Kushner, J. P., Barbuto, A. J. and Lee, G. R. (1976) An inherited enzymatic defect in porphyria cutanea tarda: decreased uroporphyrinogen decarboxylase activity. *J. Clin. Invest.* **58**, 1089–1097.

Kushner, J. P., Edwards, C. Q., Dadone, M. M. and Skolnick, M. H. (1985) Heterozygosity for HLA-linked hemochromatosis as a likely cause of the hepatic siderosis associated with sporadic porphyria cutanea tarda. *Gasteroenterol.* **88**, 1232–1238.

Lamon, J. M., Marynick, S. P., Rosenblatt, R. and Donnelly, S. (1979) Idiopathic hemochromatosis in a young female. *Gastroenterol.* **76**, 178–183.

Lee, G. R., MacDiarmid, W. D., Cartwright, G. E. and Wintrobe, M. M. (1968) Hereditary x-linked, sideroachrestic anemia. The isolation of two erythrocyte populations differing in Xg^a blood type and porphyrin content. *Blood* **32**, 59–70.

Lim, H. W., Cooper, D., Sassa, S., Dosik, H., Buchness, M. R. and Soter, N. A. (1992) Photosensitivity, abnormal porphyrin profile, and sideroblastic anemia. *J. Am. Acad. Dermatol.* **27**, 287–292.

Lipschitz, D. A., Bothwell, T. H., Seftel, H. C., Wapnick, A. A. and Charlton, R. W. (1971) The role of ascorbic acid in the metabolism of storage iron. *Br. J. Haematol.* **20**, 155–163.

Losowsky, M. S. and Hall, R. (1965) Hereditary sideroblastic anaemia. *Br. J. Haematol.* **11**, 70–85.

Lucarelli, G. (1991) For debate: Bone marrow transplantation for severe thalassaemia. *Br. J. Haematol.* **78**, 300–303.

Lundvall, O. (1971) The effect of replenishment of iron stores after phlebotomy therapy in porphyria cutanea tarda. *Acta Med. Scand.* **189**, 57–63.

MacPhail, A. P., Simon, M. O., Bothwell, T. H., Torrance, J. D. and Isaacson, C. (1979) Changing patterns of dietary iron overload in black South Africans. *Am. J. Clin. Nutr.* **32**, 1272–1278.

Marcus, R. E., Davies, S. C., Bantock, H. M., Underwood, S. R., Walton, S. and Huehns, E. R. (1984) Desferrioxamine to improve cardiac function in iron-overloaded patients with thalassaemia major. *Lancet* **i**, 392–393.

McCarthy, J. T., Johnson, W. J., Nixon, D. E., Jenson, B. M. and Moyer, T. P. (1989) Transfusional iron overload in patients undergoing dialysis: treatment with erythropoietin and phlebotomy. *J. Lab. Clin. Med.* **114**, 193–199.

McLellan, T., Pryor, M. A., Kushner, J. P., Eddy, R. L. and Shows, T. B. (1985) Assignment of uroporphyrinogen decarboxylase (URO-D) to the pter-p21 region of chromosome 1. *Cytogenet. Cell Genet.* **39**, 224–227.

McShane, M. A., Hammans, S. R., Sweeney, M. *et al.* (1991) Pearson syndrome and mitochondrial encephalomyopathy in a patient with a deletion of mtDNA. *Am. J. Hum. Genet.* **48**, 39–42.

306   M. J. PIPPARD

Mihas, A. A. and Tavassoli, M. (1991) The effect of ethanol on the uptake, binding, and desialylation of transferrin by rat liver endothelium: implications in the pathogenesis of alcohol-associated hepatic siderosis. *Am. J. Med. Sci.* **301**, 299–304.
Modell, B. (1977) Total management of thalassaemia major. *Arch. Dis. Child.* **52**, 489–500.
Modell, B. (1979) Advances in the use of iron-chelating agents for the treatment of iron overload. *Progress in Hematology* **11**, 267–312.
Mohler, D. H. and Wheby, M. S. (1986) Hemochromatosis heterozygotes may have significant iron overload when they also have hereditary spherocytosis. *Am. J. Med. Sci.* **292**, 320–324.
Mukerji, S. K., Pimstone, N. R. and Burns, M. (1984) Dual mechanism of inhibition of rat liver uroporphyrinogen decarboxylase activity by ferrous iron: its potential role in the genesis of porphyria cutanea tarda. *Gastroenterol.* **87**, 1248–1254.
Murakami, R., Takumi, T., Gouji, J., Nakamura, H. and Kondou, M. (1991) Sideroblastic anemia showing unique response to pyridoxine. *Am. J. Ped. Hematol. Oncol.* **13**, 345–350.
Nienhuis, A. W. (1981) Vitamin C and iron. *N. Engl. J. Med.* **304**, 170–171.
Nienhuis, A. W., Delea, C., Aamodt, R., Bartler, F. and Anderson, W. F. (1976) Evaluation of desferrioxamine and ascorbic acid for the treatment of chronic iron overload. In: *Iron Metabolism and Thalassemia. Birth Defects: Original Article Series XII* (eds D. Bergsma, A. Cerami, C. M. Peterson and J. H. Graziano), Alan R. Liss, New York, pp. 177–185.
Nienhuis, A. W., Benz, E. J., Propper, R. *et al.* (1979) Thalassemia major: molecular and clinical aspects. *Ann. Int. Med.* **91**, 883–897.
Nusbaum, N. J. (1991) Concise review: genetic bases for sideroblastic anemia. *Am. J. Hematol.* **37**, 41–44.
Olivieri, N. F., Wayne, A., Davis, S. *et al.* (1991) The impact of early initiation of subcutaneous deferoxamine on iron-related cardiac disease in thalassemia major. *Blood* **78** (Suppl. 1), 196a.
Olivieri, N. F., Koren, G., Matsui, D. *et al.* (1992) Reduction of tissue iron stores and normalization of serum ferritin during treatment with the oral iron chelator L1 in thalassemia intermedia. *Blood* **79**, 2741–2748.
Parfrey, P. S., Barnett, M., Sachs, J. A., Pollock, D. J. and Turnbull, A. L. (1981) Iron overload in β-thalassaemia minor. A family study. *Scand. J. Haematol.* **27**, 294–302.
Peto, T. E. A., Pippard, M. J. and Weatherall, D. J. (1983) Iron overload in mild sideroblastic anaemias. *Lancet* **i**, 375–378.
Pippard, M. J. (1987) Iron overload and iron chelation therapy in thalassaemia and sickle cell haemoglobinopathies. *Acta Haematol.* **78**, 206–211.
Pippard, M. J. (1989) Desferrioxamine-induced iron excretion in humans. *Baillière's Clin. Haematol.* **2**, 323–343.
Pippard, M. J. (1993) Iron chelation therapy and the treatment of iron overload. In: *Development of Iron Chelators for Clinical Use*, CRC Press, Boca Raton, in press.
Pippard, M. J. and Wainscoat, J. S. (1987) Erythrokinetics and iron status in heterozygous β thalassaemia, and the effect of interaction with α thalassaemia. *Br. J. Haematol.* **66**, 123–127.
Pippard, M. J. and Weatherall, D. J. (1984) Iron absorption in non-transfused iron loading anaemias: prediction of risk for iron loading and response to iron chelation treatment, in β thalassaemia intermedia and congenital sideroblastic anaemias. *Haematologia* **17**, 2–24.
Pippard, M. J., Letsky, E. A., Callender, S. T. and Weatherall, D. J. (1978a) Prevention of iron loading in transfusion-dependent thalassaemia. *Lancet* **i**, 1178–1180.
Pippard, M. J., Callender, S. T. and Weatherall, D. J. (1978b) Intensive iron-chelation therapy with desferrioxamine in iron-loading anaemias. *Clin. Sci. Mol. Med.* **54**, 99–106.
Pippard, M. J., Callender, S. T., Warner, G. T. and Weatherall, D. J. (1979) Iron absorption and loading in beta-thalassaemia intermedia. *Lancet* **ii**, 819–821.
Pippard, M. J., Callender, S. T. and Finch, C. A. (1982a) Ferrioxamine excretion in iron-loaded man. *Blood* **60**, 288–294.
Pippard, M. J., Rajagopalan, B., Callender, S. T. and Weatherall, D. J. (1982b) Iron loading, chronic anaemia, and erythroid hyperplasia as determinants of the clinical features of β-thalassaemia intermedia. In: *Advances in Red Blood Cell Biology* (eds D. J. Weatherall, G. Fiorelli and S. Gorini), Raven Press, New York, pp. 103–113.
Pippard, M. J., Jackson, M. J., Hoffman, K., Petrou, M. and Modell, C. B. (1986) Iron chelation using subcutaneous infusions of diethylene triamine penta-acetic acid (DTPA). *Scand. J. Haematol.* **36**, 466–472.

Pippard, M. J., Hughes, R. T. and Cotes, P. M. (1992) Erythropoietin. In: *Recent Advances in Haematology 6* (eds A. V. Hoffbrand and M. K. Brenner), Churchill Livingstone, London, pp. 1–18.

Pootrakul, P., Rugkiatsakul, R. and Wasi, P. (1980) Increased transferrin iron saturation in splenectomized thalassaemic patients. *Br. J. Haematol.* **46**, 143–145.

Pootrakul, P., Kitcharoen, K., Yansukon, P. *et al.* (1988) The effect of erythroid hyperplasia on iron balance. *Blood* **71**, 1124–1129.

Porter, J. B. and Huehns, E. R. (1989) Toxic effects of desferrioxamine. *Baillière's Clin. Haematol.* **2**, 459–474.

Porter, J. B., Jaswon, M. S., Huehns, E. R., East, C. A. and Jonathan, W. P. (1989) Desferrioxamine ototoxicity: evaluation of risk factors in thalassaemic patients and guidelines for safe dosage. *Br. J. Haematol.* **73**, 403–409.

Powell, L. W., Bassett, M. L., Axelsen, E., Ferluga, J. and Halliday, J. W. (1988) Is all genetic (hereditary) hemochromatosis HLA-associated. *Ann. NY Acad. Sci.* **526**, 23–33.

Propper, R. D., Shurin, S. B. and Nathan, D. G. (1976) Reassessment of the use of desferrioxamine B in iron overload. *N. Engl. J. Med.* **294**, 1421–1423.

Raja, K. B., Pippard, M. J., Simpson, R. J. and Peters, T. J. (1986) Relationship between erythropoiesis and the enhanced intestinal uptake of ferric iron in hypoxia in the mouse. *Br. J. Haematol.* **64**, 587–593.

Raja, K. B., Simpson, R. J., Pippard, M. J. and Peters, T. J. (1988) In vivo studies on the relationship between intestinal iron (Fe^{3+}) absorption, hypoxia and erythropoiesis in the mouse. *Br. J. Haematol.* **68**, 373–378.

Raja, K. B., Simpson, R. J. and Peters, T. J. (1989) Effect of exchange transfusion of reticulocytes on in vitro and in vivo intestinal iron (Fe^{3+}) absorption in mice. *Br. J. Haematol.* **73**, 254–259.

Ramsay, C. A., Magnus, I. A., Turnbull, A. and Baker, H. (1974) The treatment of porphyria cutanea tarda by venesection. *Quart. J. Med.* **43**, 1–24.

Riley, A. L., Ryan, L. M. and Roth, D. A. (1977) Renal proximal tubular dysfunction and paroxysmal nocturnal hemoglobinuria. *Am. J. Med.* **62**, 125–129.

Roberts, A. G., Elder, G. H., Newcombe, R. G., de Salamanca, R. E. and Munoz, J. J. (1988) Heterogeneity of familial porphyria cutanea tarda. *J. Med. Genet.* **25**, 669–676.

Roeser, H. P. (1983) The role of ascorbic acid in the turnover of storage iron. *Semin. Hematol.* **20**, 91–100.

Rocchi, E., Gibertini, P., Cassanelli, M. *et al.* (1986) Iron removal therapy in porphyria cutanea tarda: phlebotomy versus slow subcutaneous desferrioxamine infusion. *Br. J. Dermatol.* **114**, 621–629.

Rotig, A., Cormier, V., Blanche, S. *et al.* (1990) Pearson's marrow-pancreas syndrome. A multisystem mitochondrial disorder in infancy. *J. Clin. Invest.* **86**, 1601–1608.

Rundles, R. W. and Falls, H. F. (1946) Hereditary (? sex-linked) anemia. *Am. J. Med. Sci.* **211**, 641–658.

Schafer, A. I., Cheron, R. G., Dluhy, R. *et al.* (1981) Clinical consequences of acquired transfusional iron overload in adults. *N. Engl. J. Med.* **304**, 319–324.

Sears, D. A., Anderson, P. R., Foy, A. L., Williams, H. L. and Crosby, W. H. (1966) Urinary iron excretion and renal metabolism of hemoglobin in hemolytic diseases. *Blood* **28**, 708–725.

Seftel, H. C., Keeley, K. J., Isaacson, C. and Bothwell, T. H. (1961) Siderosis in the Bantu: the clinical incidence of hemochromatosis in diabetic subjects. *J. Lab. Clin. Med.* **58**, 837–844.

Seftel, H. C., Malkin, C., Schmaman, A. *et al.* (1966) Osteoporosis, scurvy, and siderosis in Johannesburg Bantu. *Br. Med. J.* **1**, 642–646.

Seymour, D. G., Elder, G. H., Fryer, A., Jacobs, A. and Williams, G. T. (1990) Porphyria cutanea tarda and haemochromatosis: a family study. *Gut* **31**, 719–721.

Short, E. M., Winkle, R. A. and Billingham, M. E. (1981) Myocardial involvement in idiopathic hemochromatosis. *Am. J. Med.* **70**, 1275–1279.

Siersema, P. D., van Helvoirt, R. P., Cleton-Soeteman, M. I., De Bruijn, W. C., Wilson, J. H. and van Eijk, H. G. (1992) The role of iron in experimental porphyria and porphyria cutanea tarda. *Biological Trace Element Research* **35**, 65–72.

Simon, M. (1985) Secondary iron overload and the haemochromatosis allele. *Br. J. Haematol.* **60**, 1–5.

Simon, M., Bourel, M., Genetet, B., Fauchet, R., Edran, G. and Brissot, P. (1977a) Idiopathic hemochromatosis and iron overload in alcoholic liver disease: differentiation by HLA phenotype. *Gastroenterol.* **73**, 655–658.

Simon, M., Bourel, M., Genetet, B. and Fauchet, R. (1977b) Idiopathic hemochromatosis. Demonstration of recessive inheritance and early detection by family HLA typing. *N. Engl. J. Med.* **297**, 1017–1021.

Simon, M., Fauchet, R., Hespel, J. P. *et al.* (1980) Idiopathic hemochromatosis: a study of biochemical expression in 247 heterozygous members of 63 families: evidence for a single major HLA-linked gene. *Gastroenterol.* **78**, 703–708.

Simon, M., Beaumont, C., Briere, J. *et al.* (1985) Is the HLA-linked haemochromatosis allele implicated in idiopathic refractory sideroblastic anaemia? *Br. J. Haematol.* **60**, 75–80.

Skikne, R. S. and Cook, J. D. (1992) Effect of enhanced erythropoiesis on iron absorption. *J. Lab. Clin. Med.* **20**, 746–751.

Solomon, L. R., Hillman, R. S. and Finch, C. A. (1981) Serum ferritin in refractory anemias. *Acta Haematol.* **66**, 1–5.

Sonakul, D., Sook-aneak, M. and Pacharee, P. (1978) Pathology of thalassemic diseases in Thailand. *J. Med. Assoc. Thai.* **61**, 72.

Speight, A. N. and Cliff, J. (1974) Iron storage disease of the liver in Dar es Salaam: a preliminary report on venesection therapy. *East Afr. Med. J.* **51**, 895–902.

Stibler, H. (1991) Carbohydrate-deficient transferrin in serum: a new marker of potentially harmful alcohol consumption reviewed. *Clin. Chem.* **37**, 2029–2037.

Sturgeon, P. and Finch, C. A. (1957) Erythrokinetics in Cooley's anemia. *Blood* **12**, 64–73.

Taccone-Gallucci, M., Di Nucci, G., Meloni, C. *et al.* (1987) Risk of iron overload and 'hemochromatosis allele(s)' in patients on maintenance hemodialysis. *Am. J. Nephrol.* **7**, 28–32.

Turnbull, A., Baker, H., Vernon-Roberts, B. and Magnus, I. A. (1973) Iron metabolism in porphyria cutanea tarda and in erythropoietic protoporphyria. *Q. J. Med.* **42**, 341–355.

Verwilghen, R. L. (1976) Congenital dyserythropoietic anaemia type II (Hempas). In: *Congenital Disorders of Erythropoiesis*, Ciba Foundation Symposium 37, Elsevier, Amsterdam, pp. 151–203.

Wang, W. C., Ahmed, H. and Hanna, M. (1986) Non-transferrin-bound iron in long-term transfusion in children with congenital anemias. *J. Pediatr.* **108**, 552–557.

Wapnick, A. A., Lynch, S. R., Charlton, R. W., Seftel, H. C. and Bothwell, T. H. (1969) The effect of ascorbic acid deficiency on desferrioxamine-induced urinary iron excretion. *Br. J. Haematol.* **17**, 563–568.

Weatherall, D. J. and Clegg, J. B. (1981) *The Thalassaemia Syndromes*, 3rd edn, Blackwell Scientific Publications, Oxford.

Weatherall, D. J. and Pembrey, M. E. (1970) Familial sideroblastic anaemia: problem of Xg and X chromosome inactivation. *Lancet* **ii**, 744–748.

Weaver, G. A., Rahbar, S., Ellsworth, C. A., de Alarcon, P. A., Forbes, G. B. and Beutler, E. (1984) Iron overload in three generations of a family with hemoglobin Olympia. *Gastroenterol.* **87**, 695–702.

Weintraub, L. R., Conrad, M. F. and Crosby, W. H. (1966) Iron-loading anemia. Treatment with repeated phlebotomies and pyridoxine. *N. Engl. J. Med.* **275**, 169–176.

Wheby, M. S. and Umpierre, G. (1964) Effect of transferrin saturation on iron absorption in man. *N. Engl. J. Med.* **271**, 1391–1395.

Wickramasinghe, S. N. and Pippard, M. J. (1986) Studies of erythroblast function in congenital dyserythropoietic anaemia, type I: evidence of impaired DNA, RNA, and protein synthesis and unbalanced chain synthesis in ultrastructurally abnormal cells. *J. Clin. Pathol.* **39**, 881–890.

Witzleben, C. L. and Uri, A. (1970) Perinatal hemochromatosis entity or end result? *Hum. Pathol.* **20**, 335–340.

Wolfe, L., Olivieri, N., Sallan, D. *et al.* (1985) Prevention of cardiac disease by subcutaneous deferoxamine patients with thalassemia major. *N. Engl. J. Med.* **312**, 1600–1603.

Wolman, I. J. (1964) Transfusion therapy in Cooley's anemia: growth and health as related to long-range hemoglobin levels. A progress report. *Ann. NY Acad. Sci.* **119**, 737–747.

Wonke, B., Hoffbrand, A. V., Aldouri, M. *et al.* (1989) Reversal of desferrioxamine induced auditory neurotoxicity during treatment with Ca-DTPA. *Arch. Dis. Child.* **64**, 77–82.

Worwood, M., Cragg, S. J., Jacobs, A., McLaren, C., Ricketts, C. and Economidou, J. (1980) Binding of serum ferritin to concanavalin A: patients with homozygous β thalassaemia and transfusional iron overload. *Br. J. Haematol.* **46**, 409–416.

Zurlo, M. G., Destefano, P., Borgna-Pignatti, C. *et al.* (1989) Survival and causes of death in thalassaemia major. *Lancet* **i**, 27–30.

10. Mechanisms of Iron Toxicity

R. S. BRITTON[1], A. S. TAVILL[2] AND B. R. BACON[1]

[1]Division of Gastroenterology and Hepatology, St Louis University Health Sciences Center, St Louis, Missouri 63110, USA
[2]The Maurice and Sadie Friedman Center for Digestive and Liver Disorders, Mount Sinai Medical Center, Case Western Reserve University, Cleveland, Ohio 44106, USA

I. INTRODUCTION

Iron overload has important health consequences because of the toxic effects of excess iron and the number of people affected worldwide. In studies of various Caucasian population groups from around the world (Europe, Australia, Canada and the United States), it has been estimated that 0.25–0.5% of individuals of Northern European origin have a genetically determined form of iron loading called hereditary haemochromatosis (HHC) (Bassett *et al.*, 1982; Dadone *et al.*, 1982; Borwein *et al.*, 1983; Olsson *et al.*, 1983; Edwards *et al.*, 1988, 1989) (see Chapter 8). In addition, there are thousands of individuals worldwide who have iron overload associated with refractory and transfusion-dependent anaemias such as thalassaemia major (Modell and Berdoukas, 1984; Gordeuk *et al.*, 1987) (see Chapter 9). In sub-Saharan Africa, an inherited form of iron overload, which is genetically distinct from HHC, can be exacerbated by the ingestion of home-brewed beer, which is rich in iron (Gordeuk *et al.*, 1986, 1992; Bacon, 1992). In addition, the clinical course of patients with porphyria cutanea tarda (Lundvall *et al.*, 1970; Bonkovsky, 1991), some patients with chronic liver disease (Chapman *et al.*, 1982; Di Bisceglie *et al.*, 1992), some individuals with chronic renal failure on haemodialysis (Curtis *et al.*, 1969), and patients with a number of other uncommon metabolic disorders (e.g. congenital atransferrinaemia, Kaschin-Beck disease, hereditary tyrosinaemia, Zellweger's cerebrohepatorenal syndrome, etc.) are frequently complicated by significant degrees of iron overload (Bothwell *et al.*, 1979; McLaren *et al.*, 1983; Gordeuk *et al.*, 1987; Nichols and Bacon, 1989).

This chapter will highlight the pertinent clinical and hepatic observations in iron overload states in humans and will examine, in detail, the various theories of cellular toxicity and tissue damage due to excess iron, emphasizing the potential role of iron-induced lipid peroxidation and associated organelle dysfunction leading to hepatic fibrogenesis. An understanding of the mechanisms of cellular injury and fibrogenesis in iron overload is important in many clinical entities, since oxyradical-mediated cellular and tissue injury are increasingly recognized cytopathologic processes, and iron is an important catalyst of these reactions (Halliwell and Gutteridge, 1990).

2. HEPATIC PATHOLOGY

The clinicopathological consequences of iron overload in humans are discussed elsewhere in this book (Chapters 8 and 9). Patients with HHC may present with a wide spectrum of symptoms and physical findings depending upon the reasons for initial clinical evaluation and the degree of total body iron accumulation. For example, young patients with HHC who are identified as a result of screening studies on relatives of a proband may be asymptomatic with no physical signs and only laboratory abnormalities. In contrast, older patients with fully developed HHC may present with a constellation of end-stage manifestations of the disease including cirrhosis of the liver, skin pigmentation, diabetes, heart failure and hypogonadism. Men typically present at age 40–50 years, whereas women, partly because of physiological losses of iron from menstruation and pregnancy, present approximately ten years later (Tavill and Bacon, 1990).

Hepatic involvement is found in all patients with iron overload, and thus histological interpretation and quantitative assessment of hepatic iron are necessary for the precise diagnosis and management of patients with haemochromatosis. In patients with early HHC, iron stains (Perls' Prussian blue) show deposition virtually entirely in parenchymal cells in a periportal (Rappaport zone 1) distribution (Plate 1) with very little inflammation. Later, in severe iron overload, iron deposition is found in hepatocytes throughout the hepatic lobule, although the periportal (zone 1) to pericentral (zone 3) gradient is maintained (Plate 2) (Deugnier et al., 1992). Also, at this stage, iron deposits can be found in bile duct epithelial cells (Plate 2) and occasionally in Kupffer cells (Deugnier et al., 1992). Typically, in HHC, excess iron is not found in the reticuloendothelial (RE) cells of the liver, bone marrow, or spleen (Brink et al., 1976). In contrast, in transfusional iron overload, where much of the excess iron burden is produced by repeated red blood cell transfusions, there is excessive deposition of iron in the RE cells in the liver (Kupffer cells) (Plate 3), spleen and bone marrow. Plates 1, 2 and 3 compare the appearances of the liver in HHC and transfusional iron overload in humans as a basis for comparison with the appearances in experimental iron overload. Ultrastructurally, iron in hepatocytes is found predominantly as haemosiderin in secondary lysosomes and as ferritin in the cytosol (Munro and Linder, 1978; Wixom et al., 1980; Bacon and Tavill, 1984; Richter, 1984; Alt et al., 1990).

In HHC, histological findings on liver biopsy (other than iron deposition) are variable and range from normal morphology to minimal periportal or perilobular fibrosis to micronodular cirrhosis (Plate 4). Bassett et al. (1986) suggested that the presence of fibrosis and cirrhosis in the majority of patients with HHC depends on a combination of factors which include the hepatic iron concentration and the duration of time that the liver has been exposed to high iron concentrations. They demonstrated that, in the absence of coexistent alcoholic liver disease, fibrosis and/or cirrhosis do not occur until the hepatic iron concentration exceeds 22 000 $\mu g/g$ (dry wt). However, other investigators have questioned the existence of a clear-cut iron concentration threshold for the development of fibrosis and/or cirrhosis (Sallie et al., 1991; Deugnier et al., 1992). Use of the hepatic iron concentration to assist in patient evaluation is carried one step further by the calculation of the hepatic iron index (HII). The HII is useful in differentiating patients with homozygous haemochromatosis from heterozygotes or from patients with chronic liver disease and secondary iron overload (Bassett et al., 1986; Bonkovsky et al., 1990; Olynyk et al., 1990; Summers et al., 1990; Sallie et al., 1991) (see Chapters 8 and 14).

3. ANIMAL MODELS OF IRON OVERLOAD

It is difficult to mimic the pathology and pathophysiology of a human disease with an animal 'model'. In the case of HHC, there may never be a true 'model', since the disease is a genetic one which occurs in humans and takes, on average, 40–50 years for full expression. Nonetheless, in order to understand the biochemistry of iron overload and the mechanisms of tissue injury resulting from chronic iron overload, several experimental 'models' have been developed. These include administration of parenteral iron chelates such as iron-dextran or iron-sorbitol, and the infusion of heat-treated red blood cells, both of which approximate the hepatic distribution of iron seen in parenteral or transfusional iron overload. Enteral models of iron overload include the supplementation of diets with carbonyl iron or ferrocene, and a cyclic feeding and starvation protocol using a diet containing large amounts of ferric ammonium citrate. The congenital hypotransferrinaemic mouse model has provided insights into the role of circulating nontransferrin-bound iron in iron overload. Naturally occurring iron overload in animals is found in mynah birds, quetzals, birds of paradise, starlings and reindeer. For all of the experimental models of hepatic iron overload, the ultimate demonstration of fibrosis and/or cirrhosis would be ideal, since this represents the full pathological expression of the hepatic manifestations of haemochromatosis in humans.

3.1. Use of Iron Chelates

Various types of iron chelates have been utilized to produce chronic hepatic iron overload, the two most common being iron-dextran and iron-sorbitol. After administration of iron chelates, iron is initially found predominantly in Kupffer cells in the liver in a panlobular distribution (Plate 5), whereas, at later time periods, there is a significant increase in the amount of iron within hepatocytes (Golberg *et al.*, 1957; Pechet, 1969).

Typically, use of parenteral iron chelates to study the hepatic biochemistry and pathophysiology of chronic iron overload has been limited by the fact that the iron deposition within Kupffer cells is relatively non-toxic, and long-term complications (fibrosis, cirrhosis) are difficult to produce. Recently, Carthew *et al.* (1991b) have shown that fibrosis and cirrhosis develop in gerbils just three months after a single injection of iron-dextran. The susceptibility of gerbils to iron-induced fibrosis was first observed when chronic exposure to endotoxin led to intrahepatic haemorrhage with subsequent iron deposition (Carthew *et al.*, 1991a). The mechanisms responsible for the strong profibrogenic effect of iron in the livers of gerbils are not known.

Iron administered as ferric nitrilotriacetate (FeNTA) has also been used as a model of iron overload (Awai *et al.*, 1979; May *et al.*, 1980; Bacon *et al.*, 1983b; Preece *et al.*, 1989). Here, hepatic storage iron is found in both hepatocytes and RE cells. Injection regimens are usually five out of seven days per week and result in moderate degrees of hepatic iron overload with associated lipid peroxidation (Bacon *et al.*, 1983b; Preece *et al.*, 1989). The glucosuria demonstrated with FeNTA treatment is not due to pancreatic iron deposition with subsequent destruction of β-cells and reduction in insulin release, but, rather, is due to nephrotoxicity through a peroxidative mechanism (Hamazaki *et al.*, 1985; Toyokuni *et al.*, 1990). Additionally, with chronic FeNTA treatment, renal adenocarcinoma develops, and several studies on the carcinogenic potential of this compound have been performed (Okada *et al.*, 1983; Ebina *et al.*, 1986; Li *et al.*, 1987). This form of iron loading is no longer used to study hepatic pathology, because it is tedious (daily injection regimen), hepatic iron levels do not reach those seen in haemochromatosis, and abdominal wall and intraabdominal abscesses frequently develop.

3.2. Dietary Iron Overload

Since iron accumulation in HHC results from an increase in intestinal iron absorption, several experimental models have been based on the approach of increasing the amount of iron in the diet, thereby increasing the total amount of iron absorbed from the gastrointestinal tract. Richter (1974) described experiments in which rats were fed a diet supplemented with ferric ammonium citrate in a cyclic starvation and refeeding regimen over a six-month period of time. This resulted in hepatic iron concentrations roughly comparable to those seen in human HHC, and iron was found in a periportal distribution predominantly in hepatocytes, but was also present in Kupffer cells and sinusoidal cells. No biochemical studies were performed, and no fibrosis occurred.

Longueville and Crichton (1986) have used a ferrocene derivative (3,5,5-trimethyl-hexanoyl ferrocene) added to diets to produce massive hepatic iron overload, again with a lobular and cellular distribution comparable to that seen in human HHC. An advantage of the ferrocene model is that very high hepatic iron concentrations can be achieved over a short time period without substantial growth retardation. The ferrocene model results in an increased number of iron-loaded lysosomes within hepatocytes, and there is an increase in lysosomal enzyme activities and fragility (Ward et al., 1991). Düllmann et al. (1992) have recently reported that long-term dietary supplementation with ferrocene-iron results in significant perisinusoidal fibrosis as well as portal fibrosis in rats.

Perhaps the model that has been used most over the last ten years is the carbonyl iron-loading model first described by Bacon et al. (1983b). Carbonyl iron is a form of elemental iron (Fe°) in microspheres ($<5\,\mu$m) and has been used as a food supplement. Bioavailability of carbonyl iron is higher than with other forms of elemental iron (Sacks and Houchin, 1978), and absorption studies have shown that gastric acid is necessary to solubilize the iron in the stomach and upper gut (Heubers et al., 1986). Intestinal iron absorption is increased, presumably via normal pathways, resulting in fully saturated transferrin and the presence of nontransferrin-bound iron in the portal circulation. No evidence of persorption or transfer of intact elemental iron as carbonyl iron across the gut has been demonstrated.

When diets supplemented with carbonyl iron are administered to weanling rats, hepatic iron deposition occurs quickly, resulting in a periportal or perilobular distribution with iron found predominantly in hepatocytes (Plate 6) (Bacon et al., 1983b; Park et al., 1987). With a three- to four-month period of feeding, concentrations comparable to that seen in human disease are readily achieved (Fig. 10.1). After longer periods of dietary supplementation with carbonyl iron, siderotic nodules comprised of necrotic iron-loaded hepatocytes, macrophages and Kupffer cells are found (Plate 7) (Park et al., 1987); these siderotic nodules are not seen in human HHC. Additionally, splenic iron overload occurs, which is another feature not seen in HHC. At 8 and 12 months, fibrosis and early cirrhosis are present (Plate 8) (Park et al., 1987). In studies by Pietrangelo et al. (1990b), histological evidence of septal fibrosis and increased levels of procollagen I mRNA were demonstrated after only two months of iron loading in female Wistar rats, suggesting that there may be a strain- or sex-dependent sensitivity to iron overload.

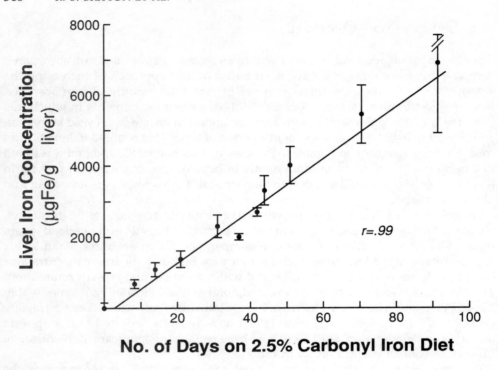

Fig. 10.1 Hepatic iron concentrations in dietary carbonyl iron overload in the rat. Hepatic iron levels increase with the duration of feeding on the iron-supplemented diet.

Numerous biochemical studies have been performed using this model of iron overload and are described elsewhere in this chapter. The advantage of this model is that the route of iron loading is enteral, which is analogous to the situation in human HHC, and the lobular and cellular distribution of iron and the hepatic iron concentrations are all comparable to those seen in HHC. A disadvantage is that there is growth retardation in the iron-supplemented animals and thus appropriate controls must be included in all studies.

3.3. Congenital Hypotransferrinaemic Mouse

Kaplan and coworkers have described the pathological features of congenitally hypotransferrinaemic mice (Craven et al., 1987; Kaplan et al., 1988). Over time, iron deposition occurs in parenchymal cells of the liver, pancreas and heart. Iron also accumulates in the renal tubules and in medullary cells of the adrenal glands. This pattern of distribution of tissue iron mimics that seen in patients with HHC and suggests that a major pathway by which parenchymal cells become iron loaded is through the uptake of non-transferrin-bound iron. Morphologic studies and studies of iron metabolism have been performed in these animals, but no studies of biochemical hepatotoxicity have been reported, and fibrosis has not been demonstrated.

3.4. Naturally Occurring Iron Overload

Mynah birds, starlings, birds of paradise, quetzals and Svalbard reindeer have been shown to develop iron overload in nature (Lowestine and Petrak, 1978; Randell et al., 1981; Gosselin and Kramer, 1983; Gosselin et al., 1983; Borch-Iohnsen et al., 1988). The reasons for this are unclear but are thought to be due to dietary ingestion of iron-containing materials. Hepatic fibrosis and hepatocellular carcinoma are commonly associated with iron overload in birds. No toxicity studies have been performed, and it is unlikely that prospective controlled studies of toxicity and fibrogenesis will be undertaken in these species.

3.5. Summary

In summary, several types of animal models have been utilized to study the consequences of iron overload. When iron chelates such as iron-dextran are used, iron is found predominantly in Kupffer cells in the liver, and little toxicity results. Models of dietary iron overload result in hepatic parenchymal iron deposition with a periportal predominance. This more closely mimics hepatic iron overload in hereditary haemochromatosis. The dietary carbonyl iron loading method has been widely used to study hepatic iron metabolism, hepatotoxicity and fibrogenesis.

4. PROPOSED MECHANISMS OF IRON TOXICITY

Clinical evidence for tissue damage caused by iron excess has been provided by studies of patients with HHC (Bomford and Williams, 1976; Powell et al., 1980; Niederau et al., 1985; Bassett et al., 1986; Tavill and Bacon, 1986), African iron overload (Isaacson et al., 1961; Bothwell and Isaacson, 1962), and secondary iron overload due to β-thalassaemia (Barry et al., 1974; Risdon et al., 1975; Cohen et al., 1984a,b). In these conditions, correlation between liver iron concentration and the occurrence of liver injury has been demonstrated, and therapeutic reduction of hepatic iron by either phlebotomy or chelation therapy has resulted in clinical improvement. In addition to the known association of chronic iron overload with hepatic fibrosis and cirrhosis, there is now sufficient clinical evidence to support an association between cirrhosis due to haemochromatosis and the development of hepatocellular carcinoma (Bradbear et al., 1985; Niederau et al., 1985). Despite the convincing clinical evidence for the hepatotoxicity of excess iron, the specific pathophysiological mechanisms for hepatocellular injury, hepatic fibrosis and hepatocellular carcinoma in hepatic iron overload are poorly understood (see Chapter 11).

4.1. Lipid Peroxidation and Free Radical-mediated Injury

Several mechanisms whereby excess hepatic iron causes cellular injury with resultant fibrosis and cirrhosis have been proposed (Fig. 10.2). Iron-induced peroxidative injury

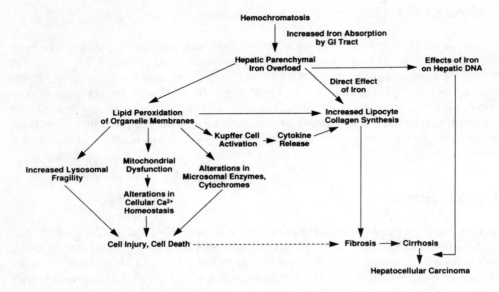

Fig. 10.2 Proposed mechanisms of hepatic injury in chronic iron overload.

to polyunsaturated fatty acids of membrane phospholipids is a potentially unifying mechanism underlying the several major theories of cellular injury and fibrogenesis in chronic iron overload (Bacon and Britton, 1989, 1990).

4.1.1. *Subcellular Organelles In Vitro*

It is clear from work *in vitro* that ionic iron (usually with a reductant present) stimulates lipid peroxidation. When isolated subcellular organelles are incubated with ionic iron, extensive structural and functional damage is produced by iron-induced peroxidative decomposition of membrane lipids. Some of the wide-ranging effects of iron-induced lipid peroxidation on isolated lysosomes, microsomes and mitochondria are summarized in Table 10.1. The two main consequences of lipid peroxidation which cause these multiple effects appear to be (a) membrane disruption and distortion which alters permeability and changes the activity of membrane-dependent enzymes and (b) the toxicity of lipid peroxides and their aldehydic breakdown products.

4.1.2. *Isolated Hepatocytes*

When isolated hepatocytes in suspension are incubated with iron salts, lipid peroxidation begins quickly (Table 10.2). However, decreases in viability (indicated by release of enzymes or uptake of trypan blue dye) may not occur until more than 2 h after the start of lipid peroxidation. Therefore, in experiments in which short incubation times are used, there is an apparent dissociation between the occurrence of lipid peroxidation and a decrease in viability, and this has led some investigators to question whether lipid peroxidation is cytotoxic. However, it is now clear from

Table 10.1. Iron-induced lipid peroxidation: effects on organelles *in vitro*

Organelle	Observation	References
Lysosomes	Decreased lysosomal latency	Fong *et al.*, 1973; Mak and Weglicki, 1985
Microsomes	Decreased cytochrome P-450	De Matteis and Sparks, 1973; Högberg *et al.*, 1973; Levin *et al.*, 1973; Cheeseman *et al.*, 1984
	Decreased drug metabolizing activities	Wills, 1972; Högberg *et al.*, 1973
	Decreased calcium sequestration	Lowrey *et al.*, 1981; Waller *et al.*, 1983
	Fragmentation	Högberg *et al.*, 1973
Mitochondria	Decreased respiratory control ratio	McKnight and Hunter, 1966; Bacon *et al.*, 1986b
	Uncoupling	McKnight and Hunter, 1966; Pfeifer and McCay, 1972
	Decreased transmembrane potential	Marshansky *et al.*, 1983; Masini *et al.*, 1985
	Increased potassium efflux	Vladimirov *et al.*, 1980
	Increased calcium release	Masini *et al.*, 1985
	Swelling	Hunter *et al.*, 1963; Pfeifer and McCay, 1972; Vladimirov *et al.*, 1980

experiments carried out for longer periods of time that exposure of hepatocytes to iron can reduce hepatocyte viability (Table 10.2). This decrease in viability seems to be the result of lipid peroxidation, since the effects of iron on both lipid peroxidation and viability were attenuated in hepatocytes isolated from rats which had been pretreated with α-tocopherol (Poli *et al.*, 1986).

A study using hepatocytes isolated from carbonyl iron-loaded rats (Plate 9) has shown strong correlations between increased lipid peroxidation (production of malondialdehyde) and hepatocyte cytotoxicity as measured by enzyme leakage and loss of cell viability (Sharma *et al.*, 1990). In these experiments, increased lipid peroxidation was apparent after 2 h of incubation, a time at which viability was still normal. At 3 and 4 h, however, lipid peroxidation had increased further, and viability was reduced to approximately 40% of control. When iron chelators (desferrioxamine or apotransferrin) or an antioxidant (α-tocopherol) were added to the isolated iron-loaded hepatocytes, there was attenuation of lipid peroxidation, reduction in enzyme leakage and improvement in cell viability to control values. Fletcher *et al.* (1989) have also observed increased malondialdehyde production by hepatocytes isolated from carbonyl iron-loaded rats and placed in culture.

The delayed effect of iron-induced lipid peroxidation on the viability of isolated hepatocytes could be explained in a number of ways. Intact cells, as opposed to isolated organelles, may be able to repair peroxidative damage to lipids by energy-dependent processes (e.g. reacylation pathways) (Ungemach, 1987); the capacity for repair may need to be overwhelmed before damage becomes evident. Alternatively, lipid peroxidation may be responsible for creating a situation in which a secondary mechanism occurs which is ultimately responsible for loss of cell viability. Studies by Ungemach (1985, 1987) have shown an increase in phospholipase A_2 activity following iron-induced peroxidative damage to hepatocyte lipids. The resultant

Table 10.2 Effects of iron on isolated rat hepatocytes*

Form of iron	Concentration	Duration of experiment	Observations	References
Fe^{3+}/ADP	0.1/2.5 mM (Fe^{3+}/ADP)	4 h	Increased TBA-reactants Increased LDH release (only at 2–4 h) Both of these effects were attenuated when the rat was pretreated with α-tocopherol	Poli et al., 1986
	45/750 µM	2 h	Increased TBA-reactants Increased lipid conjugated dienes Decreased viability (trypan blue staining) Decreased intracellular K^+ Decreased unsaturated fatty acid content Increased lysophosphatide content	Ungemach, 1985
	0.187/5 mM	20–60 min	Increased TBA-reactants Decreased LDH latency Decreased glucose-6-phosphatase Decreased alprenolol metabolism No change in cytochrome P-450 No change in NADPH-cytochrome c reductase	Högberg et al., 1975a,b
	0.2/5 mM	1 h	Increased TBA-reactants Increased lipid conjugated dienes Decreased viability (trypan blue staining) Increased LDH release Decreased glucose-6-phosphatase	Poli et al., 1983
	0.1/2.5 mM	1 h	Increased TBA-reactants No change in viability (trypan blue staining) No change in LDH release No change in glucose-6-phosphatase	Poli et al., 1983
	0.08/6.7 mM	15 or 30 min	Increased TBA-reactants Increased lipid conjugated dienes (30 min) No change in ALT release	Stacey and Priestley, 1978

Compound	Concentration	Time	Effects	Reference
Fe³⁺	100 μM	1 h	Increased TBA-reactants No change in viability (trypan blue staining)	Poli et al., 1983 Poli et al., 1983
			Decreased cytochrome P-450[†] Decreased lipoprotein secretion[†] No change in glucose-6-phosphatase No change in ornithine decarboxylase No change in protein secretion	Poli et al., 1983 Poli and Gravela, 1982 Poli and Gravela, 1982 Poli and Gravela, 1982 Poli and Gravela, 1982
	100 μM	3 h	Increased TBA reactants No change in viability (trypan blue staining) Increased cytosolic free Ca²⁺ Increased total cell Ca²⁺ No change in Ca²⁺-ATPase activity Decreased mitochondrial membrane potential These effects were attenuated by anti-oxidants	Albano et al., 1991
	200, 400 or 1000 μM	20 or 45 min	Increased TBA-reactants No change in AST release Decreased intracellular K⁺ (1000 μM Fe³⁺ at 45 min)	Stacey and Klaassen, 1981
Fe³⁺-NTA	100 μM	1 h	Increased TBA-reactants Increased ethane and chemiluminescence Little change (<10%) in viability (trypan blue staining) (at times beyond 1 h, there was a concentration-dependent decrease in viability)	Goddard et al., 1986
	5, 20 or 100 μM	1–48 h	Increased TBA-reactants Increased LDH release Increased AST release Increased ALT release	Morel et al., 1990
Iron/ascorbate	0.4/1.0 mM	2 h	Increased TBA-reactants No change in LDH release Small decrease in glutathione	Rush et al., 1985

*ALT, alanine aminotransferase; AST, aspartate aminotransferase; LDH, lactate dehydrogenase; NTA, nitrilotriacetate; TBA, thiobarbituric acid. [†]These effects were not changed in the presence of promethazine, which blocks the increase in TBA-reactants. Adapted from Bacon and Britton (1989).

increase in lysophosphatides which lags behind the lipid peroxidation may be involved in the loss of cellular viability.

Thus, addition of iron to either isolated subcellular organelles or to isolated hepatocytes clearly causes lipid peroxidation with associated functional abnormalities (Tables 10.1 and 10.2). Evidence for iron-induced lipid peroxidation with functional consequences in humans with iron overload or in experimental iron overload will be described in greater detail.

4.1.3. Evidence for Lipid Peroxidation in Humans with Iron Overload

There is a paucity of data regarding lipid peroxidation in patients with iron overload. Peters et al. (1985a) reported elevated plasma levels of thiobarbituric acid (TBA)-reactants in patients with iron overload who had detectable 'catalytic' or 'free' iron in their plasma (six of 14 patients studied). However, other indices of lipid peroxidation (diene and triene conjugates, fluorescence in lipid extracts) were not changed in the plasma of these patients. Young et al. (1992) have compared the plasma levels of malondialdehyde and antioxidants in 15 patients with HHC and 15 matched controls. Plasma malondialdehyde levels were increased in the HHC group, while the plasma concentrations of α-tocopherol, retinol and ascorbate were decreased. These data support the concept that patients with HHC have increased oxidant stress.

Heys and Dormandy (1981) observed that homogenates of iron-loaded spleens from patients with thalassaemia produced greater amounts of TBA-reactants and fluorescent products than those from patients without iron overload, when incubated in vitro. The iron concentrations in the overloaded spleens were elevated by 2- to 30-fold; homogenates with a low α-tocopherol content showed a greater tendency to peroxidize. These results do not allow conclusions to be drawn as to whether lipid perodixation occurred in vivo in these iron-loaded spleens. Interestingly, the authors noted that, in five of the six iron-loaded spleens, there was an inverse correlation between iron content and the α-tocopherol concentration. This suggests that there was an association between iron overload and depletion of tissue α-tocopherol in these patients, but whether iron-induced lipid peroxidation played a role in the α-tocopherol depletion is not known.

Several studies have shown that erythrocytes from iron-loaded thalassaemic patients show an increased susceptibility to in vitro lipid peroxidation when exposed to a peroxide challenge (Stocks et al., 1972; Zannos-Mariolea et al., 1974; Rachmilewitz, 1976; Rachmilewitz et al., 1976). Although an elevated iron content may contribute to this susceptibility (Rachmilewitz, 1976), other factors such as an increase in lipid content, the presence of precipitated haemoglobins, and low α-tocopherol levels may also be important (Rachmilewitz et al., 1976). It is not known if lipid peroxidation occurs in vivo in erythrocytes of these patients. However, serum α-tocopherol levels are reduced in some patients with thalassaemia (Stocks et al., 1972; Zannos-Mariolea et al., 1974; Rachmilewitz et al., 1976), and the possibility of therapeutic supplementation with α-tocopherol to improve erythrocyte stability has been suggested (Zannos-Mariolea et al., 1974; Rachmilewitz, 1976). The observation that arachidonate makes up a smaller percentage of erythrocyte fatty acids in thalassaemic patients (Rachmilewitz et al., 1976) is in agreement with the concept of increased peroxidation, but could also be explained as a constitutive change in membrane composition unrelated to lipid peroxidation.

Despite these data, the key question of whether lipid peroxidation occurs *in vivo* in the tissues of patients with iron overload has not been fully resolved. A number of approaches might prove useful to address this question. Ethane and pentane exhalation could be measured in patients with iron overload and might serve as a useful index of lipid perodixation after appropriate correction for the metabolic disposition of these gases. This approach has been used in alcoholic patients (Moscarella *et al.*, 1984). If tissue samples are available from surgical procedures, they could be frozen rapidly and analysed for their content of lipid conjugated dienes, fluorescent products, and lipid hydroperoxides and hydroxy acids. This technique has recently provided data supportive of peroxidative damage in hepatic copper overload (Sokol *et al.*, 1992). The new sensitive and specific methods for measuring lipid hydroperoxides and hydroxy acids may allow analysis of small tissue samples such as liver biopsies and may be able to detect low levels of these products if they circulate in the blood (Thomas *et al.*, 1991). In addition, specific antibodies against aldehyde–protein adducts have been used to detect elevated levels of these complexes in plasma and liver samples from iron-loaded rats (Houglum *et al.*, 1990) and could be used with human samples.

4.1.4. *Evidence for Lipid Peroxidation in Experimental Iron Overload*

The evidence indicating that lipid peroxidation occurs *in vivo* in experimental iron overload is substantial (Table 10.3) and includes the detection of a number of different peroxidation products.

(a) *Lipid conjugated dienes.* The polyunsaturated fatty acids of membrane phospholipids can be readily attacked by free radicals, initiating the process of lipid peroxidation. The hydrogen atoms on the methylene carbons separating the double bonds in polyunsaturated fatty acids are particularly susceptible to abstraction by free radicals (Holman, 1954), generating a lipid free radical (L$^{\cdot}$). A proportion of these lipid free radicals can undergo a resonance shift of the free radical electron, before reacting with molecular oxygen to form a lipid peroxyl free radical (LOO$^{\cdot}$). This resonance shift generates lipid species with a conjugated diene structure which are quite stable (Srinivasan and Recknagel, 1971; Bacon *et al.*, 1983a). Conjugated dienes can be detected spectrophotometrically in lipids extracted from biological samples by a characteristic increase in absorption in the 230–235 nm region (Recknagel and Glende, 1984). An advantage of this procedure is that it allows the sites of *in vivo* lipid peroxidation to be localized down to the level of the subcellular organelles. For example, after carbon tetrachloride administration, high levels of lipid conjugated dienes are found in the hepatic microsomal fraction, while levels in the mitochondrial fraction are low (Rao and Recknagel, 1968).

The lipid conjugated diene technique has been used to examine whether lipid peroxidation occurs *in vivo* in hepatic mitochondria and microsomes in experimental iron overload (Bacon *et al.*, 1983a,b, 1985, 1986a, 1989; Masini *et al.*, 1989; Wu *et al.*, 1990). Bacon *et al.* (1983a,b) initially used two methods to achieve chronic iron overload in rats: (1) daily intraperitoneal injection of FeNTA and (2) dietary supplementation with carbonyl iron. With both treatment protocols, increased

Table 10.3 Lipid perodixation in experimental iron overload

Model	Organ	Observations*	References
Dietary carbonyl iron	Liver	Conjugated dienes	Bacon et al., 1983a,b, 1985, 1986a, 1989; Masini et al., 1989; Wu et al., 1990
		TBA-reactants	Fletcher et al., 1989; Britton et al., 1990b; Houglum et al., 1990; Myers et al., 1991
		4-hydroxynonenal	Brown et al., 1991
		MDA–protein adducts	Houglum et al., 1990
		Fluorescent products	Houglum et al., 1990; Parkkila et al., 1992
	Plasma	MDA–protein adducts	Houglum et al., 1990
		HNE–protein adducts	Houglum et al., 1990
	Urine	TBA-reactants	Wu et al., 1990
Dietary iron–fumarate	Liver	Ethane	Younes et al., 1989
		TBA-reactants	Younes et al., 1990
Parenteral iron chelates	Liver	Ethane, pentane	Dillard and Tappel, 1979
		Conjugated dienes	Bacon et al., 1983a
		TBA-reactants	Golberg et al., 1962; Hultcrantz et al., 1984b
	Kidney	TBA-reactants	Golberg et al., 1962; Hultcrantz et al., 1984b
	Muscle	TBA-reactants	Golberg et al., 1962
	Skin	TBA-reactants	Golberg et al., 1962

*HNE, 4-hydroxynonenal; MDA, malondialdehyde; TBA, thiobarbituric acid.

amounts of lipid conjugated dienes were observed in hepatic mitochondria; evidence for increased microsomal lipid peroxidation was observed at higher hepatic iron concentrations which were only reached with the carbonyl iron-supplemented diet (Bacon et al., 1983a,b).

The relationship between hepatic non-haem iron concentration and the presence of lipid peroxidation was examined in rats fed dietary carbonyl iron for increasing lengths of time in order to achieve a wide range of hepatic iron levels (Bacon et al., 1983a,b, 1985, 1986a). In these studies, mitochondrial lipid peroxidation occurred in animals when the hepatic non-haem iron concentration exceeded 1000 μg/g (wet wt). In contrast, elevated levels of lipid conjugated dienes were not found in microsomes until the hepatic iron concentration exceeded 2000 μg/g. These results support the concept that a critical threshold of hepatic parenchymal iron loading must be exceeded before lipid peroxidation occurs and indicate that hepatic mitochondria undergo peroxidation at lower hepatic iron concentrations than do microsomes. Masini et al. (1989) have also found increased levels of conjugated dienes in mitochondrial lipids isolated from the livers of rats with dietary iron overload.

Tangerås (1983) did not find an increase in lipid conjugated dienes in hepatic mitochondria from rats treated with Jectofer or FeNTA. These results may be explained by the fact that the mean hepatic non-haem iron concentrations were only 924 and 722 μg/g wet wt, respectively, which were below the threshold level reported for mitochondrial lipid peroxidation (Bacon et al., 1983a,b). Wu et al. (1990) have confirmed the presence of elevated levels of conjugated dienes in hepatic microsomes and also reported increased amounts of urinary thiobarbituric acid-reactants in rats fed dietary carbonyl iron. Mitochondrial lipid peroxidation was not examined in this study.

(b) *Thiobarbituric acid-reactive products and 4-hydroxynonenal.* The thiobarbituric acid (TBA) test has been used to estimate the extent of lipid peroxidation in tissues, isolated cells and organelles. This assay involves reacting a sample with TBA under acid conditions and elevated temperatures (80–100°C) and measuring the absorbance at 530–535 nm. In biological systems, malondialdehyde (a breakdown product of lipid peroxidation) appears to be the predominant TBA-reactant, although other substances can react with TBA and contribute to the absorbance at 535 nm (Halliwell and Gutteridge, 1990).

Four research groups have reported increased hepatic levels of TBA-reactants in rats fed dietary carbonyl iron (Fletcher et al., 1989; Britton et al., 1990b; Houglum et al., 1990; Myers et al., 1991). While Britton et al. (1990b) and Houglum et al. (1990) assayed whole liver tissue, Fletcher et al. (1989) measured levels in isolated hepatocytes, and Myers et al. (1991) determined the TBA-reactant levels in hepatic lysosomes. Brown et al. (1991) have used a gas chromatographic/mass spectrophotometric method to measure the hepatic levels of 4-hydroxynonenal, an aldehydic product of lipid peroxidation, in rats with dietary carbonyl overload: the hepatic concentration of this aldehyde was elevated several-fold.

Golberg et al. (1962) observed that mice and rats given repeated intramuscular injections of iron-dextran (total dose of 0.8–1.0 g Fe/kg) had elevated levels of TBA-reactants in liver, kidney, muscle and skin. No increases were seen at a lower dose of iron-dextran (30 mg Fe/kg). Tissue levels of iron were not reported in this study. Although these results suggest that iron-dextran, at a high enough dose, has a pro-oxidant action *in vivo*, the authors note that the diet used had a 'somewhat low tocopherol content' which might have increased the sensitivity of the animals to iron. This possibility is supported by the work of Fletcher *et al.* (1989) who used an α-tocopherol-replete diet and did not find an increase in TBA-reactants in hepatocytes isolated from rats injected with iron-dextran (total dose of approximately 1 g Fe/kg).

In rats receiving 15 intramuscular injections of iron–sorbitol–citric acid complex (Jectofer) with a total dose of 0.5 g Fe/kg, Hultcrantz *et al.* (1984b) found increased amounts of TBA-reactants in liver and kidney, but not in spleen. One group of animals was iron-depleted by weekly phlebotomies for a two-month period after the iron injections; this procedure reduced both the levels of iron and TBA-reactants in the liver, suggesting that iron was causally responsible for the production of the TBA-reactants.

Hanstein *et al.* (1975, 1981) reported elevated levels of TBA-reactants and iron in hepatic mitochondrial fractions isolated by differential centrifugation from rats treated with iron-dextran. In contrast, Tangerås (1983) did not find any difference in the amount of TBA-reactants in hepatic mitochondria isolated by density gradient centrifugation from rats injected with Jectofer or FeNTA. Tangerås went on to demonstrate that mitochondrial fractions prepared by differential centrifugation from the livers of iron-loaded rats were contaminated with iron-loaded lysosomes, while with density gradient centrifugation, a mitochondrial fraction could be isolated which had less lysosomal contamination and a much lower iron content (Tangerås, 1983). Therefore, it seems likely that, in the studies of Hanstein *et al.* (1975, 1981), the markedly increased non-haem iron content of the mitochondrial fraction from the iron-loaded rats was primarily due to contamination with iron-rich lysosomes. This additional iron in the mitochondrial fraction may have stimulated lipid peroxidation during the TBA assay itself, contributing to the increased level of TBA-reactants observed (Kirkpatrick *et al.*, 1986).

(c) *Aldehyde–protein adducts*. Lipid peroxidation can produce reactive aldehydic products such as malondialdehyde (MDA) and 4-hydroxynonenal (HNE), which can then form covalent bonds to proteins, phospholipids, and DNA (Esterbauer, 1985). In proteins, these aldehydes often bind to lysine residues. Houglum *et al.* (1990) have used antisera specific for MDA–lysine and HNE–lysine adducts to investigate whether these compounds are present in rats fed a diet containing carbonyl iron. They demonstrated by immunohistochemistry the presence of MDA–protein adducts in the cytosol of periportal hepatocytes, which co-localized with iron. In addition, MDA– and HNE–lysine adducts were detected in plasma proteins of the iron-loaded rats. It is not known whether aldehyde–protein adduct formation leads to cellular injury, but *in vitro*, the binding of aldehydes to some proteins can inhibit their function (Esterbauer, 1985).

(d) *Fluorescent products*. Lipid peroxidation results in the production of fluorescent products, derived mainly from cross-linked phospholipids (Fletcher *et al.*, 1973). In rats with dietary iron overload, an increase in fluorescent products has been demonstrated within the liver in the areas of greatest iron deposition (periportal) (Houglum *et al.*, 1990; Parkkila *et al.*, 1992), and the amount of these products was reduced by α-tocopherol supplementation (Parkkila *et al.*, 1992).

(e) *Ethane and pentane*. Ethane and pentane are volatile products produced during lipid peroxidation by the breakdown of Ω-3- and Ω-6-unsaturated fatty acid hydroperoxides, respectively (Dumelin and Tappel, 1977). Measurement of ethane

(a)

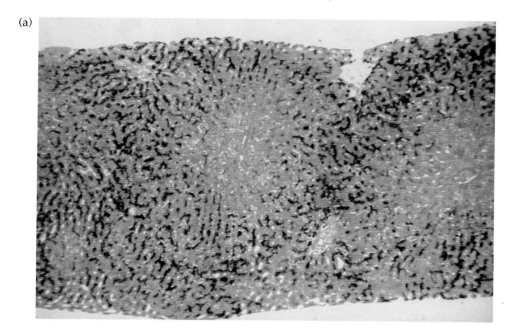

(b)

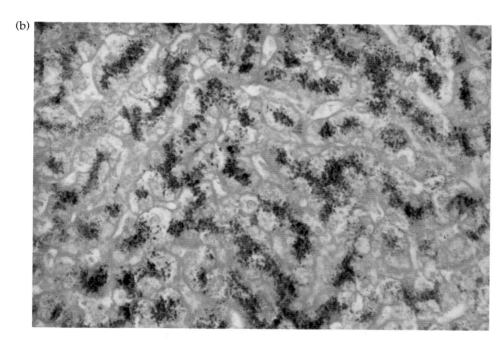

Plate 1 Hepatic iron distribution in early hereditary haemochromatosis. These photomicrographs are from a liver biopsy from a 32-year-old male with newly diagnosed HHC. The hepatic iron concentration was 17 300 μg/g (dry wt). (a) Excess storage iron is found in a periportal distribution (Perls' Prussian blue, ×100). (b) The iron is located primarily within hepatocytes (Perls' Prussian blue, ×400).

(a)

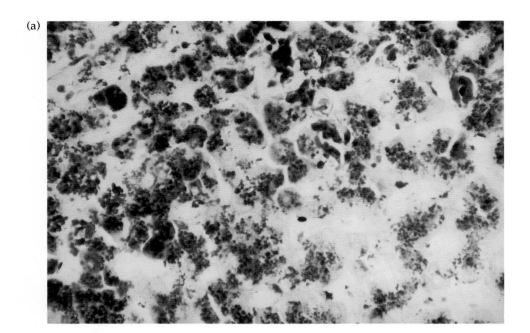

(b)

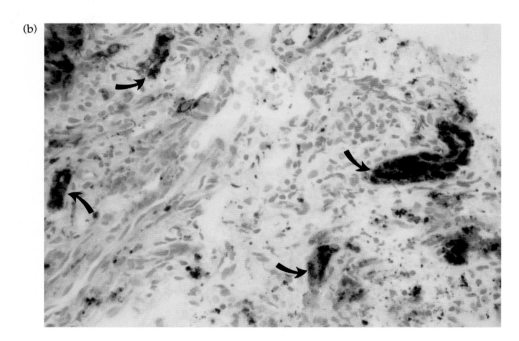

Plate 2 Hepatic iron distribution in advanced hereditary haemochromatosis. This photomicrograph (2a) is from a liver biopsy from a 58-year-old male with newly diagnosed HHC. The hepatic iron concentration was 41 040 µg/g (dry wt). (a) Iron deposition is found in hepatocytes throughout the hepatic lobule, but the periportal to pericentral gradient is maintained (Perls' Prussian blue, ×400). (b) Iron is present in bile ductular cells (arrows) within the fibrous septa of a cirrhotic liver (see Plate 4) (Perls' Prussian blue, ×100).

(a)

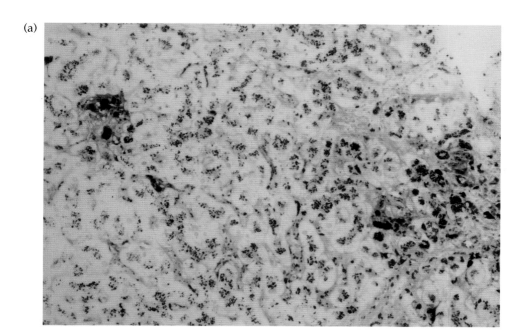

(b)

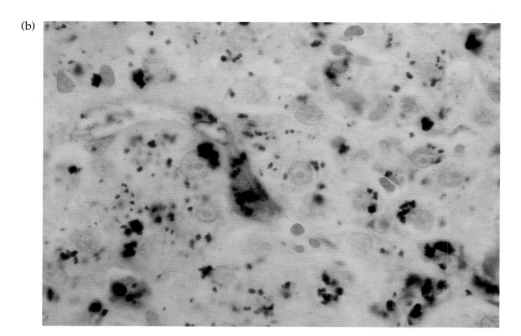

Plate 3 Hepatic iron distribution in transfusional iron overload. These photomicrographs are from a liver biopsy from a 19-year-old male with sickle cell anaemia, who had received multiple blood transfusions. The hepatic iron concentration was 20 400 µg/g (dry wt). (a) Excess storage iron is seen in a panlobular distribution and (b) is found predominantly in Kupffer cells (Perls' Prussian blue, ×100, ×400, respectively).

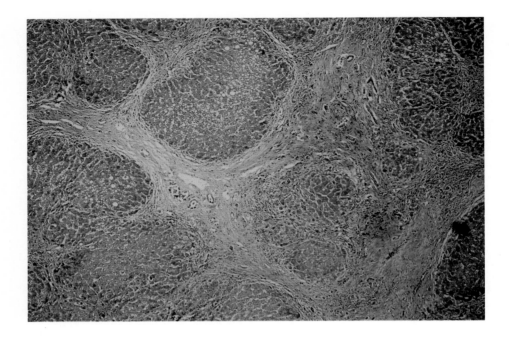

Plate 4 Micronodular cirrhosis in hereditary haemochromatosis (Masson-trichrome stain ×40). This photomicrograph is from an explant liver from a 56-year-old woman who underwent successful orthoptic liver transplantation for HHC.

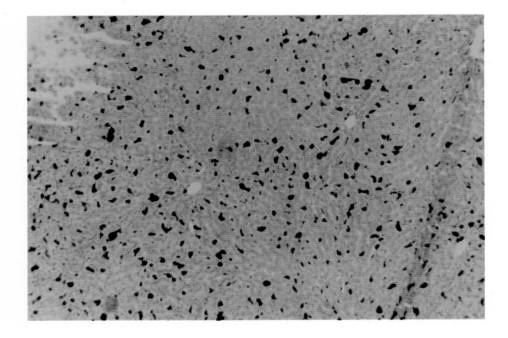

Plate 5 Hepatic iron distribution after iron–dextran administration in the rat. Storage iron is found predominantly in Kupffer cells, 48 hours after intraperitoneal administration of iron–dextran (Perls' Prussian blue, ×100).

(a)

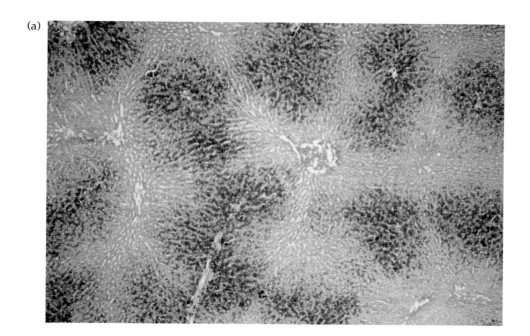

(b)

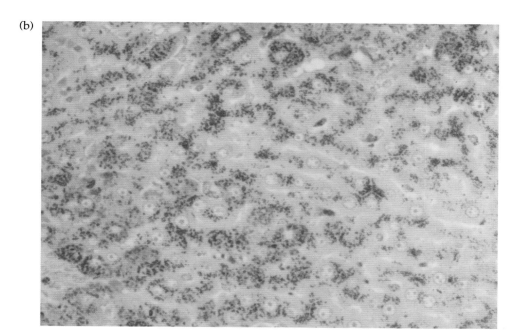

Plate 6 Hepatic iron overload after dietary carbonyl iron in the rat. This animal received a diet supplemented with 2.5% (w/w) carbonyl iron for 8 weeks. The hepatic iron concentration was 3245 µg/g (wet wt) or 9735 µg/g (dry wt). (a) Storage iron is seen in a periportal distribution and (b) is primarily within hepatocytes (Perls' Prussian blue, ×100, ×400, respectively).

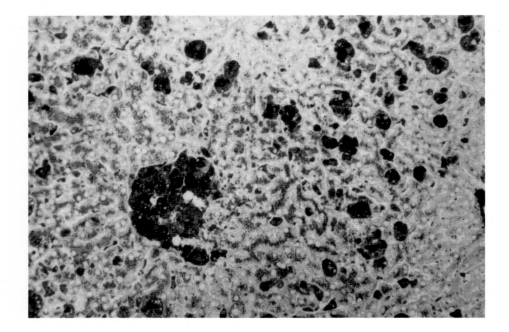

Plate 7 Siderotic nodules in rat liver after chronic dietary carbonyl iron overload. These animals (Plates 7 and 8) received the carbonyl iron-supplemented diet for 12 months. The hepatic iron concentration was 8340 µg/g (wet wt) or 25 020 µg/g (dry wt). After long-term dietary iron overload, siderotic nodules comprised of necrotic iron-loaded hepatocytes, macrophages and Kupffer cells are found in rat liver (Perls' Prussian blue, ×100).

(a)

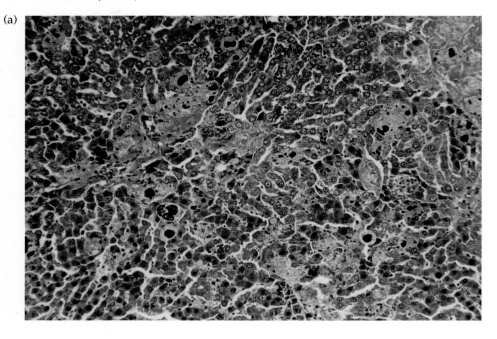

Plate 8a *Caption opposite.*

(b)

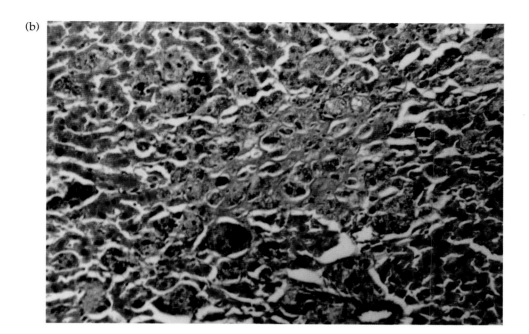

(c)

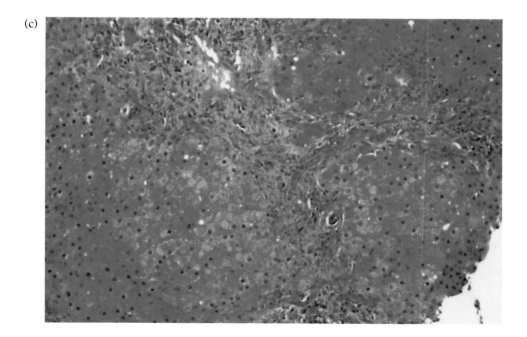

Plate 8 Hepatic fibrosis after chronic dietary carbonyl iron overload in the rat. After 8 to 12 months of iron loading, (a) hepatic fibrosis is seen in portal areas, (b) encircling hepatocytes, and (c) forming early cirrhosis (Masson-trichrome stain, ×100, ×400, ×100, respectively).

(a)

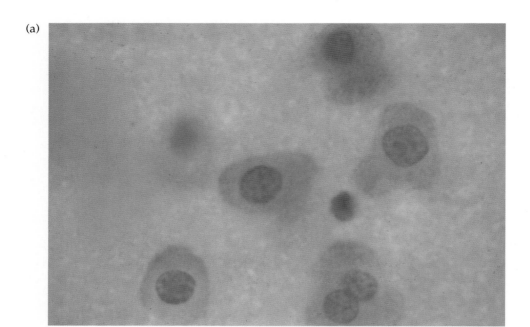

(b)

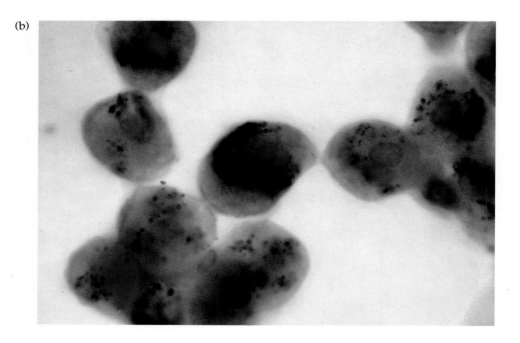

Plate 9 Storage iron in isolated hepatocytes from (a) control and (b) carbonyl iron-loaded rats. In the iron-loaded hepatocytes, storage iron has a punctate distribution, representing heavily iron-loaded lysosomes (siderosomes) (Perls' Prussian blue, ×400, ×400, respectively).

and/or pentane levels in expired air has been used as an index of *in vivo* lipid peroxidation. Since these gases are metabolized, appropriate experiments are necessary to demonstrate that an increase in exhaled alkanes is due to an increase in production rather than to a decrease in metabolic elimination (Frank *et al.*, 1980; Filser *et al.*, 1983). Because pentane is metabolized more rapidly than ethane in rats, exhaled levels of pentane are more sensitive to factors which influence its metabolism; for this reason, ethane exhalation may be a more reliable indicator of lipid peroxidation in the rat (Filser *et al.*, 1983). While measurement of alkane exhalation allows the investigator to monitor lipid peroxidation in the living animal, it has the limitation that any observed increase in lipid peroxidation cannot easily be localized to specific sites (organ or organelle) in the body.

Dillard and Tappel (1979) reported that rats fed a standard laboratory diet and given multiple injections of iron-dextran (total dose 4.6 g Fe/kg) exhaled much more ethane and pentane than controls. Although metabolic elimination of these alkanes was not measured, the magnitude of the increases seen (four- to six-fold) argues for an increase in production. The effect of iron overload on alkane evolution was a prolonged one, lasting for several weeks after the last injection. This study clearly demonstrates that iron overload produced by large parenteral doses of iron-dextran increases lipid peroxidation in rats fed a diet containing an adequate level of α-tocopherol.

Tappel and his coworkers went on to show that α-tocopherol deficiency sensitizes rats to the pro-oxidant action of iron-dextran (Dillard *et al.*, 1984; Gavino *et al.*, 1985). Animals fed a diet deficient in α-tocopherol and injected with iron-dextran exhaled much greater amounts of alkanes than rats fed the same diet supplemented with α-tocopherol (Dillard *et al.*, 1984; Gavino *et al.*, 1985) or the synthetic antioxidants N,N'-diphenyl-p-phenylene-diamine or ethoxyquin (Dillard *et al.*, 1984). However, it is not clear if antioxidant supplementation of a diet already containing adequate levels of α-tocopherol would further dampen the ability of iron-dextran to stimulate lipid perodixation.

(f) *In vitro susceptibility to lipid peroxidation*. Incubation of liver homogenates from rats fed an iron-supplemented diet produced greater amounts of TBA-reactants than those from controls (Lee *et al.*, 1981). Isolated hepatic mitochondria from rats injected with iron–gluconate also exhibited increased rates of *in vitro* lipid peroxidation (Masini *et al.*, 1985). Homogenates of liver, kidney, muscle and skin (Golberg *et al.*, 1962) as well as isolated hepatic microsomes (Wills, 1972; Dillard and Tappel, 1979) from animals injected with iron-dextran peroxidized more rapidly than those from controls. Tissue slices of liver, kidney, heart, lung, diaphragm and testes (but not those from brain and intestine) taken from α-tocopherol-deficient rats injected with iron-dextran all released more ethane and pentane than those from controls when incubated *in vitro* (Gavino *et al.*, 1984). While showing that iron overload results in an increase in *in vitro* susceptibility to lipid peroxidation, these studies do not allow conclusions to be drawn as to whether iron-induced peroxidation had occurred *in vivo*.

4.2. Subcellular Damage in Liver

4.2.1. *Iron Overload in Humans*

Peters and coworkers have proposed that iron overload results in an acquired lysosomal storage disease wherein iron accumulation in lysosomes increases their fragility, resulting in the release of hydrolytic enzymes into the cytoplasm, with the resultant initiation of cell damage (Peters and Seymour, 1976; Seymour and Peters, 1978; Selden et al., 1980a; Peters et al., 1985b). These investigators observed that the activities of several lysosomal enzymes, including N-acetyl-β-glucosaminidase (NAGA) and acid phosphatase, are increased in liver biopsies of patients with iron overload (Peters and Seymour, 1976; Seymour and Peters, 1978). These increases may result from lysosomal proliferation and distension (Peters et al., 1985b; Stål et al., 1990). When lysosomal fragility was determined in homogenates of these biopsies, there was a reduction in latent (membrane-enclosed) NAGA activity, without a change in latent acid phosphatase activity (Peters and Seymour, 1976; Seymour and Peters, 1978), suggesting that there may be two populations of lysosomes in iron-overloaded livers: one population, rich in NAGA, which becomes more fragile, and the other, rich in acid phosphatase, which is relatively unaffected (Seymour and Peters, 1978). Interestingly, in patients with HHC who had their iron stores normalized by phlebotomy, the NAGA latency returned to normal, indicating that the increase in lysosomal fragility was iron-dependent (Seymour and Peters, 1978). Although it is not known if the lysosomal fragility observed in vitro reflects the situation in vivo, suggestive evidence comes from a study in thalassaemic patients where elevated serum NAGA levels were correlated with the degree of iron overload (as assessed by serum ferritin levels) (Frigerio et al., 1984). Stål et al. (1990) have performed ultrastructural studies on liver biopsies from patients with HHC and have observed that the lysosomal volume density in hepatocytes was increased and was correlated with the degree of iron overload: lysosomal volume density normalized following iron removal by phlebotomy.

One mechanism which may contribute to the increased lysosomal fragility found in iron overload is lipid peroxidation (O'Connell et al., 1985; Peters et al., 1985b). O'Connell et al. (1986b) have shown that ferritin iron, and especially haemosiderin iron, are increased in liver biopsies from patients with iron overload (about 10- and 100-fold, respectively). However, both ferritin and haemosiderin can stimulate lipid peroxidation in vitro at acidic pH without a reductant being necessary (O'Connell et al., 1985). Since lysosomes are an acidic organelle compartment, it is possible that intralysosomal lipid peroxidation initiated by ferritin or haemosiderin occurs in iron overload.

Haemosiderin is only about 20% as potent as ferritin in stimulating lipid peroxidation in vitro, expressed per unit iron content. On this basis, it has been suggested that conversion of ferritin to haemosiderin may have a relative cytoprotective effect by reducing the ability of iron to stimulate peroxidation (O'Connell et al., 1986b). However, in iron overload, since the total amount of haemosiderin increases disproportionately, its potential role in toxicity cannot be ruled out (Peters et al., 1985b).

Selden et al. (1980b) have also measured the concentration of glutathione and the activities of superoxide dismutase, catalase, glutathione peroxidase and glutathione reductase in liver biopsies from patients with iron overload. No significant changes in any of these were found in the biopsies from patients with HHC, in comparison with the values in histologically normal biopsies. A decrease in glutathione reductase activity was evident in liver biopsies from thalassaemic patients with secondary haemochromatosis, but glutathione levels and the activities of the other enzymes were within the normal range. Therefore, there do not appear to be major deficiencies in these 'cytoprotective' systems in the livers of patients with iron overload.

Bonkovsky *et al.* (1984) have measured antipyrine clearance and hepatic cytochrome P-450 concentrations in patients with various types of iron overload. While the numbers studied were small and some variation existed between the groups, no differences were found between iron-loaded patients and controls. There have been no studies of hepatic mitochondrial function in patients with haemochromatosis.

4.2.2. Experimental Iron Overload

Numerous studies have demonstrated alterations in a variety of biochemical functions of subcellular organelles that are dependent on intact membrane structure and that may be damaged by iron-induced lipid peroxidation in chronic iron overload. Table 10.4 summarizes the types of hepatic organelle dysfunction resulting from experimental iron overload produced by dietary carbonyl iron.

(a) *Lysosomes.* Hultcrantz *et al.* (1984a) separated two populations of lysosomes from the livers of rats injected repeatedly with the iron chelate, Jectofer. One population was heavily loaded with iron in the form of haemosiderin and ferritin and had a very low proteolytic activity as well as decreased latent acid phosphatase activity. The other population of lysosomes was less loaded with iron, had the same latent acid phosphatase as control lysosomes, and had only a slight reduction in proteolytic activity compared with controls. These results indicated that lysosomes which were heavily loaded with ferritin and haemosiderin were more fragile and had reduced proteolytic activity *in vitro*. Products of lipid peroxidation were not measured in these lysosomal fractions.

Peters *et al.* (1985b) found a decrease in latent NAGA activity in liver homogenates from rats injected with FeNTA for six weeks or more (average hepatic iron content of 1110 μg/g wet wt). Iron-loaded lysosomes isolated from the livers of these rats had a reduced content of arachidonate compared with hepatic lysosomes from controls. While this decrease in arachidonate content could be a result of lipid peroxidation in these lysosomes, the possibility of a change in constituent fatty acid composition, unrelated to lipid peroxidation, cannot be ruled out.

Lysosomal fragility has also been examined in rats fed a diet containing carbonyl iron. A decrease in latent NAGA activity was seen in liver homogenates when the hepatic iron concentration was above a threshold of about 8000 μg Fe/g dry wt ($\approx$ 2400 μg Fe/g wet wt), and the degree of fragility correlated with the hepatic iron concentration (LeSage *et al.*, 1986). Iron overload in this model also increased the activity of the lysosomal enzymes acid phosphatase (Bacon *et al.*, 1985) and NAGA (Bacon *et al.*, 1985; LeSage *et al.*, 1986) in the liver, similar to the changes seen in liver biopsies from patients with iron overload (Seymour and Peters, 1978). Biliary iron excretion is increased in iron-loaded rats (Hultcrantz and Glaumann, 1982; LeSage *et al.*, 1986), and it has been proposed that lysosomes may serve as key intermediaries in this excretory pathway (LeSage *et al.*, 1986).

Myers *et al.* (1991) have performed a detailed study examining the structure, physicochemical properties and pH of hepatic lysosomes in rats with dietary iron overload. Lysosomal iron content was increased dramatically, and the lysosomes were enlarged, misshapen and more fragile. Lysosomal membranes from the iron-loaded group had evidence of increased lipid peroxidation (malondialdehyde content), and their fluidity was decreased. The pH of lysosomes within hepatocytes

Table 10.4 Hepatic organelle dysfunction in experimental iron overload produced by dietary carbonyl iron

Organelle	Observations	References
Lysosomes	Lipid peroxidation	Myers et al., 1991
	Increased volume	LeSage et al., 1986; Iancu et al., 1987; Myers et al., 1991
	Increased fragility	LeSage et al., 1986; Iancu et al., 1987; Myers et al., 1991
	Decreased membrane fluidity	Myers et al., 1991
	Increased pH	Myers et al., 1991
	Lipid peroxidation	Bacon et al., 1983a,b, 1985, 1989, Masini et al., 1989
Mitochondria	Impaired oxidative metabolism	Bacon et al., 1985, 1989; Masini et al., 1989
	Decreased calcium sequestration	Britton et al., 1991b
	Increased calcium release	Masini et al., 1989
	Decreased content of reduced pyridine nucleotides	Masini et al., 1989
	Altered lipid composition	Pietrangelo et al., 1990a
	Decreased metabolism of malondialdehyde	Britton et al., 1990b
	Lipid peroxidation	Bacon et al., 1983a,b; 1986a; Wu et al., 1990
Endoplasmic reticulum	Decreased cytochrome P-450 levels	Bacon et al., 1986a; Irving et al., 1988; Britton et al., 1991b
	Decreased aminopyrine demethylase activity	Bacon et al., 1986a
	Decreased cytochrome b$_5$ levels	Bacon et al., 1986a
	Decreased calcium sequestration	Britton et al., 1991b
Plasma membrane	Altered lipid composition	Pietrangelo et al., 1989
Nucleus	Increased DNA strand breaks	Edling et al., 1990

isolated from the livers of iron-loaded rats was increased. The authors concluded that iron-catalysed peroxidation of lysosomal membrane lipids is likely the mechanism of these structural, physicochemical and functional disturbances.

(b) *Mitochondria*. The effect of iron overload on hepatic mitochondrial oxidative metabolism has been studied in rats fed dietary carbonyl iron and in rats to which iron was administered parenterally. In normal mitochondria, electron transport is tightly coupled to the phosphorylation of ADP; thus, in the absence of ADP (state 4), the rate of oxygen consumption is low, while with ADP present (state 3), the rate of oxygen consumption is increased. Normal mitochondria, therefore, have a high respiratory control ratio (RCR), which is calculated by dividing the state 3 respiratory rate by the state 4 respiratory rate.

Hanstein and colleagues (1975, 1981) were the first to examine mitochondrial oxidative metabolism in experimental iron overload. Decreases in the mitochondrial RCR were observed at moderate degrees of hepatic iron overload produced by injections of iron–dextran. Evidence of mitochondrial lipid peroxidation was documented by an increase in TBA-reactants in mitochondrial fractions of the iron-loaded group.

In studies by Tangerås (1983) and Masini *et al.* (1984a,b) using models of iron overload in which iron chelates were administered parenterally and in which mild degrees of iron overload were produced, minimal or no changes in mitochondrial lipid peroxidation or substrate oxidation were found. Nevertheless, Masini *et al.* (1984b) demonstrated that mitochondria from these iron-loaded rats had a significant reduction in the transmembrane potential, and they had a lower potassium content. These results suggest that some mitochondrial parameters may be more sensitive to the effects of iron overload than RCR, but whether lipid peroxidation is associated with these changes is not known, since *in vivo* lipid peroxidation was not determined in this study (Masini *et al.*, 1984b). In all of the above studies using iron chelates, more extensive functional abnormalities in hepatic mitochondria may not have been evident since much of the iron in the liver was localized in Kupffer cells, not in hepatocytes.

Hepatic mitochondria from rats given dietary carbonyl iron showed significant decreases in the state 3 respiratory rate and in the RCR for three substrates (glutamate, β-hydroxybutyrate and succinate) at moderate degrees of hepatic iron overload (Bacon *et al.*, 1985, 1989). At hepatic iron concentrations at which there were decreases in oxidative metabolism, there was also evidence of conjugated diene formation indicative of mitochondrial lipid peroxidation. These studies suggested that moderate degrees of chronic hepatic iron overload *in vivo* resulted in an inhibitory defect in the mitochondrial electron transport chain as evidenced by a decrease in state 3 respiration and RCR (Bacon *et al.*, 1985). Similar defects in oxidation were produced *in vitro* by iron-induced peroxidation of normal mitochondria (Bacon *et al.*, 1986b).

The impairment in mitochondrial oxidative capacity caused by iron overload could have a deleterious effect on the energy state of the liver. Consistent with this possibility, in rats with chronic dietary iron overload, there was a 40% decrease in hepatic ATP concentration at high hepatic iron levels (3170 μg/g wet wt) (Bacon *et al.*, 1993) and a 25% decrease in rats with mild iron overload (1640 μg/g wet wt) (Ceccarelli *et al.*, 1991) where mitochondrial injury was probably less severe. This decrease in hepatic ATP levels may disturb hepatocellular functions and compromise cellular integrity.

Further studies examining mitochondrial cytochrome levels and enzyme activities in dietary iron overload have revealed decreases in the concentrations of cytochromes a, b and c and a marked reduction in cytochrome C oxidase activity (Bacon *et al.*, 1987, 1993). Cytochrome C oxidase is functionally dependent on intact cardiolipin, a mitochondrial phospholipid which contains a high percentage of polyunsaturated fatty acids. Thus, it is possible that lipid peroxidation might damage cardiolipin and impair cytochrome C oxidase activity, or alternatively, direct peroxidative injury to the protein subunits of cytochrome C oxidase might occur concomitantly with mitochondrial lipid peroxidation in iron overload.

Given the important role that α-tocopherol plays in protecting membrane phospholipids from peroxidative decomposition, Bacon *et al.* (1989) have evaluated the effect of α-tocopherol supplementation and depletion on lipid peroxidation and on the altered mitochondrial function seen in experimental dietary iron overload. In these experiments, parenteral α-tocopherol was administered throughout the feeding period to produce a group of iron-loaded rats with elevated (three-fold) hepatic α-tocopherol levels to compare with iron-loaded rats with normal or deficient α-tocopherol levels. α-Tocopherol deficiency alone (in the absence of iron overload) did not result in mitochondrial lipid peroxidation or alterations in mitochondrial function. Significant reductions in mitochondrial RCR were seen in association with increased conjugated dienes in all iron-loaded rats regardless of the α-tocopherol status (deficient, normal or increased). Thus, in this experiment, α-tocopherol deficiency did not mimic or exacerbate iron-induced mitochondrial peroxidation or injury, and α-tocopherol supplementation by parenteral administration did not prevent this injury. Dietary α-tocopherol supplementation has been shown to reduce the hepatic levels of malondialdehyde (Britton *et al.*, 1991a) and fluorescent products (Parkkila *et al.*, 1992) in carbonyl iron-loaded rats, but its potential beneficial role on mitochondrial injury has not yet been evaluated.

Another consequence of mitochondrial dysfunction in iron overload is impaired metabolism of aldehydic products of lipid peroxidation. A significant decrease in the rate of malondialdehyde metabolism by mitochondria from iron-loaded rats has been reported (Britton *et al.*, 1990a). This decrease may be due to reductions in both the oxidative capacity of the mitochondria and the activity of mitochondrial aldehyde dehydrogenase. Thus, iron-induced mitochondrial lipid peroxidation may not only cause an increase in malondialdehyde production but may also result in impaired metabolism of malondialdehyde.

Chronic iron overload in rats also resulted in an impairment in calcium sequestration by hepatic mitochondria (Britton *et al.*, 1991b), which occurred in parallel with a decrease in substrate oxidation. Since mitochondrial calcium sequestration depends on the maintenance of the mitochondrial transmembrane potential, and because a reduction in substrate oxidation will decrease the transmembrane potential, it is likely that the defect in substrate oxidation is at least, in part, responsible for the altered mitochondrial calcium sequestration. Masini *et al.* (1989) have reported an increase in calcium release from hepatic mitochondria isolated from rats with chronic iron overload, which suggests that an increase in mitochondrial permeability may also play a role in decreasing calcium sequestration. Impairment of mitochondrial calcium sequestration by itself may have little effect on the cytosolic free calcium concentration, because mitochondrial calcium uptake is low at normal cytosolic calcium concentrations (Carafoli, 1987). However, because mitochondria can accumulate large amounts of calcium when cytosolic calcium concentrations are elevated, a defect in sequestration might potentiate any increase in the cytosolic free calcium concentration resulting from other perturbations in calcium homeostasis.

(c) *Microsomes*. Hepatic microsomal lipid peroxidation was found *in vivo* in rats with chronic dietary iron overload, when the hepatic iron content exceeded a certain threshold (Bacon *et al.*, 1986a). In addition, decreases in microsomal cytochrome P-450, aminopyrine demethylase activity and cytochrome b_5 were associated with microsomal lipid peroxidation in this model (Bacon *et al.*, 1986a). In contrast, glucose-6-phosphatase activity was not changed. This latter finding was unexpected, since glucose-6-phosphatase activity is usually decreased when microsomal lipid peroxidation occurs. One possible explanation for this apparent discrepancy is based on the report of Högberg *et al.* (1973) who demonstrated that low and high levels of iron-induced lipid peroxidation reduced glucose-6-phosphatase activity in isolated microsomes, while intermediate degrees of peroxidation had little effect. It is known that glucose-6-phosphatase is located on the inner surface of the endoplasmic reticulum and that its activity is limited by the rate of transport of glucose-6-phosphate through the membrane (Arion *et al.*, 1976). When the permeability of the endoplasmic reticulum is increased (e.g. with detergents), the transport of substrate is no longer rate-limiting and an increase in glucose-6-phosphatase activity is observed (Arion *et al.*, 1972). It is possible that intermediate levels of iron-induced lipid peroxidation result in an increase in microsomal permeability, thus removing the rate-limiting step for glucose-6-phosphatase; this effect could act to counterbalance the direct inhibitory effect of lipid peroxidation on the enzyme. With greater degrees of lipid peroxidation, the inhibitory action on this enzyme would prevail.

A number of reports have described a reduction in the levels of hepatic cytochrome P-450 (De Matteis and Sparks, 1973; Bonkovsky *et al.*, 1979, 1981; Hultcrantz and Glaumann, 1982) and microsomal drug-metabolizing enzymes (Wills, 1972; Ibrahim *et al.*, 1981) after acute or chronic parenteral iron administration. However, in none of these studies was *in vivo* lipid peroxidation measured concurrently. Studies using rats with chronic dietary iron overload showed that microsomal lipid peroxidation produced *in vivo* in this model was associated with selective decreases in cytochrome P-450 and cytochrome b_5 (Bacon *et al.*, 1986a). Although this finding does not prove direct causality, it seems likely that the loss of these cytochromes was the result of lipid peroxidation. It has been demonstrated *in vitro* that iron-induced peroxidation in hepatic microsomes causes a reduction in cytochrome P-450 levels (Schacter *et al.*, 1972; De Matteis and Sparks, 1973; Högberg *et al.*, 1973; Levin *et al.*, 1973), probably due to the destruction of haem in cytochrome P-450 (Schacter *et al.*, 1972; Levin *et al.*, 1973).

Another microsomal function which is sensitive to the damaging effects of peroxidation is calcium sequestration (Lowrey *et al.*, 1981; Waller *et al.*, 1983). Chronic dietary iron overload in rats resulted in an impairment in hepatic microsomal calcium sequestration (Britton *et al.*, 1991b), and this may alter hepatocellular calcium homeostasis and contribute to cell injury.

(d) *Nucleic acids*. Patients with long-standing HHC with cirrhosis have a 200-fold increase in risk for developing hepatocellular carcinoma (Bradbear *et al.*, 1985; Niederau *et al.*, 1985; Fargion *et al.*, 1992) (see also Chapters 8 and 11). Accordingly, it has been proposed that hepatocellular carcinoma in these patients may be a consequence of iron-induced oxidative damage to hepatic DNA, combined with the replicative stimulus provided by cirrhotic nodular regeneration. Iron salts have been shown to produce DNA strand breaks when incubated *in vitro* with either purified DNA (Takeshita *et al.*, 1978; Imlay *et al.*, 1988) or with isolated rat liver mitochondria (Hruszkewycz, 1988) or nuclei (Shires, 1982). In addition to these *in vitro* data, it has been demonstrated that endogenous iron plays a key role in the DNA damage produced by hydrogen peroxide in mammalian cells, since pretreatment with iron chelating agents diminishes this damage (Mello Filho and Meneghini, 1984; Starke and Farber, 1985; Halliwell and Gutteridge, 1990). Evidence suggests that iron-induced damage to DNA may be mediated by the hydroxyl radical, which is produced by the iron-catalysed Haber-Weiss reaction. Lipid peroxidation products in the presence of iron can also produce DNA damage *in vitro* through a mechanism that also may involve the hydroxyl radical (Park and Floyd, 1992).

Hydroxyl radicals, which are also important mediators of radiation-induced damage to DNA, can abstract hydrogen atoms from both the deoxyribose moiety (leading to single-strand nicks) and from the bases of DNA (e.g. converting thymine to hydroxymethyluracil), and can be added to nucleotides in DNA (e.g. converting guanine to 8-hydroxyguanine) (Pryor, 1988). It is thought that some iron is bound to DNA *in vivo* and that this iron, in the presence of superoxide and hydrogen peroxide, can catalyse the formation of 'site-directed' hydroxyl radicals which cause DNA damage (Halliwell and Gutteridge, 1990).

The first evidence that chronic iron overload *in vivo* results in damage to hepatic DNA was provided by a study which showed an increased number of strand breaks in hepatic DNA from carbonyl iron-fed rats (Edling *et al.*, 1990). The alkaline unwinding assay used to detect DNA strand breaks in these experiments measures net strand break frequency, which is a balance between the formation of breaks and the repair of breaks. Iron overload may result in a variety of DNA lesions including frank strand breaks, alkali labile lesions and base damage which, when acted on by excision repair, could yield transient 'repair' breaks (Cantoni *et al.*, 1986). All of these lesions are detected by the strand break assay. The induction of strand breakage in DNA has been associated with both initiation and promotion events in chemically-induced carcinogenesis (Walles and Erixon, 1984; Hartley *et al.*, 1985).

Increased oxidative damage to hepatic DNA has been demonstrated in *Ah*-responsive mice after a single subcutaneous injection of iron-dextran (Faux *et al.*, 1992). Oxidative DNA damage was evaluated using 8-hydroxydeoxyguanosine as a marker. It has been demonstrated that DNA templates containing 8-hydroxydeoxyguanosine are misread both at the modified base and at adjacent residues (Kuchino *et al.*, 1987), which could result in oxidative mutagenesis (Wood *et al.*, 1990). Interestingly, combined treatment with iron and polychlorinated biphenyls produced synergistic damage to hepatic DNA *in vivo* (Faux *et al.*, 1992); this treatment protocol also resulted in a synergistic effect on the development of hepatocellular carcinoma in this strain of mice (Smith *et al.*, 1990). These data support the oxidative stress mechanism proposed for polyhalogenated aromatic compounds in genetically-susceptible animals (Smith and De Matteis, 1990) and indicate that hepatic iron can potentiate the damaging effects of these compounds.

Additionally, FeNTA has been shown to cause transformation of cells. Repeated intraperitoneal injections of FeNTA to rats for one year resulted in renal adenocarcinoma with metastases to liver, lung and peritoneum (Okada *et al.*, 1983).

A single injection of FeNTA increased the amount of 8-hydroxydeoxyguanosine in renal DNA in rats, suggesting that oxidative damage to DNA may play a role in FeNTA-induced renal carcinogenesis (Umemura et al., 1990). Exposure of cultured rat liver epithelial cells to a high concentration of FeNTA resulted in the appearance of some cells which showed morphological transformation, grew in soft agar and induced metastatic carcinomas when injected into newborn rats (Yamada et al., 1990). The authors suggested that oxidative damage to DNA catalysed by FeNTA may play a key role in the rapid neoplastic transformation of these cells.

(e) Antioxidant enzymes. The activities of superoxide dismutase (SOD) and glutathione peroxidase have been measured in the livers of carbonyl iron-loaded animals. Fletcher et al. (1989) found that hepatic SOD activity was dramatically reduced to below 25% of control values in iron-loaded rats. In contrast, the activity of glutathione peroxidase in the liver was not affected by chronic iron overload (Fletcher et al., 1989; Kawabata et al., 1989). Variable results have been reported concerning the effect of chronic iron overload on hepatic glutathione levels, with decreases (18–32%) (Bonkovsky et al., 1987), increases (35%) (Kawabata et al., 1989) or no change (Fletcher et al., 1989; Pietrangelo et al., 1989) in the measured levels. Therefore, it appears that lipid peroxidation can occur in experimental iron overload without dramatically compromising hepatic glutathione levels.

The decrease in hepatic SOD in iron-overloaded rats might be expected to make them more susceptible to a superoxide-dependent oxidant stress. However, hepatic SOD activity was not decreased in biopsy samples from patients with iron overload (Selden et al., 1980b).

4.3. Initiation of Lipid Peroxidation in Iron Overload

The form of intracellular iron responsible for initiating hepatic lipid peroxidation in iron overload is not known. One possibility which has been suggested is that ferritin and haemosiderin are involved. These macromolecules accumulate within hepatocytes in iron overload, especially in lysosomes. In vitro, both ferritin (Wills, 1966; Gutteridge et al., 1983; O'Connell et al., 1985; Thomas et al., 1985; Koster and Slee, 1986; Reif, 1992) and haemosiderin (O'Connell et al., 1985) can initiate lipid peroxidation at neutral pH when a reductant such as ascorbate or superoxide radical is present; however, at an acidic pH similar to that seen in lysosomes, both can stimulate lipid peroxidation without a reductant (O'Connell et al., 1985; Peters et al., 1985b). The data indicate that, under these conditions, ferritin and haemosiderin release a small amount of iron which is ultimately responsible for initiating lipid peroxidation (O'Connell et al., 1985; Thomas et al., 1985; Ozaki et al., 1988). Therefore, it appears that, in the cell, ferritin and haemosiderin serve to store large amounts of iron in a form that is relatively (but not completely) unavailable to initiate lipid peroxidation. Whether when present in great excess in vivo, ferritin and/or haemosiderin can participate in the initiation of lipid peroxidation is not yet known. However, hepatic lysosomes do show evidence of lipid peroxidation in experimental dietary iron overload (Myers et al., 1991). Interestingly, O'Connell et al. (1986a) suggest that haemosiderin itself may be a product of oxidative reactions involving ferritin and lipid.

In addition to the marked increases in storage iron, it has been postulated that, in severe iron overload, there is an increase in the putative intracellular transit pool of iron, components of which could be catalytically active in stimulating lipid peroxidation. Though not rigorously proven, it is believed that non-haem, non-storage iron exists within cells in low molecular weight form(s) (Jacobs, 1977; Romslo, 1980; Mulligan et al., 1986) perhaps chelated to citrate (Morley et al., 1983; Bakkeren et al., 1985), amino acids (Morley et al., 1983) or nucleotides (Pollack et al., 1985; Weaver and Pollack, 1989). A bioassay system has been developed to investigate whether, in the livers of rats with iron overload, there is an increase in a cytosolic pool of low molecular weight iron which is catalytically active in stimulating lipid peroxidation (Britton et al., 1990a). This bioassay measured the ability of hepatic cytosolic ultrafiltrates to stimulate microsomal lipid peroxidation. The ultrafiltrates of hepatic cytosol from rats with experimental dietary iron overload had a greater prooxidant action than those from controls. This prooxidant action was completely blocked either by the addition of desferrioxamine to the assay, or by administration of desferrioxamine to animals prior to sacrifice, indicating that this activity was iron-dependent. This finding supports the concept that iron overload results in an increase in an hepatic pool of low molecular weight iron which could act to initiate lipid peroxidation.

There are several potential reactions by which certain iron chelates (either from the low molecular weight pool or iron mobilized from ferritin), in the presence of available cellular reductants (ascorbate, superoxide radical, NADPH), can initiate peroxidative injury (Aisen et al., 1990). For example, ferrous (Fe^{2+}) iron can react with preformed lipid hydroperoxides (LOOH) to form alkoxyl radicals ($LO^{\cdot}$):

$$LOOH + Fe^{2+} \rightarrow Fe^{3+} + OH^- + LO^{\cdot} \tag{1}$$

and ferric (Fe^{3+}) iron can similarly react with lipid hydroperoxides to form peroxyl radicals ($LOO^{\cdot}$):

$$LOOH + Fe^{3+} \rightarrow Fe^{2+} + H^+ + LOO^{\cdot} \tag{2}$$

Both alkoxyl and peroxyl radicals can stimulate the chain reaction of lipid peroxidation by extracting further hydrogen atoms. Alternatively, it has been proposed that hydroxyl radical ($OH^{\cdot}$) produced from hydrogen peroxide (H_2O_2) either by the Fenton reaction:

$$Fe^{2+} + H_2O_2 \rightarrow Fe^{3+} + OH^{\cdot} + OH^- \tag{3}$$

or by the iron-catalysed Haber-Weiss reaction:

$$Fe^{3+}\text{-chelate} + O_2^- \rightarrow Fe^{2+}\text{-chelate} + O_2$$
$$Fe^{2+}\text{-chelate} + H_2O_2 \rightarrow Fe^{3+}\text{-chelate} + OH^{\cdot} + OH^-$$

$$\text{Net reaction: } O_2^- + H_2O_2 \xrightarrow[\text{catalyst}]{\text{Fe-chelate}} O_2 + OH^{\cdot} + OH^- \tag{4}$$

may be the radical species responsible for initiating the peroxidative reaction.

Halliwell and Gutteridge (1990) have summarized the evidence which indicates that potential iron catalysts of hydroxyl radical formation occur *in vivo*, and they suggest that close association of iron with lipids could result in 'site-selective' production of hydroxyl radicals, with initiation of lipid peroxidation which is not inhibited by hydroxyl radical scavengers in bulk solution. Recently, Burkitt and Mason (1991) have used a secondary radical-trapping technique to demonstrate the production of hydroxyl radicals in the liver of rats given a single intragastric dose of ferrous sulfate. Aust and coworkers have questioned the involvement of hydroxyl radicals in lipid peroxidation (Aust and Svingen, 1982; Minotti and Aust, 1987) and have presented data suggesting that initiation of lipid peroxidation by Fe^{2+} and H_2O_2 is mediated by an oxidant which requires both Fe^{3+} and Fe^{2+} and has optimal activity at a ratio of about 1 Fe^{3+} : 1 Fe^{2+} (Minotti and Aust, 1987). Regardless of the initiating species, peroxidative decomposition of the polyunsaturated fatty acids of organelle membrane phospholipids can result in specific abnormalities of organelle function which are dependent on intact membrane structure. Further experimental studies will be necessary to determine more precisely the species of iron and the ultimate oxidizing species responsible for initiating or catalysing peroxidative reactions *in vivo*.

4.4. Fibrogenesis in Iron Overload

The major clinical manifestation of chronic iron overload in human disease is the development of fibrosis and cirrhosis of the liver. As mentioned previously, the development of fibrosis and/or cirrhosis in HHC is iron-concentration dependent. It appears that this is the case in experimental iron overload as well. Table 10.5 summarizes the reports of hepatic fibrosis produced by iron overload in experimental animals.

Several studies demonstrating hepatic fibrosis after chronic iron overload in animals have utilized parenteral administration of iron chelates. In these models, the iron is first distributed to RE cells and later to liver parenchymal cells, a situation mimicking transfusional iron overload in humans. Using repeated injections of saccharated iron oxide, Chang *et al.* (1959) observed portal fibrosis in iron-loaded rabbits. Lisboa (1971) found portal fibrosis and cirrhosis in dogs given long-term parenteral treatment with iron-sorbitol and iron-dextran. Brissot *et al.* (1983) demonstrated pericellular collagen deposition in areas of massive sinusoidal siderosis in the liver of baboons given chronic intramuscular injections of iron-polymaltose; in these animals, there was a slight increase in the serum aminotransferases and mild portal fibrosis associated with a moderate and transient increase in hepatic prolyl hydroxylase activity. In this model, because of the form of iron administration (parenteral iron chelate), iron overload was located essentially within Kupffer cells and sinusoidal cells. In a subsequent study by Brissot *et al.* (1987), iron overload was produced in the baboon by the administration of parenteral FeNTA over a two-year period. This approach produced hepatocellular deposition of iron, but there was still marked deposition in RE cells and in sinusoidal cells. Serum aminotransferase activities were increased, and there were foci of perisinusoidal fibrosis. Most likely, the experiments by Chang, Lisboa, Brissot and their coworkers were successful because of the high doses of iron administered and the long durations of treatment.

Table 10.5 Hepatic fibrosis in experimental iron overload

Model	Species	Observations	References
Dietary carbonyl iron	Rat	Portal fibrosis	Park et al., 1987; Pietrangelo et al., 1990b
		Increased collagen fibrils	Irving et al., 1991
		Increased collagen gene expression	Pietrangelo et al., 1990b, 1992; Irving et al., 1991
Dietary ferrocene iron	Rat	Perisinusoidal and portal fibrosis	Düllmann et al., 1992
Parenteral iron chelates	Rat	Increased hydroxyproline content	Weintraub et al., 1985
		Increased prolyl hydroxylase activity	Weintraub et al., 1985
		Increased collagen fibrils	Weintraub et al., 1985
	Dog	Portal fibrosis	Lisboa, 1971
	Rabbit	Portal fibrosis	Chang et al., 1959
	Baboon	Perisinusoidal fibrosis	Brissot et al., 1983, 1987
	Gerbil	Micronodular cirrhosis	Carthew et al., 1991b

Many other studies have been unsuccessful in producing hepatic fibrosis and cirrhosis after administration of iron to mice (Cappell, 1930), rats (Golberg et al., 1957), guinea-pigs (Buchanan, 1970), rabbits (Polson, 1933; Golberg et al., 1957), dogs (Brown et al., 1957, 1959) and rhesus monkeys (Nath et al., 1972), presumably because of an inadequate degree of parenchymal iron overload.

Weintraub et al. (1985) examined hepatic collagen levels in experimental iron overload by measuring the level of hydroxyproline, an amino acid which is found predominantly in collagen. In this experiment, iron overload in rats was produced by weekly intraperitoneal injections of iron-dextran or heat-damaged red cells for a nine-month period. Although no hepatic fibrosis or necrosis was evident in the iron-loaded animals as determined by light microscopy, there was a 50% increase in liver hydroxyproline content, and collagen fibrils were seen adjacent to hepatocytes as determined by electron microscopy. These authors also found an increase in the activity of prolyl hydroxylase, a key enzyme in the collagen biosynthetic pathway, in the livers of iron-overloaded rats. This study demonstrated that increased hepatic collagen deposition could be detected in the iron-loaded liver at a time when fibrosis was not evident by light microscopy. Weintraub et al. (1985) suggested that iron overload could result in an increase in collagen production without hepatic necrosis as a prerequisite. Iancu et al. (1977) have demonstrated ultrastructural evidence of increased hepatic collagen formation in the absence of cellular injury in thalassaemic patients with very early iron overload, thus providing additional support for iron as a direct-acting profibrogenic agent.

Recent work by Carthew et al. (1991b) indicates that gerbils are particularly sensitive to iron-induced hepatic fibrosis. After parenteral iron-dextran administration, gerbils accumulated iron as ferritin in hepatic perisinusoidal cells and developed fibrosis and micronodular cirrhosis without evident necrosis. Rats and mice given equivalent amounts of parenteral iron did not accumulate large amounts of ferritin in perisinusoidal cells and did not develop fibrosis. The authors hypothesized that excess ferritin iron in perisinusoidal cells (which may be lipocytes) may play a key role in stimulating fibrogenesis by these cells. Another possibility is that the elevated ferritin levels in these cells were a response to the presence of an increased flux of intracellular low molecular weight iron, which could be the active form responsible for triggering the fibrogenic process.

In order to examine if extensive parenchymal iron loading would result in hepatic fibrosis, rats were fed a diet supplemented with carbonyl iron for up to 12 months in which hepatic iron concentrations of approximately 8000 μg/g wet wt were achieved (Park et al., 1987). In this model of iron overload, iron deposition in the liver was initially found in periportal hepatocytes, but as time progressed, iron deposits extended to midzonal and centrilobular hepatocytes. After three months on the iron-supplemented diet, Kupffer cells and sinusoidal lining cells showed heavy iron deposition and collections of macrophages, also heavily laden with stainable iron (siderotic nodules), were frequently present in the connective tissue around portal triads and occasionally in the sinusoids. By eight months, there had been no further increase in hepatic iron concentration, but collections of iron-laden phagocytic cells were noted more frequently in the sinusoids compressing or displacing hepatocytes. Occasional foci of spotty hepatocellular necrosis with polymorphonuclear leukocytes and lymphocyte infiltration were also seen. Staining for collagen showed fine delicate strands of collagen fibres in the sinusoidal spaces around the portal siderotic or microsiderotic nodules at eight months. These changes were more accentuated at 12 months when there were foci of marked periportal fibrosis with thicker bands of fibrous tissue and entrapped hepatocytes (Plate 8).

Pietrangelo et al. (1990b) have also observed periportal fibrosis in rats with dietary carbonyl iron overload. In addition, they found increased steady-state levels of procollagen I mRNA in the liver, suggesting that iron overload may have increased procollagen gene transcription and/or decreased degradation of this message. Irving et al. (1991) have also reported increased hepatic levels of procollagen I mRNA in rats with dietary iron overload; in these animals, increased collagen fibrils were observed in the liver using electron microscopy, but fibrosis was not evident using light microscopy. Two other groups have also not found histological fibrosis in rats fed a diet supplemented with carbonyl iron (Iancu et al., 1987; Roberts et al., 1993), and in these animals the hepatic mRNA levels for procollagens I, III and IV were unaltered (Roberts et al., 1993). These results suggest that factors such as the hepatic iron levels, the age, strain and sex of the animals, and the composition of the diet may have an impact on iron-induced hepatic fibrogenesis.

In the liver, pathological fibrogenesis appears to be mediated by activation of lipocytes (Ito cells, fat-storing cells) (Friedman, 1990). When activated, lipocytes change their pattern of secreted collagens, switching from predominantly collagen III to collagen I, while at the same time increasing the total amounts of collagens I, III and IV (Friedman, 1990). In experimental dietary iron overload, Pietrangelo et al. (1992) have demonstrated that lipocytes contain preferentially increased levels of procollagen I mRNA, suggesting that these cells may have an elevated rate of collagen synthesis in iron overload. In support of this concept, Li et al. (1992) have shown that lipocytes isolated from iron-loaded rats are activated, producing increased amounts of collagen and protein in culture. The mechanisms responsible for the activation of lipocytes in chronic iron overload are not known. However, one possibility is suggested by the demonstration that aldehydic products of lipid peroxidation increase collagen gene expression and collagen production in cultured human fibroblasts (Chojkier et al., 1989). Since hepatic parenchymal iron overload causes lipid peroxidation with increased hepatic malondialdehyde levels (Britton et al., 1990b), aldehydic peroxidation products might act to stimulate collagen production by lipocytes. Alternatively, these aldehydic products might activate Kupffer cells to release profibrogenic cytokines. These hypotheses regarding the potential relationship between lipid peroxidation and fibrogenesis are currently being investigated.

5. SUMMARY AND CONCLUSIONS

There are several inherited and acquired disorders that can result in chronic iron overload in humans, and the major clinical consequences are hepatic fibrosis, cirrhosis, hepatocellular cancer, cardiac disease and diabetes. It is clear that lipid peroxidation occurs in experimental iron overload if sufficiently high levels of iron within hepatocytes are achieved. While there are few data addressing this issue in iron-loaded patients, a recent report has shown that patients with HHC have elevated plasma levels of malondialdehyde (Young et al., 1992), which could be the result of increased peroxidation. Lipid peroxidation is associated with hepatic mitochondrial and microsomal dysfunction in experimental iron overload, and lipid peroxidation may underlie the increased lysosomal fragility that has been detected in liver samples from both iron-loaded human subjects and experimental animals. Reduced cellular ATP levels, impaired cellular calcium homeostasis, and damage to DNA may all contribute to hepatocellular injury in iron overload. Long-term dietary iron overload in rats can lead to increased collagen gene expression and hepatic fibrosis. A potential link between iron-induced lipid peroxidation and the induction of fibrogenesis has been provided by the demonstration of increased collagen synthesis by human lipocytes cultured in the presence of aldehydic products of lipid peroxidation (Parola *et al.*, 1993). Further studies will be necessary to clarify if this link between lipid peroxidation and fibrogenesis occurs within the iron-loaded liver.

ACKNOWLEDGEMENTS

The authors wish to thank Careen Bresee for excellent secretarial assistance. Robert S. Britton and Bruce R. Bacon are supported by a grant from the US Public Health Service, R01-DK-41816.

REFERENCES

Aisen, P., Cohen, G. and Kang, J. O. (1990) Iron toxicosis. *Int. Rev. Exper. Pathol.* **31**, 1–46.

Albano, E., Bellomo, G., Parola, M., Carini, R. and Dianzani, M. U. (1991) Stimulation of lipid peroxidation increases the intracellular calcium content of isolated hepatocytes. *Biochim. Biophys. Acta* **1091**, 310–316.

Alt, E. R., Sternlieb, I. and Goldfischer, S. (1990) The cytopathology of metal overload. *Int. Rev. Exper. Pathol.* **31**, 165–188.

Arion, W. J., Wallin, B. K., Carlson, P. W. and Lange, A. J. (1972) The specificity of glucose-6-phosphatases of intact liver microsomes. *J. Biol. Chem.* **247**, 2558–2565.

Arion, W. J., Ballas, L. M., Lange, A. J. and Wallin, B. K. (1976) Microsomal membrane permeability and the hepatic glucose-6-phosphatase system. Interactions of the system with d-mannose 6-phosphate and d-mannose. *J. Biol. Chem.* **251**, 4901–4907.

Aust, S. D. and Svingen, B. A. (1982) The role of iron in enzymatic lipid peroxidation. In: *Free Radicals in Biology* (ed. W. A. Pryor), Vol. 5, Academic Press, New York, pp. 1–28.

Awai, M., Narasaki, M., Yamanoi, Y. and Seno, S. (1979) Induction of diabetes in animals by parenteral administration of ferric nitrilotriacetate. *Am. J. Pathol.* **95**, 663–674.

Bacon, B. R. (1992) Causes of iron overload. *N. Engl. J. Med.* **326**, 126–127.

Bacon, B. R. and Tavill, A. S. (1984) Role of the liver in normal iron metabolism. *Sem. Liver Dis.* **4**, 181–192.

Bacon, B. R. and Britton, R. S. (1989) Hepatic injury in chronic iron overload. Role of lipid peroxidation. *Chem. Biol. Interact.* **70**, 183–226.

Bacon, B. R. and Britton, R. S. (1990) The pathology of hepatic iron overload: A free radical-mediated process? *Hepatology* **11**, 127–137.

Bacon, B. R., Brittenham, G. M., Tavill, A. S., McLaren, C. E., Park, C. H. and Recknagel, R. O. (1983a) Hepatic lipid peroxidation *in vivo* in rats with chronic dietary iron overload is dependent on hepatic iron concentration. *Trans. Assoc. Am. Phys.* **96**, 146–154.

Bacon, B. R., Tavill, A. S., Brittenham, G. M., Park, C. H. and Recknagel, R. O. (1983b) Hepatic lipid peroxidation *in vivo* in rats with chronic iron overload. *J. Clin. Invest.* **71**, 429–439.

Bacon, B. R., Park, C. H., Brittenham, G. M., O'Neill, R. and Tavill, A. S. (1985) Hepatic mitochondrial oxidative metabolism in rats with chronic dietary iron overload. *Hepatology* **5**, 789–797.

Bacon, B. R., Healey, J. F., Brittenham, G. M. *et al.* (1986a) Hepatic microsomal function in rats with chronic dietary iron overload. *Gastroenterology* **90**, 1844–1853.

Bacon, B. R., O'Neill, R. and Park, C. H. (1986b) Iron-induced peroxidative injury to isolated rat hepatic mitochondria. *J. Free Rad. Biol. Med.* **2**, 339–347.

Bacon, B. R., Dalton, N. and O'Neill, R. (1987) Effects of iron overload on hepatic mitochondrial cytochromes, oxidases/reductases and oxidative metabolism. (Abstract). *Hepatology* **7**, 1027.

Bacon, B. R., Britton, R. S. and O'Neill, R. (1989) Effects of vitamin E deficiency on hepatic mitochondrial lipid peroxidation and oxidative metabolism in rats with chronic dietary iron overload. *Hepatology* **9**, 398–404.

Bacon, B. R., O'Neill, R. and Britton, R. S. (1993) Hepatic mitochondrial energy production in rats with chronic iron overload. *Gastroenterology* **105**, 1134–1140.

Bakkeren, D. L., de Jeu-Jaspars, C. M. H., van der Heul, C. and van Eijk, H. G. (1985) Analysis of iron-binding components in the low molecular weight fraction of rat reticulocyte cytosol. *Int. J. Biochem.* **17**, 925–930.

Barry, M., Flynn, D. M., Letsky, E. A. and Risdon, R. A. (1974) Long-term chelation therapy in thalassemia major: effect on liver iron concentration, liver histology and clinical progress. *Br. Med. J.* **2**, 16–20.

Bassett, M., Doran, T. J., Halliday, J. W., Bashir, H. V. and Powell, L. W. (1982) Idiopathic haemochromatosis: Demonstration of homozygous–heterozygous mating by HLA typing of families. *Hum. Genet.* **60**, 352–356.

Bassett, M. L., Halliday, J. W. and Powell, L. W. (1986) Value of hepatic iron measurements in early hemochromatosis and determination of the critical iron level associated with fibrosis. *Hepatology* **6**, 24–29.

Bomford, A. and Williams, R. (1976) Long-term results of venesection therapy in idiopathic haemochromatosis. *Q. J. Med.* **45**, 611–623.

Bonkovsky, H. L. (1991) Iron and the liver. *Am. J. Med. Sci.* **301**, 32–43.

Bonkovsky, H. L., Carpenter, S. J. and Healey, J. F. (1979) Iron and the liver: subcellular distribution of iron and decreased microsomal cytochrome P-450 in livers of iron-loaded rats. *Arch. Pathol. Lab. Med.* **103**, 21–29.

Bonkovsky, H. L., Healey, J. F., Sinclair, P. R., Sinclair, J. F. and Pomeroy, J. S. (1981) Iron and the liver: acute and long-term effects of iron-loading on hepatic haem metabolism. *Biochem. J.* **196**, 57–64.

Bonkovsky, H. L., Mitchell, W. J. and Healey, J. F. (1984) Effect of hemochromatosis on hepatic cytochrome P450 and antipyrine metabolism in humans. *Clin. Chem.* **30**, 1430–1431.

Bonkovsky, H. L., Healey, J. F., Lincoln, B., Bacon, B. R., Bishop, D. F. and Elder, G. H. (1987) Hepatic heme synthesis in a new model of experimental hemochromatosis: Studies in rats fed finely divided elemental iron. *Hepatology* **7**, 1195–1203.

Bonkovsky, H. L., Slaker, D. P., Bills, E. B. and Wolf, D. C. (1990) Usefulness and limitations of laboratory and hepatic imaging studies in iron-storage disease. *Gastroenterology* **99**, 1079–1091.

Borch-Iohnsen, B., Olsson, K. S. and Nilssen, K. J. (1988) Seasonal siderosis in Svalbard reindeer. *Ann. NY Acad. Sci.* **526**, 355–356.

Borwein, S. T., Ghent, C. N., Flanagan, P. R., Chamberlain, M. J. and Valberg, L. S. (1983) Genetic and phenotypic expression of hemochromatosis in Canadians. *Clin. Invest. Med.* **6**, 171–179.

Bothwell, T. H. and Isaacson, C. (1962) Siderosis in the Bantu. A comparison of the incidence in males and females. *Br. Med. J.* **1**, 522–524.

Bothwell, T. H., Charlton, R. W., Cook, J. D. and Finch, C. A. (1979) *Iron Metabolism in Man*, Blackwell, Oxford.

Bradbear, R. A., Bain, C., Siskind, V. *et al.* (1985) Cohort study of internal malignancy in genetic hemochromatosis and other chronic nonalcoholic liver diseases. *J. Natl. Cancer Inst.* **75**, 81–84.

Brink, B., Disler, P., Lynch, S., Jacobs, P., Charlton, R. and Bothwell, T. H. (1976) Patterns of iron storage in dietary iron overload and idiopathic hemochromatosis. *J. Lab. Clin. Med.* **88**, 725–731.

Brissot, P., Campoin, J. P., Guillouzo, A. *et al.* (1983) Experimental hepatic iron overload in the baboon: results of a two-year study. Evolution of biological and morphological hepatic parameters of iron overload. *Dig. Dis. Sci.* **28**, 616–624.

Brissot, P., Farjanel, J., Bourel, D. *et al.* (1987) Chronic liver iron overload in the baboon by ferric nitrilotriacetate: Morphologic and functional changes with special reference to collagen synthesis enzymes. *Dig. Dis. Sci.* **32**, 620–627.

Britton, R. S., Ferrali, M., Magiera, C. J., Recknagel, R. O. and Bacon, B. R. (1990a) Increased prooxidant action of hepatic cytosolic low-molecular-weight iron in experimental iron overload. *Hepatology* **11**, 1038–1043.

Britton, R. S., O'Neill, R. and Bacon, B. R. (1990b) Hepatic mitochondrial malondialdehyde metabolism in rats with chronic iron overload. *Hepatology* **11**, 93–97.

Britton, R. S., O'Neill, R., Singh, R. and Bacon, B. R. (1991a) Dietary supplementation with vitamin E suppresses hepatic malondialdehyde levels in rats with chronic iron overload. (Abstract). *Hepatology* **14**, 158A.

Britton, R. S., O'Neill, R. and Bacon, B. R. (1991b) Chronic dietary iron overload in rats results in impaired calcium sequestration by hepatic mitochondria and microsomes. *Gastroenterology* **101**, 806–811.

Brown, E. B., Jr, Dubach, R., Smith, D. E., Reynafarje, C. and Moore, C. V. (1957) Studies in iron transportation and metabolism. X. Long-term iron overload in dogs. *J. Lab. Clin. Med.* **50**, 862–893.

Brown, E. B., Jr, Smith, D. E., Dubach, R. and Moore, C. V. (1959) Lethal iron overload in dogs. *J. Lab. Clin. Med.* **53**, 591–606.

Brown, K. E., Kinter, M. T., Spitz, D. R., Savory, J. and Myers, B. M. (1991) Experimental iron overload is associated with increased levels of 4-hydroxynonenal, a toxic by-product of lipid peroxidation (Abstract). *Hepatology* **14**, 159A.

Buchanan, W. M. (1970) Experimental production of 'Bantu' siderosis using home-brewed beer. *S. Afr. J. Med. Sci.* **35**, 15–21.

Burkitt, M. J. and Mason, R. P. (1991) Direct evidence for *in vivo* hydroxyl-radical generation in experimental iron overload: An ESR spin-trapping investigation. *Proc. Natl. Acad. Sci. USA* **88**, 8440–8444.

Cantoni, O., Murray, D. and Meyn, R. E. (1986) Effect of 3-aminobenzamide on DNA strand-break rejoining and cytotoxicity in CHO cells treated with hydrogen peroxide. *Biochim. Biophys. Acta* **867**, 135–143.

Cappell, D. F. (1930) The late results of intravenous injection of colloidal iron. *J. Pathol. Bacteriol.* **33**, 175–196.

Carafoli, E. (1987) Intracellular calcium homeostasis. *Annu. Rev. Biochem.* **56**, 395–433.

Carthew, P., Edwards, R. E. and Dorman, B. M. (1991a) Hepatic fibrosis and iron accumulation due to endotoxin-induced haemorrhage in the gerbil. *J. Comp. Path.* **104**, 303–311.

Carthew, P., Edwards, R. E., Smith, A. G., Dorman, B. and Francis, J. E. (1991b) Rapid induction of hepatic fibrosis in the gerbil after the parenteral administration of iron-dextran complex. *Hepatology* **13**, 534–539.

Ceccarelli, D., Predieri, G., Muscatello, U. and Masini, A. (1991) A ^{31}P-NMR study on the energy state of rat liver in an experimental model of chronic dietary iron overload. *Biochem. Biophys. Res. Commun.* **176**, 1262–1268.

Chang, H. Y., Robbins, S. L. and Mallory, G. K. (1959) Prolonged intravenous administration of iron to normal and anemic rabbits. *Lab. Invest.* **8**, 1–18.

Chapman, R. W., Morgan, M. Y., Laulicht, M., Hoffbrand, A. V. and Sherlock, S. (1982) Hepatic iron stores and markers of iron overload in alcoholics and patients with hemochromatosis. *Dig. Dis. Sci.* **27**, 909–916.

Cheeseman, K. H., Milia, A., Chiarpotto, E. *et al.* (1984) Iron overload, lipid peroxidation and loss of cytochrome P-450: comparative studies *in vitro* using microsomes and isolated hepatocytes. *Int. Res. Commun. Sys. Med. Sci.* **12**, 61–62.

Chojkier, M., Houglum, K., Solis-Herruzo, J. and Brenner, D. A. (1989) Stimulation of collagen gene expression by ascorbic acid in cultured human fibroblasts. A role for lipid peroxidation? *J. Biol. Chem.* **264**, 16957–16962.

Cohen, A., Martin, M. and Schwartz, E. (1984a) Depletion of excessive liver iron stores with desferrioxamine. *Br. J. Haematol.* **58**, 369–373.

Cohen, A., Witzleben, C. and Schwartz, E. (1984b) Treatment of iron overload. *Semin. Liver Dis.* **4**, 228–238.

Craven, C. M., Alexander, J., Eldridge, M., Kushner, J. P., Bernstein, S. and Kaplan, J. (1987) Tissue distribution and clearance kinetics of non-transferrin-bound iron in the hypotransferrinemic mouse: A rodent model for hemochromatosis. *Proc. Natl. Acad. Sci. USA* **84**, 3457–3461.

Curtis, J. R., Eastwood, J. B., Smith, E. K. M. *et al.* (1969) Maintenance hemodialysis. *Q. J. Med.* **38**, 49–89.

Dadone, M. M., Kushner, J. P., Edwards, C. Q., Bishop, D. T. and Skolnick, M. H. (1982) Hereditary hemochromatosis: analysis of laboratory expression of the disease by genotype in 18 pedigrees. *Am. J. Clin. Pathol.* **78**, 196–207.

De Matteis, F. and Sparks, R. G. (1973) Iron-dependent loss of liver cytochrome P-450 haem *in vivo* and *in vitro*. *FEBS Lett.* **29**, 141–144.

Deugnier, Y. M., Loréal, O., Turlin, B. *et al.* (1992) Liver pathology in genetic hemochromatosis: A review of 135 homozygous cases and their bioclinical correlations. *Gastroenterology* **102**, 2050–2059.

Di Bisceglie, A. M., Axiotis, C. A., Hoofnagle, J. H. and Bacon, B. R. (1992) Measurement of iron status in patients with chronic hepatitis. *Gastroenterology* **102**, 2108–2113.

Dillard, C. J. and Tappel, A. L. (1979) Volatile hydrocarbon and carbonyl products of lipid peroxidation: a comparison of pentane, ethane, hexanal and acetone as *in vivo* indices. *Lipids* **14**, 989–995.

Dillard, C. J., Downey, J. E. and Tappel, A. L. (1984) Effects of antioxidants on lipid peroxidation in iron-loaded rats. *Lipids* **19**, 127–133.

Düllmann, J., Wulfhekel, U., Nielsen, P. and Heinrich, H. C. (1992) Iron overload of the liver by trimethylhexanoylferrocene in rats. *Acta Anatomica* **143**, 96–108.

Dumelin, E. E. and Tappel, A. L. (1977) Hydrocarbon gases produced during *in vitro* peroxidation of polyunsaturated fatty acids and decomposition of preformed hydroperoxides. *Lipids* **12**, 894–900.

Ebina, Y., Okada, S., Hamazaki, S., Ogino, F., Li, J.-L. and Midorikawa, O. (1986) Nephrotoxicity and renal cell carcinoma after use of iron- and aluminum–nitrilotriacetate complexes in rats. *J. Natl. Cancer Inst.* **76**, 107–113.

Edling, J. E., Britton, R. S., Grisham, M. B. and Bacon, B. R. (1990) Increased unwinding of hepatic double-stranded DNA (dsDNA) in rats with chronic dietary iron overload (abstract). *Gastroenterology* **98**, A585.

Edwards, C. Q., Griffen, L. M., Goldgar, D., Drummond, C., Skolnick, M. H. and Kushner, J. P. (1988) Prevalence of hemochromatosis among 11,065 presumably healthy blood donors. *N. Engl. J. Med.* **318**, 1355–1362.

Edwards, C. Q., Griffen, L. M., Kaplan, J. and Kushner, J. P. (1989) Twenty-four hour variation of transferrin saturation in treated and untreated haemochromatosis homozygotes. *J. Intern. Med.* **226**, 373–379.

Esterbauer, H. (1985) Lipid peroxidation products: formation, chemical properties and biological activities. In: *Free Radicals in Liver Injury* (eds G. Poli, K. H. Cheeseman, M. U. Dianzani and T. F. Slater), IRL Press, Oxford, pp. 2–47.

Fargion, S., Mandelli, C., Piperno, A. *et al.* (1992) Survival and prognostic factors in 212 Italian patients with genetic hemochromatosis. *Hepatology* **15**, 655–659.

Faux, S. P., Francis, J. E., Smith, A. G. and Chipman, J. K. (1992) Induction of 8-hydroxydeoxyguanosine in *Ah*-responsive mouse liver by iron and Aroclor 1254. *Carcinogenesis* **13**, 247–250.

Filser, J. G., Bolt, H. M., Muliawan, H. and Kappus, H. (1983) Quantitative evaluation of ethane and n-pentane as indicators of lipid peroxidation *in vivo*. *Arch. Toxicol.* **52**, 135–147.

Fletcher, B. L., Dillard, C. J. and Tappel, A. L. (1973) Measurement of fluorescent lipid peroxidation products in biological systems and tissues. *Anal. Biochem.* **52**, 1–9.

Fletcher, L. M., Roberts, F. D., Irving, M. G., Powell, L. W. and Halliday, J. W. (1989) Effects of iron loading on free radical scavenging enzymes and lipid peroxidation in rat liver. *Gastroenterology* **97**, 1011–1018.

Fong, K.-L., McCay, P. B., Poyer, J. L., Keele, B. B. and Misra, H. (1973) Evidence that peroxidation of lysosomal membranes is initiated by hydroxyl free radicals produced during flavin enzyme activity. *J. Biol. Chem.* **248**, 7792–7797.

Frank, H., Hintze, T., Bimboes, D. and Remmer, H. (1980) Monitoring lipid peroxidation by breath analysis: endogenous hydrocarbons and their metabolic elimination. *Toxicol. Appl. Pharmacol.* **52**, 337–344.

Friedman, S. L. (1990) Cellular sources of collagen and regulation of collagen production in liver. *Semin. Liver Dis.* **10**, 20–29.

Frigerio, R., Mela, Q., Passiu, G. *et al.*(1984) Iron overload and lysosomal stability in β-thalassemia intermedia and trait: correlation between serum ferritin and serum N-acetyl-β-D-glucosaminidase levels. *Scand. J. Haematol.* **33**, 252–255.

Gavino, V. C., Dillard, C. J. and Tappel, A. L. (1984) Release of ethane and pentane from rat tissue slices: Effect of vitamin E, halogenated hydrocarbons and iron overload. *Arch. Biochem. Biophys.* **233**, 741–747.

Gavino, V. C., Dillard, C. J. and Tappel, A. L. (1985) The effect of iron overload on urinary excretion of immunoreactive prostaglandin E_2. *Arch. Biochem. Biophys.* **237**, 322–327.

Goddard, J. G., Basford, D. and Sweeney, G. D. (1986) Lipid peroxidation stimulated by iron nitrilotriacetate in rat liver. *Biochem. Pharmacol.* **35**, 2381–2387.

Golberg, L., Smith, J. P. and Martin, L. E. (1957) The effects of intensive and prolonged administration of iron parenterally in animals. *Br. J. Exp. Pathol.* **38**, 297–311.

Golberg, L., Martin, L. E. and Batchelor, A. (1962) Biochemical changes in the tissues of animals injected with iron. 3. Lipid peroxidation. *Biochem. J.* **83**, 291–298.

Gordeuk, V. R., Boyd, R. D. and Brittenham, G. M. (1986) Dietary iron overload persists in rural sub-Saharan Africa. *Lancet* **i**, 1310–1313.

Gordeuk, V. R., Bacon, B. R. and Brittenham, G. M. (1987) Iron overload: causes and consequences. *Annu. Rev. Nutr.* **7**, 485–508.

Gordeuk, V., Mukiibi, J., Hasstedt, S. J. *et al.* (1992) Iron overload in Africa. Interaction between a gene and dietary iron content. *N. Engl. J. Med.* **326**, 95–100.

Gosselin, S. J. and Kramer, L. W. (1983) Pathophysiology of excessive iron storage in mynah birds. *J. Am. Vet. Med. Assoc.* **183**, 1238–1240.

Gosselin, S. J., Kramer, L. W., Loudy, D. E. and Giroux, E. L. (1983) Naturally occurring idiopathic hemochromatosis in birds of the starling family (Abstract). *Hepatology* **3**, 848.

Gutteridge, J. M. C., Halliwell, B., Treffry, A., Harrison, P. M. and Blake, D. (1983) Effect of ferritin-containing fractions with different iron loading on lipid peroxidation. *Biochem. J.* **209**, 557–560.

Halliwell, B. and Gutteridge, J. M. C. (1990) Role of free radicals and catalytic metal ions in human disease: An overview. *Methods Enzymol.* **186**, 1–85.

Hamazaki, S., Okada, S., Ebina, Y. and Midorikawa, O. (1985) Acute renal failure and glucosuria induced by ferric nitrilotriacetate in rats. *Toxicol. Appl. Pharmacol.* **77**, 267–274.

Hanstein, W. G., Sacks, P. V. and Müller-Eberhard, U. (1975) Properties of liver mitochondria from iron-loaded rats. *Biochem. Biophys. Res. Commun.* **67**, 1175–1184.

Hanstein, W. G., Heitmann, T. D., Sandy, A., Biesterfeldt, H. L., Liem, H. H. and Müller-Eberhard, U. (1981) Effects of hexachlorobenzene and iron loading on rat liver mitochondria. *Biochim. Biophys. Acta* **678**, 293–299.

Hartley, J. A., Gibson, N. W., Zwelling, L. A. and Yuspa, S. H. (1985) Association of DNA strand breaks with accelerated terminal differentiation in mouse epidermal cells exposed to tumor promoters. *Cancer Res.* **45**, 4864–4870.

Heys, A. D. and Dormandy, T. L. (1981) Lipid peroxidation in iron-overloaded spleens. *Clin. Sci.* **60**, 295–301.

Högberg, J., Bergstrand, A. and Jakobsson, S. V. (1973) Lipid peroxidation of rat-liver microsomes. Its effect on the microsomal membrane and some membrane-bound microsomal enzymes. *Eur. J. Biochem.* **37**, 51–59.

Högberg, J., Orrenius, S. and O'Brien, P. J. (1975a) Further studies on lipid-peroxide formation in isolated hepatocytes. *Eur. J. Biochem.* **59**, 449–455.

Högberg, J., Moldeus, P., Arborgh, B., O'Brien, P. J. and Orrenius, S. (1975b) The consequence of lipid peroxidation in isolated hepatocytes. *Eur. J. Biochem.* **59**, 457–462.

Holman, R. T. (1954) Autoxidation of fats and related substances. In *Progress in the Chemistry of Fats and Other Lipids*, Vol. 2, (eds R. T. Holman, W. O. Lundberg and T. Malkin), Academic Press, London, pp. 51–98.

Houglum, K., Filip, M., Witztum, J. L. and Chojkier, M. (1990) Malondialdehyde and 4-hydroxynonenal protein adducts in plasma and liver of rats with iron overload. *J. Clin. Invest.* **86**, 1991–1998.

Hruszkewycz, A. M. (1988) Evidence for mitochondrial DNA damage by lipid peroxidation. *Biochem. Biophys. Res. Commun.* **153**, 191–197.

Huebers, H. A., Brittenham, G. M., Csiba, E. and Finch, C. A. (1986) Absorption of carbonyl iron. *J. Lab. Clin. Med.* **108**, 473–478.

Hultcrantz, R. and Glaumann, H. (1982) Studies on the rat liver following iron overload: biochemical analysis after iron mobilization. *Lab. Invest.* **46**, 383–392.

Hultcrantz, R., Ahlberg, J. and Glaumann, H. (1984a) Isolation of two lysosomal populations from iron-overloaded rat liver with different iron concentration and proteolytic activity. *Virchows Arch. B (Cell Pathol.)* **47**, 55–65.

Hultcrantz, R., Ercisson, J. L. E. and Hirth, T. (1984b) Levels of malondialdehyde production in rat liver following loading and unloading of iron. *Virchows Arch. B (Cell Pathol.)* **45**, 139–146.

Hunter, F. E., Jr, Gebicki, J. M., Hoffsten, P. E., Weinstein, J. and Scott, A. (1963) Swelling and lysis of rat liver mitochondria induced by ferrous ions. *J. Biol. Chem.* **238**, 828–835.

Iancu, T. C., Neustein, H. B. and Landing, B. H. (1977) The liver in thalassemia major: ultrastructural observations. In: *Iron Metabolism*. Ciba Foundation Symposium, New Series, Elsevier, Amsterdam, pp. 293–307.

Iancu, T. C., Ward, R. J. and Peters, T. J. (1987) Ultrastructural observations in the carbonyl iron-fed rat, an animal model for hemochromatosis. *Virchows Arch. B. (Cell Pathol.)* **53**, 208–217.

Ibrahim, N. G., Nelson, J. C. and Levere, R. D. (1981) Control of δ-aminolaevulinate synthase and haem oxygenase in chronic iron overloaded rats. *Biochem. J.* **200**, 35–42.

Imlay, J. A., Chin, S. M. and Linn, S. (1988) Toxic DNA damage by hydrogen peroxide through the Fenton reaction *in vivo* and *in vitro*. *Science* **240**, 640–642.

Irving, M. G., Halliday, J. W. and Powell, L. W. (1988) Association between alcoholism and increased hepatic iron stores. *Alcoholism: Clin. Exp. Res.* **12**, 7–13.

Irving, M. G., Booth, C. J., Devlin, C. M., Halliday, J. W. and Powell, L. W. (1991) The effect of iron and ethanol on rat hepatocyte collagen synthesis. *Comp. Biochem. Physiol.* **100C**, 583–590.

Isaacson, C., Seftel, H., Keeley, K. J. and Bothwell, T. H. (1961) Siderosis in the Bantu. The relationship between iron overload and cirrhosis. *J. Lab. Clin. Med.* **58**, 845–853.

Jacobs, A. (1977) Low molecular weight intracellular iron transport compounds. *Blood* **50**, 433–439.

Kaplan, J., Craven, C., Alexander, J., Kushner, J., Lamb, J. and Bernstein, S. (1988) Regulation of the distribution of tissue iron. Lessons learned from the hypotransferrinemic mouse. *Ann. NY Acad. Sci.* **526**, 124–135.

Kawabata, T., Ogino, T. and Awai, M. (1989) Protective effects of glutathione against lipid peroxidation in chronically iron-loaded mice. *Biochim. Biophys. Acta* **1004**, 89–94.

Kirkpatrick, D. T., Guth, D. J. and Mavis, R. D. (1986) Detection of *in vivo* lipid peroxidation using the thiobarbituric acid assay for lipid hydroperoxides. *J. Biochem. Toxicol.* **1**, 93–104.

Koster, J. F. and Slee, R. G. (1986) Ferritin, a physiological iron donor for microsomal lipid peroxidation. *FEBS Lett.* **199**, 85–88.

Kuchino, Y., Mori, F., Kasai, H. *et al.* (1987) Misreading of DNA templates containing 8-hydroxydeoxyguanosine at the modified base and at adjacent residues. *Nature* **327**, 77–79.

Lee, Y. H., Layman, D. K., Bell, R. R. and Norton, H. W. (1981) Response of glutathione peroxidase and catalase to excess dietary iron in rats. *J. Nutr.* **111**, 2195–2202.

LeSage, G. D., Kost, L. J., Barham, S. S. and LaRusso, N. F. (1986) Biliary excretion of iron from hepatocyte lysosomes in the rat. A major excretory pathway in experimental iron overload. *J. Clin. Invest.* **77**, 90–97.

Levin, W., Lu, A. Y. H., Jacobson, M., Kuntzman, R., Poyer, J. L. and McCay, P. B. (1973) Lipid peroxidation and the degradation of cytochrome P-450 heme. *Arch. Biochem. Biophys.* **158**, 842–853.

Li, J.-L., Okada, S., Hamazaki, S., Ebina, Y. and Midorikawa, O. (1987) Subacute nephro-toxicity and induction of renal cell carcinoma in mice treated with ferric nitrilotriacetate. *Cancer Res.* **47**, 1867–1869.

Li, S. C. Y., O'Neill, R., Britton, R. S., Kobayashi, Y. and Bacon, B. R. (1992) Lipocytes from rats with chronic iron overload have increased collagen and protein production. (Abstract). *Gastroenterology* **102**, A841.

Lisboa, P. E. (1971) Experimental hepatic cirrhosis in dogs caused by chronic massive iron overload. *Gut* **12**, 363–368.

Longueville, A. and Crichton, R. R. (1986) An animal model of iron overload and its application to study hepatic ferritin iron mobilization by chelators. *Biochem. Pharmacol.* **35**, 3669–3678.

Lowenstine, L. J. and Petrak, M. L. (1978) Iron pigment in the liver of birds. In: *The Comparative Pathology of Zoo Animals* (eds R. Montali and G. Migaki), Smithsonian Press, Washington, D. C., pp. 127–135.

Lowrey, K., Glende, E. A., Jr and Recknagel, R. O. (1981) Destruction of liver microsomal calcium pump activity by carbon tetrachloride and bromotrichloromethane. *Biochem. Pharmacol.* **30**, 135–140.

Lundvall, O., Weinfeld, A. and Lundin, P. (1970) Iron storage in porphyria cutanea tarda. *Acta Med. Scand.* **188**, 37–53.

Mak, I. T. and Weglicki, W. B. (1985) Characterization of iron-mediated peroxidative injury in isolated hepatic lysosomes. *J. Clin. Invest.* **75**, 58–63.

Marshansky, V. N., Novgorodov, S. A. and Yaguzhinsky, L. S. (1983) The role of lipid peroxidation in the induction of cation transport in rat liver mitochondria. The antioxidant effect of oligomycin and dicyclohexylcarbodiimide. *FEBS Lett.* **158**, 27–30.

Masini, A., Ceccarelli-Stanzani, D., Trenti, T., Rocchi, E. and Ventura, E. (1984a) Structural and functional properties of rat liver mitochondria in hexachlorbenzene induced experimental porphyria. *Biochem. Biophys. Res. Commun.* **118**, 356–363.

Masini, A., Trenti, T., Ventura, E., Ceccarelli-Stanzani, D. and Muscatello, U. (1984b) Functional efficiency of mitochondrial membrane of rats with hepatic chronic iron overload. *Biochem. Biophys. Res. Commun.* **124**, 462–469.

Masini, A., Trenti, T., Ventura, E., Ceccarelli, D. and Muscatello, U. (1985) The effect of ferric iron complex on Ca^{2+} transport in isolated rat liver mitochondria. *Biochem. Biophys. Res. Commun.* **130**, 207–213.

Masini, A., Ceccarelli, D., Trenti, T., Corongiu, F. P. and Muscatello, U. (1989) Perturbation in liver mitochondrial Ca^{2+} homeostasis in experimental iron overload: A possible factor in cell injury. *Biochim. Biophys. Acta* **1014**, 133–140.

May, M. E., Parmley, R. T., Spicer, S. S., Ravenel, D. P., May, E. E. and Buse, M. G. (1980) Iron nitrilotriacetate-induced experimental diabetes in rats. *J. Lab. Clin. Med.* **95**, 525–535.

McLaren, G. D., Muir, W. A. and Kellermeyer, R. W. (1983) Iron overload disorders. Natural history, pathogenesis, diagnosis and therapy. *CRC Crit. Rev. Clin. Lab. Sci.* **19**, 205–266.

McKnight, R. C. and Hunter, F. E., Jr (1966) Mitochondrial membrane ghosts produced by lipid peroxidation induced by ferrous ion. II. Composition and enzymatic activity. *J. Biol. Chem.* **241**, 2757–2765.

Mello Filho, A. C. and Meneghini, R. (1984) *In vivo* formation of single strand breaks in DNA by hydrogen peroxide is mediated by the Haber-Weiss reaction. *Biochim. Biophys. Acta* **781**, 56–63.

Minotti, G. and Aust, S. D. (1987) The requirement for iron (III) in the initiation of lipid peroxidation by iron (II) and hydrogen peroxide. *J. Biol. Chem.* **262**, 1098–1104.

Modell, B. and Berdoukas, V. (1984) *The Clinical Approach to Thalassemia*. Grune and Stratton, London.

Morel, I., Lescoat, G., Cillard, J., Pasdeloup, N., Brissot, P. and Cillard, P. (1990) Kinetic evaluation of free malondialdehyde and enzyme leakage as indices of iron damage in rat hepatocyte cultures. Involvement of free radicals. *Biochem. Pharmacol.* **11**, 1647–1655.

Morley, C. G. D., Rewers, K. A. and Bezkorovainy, A. (1983) Iron metabolism pathways in the rat hepatocyte. *Clin. Physiol. Biochem.* **1**, 3–11.

Moscarella, S., Laffi, G., Buzzelli, G., Mazzanti, R., Caramelli, L. and Gentilini, P. (1984) Expired hydrocarbons in patients with chronic liver disease. *Hepato-Gastroenterology* **31**, 60–63.

Mulligan, M., Althaus, B. and Linder, M. C. (1986) Non-ferritin, non-heme iron pools in rat tissues. *Int. J. Biochem.* **18**, 791–798.

Munro, H. N. and Linder, M. C. (1978) Ferritin: structure, biosynthesis and role in iron metabolism. *Physiol. Rev.* **58**, 317–396.

Myers, B. M., Prendergast, F. G., Holman, R., Kuntz, S. M. and LaRusso, N. F. (1991) Alterations in the structure, physicochemical properties, and pH of hepatocyte lysosomes in experimental iron overload. *J. Clin. Invest.* **88**, 1207–1215.

Nath, L., Sood, S. K. and Nayak, N. C. (1972) Experimental siderosis and liver injury in the rhesus monkey. *J. Pathol.* **106**, 103–111.

Nichols, G. M. and Bacon, B. R. (1989) Hereditary hemochromatosis: Pathogenesis and clinical features of a common disease. *Am. J. Gastroenterol.* **84**, 851–862.

Niederau, C., Fischer, R., Sonnenberg, A, Stremmel, W., Trampisch, H. J. and Strohmeyer, G. (1985) Survival and causes of death in cirrhotic and in noncirrhotic patients with primary hemochromatosis. *N. Engl. J. Med.* **313**, 1256–1262.

O'Connell, M. J., Ward, R. J., Baum, H. and Peters, T. J. (1985) The role of iron in ferritin and haemosiderin-mediated lipid peroxidation in lysosomes. *Biochem. J.* **229**, 135–139.

O'Connell, M. J., Baum, H. and Peters, T. J. (1986a) Haemosiderin-like properties of free-radical-modified ferritin. *Biochem. J.* **240**, 297–300.

O'Connell, M., Halliwell, B., Moorhouse, C. P., Aruoma, O. I., Baum, H. and Peters, T. J. (1986b) Formation of hydroxyl radicals in the presence of ferritin and haemosiderin. Is haemosiderin formation a biological protective mechanism? *Biochem. J.* **234**, 727–731.

Okada, S., Hamazaki, S., Ebina, Y., Fujioka, M. and Midorikawa, O. (1983) Nephrotoxicity and induction of the renal adenocarcinoma by ferric-nitrilotriacetate (Fe-NTA) in rats. In: *Structure and Function of Iron Storage and Transport Proteins* (eds I. Urushizaki, P. Aisen, I. Listowsky and J. W. Drysdale), Elsevier, New York, pp. 473–478.

Olsson, K. S., Ritter, B., Rosen, U., Heedman, P. A. and Staugard, F. (1983) Prevalence of iron overload in central Sweden. *Acta Med. Scand.* **213**, 145–150.

Olynyk, J., Hall, P., Sallie, R., Reed, W., Shilkin, K. and Mackinnon, M. (1990) Computerized measurement of iron in liver biopsies: a comparison with biochemical iron measurement. *Hepatology* **12**, 26–30.

Ozaki, M., Kawabata, T. and Awai, M. (1988) Iron release from haemosiderin and production of iron-catalyzed hydroxyl radicals *in vitro*. *Biochem. J.* **250**, 589–595.

Park, C. H., Bacon, B. R., Brittenham, G. M. and Tavill, A. S. (1987) Pathology of dietary carbonyl iron overload in rats. *Lab. Invest.* **57**, 555–563.

Park, J.-W. and Floyd, R. A. (1992) Lipid peroxidation products mediate the formation of 8-hydroxydeoxyguanosine in DNA. *Free Rad. Biol. Med.* **12**, 245–250.

Parkkila, S., Niemelä, O., Ylä-Herttuala, S., Bacon, B. R., Singh, R. and Britton, R. S. (1992) Dietary supplementation with vitamin E decreases hepatic levels of fluorescent peroxidation products in rats with iron overload (Abstract). *Gastroenterology* **102**, A867.

Parola, M., Pinzani, M., Casini, A. *et al.* (1993) Stimulation of lipid peroxidation or 4-hydroxynonenal treatment increases procollagen alpha 1 (I) gene expression in human liver fat-storing cells. *Biochem. Biophys. Res. Commun.* **194**, 1044–1050.

Pechet, G. S. (1969) Parenteral iron overload. Organ and cell distribution in rats. *Lab. Invest.* **20**, 119–126.

Peters, T. J. and Seymour, C. A. (1976) Acid hydrolase activities and lysosomal integrity in liver biopsies from patients with iron overload. *Clin. Sci. Mol. Med.* **50**, 75–78.

Peters, T. J., Jones, B. M., Jacobs, A. and Wagstaff, J. (1985a) 'Free' iron and lipid peroxidation in the plasma of patients with iron overload. In: *Proteins of Iron Storage and Transport* (eds. G. Spik, J. Montreuil, R. R. Crichton and J. Mazurier), Elsevier, New York, pp. 321–324.

Peters, T. J., O'Connell, M. J. and Ward, R. J. (1985b) Role of free-radical mediated lipid peroxidation in the pathogenesis of hepatic damage by lysosomal disruption. In: *Free Radicals in Liver Injury* (eds G. Poli, K. H. Cheeseman, M. U. Dianzani and T. F. Slater), IRL Press, Oxford, pp. 107–115.

Pfeifer, P. M. and McCay, P. B. (1972) Reduced triphosphopyridine nucleotide oxidase-catalyzed alterations of membrane phospholipids. VI. Structural changes in mitochondria associated with inactivation of electron transport activity. *J. Biol. Chem.* **247**, 6763–6769.

Pietrangelo, A., Tripodi, A,. Carulli, N. *et al.* (1989) Lipid composition and fluidity of liver plasma membranes from rats with chronic dietary iron overload. *J. Bioenergetics Biomembranes* **21**, 527–533.

Pietrangelo, A., Grandi, R., Tripodi, A. *et al.* (1990a) Lipid composition and fluidity of liver mitochondria, microsomes and plasma membrane of rats with chronic dietary iron overload. *Biochem. Pharmacol.* **39**, 123–128.

Pietrangelo, A., Rocchi, E., Schiaffonati, L., Ventura, E. and Cairo, G. (1990b) Liver gene expression during chronic dietary iron overload in rats. *Hepatology* **11**, 798–804.

Pietrangelo, A., Gualdi, R., Geerts, A., De Bleser, P., Casalgrandi, G. and Ventura, E. (1992) Enhanced hepatic collagen gene expression in a rodent model of hemochromatosis. (Abstract). *Gastroenterology* **102**, A868.

Poli, G. and Gravela, E. (1982). Lipid peroxidation in isolated hepatocytes. In: *Free Radicals, Lipid Peroxidation and Cancer* (eds D. C. H. McBrien and T. F. Slater), Academic Press, New York, pp. 215–234.

Poli, G., Chiarpotto, E., Albano, E. *et al.* (1983) Biochemical evidence for chemical and/or topographic differences in the lipoperoxidative processes induced by CCl_4 and iron. *Chem. Biol. Interact.* **43**, 253–261.

Poli, G., Chiarpotto, E., Albano, E., Biasi, F., Cecchini, G. and Dianzani, M. U. (1986) Iron overload: experimental approach using rat hepatocytes in single cell suspension. *Front. Gastrointest. Res.* **9**, 38–49.

Pollack, S., Campana, T. and Weaver, J. (1985) Low molecular weight iron in guinea pig reticulocytes. *Am. J. Hematol.* **19**, 75–84.

Polson, C. (1933) The failure of prolonged administration of iron to cause haemochromatosis. *Br. J. Exp. Pathol.* **14**, 73–76.

Powell, L. W., Bassett, M. L. and Halliday, J. W. (1980) Hemochromatosis: 1980 update. *Gastroenterology* **78**, 374–381.

Preece, N. E., Hall, D. E., Howarth, J. A., King, L. J. and Parke, D. V. (1989) Effects of acute and sub-chronic administration of iron nitrilotriacetate in the rat. *Toxicology* **59**, 37–58.

Pryor, W. A. (1988) Why is the hydroxyl radical the only radical that commonly adds to DNA? Hypothesis: It has a rare combination of electrophilicity, high thermochemical reactivity, and a mode of production that can occur near DNA. *Free Rad. Biol. Med.* **4**, 219–223.

Rachmilewitz, E. A. (1976) The role of intracellular hemoglobin precipitation, low MCHC, and iron overload on red blood cell membrane peroxidation in thalassemia. *Birth Defects: Orig. Artic. Ser.* **12**, 123–133.

Rachmilewitz, E. A., Lubin, B. H. and Shoet, S. B. (1976) Lipid membrane peroxidation in β-thalassemia major. *Blood* **47**, 495–505.

Randell, M. G., Patnaik, A. K. and Gould, W. J. (1981) Hepatopathy associated with excessive iron storage in mynah birds. *J. Am. Vet. Med. Assoc.* **179**, 1214–1217.

Rao, K. S. and Recknagel, R. O. (1968) Early onset of lipoperoxidation in rat liver after carbon tetrachloride administration. *Exp. Mol. Pathol.* **9**, 271–278.

Recknagel, R. O. and Glende, E. A., Jr (1984) Spectrophotometric detection of lipid conjugated dienes. *Methods Enzymol.* **105**, 331–337.

Reif, D. W. (1992) Ferritin as a source of iron for oxidative damage. *Free Rad. Biol. Med.* **12**, 417–427.

Richter, G. W. (1974) Effects of cyclic starvation-feeding and of splenectomy on the development of hemosiderosis in rat livers. *Am. J. Pathol.* **74**, 481–502.

Richter, G. W. (1984) Studies of iron overload. Rat liver siderosome formation. *Lab. Invest.* **50**, 26–35.

Risdon, R. A., Barry, M. and Flynn, D. M. (1975) Transfusional iron overload: The relationship between tissue iron concentration and hepatic fibrosis in thalassemia. *J. Pathol.* **116**, 83–95.

Roberts, F. D., Charalambous, P., Fletcher, L., Powell, L. W. and Halliday, J. W. (1993) Effect of chronic iron overload on procollagen gene expression. *Hepatology* **18**, 590–595.

Romslo, I. (1980) Intracellular transport of iron. In: *Iron in Biochemistry and Medicine II* (eds A. Jacobs and M. Worwood), Academic Press, London, pp. 325–362.

Rush, G. F., Gorski, J. R., Ripple, M. G., Sowinski, J., Bugelski, P. and Hewitt, W. R. (1985) Organic hydroperoxide-induced lipid peroxidation and cell death in isolated hepatocytes. *Toxicol. Appl. Pharmacol.* **78**, 473–483.

Sacks, P. V. and Houchin, D. N. (1978) Comparative bioavailability of elemental iron powders for repair of iron deficiency anemia in rats. Studies of efficacy and toxicity of carbonyl iron. *Am. J. Clin. Nutr.* **31**, 566–573.

Sallie, R. W., Reed, W. D. and Shilkin, K. B. (1991) Confirmation of the efficacy of hepatic tissue iron index in differentiating genetic haemochromatosis from alcoholic liver disease complicated by alcoholic haemosiderosis. *Gut* **32**, 207–210.

Schacter, B. A., Marver, H. S. and Meyer, U. A. (1972) Hemoprotein catabolism during stimulation of microsomal lipid peroxidation. *Biochim. Biophys. Acta* **279**, 221–227.

Selden, C., Owen, M., Hopkins, J. M. P. and Peters, T. J. (1980a) Studies on the concentration and intracellular localization of iron proteins in liver biopsy specimens from patients with iron overload with special reference to their role in lysosomal disruption. *Br. J. Haematol.* **44**, 593–603.

Selden, C., Seymour, C. A. and Peters, T. J. (1980b) Activities of some free-radical scavenging enzymes and glutathione concentrations in human and rat liver and their relationship to the pathogenesis of tissue damage in iron overload. *Clin. Sci.* **58**, 211–219.

Seymour, C. A. and Peters, T. J. (1978) Organelle pathology in primary and secondary haemochromatosis with special reference to lysosomal changes. *Br. J. Haematol.* **40**, 239–253.

Sharma, B. K., Bacon, B. R., Britton, R. S. *et al.* (1990) Prevention of hepatocyte injury and lipid peroxidation by iron chelators and α-tocopherol in isolated iron-loaded rat hepatocytes. *Hepatology* **12**, 31–39.

Shires, T. K. (1982) Iron-induced DNA damage and synthesis in isolated rat liver nuclei. *Biochem. J.* **205**, 321–329.

Smith, A. G. and De Matteis, F. (1990) Oxidative injury mediated by the cytochrome P-450 system in conjuction with cellular iron. Effects on the pathway of haem biosynthesis. *Xenobiotica* **20**, 865–877.

Smith, A. G., Francis, J. E. and Carthew, P. (1990) Iron as a synergist for hepatocellular carcinoma induced by polychlorinated biphenyls in *Ah*-responsive C57BL/10ScSn mice. *Carcinogenesis* **11**, 437–444.

Sokol, R. J., Twedt, D., Devereaux, M. W., Karrer, F., Kam, I. and Hambidge, K. M. (1992) Role of free radicals in copper hepatotoxicity: Evidence from the Bedlington terrier and Wilson's disease patients. (Abstract). *Hepatology* **16**, 159A.

Srinivasan, S. and Recknagel, R. O. (1971) A note on the stability of conjugated diene absorption of rat liver microsomal lipids after carbon tetrachloride poisoning. *J. Lipid Res.* **12**, 766–767.

Stacey, N. and Priestly, B. G. (1978) Lipid peroxidation in isolated rat hepatocytes: relationship to toxicity of CCl_4, ADP/Fe^{3+}, and diethyl maleate. *Toxicol. Appl. Pharmacol.* **45**, 41–48.

Stacey, N. H. and Klaassen, C. D. (1981) Comparison of the effects of metals on cellular injury and lipid peroxidation in isolated rat hepatocytes. *J. Toxicol. Environ. Health* **7**, 139–147.

Stål, P., Glaumann, H. and Hultcrantz, R. (1990) Liver cell damage and lysosomal iron storage in patients with idiopathic hemochromatosis. A light and electron microscopic study. *J. Hepatol.* **11**, 172–180.

Starke, P. E. and Farber, J. L. (1985) Ferric iron and superoxide ions are required for the killing of cultured hepatocytes by hydrogen peroxide. Evidence for the participation of hydroxyl radicals formed by an iron-catalyzed Haber-Weiss reaction. *J. Biol. Chem.* **260**, 10099–10104.

Stocks, J., Offerman, E. L., Modell, C. B. and Dormandy, T. L. (1972) The susceptibility to autoxidation of human red cell lipids in health and disease. *Br. J. Haematol.* **23**, 713–724.

Summers, K. M., Halliday, J. W. and Powell, L. W. (1990) Identification of homozygous hemochromatosis subjects by measurement of hepatic iron index. *Hepatology* **12**, 20–25.

Takeshita, M., Grollman, A. P., Ohtsubo, E. and Ohtsubo, H. (1978) Interaction of bleomycin with DNA. *Proc. Natl. Acad. Sci. USA* **75**, 5983–5987.

Tangerås, A. (1983) Iron content and degree of lipid peroxidation in liver mitochondria isolated from iron-loaded rats. *Biochim. Biophys. Acta* **757**, 59–68.

Tavill, A. S. and Bacon, B. R. (1986) Hemochromatosis: How much iron is too much? *Hepatology* **6**, 142–145.

Tavill, A. S. and Bacon, B. R. (1990) Hemochromatosis: Iron metabolism and the iron overload syndromes. In: *Hepatology: A Textbook of Liver Disease* (eds D. Zakim and T. D. Boyer), W. B. Saunders, Philadelphia, pp. 1273–1299.

Thomas, C. E., Morehouse, L. A. and Aust, S. D. (1985) Ferritin and superoxide-dependent lipid peroxidation. *J. Biol. Chem.* **260**, 3275–3280.

Thomas, D. W., van Kuijk, F. J. G. M., Dratz, E. A. and Stephens, R. J. (1991) Quantitative determination of hydroxy fatty acids as an indicator of *in vivo* lipid peroxidation: Gas chromatography–mass spectrometry methods. *Anal. Biochem.* **198**, 104–111.

Toyokuni, S., Okada, S., Hamazaki, S. *et al.* (1990) Combined histochemical and biochemical analysis of sex hormone dependence of ferric nitrilotriacetate-induced renal lipid peroxidation in ddY mice. *Cancer Res.* **50**, 5574–5580.

Umemura, T., Sai, K., Takagi, A., Hasegawa, R. and Kurokawa, Y. (1990) Formation of 8-hydroxydeoxyguanosine (8-OH-dG) in rat kidney DNA after intraperitoneal administration of ferric nitrilotriacetate (Fe-NTA). *Carcinogenesis* **11**, 345–347.

Ungemach, F. R. (1985) Plasma membrane damage of hepatocytes following lipid peroxidation: involvement of phospholipase A_2. In: *Free Radicals in Liver Injury* (eds G. Poli, K. H. Cheeseman, M. U. Dianzani and T. F. Slater), IRL Press, Oxford, pp. 127–134.

Ungemach, F. R. (1987) Pathobiochemical mechanisms of hepatocellular damage following lipid peroxidation. *Chem. Phys. Lipids* **45**, 171–205.

Vladimirov, Y. A., Olenev, V. I., Suslova, T. B. and Cheremisina, Z. P. (1980) Lipid peroxidation in mitochondrial membranes. *Adv. Lipid Res.* **17**, 173–249.

Waller, R. L., Glende E. A., Jr and Recknagel, R. O. (1983) Carbon tetrachloride and bromotrichloromethane toxicity. Dual role of covalent binding of metabolic cleavage products and lipid peroxidation in depression of microsomal calcium sequestration. *Biochem. Pharmacol.* **32**, 1613–1617.

Walles, S. A. S. and Erixon, K. (1984) Single-strand breaks in DNA of various organs of mice induced by methyl methanesulfonate and dimethylsulfoxide determined by the alkaline unwinding technique. *Carcinogenesis* **5**, 319–323.

Ward, R. J., Florence, A. L., Baldwin, D. *et al.* (1991) Biochemical and biophysical investigations of the ferrocene-iron-loaded rat. An animal model of primary haemochromatosis. *Eur. J. Biochem.* **202**, 405–410.

Weaver, J. and Pollack, S. (1989) Low-Mr iron isolated from guinea pig reticulocytes as AMP-Fe and ATP-Fe complexes. *Biochem. J.* **261**, 787–792.

Weintraub, L. R., Goral, A., Grasso, J., Franzblau, C., Sullivan, A. and Sullivan, S. (1985) Pathogenesis of hepatic fibrosis in experimental iron overload. *Br. J. Haematol.* **59**, 321–331.

Wills, E. D. (1966) Mechanisms of lipid peroxide formation in animal tissues. *Biochem. J.* **99**, 667–676.

Wills, E. D. (1972) Effects of iron overload on lipid peroxide formation and oxidative demethylation by the liver endoplasmic reticulum. *Biochem. Pharmacol.* **21**, 239–247.

Wixom, R. L., Prutkin, L. and Munro, H. M. (1980) Hemosiderin: nature, formation and significance. *Int. Rev. Exp. Pathol.* **22**, 193–225.

Wood, M. L., Dizdaroglu, M., Gajewski, E. and Essigmann, J. M. (1990) Mechanistic studies of ionizing irradiation and oxidative mutagenesis: genetic effects of a single 8-hydroxyguanine (7-hydro-8-oxoguanine) residue inserted at a unique site in a viral genome. *Biochemistry* **29**, 7024–7032.

Wu, W.-H., Meydani, M., Meydani, S. N., Burklund, P. M., Blumberg, J. B. and Munro, H. H. (1990) Effect of dietary iron overload on lipid peroxidation, prostaglandin synthesis and lymphocyte proliferation in young and old rats. *J. Nutr.* **120**, 280–289.

Yamada, M., Awai, M. and Okigaki, T. (1990) Rapid *in vitro* transformation system for liver epithelial cells by iron chelate, Fe-NTA. *Cytotechnology* **3**, 149–156.

Younes, M., Eberhardt, I. and Lemoine, R. (1989) Effect of iron overload on spontaneous and xenobiotic-induced lipid peroxidation *in vivo*. *J. Appl. Toxicol.* **9**, 103–108.

Younes, M., Trepkau, H.-D. and Siegers, C.-P. (1990) Enhancement by dietary iron of lipid peroxidation in mouse colon. *Res. Commun. Chem. Pathol. Pharmacol.* **70**, 349–354.

Young, I. S., Trouton, T. G., Torney, J. J., Callender, M. E. and Trimble, E. R. (1992) Antioxidant status in hereditary haemochromatosis. (Abstract). *Free Rad. Res. Commun.* **16**, (Suppl. 1), 187.

Zannos-Mariolea, L., Tzortzatou, F., Dendaki-Svolaki, K., Katerellos, Ch., Kavallari, M. and Matsaniotis, N. (1974) Serum vitamin E levels with beta-thalassaemia major: Preliminary report. *Br. J. Haematol.* **26**, 193–199.

11. Iron in Infection, Immunity, Inflammation and Neoplasia

J. H. BROCK

University Department of Immunology, Western Infirmary, Glasgow G11 6NT, Scotland, UK

I. INTRODUCTION

Although the majority of iron in the body is found in haemoglobin, smaller quantities are present in many other molecules, in which the presence of this metal is essential to their biological activity. These have diverse functions, and include various activities associated with both specific and innate (or non-specific) immunity. Iron is also essential for the growth of nearly all microorganisms, and it is possible that its limited availability in host tissues may influence the progress of microbial infections. Iron may thus play an important role in determining the ability of the host to mount an immune response and on the outcome of infection. Furthermore, these processes, and the associated inflammatory response, induce changes in the normal pattern of iron recirculation, resulting in hypoferraemia and anaemia. Iron may also play a role in carcinogenesis, due in part to its ability to enhance tumour cell development and growth, and also to its potential role as a carcinogen.

Nevertheless, in spite of the ever-increasing body of knowledge on the subject of iron, infection and neoplasia, many aspects remain unclear and in some cases controversial. This chapter will attempt to draw together our current state of knowledge.

2. IRON, IMMUNITY AND INFECTION

There are two ways in which iron may influence the course of infection. On the one hand the iron requirement of most microorganisms coupled with a lack of readily available iron in normal body tissues means that any abnormality, such as iron overload, which makes iron unusually available may predispose to infection. On the other hand, the immune system requires iron for a number of its functions, and

Table 11.1 Potential roles of iron in immunity

Activity	Role of iron	Iron deficiency	Iron overload
(A) Non-specific (innate) immunity			
Inhibition of microbial growth	Sequestration of iron by host molecules	(Enhanced resistance to malaria?)	Possibly enhances susceptibility to some infections
Phagocytic activity of neutrophils	1. Involved in oxygen-mediated microbicidal mechanisms	Depressed microbicidal activity	—
	2. Membrane lipid peroxidation	—	Phagocytic uptake impaired
(B) Specific immunity			
Lymphocyte proliferation	DNA synthesis (ribonucleotide reductase)	Depressed cell-mediated immunity	—
T-cell subsets	Unknown	—	Decreased CD4:CD8 ratio
Macrophage cytotoxicity (immunologically-activated)	Destruction of target iron-proteins by nitric oxide	—	(Reduced tumouricidal activity?)

an inadequate supply, such as can occur in iron deficiency, may impair immune function, which in turn could also predispose to infection. Both these aspects, which are discussed below, have received considerable attention, and have been reviewed (Hershko *et al.*, 1988; Dhur *et al.*, 1989; Oppenheimer, 1989; Weinberg, 1992a; Brock, 1993). The potential role of iron in these activities is summarized in Table 11.1.

2.1. Iron and Microbial Growth

2.1.1. *The Role of Siderophores*

One of the earliest properties attributed to transferrin was its ability to inhibit bacterial growth *in vitro* due to sequestration of available iron (Schade and Caroline, 1946). This observation has been confirmed in numerous subsequent studies, and an enormous range of microorganisms is now known to be inhibited by transferrin (and lactoferrin) *in vitro*. These include numerous potential pathogens (Table 11.2).

However, many microorganisms possess mechanisms to obtain iron from host tissues, and these may contribute to microbial pathogenicity. The best characterized involves the synthesis of low molecular weight, high affinity iron chelating molecules known as siderophores, which are capable, in theory at least, of removing iron from transferrin and other non-haem host iron proteins. The majority of siderophores are derivatives of either catechol or hydroxamic acid (reviewed by Hider, 1984). The siderophore enterochelin (also known as enterobactin) (O'Brien and Gibson, 1970) is the best characterized of the former group and is produced by many enterobacteria. However, these organisms frequently also produce a hydroxamate siderophore known as aerobactin (Braun, 1981). Despite its lower affinity for iron (Harris *et al.*, 1979), production of aerobactin rather than enterochelin tends to correlate with microbial pathogenicity (Warner *et al.*, 1981; De Lorenzo and Martinez, 1988), perhaps because aerobactin is less likely to be sequestered by serum albumin (Konopka and Neilands,

Table 11.2 Pathogenic microorganisms whose growth is inhibited *in vitro* by transferrin or lactoferrin

Organism	Reference
Escherichia coli	Bullen and Rogers (1969)
	Brock *et al.* (1983)
Legionella pneumophila	Quinn and Weinberg (1988)
Candida albicans	Valenti *et al.* (1986)
Vibrio vulnificus	Bullen *et al.* (1991*a*)
Bacteroides fragilis	Rocha *et al.* (1991)
Klebsiella pneumoniae	Ward *et al.* (1986)
Pseudomonas aeruginosa	Ankenbauer *et al.* (1985)
Neisseria meningitidis	Calver *et al.* (1979)
Neisseria gonorrhoeae	Finkelstein *et al.* (1983)
Listeria monocytogenes	Cowart and Foster (1985)
Clostridium welchii	Rogers *et al.* (1970)
Yersinia enterocolitica	Brock and Ng (1983)
Staphylococcus aureus	Brock and Ng (1983)
Vibrio cholerae	Boesman-Finkelstein and Finkelstein (1985)
Salmonella typhimurium	Yancey *et al.* (1979)

1984), or is more readily able to remove iron from within host cells, thus by-passing the need to extract iron from transferrin (Brock *et al.*, 1991).

Microorganisms take up iron–siderophore complexes via specific outer membrane receptors (Braun *et al.*, 1976; Grewal *et al.*, 1982; Neilands, 1982; Lundrigan and Kadner, 1986). Some siderophores such as enterochelin are then broken down within the microorganism (Langman *et al.*, 1972), while others such as aerobactin are recycled following release of iron to the cell (Braun *et al.*, 1984). Production of siderophores and their outer membrane receptors is generally not constitutive, but is induced by low levels of available iron (Perry and San Clemente, 1979; Williams *et al.*, 1984; Fernández-Beros *et al.*, 1989; reviewed by Griffiths, 1987). Some systems, such as aerobactin and its receptor, are plasmid-linked (Williams, 1979). It is also worth noting that some bacteria such as *Campylobacter jejuni* (Baig *et al.*, 1986) and *Yersinia enterocolitica* (Brock and Ng, 1983) can utilize siderophores they themselves do not produce. This may include the *Streptomyces* siderophore desferrioxamine, which is commonly used as an iron chelating drug (Chapter 12), and its use is thus sometimes associated with an increased risk of infection (Melby *et al.*, 1982; Boelaert *et al.*, 1988). However, in other cases (Chapter 12) desferrioxamine may suppress microbial growth, and it is of interest that orally-active hydroxypyridone chelators currently being developed for clinical use show less tendency than desferrioxamine to enhance microbial growth (Brock *et al.*, 1988).

Recent studies have suggested that siderophores may also assist microbial growth indirectly, for example by interfering with iron supply to the immune system (Autenrieth *et al.*, 1991), or catalysing production of tissue-damaging hydroxyl radicals (Coffman *et al.*, 1990).

2.1.2. Microbial Transferrin Receptors

Some bacteria do not synthesize siderophores, but instead express receptors for transferrin or lactoferrin, thus enabling the organism directly to acquire iron from the host protein. Such receptors are found in *Haemophilus* (Schryvers, 1989), *Neisseria meningitidis* (Schryvers and González, 1989; Ferrón *et al.*, 1992), *Pasteurella haemolytica* (Ogunnariwo and Schryvers, 1990) and *Mycoplasma pneumoniae* (Tryon and Baseman, 1987). These receptors are generally both protein- and species-specific; thus *Neisseria meningitidis*, a human pathogen, will bind human lactoferrin, but not bovine lactoferrin or human transferrin (Schryvers and Morris, 1988), whereas the bovine pathogen *Haemophilus somnus* will bind only bovine transferrin (Yu *et al.*, 1992). The ability of bacteria to acquire iron by binding host iron-proteins has been reviewed by Otto *et al.* (1992).

Transferrin- or lactoferrin-binding proteins may also be produced by some parasites, including *Leishmania* (Voyiatzaki and Soteriadou, 1992), *Trypanosoma brucei* (Schell *et al.*, 1991), *Schistosoma mansoni* (Clemens and Basch, 1989), *Trichomonas vaginalis* (Lehker and Alderete, 1992) and *Plasmodium falciparum* (Rodríguez and Jungery, 1986). It seems likely that these serve to provide iron to parasites. However, except in the case of *Plasmodium*, in which there is some doubt about the role of transferrin as an iron source (Hershko and Peto, 1988; see also Chapter 12) little is known about iron uptake and metabolism in parasites, and the role of iron in parasitic infections has received very little attention. This is an area that deserves further study.

2.1.3. Other Microbial Iron-uptake Systems

A number of other strategies exist for microbial acquisition of host iron. Some organisms produce proteolytic enzymes that can degrade host iron-binding proteins (Carlsson et al., 1984; Döring et al., 1988), while others are able to utilize haem iron (Otto et al., 1992) which may be present in plasma in high levels during haemolytic diseases and as a result increase susceptibility to infection (Bullen et al., 1991b). In some cases the haem-binding proteins haemopexin and hapto-globin can inhibit microbial uptake of free haem or haemoglobin respectively (Eaton et al., 1982; Dyer et al., 1987), though other microorganisms can still utilize these complexed forms (Massad et al., 1991; Lee, 1991). Finally, most research has centred upon iron uptake by extracellular microorganisms, and little is known about the extent to which growth and survival of intracellular pathogens depends upon iron availability. In the case of Shigella, intracellular haem compounds may provide a source of iron for intracellular growth (Payne, 1989). On the other hand, Listeria monocytogenes probably utilizes non-haem iron within macrophages (Alford et al., 1991).

2.1.4. Microbial Iron Acquisition In Vivo

The fact that many microorganisms need to synthesize components of specific iron-uptake systems when grown in the presence of host iron-binding proteins in vitro suggests that iron sequestration by the host could be an important innate defence mechanism against infection. Evidence that microbial growth in vivo under conditions of normal iron status does indeed take place in an iron-restricted environment comes from studies showing that siderophores or microbial membrane receptors for siderophores or host iron-binding proteins are hyperexpressed during in vivo growth (Griffiths and Humphreys, 1980; Anwar et al., 1984; Holland et al., 1992).

However, it is less clear whether alterations in the iron status of the host materially affect iron-withholding mechanisms. It has often been suggested that iron overload may predispose to infection due to increased availability of host iron to micro-organisms, but as discussed later (p. 367) evidence for this is not particularly convincing. In the first place it must be remembered that both transferrin and ferritin in normal individuals possess considerable reserves of iron-binding capacity, and even a substantial increase in total body burden may not saturate either protein. It is only when transferrin in particular becomes saturated with iron that forms of extracellular iron more immediately available to microorganisms are present in plasma, and until this occurs differences in transferrin saturation are not in themselves likely to alter the availability of iron to microorganisms to any great extent (Baltimore et al., 1982; Gordeuk et al., 1986; Gordeuk and Brittenham, 1992). The many early animal studies showing that parenteral iron administration increased susceptibility to infection (reviewed by Weinberg, 1984) need to be interpreted with care, as such treatment will provide a transient pool of non-transferrin-bound extracellular iron that can provide microorganisms with a period of enhanced growth potential. As discussed later (p. 367), such unbound iron may be responsible for the clinical evidence of increased incidence of infection in infants or malnourished individuals given parenteral iron.

It is also widely considered that the hypoferraemia associated with infection and inflammation (p. 367–371) serves to restrict microbial growth *in vivo* by reducing the level of extracellular (i.e. transferrin-bound) iron. However, there is actually little experimental data to support this hypothesis. Although decreased susceptibility to infection in animals may be found after induction of an inflammatory response this could be due to mechanisms unrelated to iron availability. Moreover the relatively modest reduction in transferrin saturation, from about 30% to 15% in man, is, as discussed above, unlikely in itself to alter the availability of iron to microbial iron-sequestering mechanisms. Indeed, recovery of patients suffering from staphylococcal furunculosis actually followed alleviation of an associated anaemia by iron supplements (Weijmer *et al.*, 1990). Thus more work is needed before this role of the hypoferraemia of inflammation can be considered as established.

2.1.5. *The Antimicrobial Function of Lactoferrin*

Lactoferrin, which unlike transferrin is present mainly in external secretions and in the secondary granules of neutrophils, may play a role in the defence of secretory tissues against infection (Sánchez *et al.*, 1992). As well as exercising a bacteriostatic effect through the traditional iron-withholding mechanism (Weinberg, 1984), lactoferrin is also bactericidal for some organisms (Arnold *et al.*, 1982). This effect is probably not directly due to the iron-binding function of lactoferrin and may involve interference with transport of other cations (Ellison and Giehl, 1991), mediated by a basic region near the N-terminus of the lactoferrin molecule (Bellamy *et al.*, 1992). Lactoferrin is responsible for the *in vitro* bacteriostatic effect of human milk (Bullen *et al.*, 1972; Griffiths and Humphreys, 1977) and is thought to contribute to the increased resistance of breast-fed babies to gastrointestinal infections compared with bottle-fed babies. Although this remains an attractive hypothesis, clinical studies designed to determine whether addition of (bovine) lactoferrin to infant formula can produce a gut flora resembling that of breast-fed infants have failed to show any significant effect (Moreau *et al.*, 1983; Balmer *et al.*, 1989; Roberts *et al.*, 1992). Possibly use of human rather than bovine lactoferrin might be more effective. It has also been suggested that lactoferrin contributes to maintaining the microbiological sterility of the mammary gland, though again there is scant *in vivo* evidence and what little there is relates to cattle rather than to man (Nonnecke and Smith, 1984).

Lactoferrin in neutrophils probably contributes to the antimicrobial armoury of these cells. Saturation of neutrophil lactoferrin *in vitro* by allowing the cells to phagocytose iron-containing immune complexes reduced their bactericidal activity (Bullen and Joyce, 1982), and patients with lactoferrin-deficient neutrophils suffered from increased incidence of infection (Breton-Gorius *et al.*, 1980; Boxer *et al.*, 1982).

2.1.6. *Conclusions*

In conclusion, therefore, it seems likely that the ability of host iron-binding proteins such as transferrin to sequester 'free' extracellular iron contributes to the innate or non-specific defences against infection. Lactoferrin may fulfil a similar function at secretory surfaces, though convincing *in vivo* evidence has yet to be provided. However, the degree to which the efficacy of this defence mechanism is significantly altered either by iron overload or by the hypoferraemia of inflammation is less clear, and the ability of these conditions to alter susceptibility to infection may not be as great as is sometimes suggested.

2.2. Iron and the Immune System

The immune system consists of a complex network of cells and proteins, the activation of which by a specific antigen involves various metabolic events. Experimental investigations have shown that some of these activities are iron-dependent, and clinical and experimental studies have therefore sought to determine whether abnormalities in iron metabolism can lead to impairment of the immune system. These latter studies have, however, been hindered by the difficulty of carrying out such work in human subjects, often in developing countries, and by poor experimental design and choice of controls, and it is therefore not surprising that conflicting results have quite often been obtained.

2.2.1. The Effect of Iron Deficiency on the Immune System

The possibility that iron deficiency impairs the functioning of the immune system has been the subject of a large number of clinical studies. The problems of experimental design and adequate controls are particularly evident in this area, and have been addressed in more detail elsewhere (Brock, 1993). Consequently many of the abnormalities reported are controversial, although others appear to be more consistent.

(a) *Lymphocyte function.* The effect of iron deficiency on various aspects of lymphocyte function has been extensively investigated, and these studies and their main findings are summarized in Table 11.3. Depressed cutaneous sensitivity to appropriate model antigens in iron-deficient individuals is a fairly frequent finding, though a few contrary results have also been reported. Although this may be due simply to reduced lymphocyte numbers, this has not been reported with the same degree of consistency, suggesting that other factors are also involved. However, a reduced proportion of T-cells is commonly found. Perhaps the most likely explanation for the decreased cutaneous hypersensitivity is an impairment of T-lymphocyte proliferation, as a failure of peripheral blood mononuclear cells to respond normally to T-cell mitogens *in vitro* is one of the most consistently reported immunological defects associated with iron deficiency. Even here, three studies have nevertheless reported normal T-cell responses in iron deficient individuals, but in two of these there were complicating factors, *viz.* pregnancy (Prema *et al.*, 1982) or hookworm infection (Kulapongs *et al.*, 1974). Studies in iron deficient experimental animals have confirmed the defect in T-cell mitogen responses (Kuvibidila *et al.*, 1981, 1983b; Soyano *et al.*, 1982; Mainou-Fowler and Brock, 1985; Kuvibidila and Sarpong, 1990), and suggest that the low transferrin saturation found in such conditions may result in an inadequate supply of the metal to the activated lymphocytes, thus preventing optimal proliferation (Mainou-Fowler and Brock, 1985). Such an explanation is supported by the observation that primed T-cells from iron deficient donors function normally in iron replete recipients, whereas cells from normal individuals showed impaired activity in iron deficient recipients (Cummins *et al.*, 1978). However, iron deficiency may also lead to intrinsic defects in

Table 11.3 Effects of iron deficiency on lymphocyte function

Function	References No. Depressed	Normal
Cutaneous hypersensitivity	3,8,10,11,14,18	1,15
Total lymphocytes	2,6,8	1,3,9,10,13,14
Total T-cells	1,2,8,9	3
Proportion of T-cells	1[†],3,6,8,9,13,14,17,18	2
In vitro T-cell proliferation	4–8,10,11,13–16,19	3,9,12
Total B-cells	2,9	1,3,8,17
Immunoglobulin levels	20	3,9,10,15,17
Antibody response to vaccination	21*	14,21*

References
1. Berger et al. (1992)
2. Santos and Falcão (1990)
3. Moraes-de-Souza et al. (1984)
4. Wakabayashi et al. (1988)
5. Srikantia et al. (1976)
6. Sawitsky et al. (1976)
7. Hoffbrand et al. (1976)
8. Krantman et al. (1982)
9. Prema et al. (1982)
10. MacDougall et al. (1975)
11. Joynson et al. (1972)
12. Kulapongs et al. (1974)
13. Bhaskaram and Reddy (1975)
14. Chandra (1975)
15. Gross et al. (1975)
16. Fletcher et al. (1975)
17. Bagchi et al. (1980)
18. Kemahli et al. (1988)
19. Jacobs and Joynson (1974)
20. Galán et al. (1988)
21. MacDougall and Jacobs (1978)

[†]Helper subset decreased, suppressor/cytotoxic subset unchanged.
*Response varied with different vaccines (see text).

lymphocytes, as electron microscopy has revealed mitochondrial abnormalities in cells from iron deficient individuals (Jarvis and Jacobs, 1974; Jiménez et al., 1982).

Evidence for impairment of B-cell function in iron deficiency is less convincing. Both normal and reduced B-cell numbers have been reported in iron deficient individuals, but immunoglobulin levels have generally been reported as normal, suggesting that B-cell function is not unduly affected. Clinically, the response to vaccination is probably also normal, and one study reporting an impaired response (MacDougall and Jacobs, 1978) is difficult to interpret as antibody responses were depressed to diphtheria toxoid but normal to typhoid. However, studies in iron deficient experimental animals have generally found an impaired response to vaccination (Nalder et al., 1972; Kochanowski and Sherman, 1985; Dhur et al., 1990). Thus although there is some evidence that B-cell activation is less iron-dependent than T-cell activation (see below), further work is required in this area.

(b) Macrophage function. The rather limited studies on macrophage function in iron deficiency suggest that some activities may be impaired. Although one clinical study of iron deficiency reported normal cytotoxic activity and IL1 release by monocytes activated in vitro (Bhaskaram et al., 1989), studies in animals in which macrophages were activated in vivo reported decreased production of IL1 (Helyar and Sherman, 1987) and α-interferon (Hallquist and Sherman, 1989), and reduced tumouricidal activity (Kuvibidila et al., 1983a). Clearance of polyvinylpyrrolidone in iron deficient rats is reduced (Kuvibidila and Wade, 1987), though whether this is due to a defect in macrophage function is unclear. However, the paucity of studies, particularly in man, make it difficult to draw any firm conclusions regarding the effect of iron deficiency on macrophage function.

(c) *Neutrophil function*. There is rather more information about the effect of iron deficiency on neutrophil activity. A number of clinical studies have shown that although phagocytic uptake is generally normal (Arbeter *et al.*, 1971; Chandra 1973, 1975; MacDougall *et al.*, 1975; Walter *et al.*, 1986), intracellular killing mechanisms are usually defective (Chandra, 1975; MacDougall *et al.*, 1975; Srikantia *et al.*, 1976; Yetgin *et al.*, 1979; Walter *et al.*, 1986), a finding that can probably be linked to a defect in the generation of reactive oxygen intermediates (Celada *et al.*, 1979; Prasad, 1979; Mackler *et al.*, 1984; Turgeon-O'Brien *et al.*, 1985; Murakawa *et al.*, 1987; Hasan *et al.*, 1989; Sullivan *et al.*, 1989). Similar findings have been reported in iron deficient rats (Moore and Humbert, 1984). However, two clinical studies failed to detect any abnormality in neutrophil function (Kulapongs *et al.*, 1974; Van Heerden *et al.*, 1983). Other neutrophil activities appear to be unaffected: lysozyme production and chemotaxis were both normal (MacDougall *et al.*, 1975; Van Heerden *et al.*, 1983), although a decreased recruitment of neutrophils into the lung and peritoneum was noted in iron deficient rats (Sullivan *et al.*, 1989).

(d) *Other immunological mechanisms*. Studies of the effect of iron deficiency on other aspects of the immune system are relatively few. In one study antibody-dependent lymphocyte cytotoxicity was impaired in iron deficient patients, but the defect was not corrected after iron depletion (Santos and Falcão, 1990). Defective natural killer cell activity was found in iron deficient rodents (Sherman and Lockwood, 1987; Hallquist and Sherman, 1989; Hallquist *et al.*, 1992; Spear and Sherman, 1992), but this may have been a secondary effect resulting from impaired γ-interferon production by macrophages (Hallquist and Sherman, 1989).

2.2.2. The Effect of Iron Overload on the Immune System

The degree to which iron overload affects the immune system has received less attention than iron deficiency, and the current state of knowledge, reviewed by De Sousa (1989), is somewhat sketchy. Most studies have been carried out with patients suffering from hereditary haemochromatosis, or from transfusional iron overload associated with conditions such as β-thalassaemia.

(a) *Lymphocyte function*. Particular attention has been paid to abnormalities in the proportions of T-lymphocyte subsets associated with iron overload. A frequent finding in β-thalassaemia is a reduced CD4:CD8 T-lymphocyte ratio (Guglielmo *et al.*, 1984; Grady *et al.*, 1985; Dwyer *et al.*, 1987; Nualart *et al.*, 1987). However, it is quite possible that chronic alloantigenic stimulation arising from repeated blood transfusions, rather than iron overload, may be responsible for these changes (Kaplan *et al.*, 1984; Grady *et al.*, 1985). Unfortunately the situation in hereditary haemochromatosis, in which this complication does not arise, is unclear, both normal and decreased CD4:CD8 ratios having been reported by the same group (Bryan *et al.*, 1984, 1991). In contrast, increased expression of CD2, a molecule involved in cell adhesion, has been reported in haemochromatosis (Bryan *et al.*, 1984, 1991) but appears not to have been noted in transfusional iron overload. The reason for this is unknown, and paradoxically exposure of normal T-lymphocytes to non-transferrin-bound iron *in vitro* causes a decrease rather than an increase in CD2 reactivity (De Sousa and Nishiya, 1978; Carvalho and de Sousa, 1988). Abnormally high expression of CD1 has been reported in thalassaemia intermedia (Guglielmo *et al.*, 1984), and is thought to be due to a maturation defect. The effect of iron overload on B-lymphocytes is also unclear: normal numbers were found in haemochromatosis patients (Bryan *et al.*, 1991), and although there is a report of elevated B-cell numbers in children with β-thalassaemia (Dwyer *et al.*, 1987) there was no correlation with serum ferritin levels, which again suggests that iron overload *per se* was not the cause. Increased spontaneous *in vitro* production of immunoglobulin by B-cells has been found in both thalassaemia and haemochromatosis (Bryan *et al.*, 1984; Nualart *et al.*, 1987), but serum immunoglobulin levels, though increased in thalassaemia (Dwyer *et al.*, 1987), were normal in haemochromatosis (Bryan *et al.*, 1984).

As with iron deficiency, there are reports, particularly in thalassaemia, of reduced skin test responses (Dwyer *et al.*, 1987) and *in vitro* T-cell responses to mitogens (Munn *et al.*, 1981; Dwyer *et al.*, 1987; Pattanapanyasat, 1990), though here again the relative importance of iron overload versus chronic alloantigen stimulation remains to be established. In haemochromatosis there are again conflicting reports, with both normal (Bryan *et al.*, 1991) and depressed (Bryan *et al.*, 1984) responses to mitogens being found. It is, however, worth noting that the mitogen responses of T-cells from iron-overloaded mice, as determined by release of IL2, were also reduced (Good *et al.*, 1987).

Decreased NK cell activity has been reported in thalassaemia patients (Gascón *et al.*, 1984; Kaplan *et al.*, 1984; Akbar *et al.*, 1986), but although desferrioxamine was able to restore activity *in vitro* (Akbar *et al.*, 1987), it had no effect when administered *in vivo* (Gascón *et al.*, 1984), and furthermore no defect in NK activity was found in haemochromatosis patients (Chapman *et al.*, 1988). A proposal that the transferrin receptor might function as an iron-regulated recognition molecule on NK-sensitive target cells (Vodinelich *et al.*, 1983) has now been discounted (Borysiewicz *et al.*, 1986; Shau *et al.*, 1986). Cytotoxic T-cell activity was found to be reduced in iron-overloaded mice, but as with impaired mitogen responses this was due to decreased IL2 production (Good *et al.*, 1987).

(b) *Phagocytic function*. As discussed in Chapter 8, an abnormality in macrophage iron handling may play a role in the development of hereditary haemochromatosis. Despite this, little work has been carried out to determine whether other macrophage functions, particularly those of a more immunological nature, are also altered. There are two reports of defective *in vitro* phagocytosis of bacteria by monocytes from haemochromatosis patients, which was corrected by phlebotomy (Van Asbeck *et al.*, 1982, 1984). Intracellular killing of microorganisms (but not their ingestion) was defective in thalassaemia and other transfusional iron-overload conditions (Van Asbeck *et al.*, 1984; Ballart *et al.*, 1986). Several studies have reported defective neutrophil phagocytosis associated with transfusional iron overload (Martino *et al.*, 1984; Waterlot *et al.*, 1985; Flament *et al.*, 1986; Cantinieaux *et al.*, 1987, 1990) but this function appears to be normal in haemochromatosis (Van Asbeck *et al.*, 1982, 1984).

At present the limited and often contradictory data on immune function in iron overload makes it difficult to decide whether impaired immunocompetence is a serious consequence of this condition. The problem is complicated by the fact iron overload is invariably associated with other conditions or events that may themselves have immunomodulatory effects, such as diabetes, or abnormal macrophage function in hereditary haemochromatosis, and chronic allogeneic stimulation and/or splenectomy in transfusional iron overload. Unfortunately, few animal studies of immune function in iron overload, in which such complications would be avoided, have been carried out.

2.2.3. The Role of Iron in Immune Cell Function

From the foregoing it is evident that despite uncertainties in some areas, abnormal iron status can affect immune function. In some cases it is fairly clear why such defects may occur. In others no obvious mechanisms present themselves, while in some instances biochemical and cell biological studies have suggested a potentially critical role of iron in certain immunological mechanisms which have not so far manifested themselves in clinical and experimental studies of immune function.

(a) *The effect of iron on lymphocyte activation*. The critical role of iron in lymphocyte activation, and in particular T-cell proliferation, appears to be mainly due to the fact that the enzyme ribonucleotide reductase, which is involved in DNA synthesis, is dependent upon a continuous supply of iron (Hoffbrand *et al.*, 1976). It is well established that mitogen-stimulated T-cell proliferation will not proceed if cells are cultured in iron-poor media (Brock and Mainou-Fowler, 1983; Seligman *et al.*, 1992), or iron supply is interrupted by the addition of a high affinity chelator such as desferrioxamine (Bowern *et al.*, 1984) or desferrithiocin (Bierer and Nathan, 1990). Moreover, transferrin is important as a donor, iron being taken up by receptor-mediated endocytosis of the transferrin ligand, as described in Chapter 3, and expression of transferrin receptors on T-lymphocytes markedly increases following activation (Larrick and Cresswell, 1979). When lectin-type mitogens are used, transferrin receptor expression is dependent upon prior activation by IL2 (Hamilton, 1982; Neckers and Cossman, 1983; Pelosi-Testa *et al.*, 1988), but if T-cells are activated with phorbol esters, transferrin receptor expression occurs at an earlier stage in the activation process and is IL2-independent (Kumagai *et al.*, 1988; Teixeira and Kühn, 1991). This early expression of transferrin receptors, well before DNA synthesis occurs, may signify that iron is also critical for other metabolic events apart from DNA synthesis, and it may be relevant that protein kinase C activation is impaired in iron deficiency (Kuvibidila *et al.*, 1991). It is also possible that T-cell subsets differ in their dependence upon iron, as iron deprivation had a greater inhibitory effect upon the proliferation of cloned murine lymphocytes corresponding to the TH_1 helper subset than on clones of the TH_2 helper subset (Thorson *et al.*, 1991). This suggests that changes in iron status could exert subtle effects on immune function by altering the relative activity of different lymphocyte subpopulations.

The role of iron in B-lymphocyte activation is less clear. Although proliferation in response to mitogens such as bacterial lipopolysaccharide is iron-dependent (Brock, 1981; Neckers and Cossman, 1983), other activities, notably immunoglobulin synthesis, may be less so, as it may occur prior to expression of transferrin receptors (Neckers *et al.*, 1984). This may explain why clinical studies of iron deficiency suggest that B-cell function is less affected than T-cell activity. Nevertheless, others have reported that transferrin receptor expression is a very early event in B-cell activation (Futran *et al.*, 1989), suggesting that B-cells may, like T-cells, require iron for processes that precede proliferation. Indeed, transferrin appears to be necessary for *in vitro* synthesis of IgE (and to a lesser extent IgM) by blood mononuclear cells (Van der Pouw-Kraan *et al.*, 1991).

In contrast to the stimulatory effect of transferrin-bound iron on lymphocyte proliferation, and perhaps other activities, iron in other forms, particularly when presented as hydrophilic chelates such as citrate or nitrilotriacetate, may inhibit *in vitro* proliferation (Soyano *et al.*, 1985; Djeha and Brock, 1992a,b; Pons *et al.*, 1992). The CD4 subset is more sensitive than the CD8 (Djeha and Brock, 1992b), which accords with the reduced CD4:CD8 ratio noted in iron-overload disease. The inhibitory effect of these compounds seems to be due partly to excessive uncontrolled uptake into lymphocytes, which appear to have a limited capacity to synthesize ferritin in these conditions (Djeha and Brock, 1992a), and also to membrane binding of iron polymers (Pons *et al.*, 1992), which may cause membrane damage. The inhibitory effect of non-transferrin-bound iron can be reversed by apolactoferrin (Djeha and Brock, 1992b), which may account for some of the immunoregulatory effects of lactoferrin, discussed later (p. 365). Iron citrate also decreases reactivity of normal T-cells to anti-CD2 antibodies (Carvalho and De Sousa, 1988), though whether this is due to reduced expression of CD2 or simply to its occlusion by membrane-bound iron citrate is unclear. Either mechanism could explain the inhibitory effect of such compounds on proliferation, in which CD2 plays a critical role.

(b) *Interaction of ferritin with lymphocytes*. Another factor that may contribute to impairment of lymphocyte function in iron overload is the raised level of serum ferritin. Lymphocyte proliferation *in vitro* is inhibited by ferritin (Matzner *et al.*, 1979, 1985) and an immunosuppressive effect *in vivo* has also been reported (Harada *et al.*, 1987). Ferritin molecules, particularly those rich in heavy (H) subunits, bind to activated T-cells (Pattanapanyasat *et al.*, 1987), and H-ferritin receptors (see Chapter 4) are expressed by T-cell lines (Konijn *et al.*, 1990; Moss *et al.*, 1992). How ferritin exerts its antiproliferative effect is unknown, though it might be connected with the proposed myelosuppressive effects of 'acidic isoferritins' discussed on p. 365. Moreover, ferritin binding to unstimulated human peripheral blood mononuclear cells occurs mainly to B-lymphocytes rather than T-lymphocytes (Cragg *et al.*, 1984), but there appear to be no reports of ferritin inhibiting B-cell function. Finally, despite its apparently inhibitory effect on lymphocytes, ferritin has been found to protect mice against experimental *E. coli* infection, though the mechanism involved is unknown (Lipinski *et al.*, 1991). In order to clarify its potential immunoregulatory role more needs to be known about the mechanisms by which ferritin can modulate the function of cells of the immune system.

(c) *The role of iron in cytotoxic mechanisms*. There is little evidence that iron plays a direct role in lymphocyte cytotoxicity, and it seems likely that the inhibitory effect of both iron overload and iron deficiency on NK activity or cytotoxic T-cells is secondary to alterations in cytokine production, as discussed above. However, it is becoming apparent that iron plays a critical role in the cytotoxic activity of activated macrophages. Such activity has generally been related to the production of reactive oxygen species such as hydrogen peroxide, superoxide, and in particular hydroxyl radicals. Iron is required for the catalytic production of the last of these from the other two (Halliwell, 1989), and may explain why in some cases iron-rich microorganisms may be more readily killed than those with a low iron content (Hoepelman *et al.*, 1990), though this is not true in all cases (Byrd and Horwitz, 1990; Lane *et al.*, 1991). Furthermore, although iron-rich macrophages show reduced killing of *Listeria monocytogenes*, reduction of macrophage iron levels below a critical point also reduces listericidal activity (Alford et al., 1991), suggesting a critical role for iron in the production of microbicidal compounds.

It is now apparent that many cytotoxic effects of activated macrophages, including some previously ascribed to reactive oxygen compounds, are in fact mediated by nitric oxide, which is generated enzymatically from L-arginine (Granger et al., 1991; Liew and Cox, 1991). Nitric oxide induces loss of iron from enzymes containing iron–sulfur clusters (Lancaster and Hibbs, 1990; Drapier et al., 1991), and may have a similar effect on other iron-containing proteins as it also induces iron release from ferritin (Reif and Simmons, 1990). These findings almost certainly explain the results of earlier studies of macrophage-induced tumour cell cytotoxicity in which cell death was preceded by a loss of iron from the target cells (Hibbs et al., 1984; Klostergaard, 1987; Wharton et al., 1988). A similar mechanism is probably responsible for macrophage-mediated killing of some parasites, including schistosomes (James and Glaven, 1989), Entamoeba histolytica (Denis and Ghadirian, 1992), Leishmania (Mauel et al., 1991) and Trypanosoma musculi (Vincendeau and Daulouede, 1991), as excess iron reduces parasite killing. Thus the efficacy of the nitric oxide cytotoxic system may depend upon the iron status of the target cells, and the degree to which exogenous iron is available to replenish that lost through the action of nitric oxide. Further studies will need to examine the role of iron status in this mechanism, and also determine its importance in man, as to date the role of the inducible nitric oxide system in the cytotoxic activity of macrophages has been clearly established only in rodents. However, a human inducible NO synthase closely resembling the murine macrophage enzyme has recently been cloned from human hepatocytes (Geller et al., 1993). It is also worth noting that nitric oxide can increase the affinity of the iron-responsive element-binding protein (IRE-BP; see Chapter 5) for transferrin receptor and ferritin mRNAs (Weiss et al., 1993), suggesting that nitric oxide may have a role as a mediator of cellular iron homeostasis. This may be important in inflammation, as discussed on p. 370.

The role of iron in neutrophil function has been less well studied, probably because of the short life-span of these cells in culture. One of the key microbicidal mechanisms is the myeloperoxidase halide system, which results in the enzymatic production of toxic oxyhalide species. Myeloperoxidase is a haem-containing enzyme and animal studies have shown reduced activity in iron deficiency (Murakawa et al., 1987; Sullivan et al., 1989), although there is little direct evidence that lack of iron is directly responsible for reduced cellular levels of the enzyme.

The defect in neutrophil phagocytosis noted in iron overload may be caused by binding of iron to the cell membrane, as iron compounds were found to damage neutrophils in vitro due to production of toxic oxygen intermediates at the cell membrane (Hoepelman et al., 1988a,b, 1989). The serum factor thought to be responsible for the defect in intracellular killing by neutrophils from patients with transfusional iron overload is probably non-transferrin-bound iron (Cantinieaux et al., 1990).

(d) Immunoregulatory activity of ferritin and lactoferrin. As discussed above, transferrin and iron itself mediate fairly well-defined effects on the function of cells of the immune system. Immunoregulatory roles have also been proposed for the iron-binding proteins ferritin and lactoferrin, though the nature of these activities is much less understood. These iron-binding proteins may be involved in regulating the production of neutrophils and monocytes, as both ferritin and lactoferrin have been reported to inhibit myelopoiesis. This complex and somewhat controversial area is reviewed in detail elsewhere (Broxmeyer, 1989; Fletcher, 1989). In brief, H-rich ferritin molecules (the so-called 'acidic isoferritins') have been found to suppress CFU-GM, BFU-E and CFU-GEMM colony formation (Broxmeyer *et al.*, 1981, 1982; Bognacki *et al.*, 1981; Lu *et al.*, 1983; Dezza *et al.*, 1986). The mechanism is unknown and appears not to involve other cell types; it may be linked to the ferroxidase activity of ferritin (Broxmeyer *et al.*, 1991), and the decrease in proliferation of progenitor cells may be due to their more rapid differentiation (Guimaraes *et al.*, 1988). Lactoferrin is reported to inhibit colony-stimulating activity, probably as a result of interaction with monocytes and inhibition of production of IL1 (Zucali *et al.*, 1989; Crouch *et al.*, 1992). Lactoferrin may therefore act as a feedback regulator of granulopoiesis. However, the role of both ferritin (Sala *et al.*, 1986) and lactoferrin (Stryckmans *et al.*, 1984) as regulators of myelopoiesis has been challenged, and the exact mechanisms involved remain to be established. Lactoferrin has also been implicated in the regulation of a number of other immune functions, including antibody production (Duncan and McArthur, 1981), T-cell maturation (Zimecki *et al.*, 1991), complement activity (Kulics and Kijlstra, 1987), production of various cytokines (Kijlstra and Broersma, 1984; Crouch *et al.*, 1992) and NK cell cytotoxicity (Horwitz *et al.*, 1984; McCormick *et al.*, 1991; Shau *et al.*, 1992). As discussed in detail elsewhere (Sánchez *et al.*, 1992; Brock, 1993), the mechanisms involved in these activities, and in particular the role of iron, are largely unknown.

2.3. Iron and Infection – Clinical Evidence

The preceding sections clearly show that iron can affect microbial growth and certain immunological mechanisms. However, evidence that iron status affects susceptibility to infection is much harder to come by, and is complicated by the fact that many of the study groups are from third-world countries where the incidence of infection is high and it is difficult to make a properly-controlled study. These problems have been discussed in detail by Hershko *et al.* (1988) and Oppenheimer (1989).

Despite the strong evidence for impaired T-cell function in iron deficiency, evidence of increased susceptibility to infection associated with iron deficiency is far from abundant. Two studies reported that the incidence of respiratory infections in iron deficient children decreased after oral iron administration (Mackay, 1928; Andelman and Sered, 1966), but these studies were not well controlled, and a third reported no difference (Burman, 1972). However, iron deficiency was found to exacerbate chronic mucocutaneous candidiasis, resistance to which is thought to involve principally cell-mediated immunity (Higgs and Wells, 1972), and a more recent study found increased incidence of upper respiratory tract and gastrointestinal infections in iron deficient infants with depressed levels of T-helper cells (Berger *et al.*, 1992). A link between increased incidence of infection following abdominal surgery and low serum ferritin has also been reported (Harju, 1988).

There have been suggestions that iron deficiency may actually decrease the incidence of infection, due to reduced availability of iron to the invading micro-organisms. One report (Masawe *et al.*, 1974) which reported such findings is of doubtful significance because the control group were suffering from other types of anaemias, but in another study iron-deficient Somali nomads showed a lower incidence of infection than controls of normal iron status (Murray *et al.*, 1978). An experimental study also reported reduced mortality associated with nutritional iron deficiency in experimental *Salmonella typhimurium* infection in mice (Puschmann and Ganzoni, 1977). However, the proposal that iron deficiency may protect against malaria (Murray *et al.*, 1975) remains doubtful (Hershko *et al.*, 1988; Snow *et al.*, 1991). Thus the effect of iron deficiency on susceptibility to infection remains controversial.

Despite the fact that iron clearly enhances bacterial growth in serum *in vitro*, there is surprisingly little evidence that iron overload in itself predisposes to infection. There are a few reports of infections with organisms such as *Pasteurella pseudo-tuberculosis* (Marlon *et al.*, 1971; Yamashiro *et al.*, 1971) or *Yersinia enterocolitica* (Rabson *et al.*, 1975) associated with hereditary haemochromatosis, and these organisms can also cause infections in other iron-overload conditions (Melby *et al.*, 1982; Boelaert *et al.*, 1987). However, infection seems to be a surprisingly infrequent complication of hereditary haemochromatosis (Higginson *et al.*, 1953). In contrast, increased susceptibility to infection has often been noted in iron-overloaded patients suffering from β-thalassaemia, but this correlates more closely with splenectomy than with the degree of iron overload (Smith *et al.*, 1964; Eraklis and Filler, 1972). An increased incidence of infection has also been reported in infants with sickle cell anaemia (Powars, 1975), in which free haemoglobin resulting from haemolysis may play a role. Episodes of sepsis have been reported in patients undergoing chemotherapy for non-lymphocytic leukaemia, in whom serum transferrin was fully saturated and non-transferrin-bound iron was present (Gordeuk *et al.*, 1986; Gordeuk and Brittenham, 1992). Nevertheless, on the available evidence it seems likely that infection is not one of the most important complications arising from iron overload disease.

In contrast, injudicious use of iron supplements can markedly increase the risk of infection. Polynesian infants given intramuscular iron-dextran prophylactically showed an increased incidence of neonatal sepsis (Barry and Reeve, 1974, 1977, 1988; Becroft *et al.*, 1977), and this treatment may also exacerbate malaria (Oppenheimer, 1989). Increased pyuria in chronic pyelonephritis has been associated with the use of intramuscular iron (Briggs *et al.*, 1963). It seems likely that in these cases it is the transient presence of these relatively labile iron compounds, rather than iron overload *per se*, that provides microorganisms with an opportunity for more rapid growth. A similar effect of oral iron supplementation has also been reported in Somali nomads (Murray *et al.*, 1978), in whom the incidence of certain infections, particularly malaria, increased after iron supplementation. It is possible that in these severely malnourished individuals a combination of low serum transferrin and a large rise in serum iron following treatment may have enhanced iron availability to microorganisms.

3. IRON AND INFLAMMATION

A characteristic feature of inflammation is an alteration in the metabolism of several trace elements, particularly iron. The main features are a modest decrease in serum iron and transferrin, but unlike true iron deficiency, serum ferritin is usually not reduced. This reflects the key feature of the condition, namely an increase in storage iron, particularly in macrophages of the liver, spleen and bone marrow. In chronic inflammation anaemia develops, the so-called anaemia of chronic disease (Lee, 1983; Sears, 1992). This is normally a normocytic, normochromic anaemia, although when prolonged it can become hypochromic and occasionally microcytic. Almost any inflammatory condition, ranging from infection through neoplasia to surgery and trauma, can provoke this condition, although the anaemias associated with renal, hepatic or endocrinological disorders probably have a different aetiology. A study of over 16 000 individuals in the USA concluded that inflammation may be a more common explanation of anaemia in infants and the elderly than was previously thought to be the case (Yip and Dallman, 1988). However, despite the frequency with which the hypoferraemia and anaemia of inflammation occur, the mechanisms involved, and the physiological function of these changes remain unclear. Some of the features of iron metabolism in the anaemia of chronic disease are shown in Table 11.4, and the laboratory investigations which are useful diagnostically, particularly in distinguishing this condition from mild iron deficiency anaemia, are considered in more detail in Chapters 7 and 14. Epidemiological aspects are discussed in Chapter 13.

3.1. Erythropoiesis

Two main mechanisms have been proposed to account for decreased erythropoiesis in the anaemia of chronic disease. Firstly, it is possible that inadequate erythropoiesis results from reduced levels and/or activity of erythropoietin. This is supported by studies showing decreased urinary erythropoietin levels in patients with anaemia of chronic disease (Zucker et al., 1974; Douglas and Adamson, 1975). A more recent study of the anaemia of rheumatoid arthritis showed that serum erythropoietin levels were low compared with those of patients with anaemias not related to a chronic inflammatory disorder (Baer et al., 1987). In rats hypoxia could restore decreased

Table 11.4 Iron metabolism in inflammatory disease

Body iron compartment	Test	Result	Typical values
Iron stores	Bone marrow iron	N or I	*
	Serum ferritin	N or I	*
	Total iron-binding capacity/ transferrin	N or R	40–60 μmol/l
Tissue iron supply	Serum iron	N or R	5–12 μmol/l
	Transferrin saturation	N or R	10–20%
	Red cell Zn-protoporphyrin	N or I	>80 μmol/mol haem
Functional iron	Haemoglobin	N or R	8–12 g/dl*
	Red cell MCV	N or R	70–85 fl

*In the absence of blood loss, any anaemia is associated with movement of iron from circulating haemoglobin into macrophage iron stores, with a consequent rise in serum ferritin. Stimulation of the synthesis of ferritin protein, as an acute phase reactant, will also increase serum concentrations independently of iron stores. This means that serum concentrations of up to 100 μg/l, well above the lower limit of 10 μg/l in normals, may still be associated with absent iron stores. A dissociation between normal or increased iron stores and reduced transport iron (eventually giving rise to iron-deficient erythropoiesis) is characteristic of the anaemia of chronic disease (ACD). This is useful diagnostically for distinguishing ACD from uncomplicated iron deficiency (see Chapters 7 and 14). N, normal; R, reduced; I, increased.

erythropoietin levels, although not to the extent that would be expected in non-inflammatory conditions (Lukens, 1973), and a more recent clinical study of patients with the anaemia of cancer also found that the depressed response to erythropoietin was restored if the patients had hypoxaemia (Miller *et al.*, 1990). Evidence that the response to erythropoietin is defective comes from studies showing that erythropoietin could increase the number of CFU-Es in normal mice but not in mice with turpentine-induced inflammation (Reissman and Udupa, 1978), and that endotoxin inhibited the response to erythropoietin in polycythaemic mice (Schade and Fried, 1976). Moreover, clinical trials of recombinant erythropoietin produced only a modest alleviation of the anaemia associated with rheumatoid arthritis, a classic example of the anaemia of chronic disease (Pincus *et al.*, 1990; Smith *et al.*, 1992). This contrasts with the anaemia of renal failure, which is readily corrected by recombinant erythropoietin (Adamson and Eschbach, 1990). As reviewed by Means and Krantz (1992), some cytokines such as IL1 (Johnson *et al.*, 1989) and γ-interferon (Zoumbos *et al.*, 1984) can directly suppress erythropoiesis, and TNFα may have a similar, albeit indirect, effect (Means *et al.*, 1990).

3.2. Iron Retention and Hypoferraemia

The association of anaemia with decreased serum iron levels and increased iron storage strongly suggests that a defect in erythropoietin *per se* is not solely responsible, and that a failure to deliver iron to the erythron may be a critical defect. Various studies in man and experimental animals, reviewed by Lee (1983), have shown that the rate of iron release to plasma is decreased in inflammation. Moreover, there is a small but consistent reduction in erythrocyte lifespan (Dinant and De Maat, 1978), which if not compensated by increased release of iron to plasma would further increase levels of storage iron. There is good evidence both *in vivo* (Quastel and Ross, 1966; Fillet *et al.*, 1989), and *in vitro* (Esparza and Brock, 1981; Alvarez-Hernández *et al.*, 1986) that inflammation reduces iron release from the reticuloendothelial (macrophage–monocyte) system (reviewed by Konijn and Hershko, 1989).

The cause of the decreased release of iron from storage sites, particularly macrophages, in inflammation is still not known. One proposal that has received much attention is that lactoferrin released by degranulating neutrophils may remove iron from transferrin and short-circuit the metal back to macrophages, which are able to bind lactoferrin (Van Snick *et al.*, 1974). However, there are a number of objections to this mechanism; under physiological conditions iron exchange between proteins of the transferrin class is extremely slow, and even during inflammation the plasma concentration of lactoferrin is several orders of magnitude lower than that of transferrin. Indeed, plasma iron turnover appears to be unaffected during infection (Letendre and Holbein, 1983). Furthermore, although it is indeed well established that lactoferrin can bind to macrophages (Birgens, 1991), subsequent delivery of iron is either extremely slow (Birgens *et al.*, 1988) or non-existent (Oria *et al.*, 1988). In addition, hypoferraemia still occurs in conditions where levels of neutrophils, the source of plasma lactoferrin, are much reduced (Gordeuk *et al.*, 1988; Baynes *et al.*, 1990). It thus seems highly unlikely that lactoferrin plays any role in systemic hypoferraemia, though it might conceivably contribute to local accumulation of iron in macrophages at inflammatory sites, such as the rheumatoid joint (Muirden, 1970) or the inflamed lung (Corhay et al., 1992). At such sites the lower pH and higher lactoferrin:transferrin ratio might allow some iron transfer to occur between these proteins.

A more plausible explanation for increased retention of iron involves an increase in ferritin synthesis, stimulated not by iron but by some inflammatory mediator (Konijn and Hershko, 1977; Konijn et al., 1981; Campbell et al., 1989). The increased ferritin levels would lead to storage of iron that would otherwise have been released by the cells. The nature of the inflammatory stimulus is unresolved, but is probably a cytokine. Early observations that a serum factor named leucocyte endogenous mediator (LEM) could induce hypoferraemia (reviewed by Lee, 1983) have been followed by studies indicating that recombinant IL1, thought to be the main component of LEM, can induce hypoferraemia in vivo (Westmacott et al., 1986; Gordeuk et al., 1988) and induce ferritin transcription in vitro (Rogers et al., 1990; Wei et al., 1990). Preliminary evidence suggests that IL1 also exerts translational control over ferritin synthesis via a stem-loop structure of a type present in the mRNAs of several acute-phase proteins (Rogers et al., 1993).

However, there is increasing evidence that IL1 may not be the only, or even the most important cytokine involved in iron retention. In mice, tumour necrosis factor (TNFα), but not IL1, induced hypoferraemia and altered handling of iron by macrophages in vitro (Tanaka et al., 1987; Alvarez-Hernández et al., 1989), and the IL1-receptor-antagonist (IL1ra) failed to prevent hypoferraemia in rats given an inflammatory stimulus even though it reduced fever (Thomas et al., 1991). TNFα can also stimulate ferritin synthesis (Miller et al., 1991). Studies in man (Baynes et al., 1990) and animals (Van Miert et al., 1990) suggest that α-interferon can induce hypoferraemia, and there is preliminary evidence of a role for IL6 (Sakata et al., 1991) and IL8 (Bharadwaj et al., 1991). However, γ-interferon has the opposite effect, i.e. it induces iron release from macrophages (Taetle and Honeysett, 1988). This is probably linked to the recently-reported ability of nitric oxide, synthesis of which is induced by γ-interferon, to convert the IRE-BP (see Chapter 5) to the high-affinity form (Weiss et al., 1993), which would result in an increased transferrin receptor synthesis and a decrease in ferritin. It therefore seems likely that several cytokines can induce changes in iron metabolism that would give rise to the hypoferraemia of inflammation, while γ-interferon may have a counterbalancing effect.

Thus although some advances have been made in understanding the mechanisms of the hypoferraemia of inflammation, particularly the role of cytokines, much remains to be explained. It seems likely that iron retention by macrophages and a direct reduction in erythropoiesis both play a role. The demonstration that ferritin behaves as a heat-shock protein in erythrocytes (Atkinson et al., 1990) further emphasizes the important role of changes in ferritin synthesis in pathological conditions.

3.3. The Role of Hypoferraemia in Inflammation

The physiological function of these changes in iron metabolism is still uncertain. As discussed above (pp. 357–358), there is little evidence for the widely-held notion that such changes can decrease the growth of invading microorganisms. Likewise, a decrease in serum iron seems more likely to inhibit than enhance the function of the immune system, although it is possible that increased macrophage iron release in response to

γ-interferon (Taetle and Honeysett, 1988) coupled with increased transferrin synthesis by macrophages and lymphocytes (Lum *et al.*, 1986; Djeha *et al.*, 1992) might provide an alternative supply of iron to activated lymphocytes. An interesting recent suggestion is that hypoferraemia may serve to increase the activity of γ-interferon, which plays a critical role in macrophage activation (Weiss *et al.*, 1992). Perhaps the old idea of a diversion of iron and iron-related precursors away from erythropoiesis into inflammatory mechanisms should be re-evaluated.

4. IRON AND NEOPLASIA

The idea that iron, and in particular iron overload, plays a role in the development of neoplasia has aroused considerable interest. Nevertheless, despite some persuasive arguments that iron overload favours development of cancer (Weinberg, 1984, 1992a,b), much of this area remains controversial.

4.1. Hepatoma and Severe Iron Overload

It now widely recognized that in individuals with severe iron overload, such as is found in hereditary haemochromatosis, there is an increased incidence of hepatocellular carcinoma, and indeed this is a significant cause of death in such patients, particularly when cirrhosis is present (Bomford and Williams, 1976; Bradbear *et al.*, 1985; Niederau *et al.*, 1985; Fargion *et al.*, 1992; see also Chapter 8). In addition, development of sarcoma has been reported at the site of injection in animals receiving parenteral iron-dextran (Richmond, 1959; Magnusson *et al.*, 1977).

In both these situations severe general or local iron overload occurs, and iron will be present in plasma and tissue in abnormal forms which may allow it to catalyse the production of oxygen radicals which are proximate carcinogens (Ames, 1983; Halliwell and Gutteridge, 1984; see also Chapter 10). In addition, *in vitro* studies suggest that tumour cells show a greater ability than normal cells to grow and/or survive in the presence of high levels of extracellular iron. Some tumour cells possess mechanisms that allow them to acquire and utilize non-transferrin-bound iron (Taetle *et al.*, 1985; Bassett *et al.*, 1986; Sturrock *et al.*, 1990), which in contrast tends to be toxic for normal cells (Djeha and Brock, 1992a,b). Thus excess iron may not only initiate the carcinogenic process, but also favour growth of tumour cells over others, such as cells of the immune system, that might otherwise help to limit tumour development.

4.2. Cancer in Relation to Iron Status

While there is a clear correlation between severe iron overload and the incidence of neoplasia, an association between other types of cancer and iron overload is much less conclusive. Furthermore, there is controversy over whether individuals with levels of storage iron at the upper end of the normal range, such as may arise from dietary habits, run a risk of a higher incidence of neoplasia. In haemochromatosis patients the death rate due to cancer of tissues other than the liver was no greater than normal (Niederau *et al.*, 1985; Fargion *et al.*, 1992), although in other studies a higher than normal incidence of extrahepatic cancers has been reported (Bomford and Williams, 1976; Ammann *et al.*, 1980; Adams *et al.*, 1991).

Nevertheless, there is epidemiological evidence of an association between moderately increased iron stores and cancer risk. Stevens *et al.* (1986) found that the development of cancer of all types was significantly correlated with elevated serum ferritin and decreased serum transferrin levels prior to diagnosis of the disease, although it should be emphasized that storage iron was not measured directly in the subjects studied. In a subsequent large epidemiological study of over 14 000 adults (Stevens *et al.*, 1988) an association between development of cancer and iron status was found in men, but such a correlation was not detected in women. Further analysis of this data (Stevens *et al.*, 1993) showed a significant positive correlation between serum transferrin saturation and cancer risk for men and women combined. In another large study the incidence of lung cancer was lower than normal in iron-depleted women (Selby and Friedman, 1988), though it is possible that the confounding effect of smoking was not totally eliminated in this survey.

In animal models, both transplantable (Hann *et al.*, 1988) and spontaneous (Hann *et al.*, 1991) mammary tumours grew more slowly in mice fed a low iron diet, although in another study this protective effect of iron deficiency disappeared once haematocrit and body weight were restored to normal (Thompson *et al.*, 1991). Animals fed high iron diets have been reported to show increased tumour development (Nelson *et al.*, 1989; Thompson *et al.*, 1991), and it has been hypothesized that dietary fibre might protect against colorectal cancer by sequestering iron from the diet (Nelson, 1992). It has been suggested that transfusion of cancer patients undergoing surgery may increase the risk of recurrence due to the additional iron loading (Weinberg, 1992b), though there is no direct evidence for such a mechanism and immunological abnormalities may be of greater importance. It has also been proposed (Blumberg *et al.*, 1981; Stevens *et al.*, 1983, 1986) that the increased iron stores found in chronic carriers of hepatitis B may be the reason why these individuals have a 200-fold excess risk for hepatocellular carcinoma (Beasley *et al.*, 1981).

While there are clear mechanistic explanations for the high incidence of hepatoma in individuals with severe iron overload, it is less easy to see how modest amounts of iron can increase, or iron deficiency reduce, the incidence of cancer. It is well established that transferrin can support the growth of many tumour cells *in vitro* through donation of iron (Sussman, 1992). Nevertheless, as argued in relation to microbial growth (see above), modest changes in transferrin saturation are unlikely significantly to alter iron availability to tumour cells, and suggestions that transferrin may be a specific tumour cell growth factor (Riss and Sirbasku, 1987; Cavanaugh and Nicolson, 1991) are difficult to sustain since transferrin is also essential for growth and development of normal cells. However, the ability of tumour cells to synthesize transferrin might confer a growth advantage when tumours are starved of circulating transferrin by poor vascularization (Vostrejs *et al.*, 1988; Vandewalle *et al.*, 1991).

One anti-tumour mechanism that might conceivably be impaired by modest iron overload is the cytotoxic activity of activated macrophages. As discussed above (p. 365), an initial step in the cytotoxic mechanism is loss of iron from the target cells, and it has been shown that macrophage cytotoxic activity is impaired by excess iron

(Green *et al.*, 1988; Huot *et al.*, 1990). Furthermore, as mentioned above, iron reduces the activity of γ-interferon, and could thus interfere with the development of tumouricidal activated macrophages (Weiss *et al.*, 1992). Further research, particularly with respect to the role of nitric oxide in tumouricidal activity, may clarify this area.

4.3. Iron and Cancer Therapy

The fact that tumour cells express large numbers of transferrin receptors has suggested that this molecule might be a suitable target for delivery of antitumour drugs. Antitransferrin receptor monoclonal antibodies, either alone or conjugated to toxins, could inhibit growth of tumour cells *in vitro* and *in vivo* (Trowbridge and Domingo, 1981; Sauvage *et al.*, 1987; White *et al.*, 1990; reviewed by Trowbridge, 1989). Combination of such antibodies with desferrioxamine treatment has also been proposed (Taetle *et al.*, 1989; Kemp *et al.*, 1992). However, a basic problem with this type of treatment is that interference with iron delivery to tumour cells by antitransferrin receptor antibodies will also have a similar effect on normal cells such as erythroid precursors and lymphocytes (Mendelsohn *et al.*, 1983). Nevertheless, future investigations may reveal differences in cellular iron metabolism between tumour cells and normal cells that might be exploited in this type of therapy.

There is evidence that body iron stores may play a role in prognosis after cancer diagnosis (Hann *et al.*, 1989). This has led to preliminary trials of iron chelation therapy and antioxidant therapy in the treatment of established cancer (Donfrancesco *et al.*, 1990; Weitman *et al.*, 1991). Diets containing such nutrients as α-tocopherol, carotenoids and ascorbic acid may be protective due to their antioxidant properties (Willett and MacMahon, 1984).

5. CONCLUSIONS AND FUTURE PERSPECTIVES

Over the past 20 years it has become apparent that iron metabolism plays a role in immune function, inflammation and neoplasia. Consequently, it is not unreasonable to propose that a relationship may exist between iron status, the outcome of infection and prognosis in neoplasia. While some progress has been made, particularly in understanding underlying mechanisms, the results of clinical investigations are often contradictory. This is especially true with respect to the role of iron deficiency and iron overload in resistance to infection, and the degree to which iron status effects cancer other than hepatoma. One may conclude that normal iron status ensures ready availability of iron for metabolic activity, including function of the immune system, while at the same time impeding uptake by microorganisms and denying growth advantages to tumour cells. How far one can go to either side of the 'normal' situation without upsetting this balance is perhaps the critical factor in understanding whether changes in iron status can predispose to infectious, inflammatory or neoplastic disease.

REFERENCES

Adams, P. C., Speechley, M. and Kertesz, A. E. (1991) Long-term survival analysis in hereditary hemochromatosis. *Gastroenterology* **101**, 368–372.

Adamson, J. W. and Eschbach, J. W. (1990) Treatment of the anemia of chronic renal failure with recombinant human erythropoietin. *Ann. Rev. Med.* **41**, 349–360.

Akbar, A. N., Fitzgerald-Bocarsly, P. A., De Sousa, M., Giardina, P. J., Hilgartner, M. W. and Grady, R. W. (1986) Decreased natural killer activity in thalassemia major: a possible consequence of iron overload. *J. Immunol.* **136**, 1635–1640.

Akbar, A. N., Fitzgerald-Bocarsly, P. A., Giardina, P. J., Hilgartner, M. W. and Grady, R. W. (1987) Modulation of the defective natural killer activity seen in thalassaemia major with desferrioxamine and α-interferon. *Clin. Exp. Immunol.* **70**, 345–353.

Alford, C. E., King, T. E. and Campbell, P. A. (1991) Role of transferrin, transferrin receptors, and iron in macrophage listericidal activity. *J. Exp. Med.* **174**, 459–466.

Alvarez-Hernández, X., Felstein, M. V. and Brock, J. H. (1986) The relationship between iron release, ferritin synthesis and intracellular iron distribution in mouse peritoneal macrophages. Evidence for a reduced level of metabolically available iron in elicited macrophages. *Biochim. Biophys. Acta* **886**, 214–222.

Alvarez-Hernández, X., Licéaga, J., McKay, I. C. and Brock, J. H. (1989) Induction of hypoferremia and modulation of macrophage iron metabolism by tumor necrosis factor. *Lab. Invest.* **61**, 319–322.

Ames, B. N. (1983) Dietary carcinogens and anticarcinogens. *Science* **221**, 1256–1264.

Ammann, R. W., Muller, E., Bansky, J., Schuler, G. and Hacki, W. H. (1980) High incidence of extrahepatic carcinomas in idiopathic haemochromatosis. *Scand. J. Gastroenterol.* **15**, 733–736.

Andelman, M. B. and Sered, B. R. (1966) Utilization of dietary iron by term infants: a study of 1048 infants from a low socioeconomic population. *Amer. J. Dis. Child.* **111**, 45–55.

Ankenbauer, R., Sriyosachati, S. and Cox, C. D. (1985) Effect of siderophores on the growth of *Pseudomonas aeruginosa* in human serum and transferrin. *Infect. Immunity* **49**, 132–140.

Anwar, H., Brown, M. R. W., Day, A. and Weller, P. H. (1984) Outer membrane antigens of mucoid *Pseudomonas aeruginosa* isolated directly from the sputum of a cystic fibrosis patient. *FEMS Microbiol. Lett.* **24**, 235–239.

Arbeter, A., Echeverri, L., Franco, D., Munson, D., Vélez, H. and Vitale, J. J. (1971) Nutrition and infection. *Fed. Proc.* **30**, 1421–1428.

Arnold, R. R., Russell, J. E., Champion, W. J., Brewer, M. and Gauthier, J. J. (1982) Bactericidal activity of human lactoferrin: differentiation from the stasis of iron deprivation. *Infect. Immunity* **35**, 792–799.

Atkinson, B. G., Blaker, T. W., Tomlinson, J. and Dean, R. L. (1990) Ferritin is a translationally regulated heat shock protein of avian erythrocytes. *J. Biol. Chem.* **265**, 14156–14162.

Autenrieth, I., Hantke, K. and Heeseman, J. (1991) Immunosuppression of the host and delivery of iron to the pathogen: a possible dual role of siderophores in the pathogenesis of microbial infections. *Med. Microbiol. Immunol.* **180**, 135–141.

Baer, A. N., Dessypris, E. N., Goldwasser, E. and Krantz, S. B. (1987) Blunted erythropoietin response to anaemia in rheumatoid arthritis. *Brit. J. Haematol.* **66**, 559–564.

Bagchi, K., Mohanram, M. and Reddy, V. (1980) Humoral immune response in children with iron deficiency. *Br. Med. J.* **280**, 1249–1251.

Baig, B. H., Wachsmuth, I. K. and Morris, G. K. (1986) Utilization of exogenous siderophores by *Campylobacter* species. *J. Clin. Microbiol.* **23**, 431–433.

Ballart, I. J., Estevez, M. E., Sen, L. *et al.* (1986) Progressive dysfunction of monocytes associated with iron overload and age in patients with thalassemia major. *Blood* **67**, 105–109.

Balmer, S. E., Scott, P. H. and Wharton, B. A. (1989) Diet and faecal flora in the newborn: lactoferrin. *Arch. Dis. Childh.* **64**, 1685–1690.

Baltimore, R. S., Shedd, D. G. and Pearson, H. A. (1982) Effect of iron saturation on the bacteriostasis of human serum: in vivo does not correlate with in vitro saturation. *J. Pediatr.* **101**, 519–523.

Barry, D. M. J. and Reeve, A. W. (1974) Iron and infection in the newborn. *Lancet* ii, 1385.

Barry, D. M. J. and Reeve, A. W. (1977) Increased incidence of Gram-negative neonatal sepsis with intramuscular iron administration. *Pediatrics* **60**, 908–912.

Barry, D. M. J. and Reeve, A. W. (1988) Iron and infection. *Brit. Med. J.* **296**, 1736.

Basset, P., Quesneau, Y. and Zwiller, J. (1986) Iron-induced L1210 cell growth – evidence of a transferrin-independent iron transport. *Cancer Res.* **46**, 1644–1647.

Baynes, R. D., Bezwoda, W. R., Dajee, D., Lamparelli, R. D. and Bothwell, T. H. (1990) Effects of alpha-interferon on iron-related measurements in human subjects. *S. Afr. Med. J.* **78**, 627–628.

Beasley, R. P., Lin, C. C., Hwang, L. Y. (1981) Hepatocellular carcinoma and hepatitis B virus. *Lancet* **ii**, 1129–1133.

Becroft, D. M. O., Dix, M. R. and Farmer, K. (1977) Intramuscular iron dextran and susceptibility of neonates to bacterial infections. *Arch. Dis. Childh.* **52**, 778–781.

Bellamy, W., Takase, M., Yamauchi, K., Wakabayashi, H., Kawase, K. and Tomita, M. (1992) Identification of the bactericidal domain of lactoferrin. *Biochim. Biophys. Acta* **1121**, 235–240.

Berger, J., Schneider, D., Dyck, J. L. *et al.* (1992) Iron deficiency, cell-mediated immunity and infection among 6–36 month old children living in rural Togo. *Nutr. Res.* **12**, 39–49.

Bharadwaj, M., Khanna, N., Mathur, A. and Chaturvedi, U. C. (1991) Effect of macrophage-derived factor on hypoferraemia induced by Japanese encephalitis virus in mice. *Clin. Exp. Immunol.* **83**, 215–218.

Bhaskaram, C. and Reddy, V. (1975) Cell-mediated immunity and iron- and vitamin-deficient children. *Br. Med. J.* **3**, 522.

Bhaskaram, P., Sharada, K., Sivakumar, B., Rao, K. V. and Nair, M. (1989) Effect of iron and vitamin A deficiencies on macrophage function in children. *Nutr. Res.* **9**, 35–45.

Bierer, B. E. and Nathan, D. G. (1990) The effect of desferrithiocin, an oral iron chelator, on T-cell function. *Blood* **76**, 2052–2059.

Birgens, H. S. (1991) The interaction of lactoferrin with human monocytes. *Dan. Med. Bull.* **38**, 244–252.

Birgens, H. S., Kristensen, L. Ø., Borregaard, N., Karle, H. and Hansen, N. E. (1988) Lactoferrin-mediated transfer of iron to intracellular ferritin in human monocytes. *Eur. J. Haematol.* **41**, 52–57.

Blumberg, B. S., Lustbader, E. D. and Whitford, P. L. (1981) Changes in serum iron levels due to infection and hepatitis B virus. *Proc. Natl. Acad. Sci. USA* **78**, 3222–3224.

Boelaert, J. R., Van Landuyt, H. W., Valcke, Y. J. *et al.* (1987) The role of iron overload in *Yersinia enterocolitica* and *Yersinia paratuberculosis* bacteremia in hemodialysis patients. *J. Infect. Dis.* **156**, 384–387.

Boelaert, J. R., Van Roost, G. F., Vergauwe, P. L., Verbanck, J. J., De Vroey, C. and Segaert, M. F. (1988) The role of desferrioxamine in dialysis-associated mucormycosis: report of three cases and review of the literature. *Clin. Nephrol.* **29**, 261–266.

Boesman-Finkelstein, M. and Finkelstein, R. A. (1985) Antimicrobial effects of human milk: inhibitory activity on enteric pathogens. *FEMS Microbiol. Lett.* **27**, 167–174.

Bognacki, J., Broxmeyer, H. E. and Lobue, J. (1981) Isolation and biochemical characterization of leukaemia-associated inhibitory activity that suppresses colony and cluster formation of cells. *Biochim. Biophys. Acta* **672**, 176–190.

Bomford, A. and Williams, R. (1976) Long term results of venesection therapy in idiopathic haemochromatosis. *Q. J. Med.* **180**, 611–623.

Borysiewicz, L. K., Graham, S. and Sissons, J. G. P. (1986) Human natural killer cell lysis of virus-infected cells. Relationship to expression of the transferrin receptor. *Eur. J. Immunol.* **16**, 405–411.

Bowern, N., Ramshaw, I. A., Badenoch-Jones, P. and Doherty, P. C. (1984) Effect of an iron-chelating agent on lymphocyte proliferation. *Austr. J. Exp. Biol. Med. Sci.* **62**, 743–754.

Boxer, L. A., Coates, T. D., Haak, R. A., Wolach, J. B., Hoffstein, S. and Baehner, R. L. (1982) Lactoferrin deficiency associated with altered granulocyte function. *New Engl. J. Med.* **303**, 404–410.

Bradbear, R. A., Bain, C., Siskind, V. *et al.* (1985) Cohort study of internal malignancy in genetic hemochromatosis and other chronic non-alcoholic liver disease. *J. Nat. Cancer Inst.* **75**, 81–84.

Braun, V. (1981) *Escherichia coli* cells containing the plasmid Col V produce the ionophore aerobactin. *FEMS Microbiol. Lett.* **11**, 225–228.

Braun, V., Hancock, R. E., Hantke, K. and Hartmann, A. (1976) Functional organization of the outer membrane of *Escherichia coli*: phage and colicin receptors as components of iron uptake systems. *J. Supramol. Struct.* **5**, 37–58.

Braun, V., Brazel-Faisst, C. and Schneider, R. (1984) Growth stimulation of *Escherichia coli* in serum by iron(III) aerobactin. Recycling of aerobactin. *FEMS Microbiol. Lett.* **21**, 99–103.

Breton-Gorius, J., Mason, D. Y., Buriot, D., Vilde, J. L. and Griscelli, C. (1980) Lactoferrin deficiency as a consequence of a lack of specific granules in neutrophils from a patient with recurrent infections. *Am. J. Pathol.* **99**, 413–428.

Briggs, J. D., Kennedy, A. C. and Goldberg, A. (1963) Urinary white cell excretion after iron-sorbitol-citric acid. *Brit. Med. J.* **2**, 352–354.

Brock, J. H. (1981) The effect of iron and transferrin on the response of serum-free cultures of mouse lymphocytes to concanavalin A and lipopolysaccharide. *Immunology* **43**, 387–392.

Brock, J. H. (1993) Iron and immunity. *J. Nutr. Immunol.*, in press.

Brock, J. H. and Mainou-Fowler, T. (1983) The role of iron and transferrin in lymphocyte transformation. *Immunol. Today* **4**, 347–351.

Brock, J. H. and Ng, J. (1983) The effect of desferrioxamine on the growth of *Staphylococcus aureus*, *Yersinia enterocolitica* and *Streptococcus faecalis* in human serum: uptake of desferrioxamine-bound iron. *FEMS Microbiol. Lett.* **20**, 439–442.

Brock, J. H., Pickering, M. G., McDowall, M. G. and Deacon, A. G. (1983) Role of antibody and enterobactin in controlling growth of *Escherichia coli* in human milk and acquisition of lactoferrin- and transferrin-bound iron. *Infect. Immunity* **40**, 453–459.

Brock, J. H., Licéaga, J. and Kontoghiorghes, G. J. (1988) The effect of synthetic iron chelators on bacterial growth in human serum. *FEMS Microbiol. Immunol.* **47**, 55–60.

Brock, J. H., Williams, P. H. Licéaga, J. and Wooldridge, K. G. (1991) Relative availability of transferrin-bound iron and cell-derived iron to aerobactin-producing and enterochelin-producing strains of *Escherichia coli* and to other microorganisms. *Infect. Immunity* **59**, 3185–3190.

Broxmeyer, H. E. (1989) Iron-binding proteins and the regulation of hematopoietic cell proliferation/differentiation. In: *Iron in Immunity, Cancer and Inflammation* (eds M. De Sousa and J. H. Brock), John Wiley, Chichester, pp. 199–221.

Broxmeyer, H. E., Smithyman, A., Eger, R. R., Meyers, P. A. and De Sousa, M. (1978) Identification of lactoferrin as the granulocyte-derived inhibitor of colony stimulating activity (CSA)-production. *J. Exp. Med.* **148**, 1052–1067.

Broxmeyer, H. E., Bognacki, J., Dörner, M. H. and De Sousa, M. (1981) The identification of leukemia-associated inhibitory activity (LIA) as acidic isoferritins: a regulatory role for acidic isoferritins in the production of granulocytes and macrophages. *J. Exp. Med.* **153**, 1426–1444.

Broxmeyer, H. E. Bognacki, J., Ralph, P., Dörner, M. H., Lu, L. and Castro-Malaspina, H. (1982) Monocyte–macrophage-derived acidic isoferritins: normal feedback regulators of granulocyte–macrophage progenitor cells in vitro. *Blood* **60**, 595–607.

Broxmeyer, H. E., Cooper, S., Levi, S. and Arosio, P. (1991) Mutated recombinant human heavy-chain ferritins and myelosuppression *in vitro* and *in vivo* – a link between ferritin ferroxidase activity and biological function. *Proc. Natl. Acad. Sci. USA* **88**, 770–774.

Bryan, C. F., Leech, S. H., Ducos, R. *et al.* (1984) Thermostable erythrocyte rosette-forming lymphocytes in hereditary hemochromatosis. I. Identification in peripheral blood. *J. Clin. Immunol.* **4**, 134–142.

Bryan, C. F., Leech, S. H., Kumar, P., Gaumer, R., Bozelka, B. and Morgan, J. (1991) The immune system in hereditary hemochromatosis: a quantitative and functional assessment of the cellular arm. *Amer. J. Med. Sci.* **301**, 55–61.

Bullen, J. J. and Joyce, P. R. (1982) Abolition of the bacterial function of polymorphs by ferritin–antiferritin complexes. *Immunology* **46**, 497–505.

Bullen, J. J. and Rogers, H. J. (1969) Bacterial iron metabolism and immunity to *Pasteurella septica* and *Escherichia coli*. *Nature (Lond.)* **224**, 380–382.

Bullen, J. J., Rogers, H. J. and Leigh, L. (1972) Iron-binding proteins in milk and resistance to *Escherichia coli* infections in infants. *Br. Med. J.* **1**, 69–75.

Bullen, J. J., Spalding, P. B., Ward, C. G. and Gutteridge, J. M. C. (1991a) Hemochromatosis, iron, and septicemia caused by *Vibrio vulnificus*. *Arch. Intern. Med.* **151**, 1606–1609.

Bullen, J. J., Ward, C. G. and Rogers, H. J. (1991b) The critical role of iron in some clinical infections. *Eur. J. Clin. Microbiol. Infect. Dis.* **10**, 613–617.

Burman, D. (1972) Haemoglobin levels in normal infants aged 3–24 months and the effect of iron. *Arch. Dis. Childh.* **47**, 261–271.

Byrd, T. F. and Horwitz, M. A. (1990) Interferon-gamma activated human monocytes downregulate transferrin receptors and inhibit the intracellular multiplication of *Legionella pneumophila* by limiting the availability of iron. *J. Clin. Invest.* **83**, 1457–1465.

Calver, G. A., Kenny, C. P. and Kushner, D. J. (1979) Inhibition of the growth of *Neisseria meningitidis* by reduced ferritin and other iron-binding agents. *Infect. Immunity* **25**, 880–890.

Campbell, C. H., Solgonick, R. M. and Linder, M. C. (1989) Translational regulation of ferritin synthesis in rat spleen: effects of iron and inflammation. *Biochem. Biophys. Res. Comm.* **160**, 453–459.

Cantinieaux, B., Hariga, C., Ferster, A., de Maertelaere, E., Toppet, M. and Fondu, P. (1987) Neutrophil dysfunctions in thalassaemia major: the role of cell iron overload. *Eur. J. Haematol.* **39**, 28–34.

Cantinieaux, B., Hariga, C., Ferster, A., Toppet, M. and Fondu, P. (1990) Desferrioxamine improves neutrophil phagocytosis in thalassemia major. *Am. J. Hematol.* **35**, 13–17.

Carlsson, J., Höfling, J. F. and Sundqvist, G. K. (1984) Degradation of albumin, haemopexin, haptoglobin and transferrin by black-pigmented *Bacteroides* species. *J. Med. Microbiol.* **18**, 39–46.

Carvalho, G. S. and De Sousa, M. (1988) Iron exerts a specific inhibitory effect on CD2 expression of human PBL. *Immunol. Lett.* **19**, 163–168.

Cavanaugh, P. G. and Nicolson, G. L. (1991) Lung-derived growth factor that stimulates the growth of lung-metastasizing tumor cells: identification as transferrin. *J. Cell. Biochem.* **47**, 261–271.

Celada, A., Herreros, V., Pugin, P. and Rudolf, M. (1979) Reduced leucocyte alkaline phosphatase activity and decreased NBT reduction test in induced iron deficiency. *Br. J. Haematol.* **43**, 457–463.

Chandra, R. K. (1973) Reduced bactericidal capacity of polymorphs in iron deficiency. *Arch. Dis. Childh.* **48**, 864–866.

Chandra, R. K. (1975) Impaired immunocompetence associated with iron deficiency. *J. Pediatr.* **86**, 899–902.

Chapman, D. E., Good, M. F., Powell, L. W. and Halliday, J. W. (1988) The effect of iron, iron-binding proteins and iron-overload on human natural killer cell activity. *J. Gastroenterol. Hepatol.* **3**, 9–17.

Clemens, L. E. and Basch, P. F. (1989) *Schistosoma mansoni*: effect of transferrin and growth factors on development of schistosomula in vitro. *J. Parasitol.* **75**, 417–421.

Coffman, T. J., Cox, C. D., Edeker, B. L. and Britigan, B. E. (1990) Possible role of bacterial siderophores in inflammation. Iron bound to the *Pseudomonas* siderophore pyochelin can function as a hydroxyl radical catalyst. *J. Clin. Invest.* **86**, 1030–1037.

Corhay, J. L., Weber, G., Bury, T., Mariz, S., Roelandts, I. and Radermecker, M. F. (1992) Iron content in human alveolar macrophages. *Eur. Respir. J.* **5**, 804–809.

Cowart, R. E. and Foster, B. G. (1985) Differential effects of iron on the growth of *Listeria monocytogenes*: minimum requirements and mechanism of acquisition. *J. Infect. Dis.* **151**, 721–730.

Cragg, S. J., Hoy, T. G. and Jacobs, A. (1984) The expression of cell surface ferritin by peripheral blood lymphocytes and monocytes. *Br. J. Haematol.* **57**, 679–684.

Crouch, S. P. M., Slater, K. J. and Fletcher, J. (1992) Regulation of cytokine release from mononuclear cells by the iron-binding protein lactoferrin. *Blood* **80**, 235–240.

Cummins, A. G., Duncombe, V. M., Bolin, T. D., Davis, A. E. and Kelly, J. D. (1978) Suppression of rejection of *Nippostrongylus brasiliensis* in iron and protein deficient rats: effect of syngeneic lymphocyte transfer. *Gut* **19**, 823–826.

De Lorenzo, V. and Martínez, J. L. (1988) Aerobactin production as a virulence factor: a reevaluation. *Eur. J. Clin. Microbiol. Infect. Dis.* **7**, 621–629.

Denis, M. and Ghadirian, E. (1992) Activated mouse macrophages kill *Entamoeba histolytica* trophozoites by releasing reactive nitrogen intermediates. *Microb. Pathogenesis* **12**, 193–198.

De Sousa, M. (1989) Immune cell function in iron overload. *Clin. Exp. Immunol.* **75**, 1–6.

De Sousa, M. and Nishiya, K. (1978) Inhibition of E-rosette formation by two iron salts. *Cell. Immunol.* **38**, 203–208.

Dezza, L., Cazzola, M., Piacibello, W., Arosio, P., Levi, S. and Aglietta, M. (1986) Effect of acidic and basic isoferritins on in vitro growth of human granulocyte–monocyte progenitors. *Blood* **67**, 789–795.

Dhur, A., Galán, P. and Hercberg, S. (1989) Iron status, immune capacity and resistance to infections. *Comp. Biochem. Physiol.* **94A**, 11–19.

Dhur, A., Galán, P., Hannoun, C., Huot, K. and Hercberg, S. (1990) Effects of iron deficiency upon the antibody response to influenza virus in rats. *J. Nutr. Biochem.* **1**, 629–634.

Dinant, H. J. and De Maat, C. E. M. (1978) Erythropoiesis and mean red cell life span in normal subjects and in patients with the anaemia of active rheumatoid arthritis. *Br. J. Haematol.* **39**, 437–444.

Djeha, A. and Brock, J. H. (1992a) Uptake and intracellular handling of iron from transferrin and iron chelates by mitogen stimulated mouse lymphocytes. *Biochim. Biophys. Acta* **1133**, 147–152.

Djeha, A. and Brock, J. H. (1992b) Effect of transferrin, lactoferrin and chelated iron on human T-lymphocytes. *Br. J. Haematol.* **80**, 235–241.

Djeha, A., Pérez-Arellano, J. L., Hayes, S. L. and Brock, J. H. (1992) Transferrin synthesis by macrophages: up-regulation by γ-interferon and effect on lymphocyte proliferation. *FEMS Microbiol. Immunol.* **105**, 279–282.

Donfrancesco, A., Deb, G., Dominici, C., Pileggi, D., Castello, M. A. and Helson, L. (1990) Effects of a single course of deferoxamine in neuroblastoma patients. *Cancer Res.* **50**, 4929–4930.

Döring, G., Pfestorf, M., Botzenhart, K. and Abdallah, M. A. (1988) Impact of proteases on iron uptake of *Pseudomonas aeruginosa* pyoverdin from transferrin and lactoferrin. *Infect. Immunity* **56**, 291–293.

Douglas, S. W. and Adamson, J. W. (1975) The anemia of chronic disorders: studies of marrow regulation and iron metabolism. *Blood* **45**, 55–65.

Drapier, J. C., Pellat, C. and Henry, Y. (1991) Generation of EPR-detectable nitrosyl–iron complexes in tumor target cells cocultured with activated macrophages. *J. Biol. Chem.* **266**, 10162–10167.

Duncan, R. L. and McArthur, W. P. (1981) Lactoferrin-mediated modulation of mononuclear cell activities. 1. Suppression of the murine *in vitro* primary antibody response. *Cell. Immunol.* **63**, 308–320.

Dwyer, J., Wood, C., McNamara, J. *et al.* (1987) Abnormalities in the immune system of children with beta-thalassaemia major. *Clin. Exp. Immunol.* **68**, 621–629.

Dyer, D. W., West, E. P. and Sparling, P. F. (1987) Effects of serum carrier proteins on the growth of pathogenic *Neisseriae* with heme-bound iron. *Infect. Immunity* **55**, 2171–2175.

Eaton, J. W., Brandt, P., Mahoney, J. R. and Lee, J. T. (1982) Haptoglobin: a natural bacteriostat. *Science* **215**, 691–693.

Ellison, R. T. and Giehl, T. J. (1991) Killing of Gram-negative bacteria by lactoferrin and lysozyme. *J. Clin. Invest.* **88**, 1080–1091.

Eraklis, A. J. and Filler, R. M. (1972) Splenectomy in childhood: a review of 1413 cases. *J. Pediat. Surg.* **7**, 382–388.

Esparza, I. and Brock, J. H. (1981) Release of iron by resident and stimulated mouse peritoneal macrophages following ingestion and degradation of transferrin–antitransferrin immune complexes. *Br. J. Haematol.* **49**, 603–614.

Fargion, S., Mandelli, C., Piperno, A. *et al.* (1992) Survival and prognostic factors in 212 Italian patients with genetic hemochromatosis. *Hepatology* **15**, 655–659.

Fernández-Beros, M. E., González, C., McIntosh, M. A. and Cabello, F. C. (1989) Immune response to the iron-deprivation-induced proteins of *Salmonella typhi* in typhoid fever. *Infect. Immunity* **57**, 1271–1275.

Ferrón, L., Ferreiros, C. M., Criado, M. T. and Pintor, M. (1992) Immunogenicity and antigenic heterogeneity of a human transferrin-binding protein from *Neisseria meningitidis*. *Infect. Immunity* **60**, 2887–2892.

Fillet, G., Beguin, G. and Baldelli, L. (1989) Model of reticuloendothelial iron metabolism in humans: abnormal behaviour in idiopathic hemochromatosis and in inflammation. *Blood* **74**, 844–851.

Finkelstein, R. A., Sciortino, C. V. and McIntosh, M. A. (1983) Role of iron in microbe–host interactions. *Rev. Infect. Dis.* **5**, S759–S777.

Flament, J., Goldman, M., Waterlot, Y., Dupont, E., Wybran, J. and Vanherweghem, J.-L. (1986) Impairment of phagocytic oxidative metabolism in hemodialyzed patients with iron overload. *Clin. Nephrol.* **25**, 227–230.

Fletcher, J. (1989) Iron, the iron-binding proteins and bone marrow cell differentiation. In: *Iron in Immunity, Cancer and Inflammation* (eds M. De Sousa and J. H. Brock), John Wiley, Chichester, pp. 223–244.

Fletcher, J., Mather, J., Lewis, M. J. and Whiting, G. (1975) Mouth lesions in iron-deficient anemia: relationship to *Candida albicans* in saliva and to impairment of lymphocyte transformation. *J. Infect. Dis.* **131**, 44–50.

Futran, J., Kemp, J. D., Field, E. H., Vora, A. and Ashman, R. F. (1989) Transferrin receptor synthesis is an early event in B-cell activation. *J. Immunol.* **143**, 787–792.

Galán, P., Davila, M., Mekki, N. and Hercberg, S. (1988) Iron deficiency, inflammatory processes and humorol immunity in children. *Int. J. Vit. Nutr. Res.* **58**, 225–230.

Gascón, P., Zoumbos, N. C. and Young, N. S. (1984) Immunological abnormalities in patients receiving multiple blood transfusions. *Ann. Intern. Med.* **100**, 173–177.

Geller, D. A., Lowenstein, C. J., Shapiro, R. A. *et al.* (1993) Molecular cloning and expression of inducible nitric oxide synthase from human hepatocytes. *Proc. Nat. Acad. Sci. USA* **90**, 3491–3495.

Good, M. F., Chapman, D. E., Powell, L. W. and Halliday, J. W. (1987) The effect of experimental iron-overload on splenic T cell function: analysis using cloning techniques. *Clin. Exp. Immunol.* **68**, 375–383.

Gordeuk, V. R. and Brittenham, G. M. (1992) Bleomycin-reactive iron in patients with acute non-lymphocytic leukemia. *FEBS Lett.* **308**, 4–6.

Gordeuk, V. R., Brittenham, G. M., McLaren, G. D. and Spagnuolo, P. J. (1986) Hyperferremia in immunosuppressed patients with acute nonlymphocytic leukemia and the risk of infection. *J. Lab. Clin. Med.* **108**, 466–472.

Gordeuk, V. R. Prithviraj, P., Dolinar, T. and Brittenham, G. M. (1988) Interleukin 1 administration in mice produces hypoferremia despite neutropenia. *J. Clin. Invest.* **82**, 1934–1938.

Grady, R. W., Akbar, A., Giardina, P. J., Hilgartner, M. W. and De Sousa, M. (1985) Disproportionate lymphoid cell subsets in thalassaemia major: the relative contributions of transfusion and splenectomy. *Br. J. Haematol.* **72**, 361–367.

Granger, D. L., Hibbs, J. R., Perfect, J. R. and Durack, D. T. (1991) Specific amino acid (L-arginine) requirement for the microbiostatic activity of murine macrophages. *J. Clin. Invest.* **81**, 1129–1136.

Green, R., Esparza, I. and Schreiber, R. (1988) Iron inhibits the non-specific tumoricidal activity of macrophages: a possible contributory mechanism for neoplasia in hemochromatosis. *Ann. NY Acad. Sci.* **526**, 301–309.

Grewal, K. K., Warner, P. J. and Williams, P. H. (1982) An inducible outer membrane protein involved in aerobactin-mediated iron transport by ColV strains of *Escherichia coli. FEBS Lett.* **140**, 27–30.

Griffiths, E. (1987) The iron uptake systems of pathogenic bacteria. In: *Iron and Infection* (eds J. J. Bullen and E. Griffiths), John Wiley, Chichester, pp. 69–137.

Griffiths, E. and Humphreys, J. (1977) Bacteriostatic effect of human milk and bovine colostrum on *Escherichia coli*: importance of bicarbonate. *Infect. Immunity* **15**, 396–401.

Griffiths, E. and Humphreys, J. (1980) Isolation of enterochelin from the peritoneal washings of guinea pigs lethally infected with *Escherichia coli. Infect. Immunity* **28**, 286–289.

Gross, R. L., Reid, J. V. O., Newberne, P. M., Burgess, B., Marston, R. and Hift, W. (1975) Depressed cell-mediated immunity in megaloblastic anemia due to folic acid deficiency. *Am. J. Clin. Nutr.* **28**, 225–232.

Guglielmo, P., Cunsolo, F., Lombardo, T. *et al.* (1984) T-subset abnormalities in thalassaemia intermedia: possible evidence for a thymus functional deficiency. *Acta Haematol.* **72**, 361–367.

Guimaraes, J. E. T. E., Berney, J. J., Broxmeyer, H. E., Hoffbrand, A. V. and Francis, G. E. (1988) Acidic isoferritin stimulates differentiation of normal granulomonocytic progenitors. *Leukemia* **2**, 466–471.

Halliwell, B. (1989) Free radicals, reactive oxygen species and human disease: a critical review with special reference to atherosclerosis. *Brit. J. Exp. Path.* **70**, 737–757.

Halliwell, B. and Gutteridge, J. M. C. (1984) Oxygen toxicity, oxygen radicals, transition metals and disease. *Biochem. J.* **219**, 1–14.

Hallquist, N. A. and Sherman, A. R. (1989) Effect of iron deficiency on the stimulation of natural killer cells by macrophage-produced interferon. *Nutr. Res.* **9**, 283–292.

Hallquist, N. A., McNeil, L., Lockwood, J. F. and Sherman, A. R. (1992) Maternal-iron-deficiency effect on peritoneal macrophage and peritoneal natural-killer-cell cytotoxicity in rat pups. *Amer. J. Clin. Nutr.* **55**, 741–746.

Hamilton, T. A. (1982) Regulation of transferrin receptor expression in concanavalin A stimulated and Gross virus transformed rat lymphoblasts. *J. Cell. Physiol.* **113**, 40–46.

Hann, H.-W. L., Stahlhut, M. W. and Blumberg, B. S. (1988) Iron nutrition and tumor growth: decreased tumor growth in iron-deficient mice. *Cancer Res.* **48**, 4168–4170.

Hann, H.-W. L., Kim, C. Y., London, W. Y. and Blumberg, B. S. (1989) Increased serum ferritin in chronic liver disease: a risk factor for primary hepatocellular carcinoma. *Int. J. Cancer* **43**, 376–379.

Hann, H.-W. L., Stahlhut, M. W. and Menduke, H. (1991) Iron enhances tumor growth: observation on spontaneous mammary tumors in mice. *Cancer* **68**, 2407–2410.

Harada, T., Baba, M., Torii, I. and Morikawa, S. (1987) Ferritin selectively suppresses delayed-type hypersensitivity responses at induction or effecter phase. *Cell. Immunol.* **109**, 75–88.

Harju, E. (1988) Empty iron stores as a significant risk factor in abdominal surgery. *J. Parenteral Enteral Nutr.* **12**, 282–285.

Harris, W. R., Carrano, C. J. and Raymond, K. N. (1979) Coordination chemistry of microbial iron transport compounds. 16. Isolation, characterization and formation constants of ferric aerobactin. *J. Am. Chem. Soc.* **101**, 2722–2727.

Hasan, S. M., Aziz, M., Ahmad, P. and Aggarwal, M. (1989) Phagocyte metabolic functions in iron deficiency anaemia of Indian children. *J. Trop. Pediat.* **35**, 6–9.

Helyar, L. and Sherman, A. R. (1987) Iron deficiency and interleukin 1 production by rat leukocytes. *Am. J. Clin. Nutr.* **46**, 346–352.

Hershko, C. and Peto, T. E. A. (1988) Deferoxamine inhibition of malaria is independent of host iron status. *J. Exp. Med.* **168**, 375–387.

Hershko, C., Peto, T. E. A. and Weatherall, D. J. (1988) Iron and infection. *Brit. Med. J.* **296**, 660–664.

Hibbs, J. B., Taintor, R. R. and Vavrin, Z. (1984) Iron depletion: possible cause of tumor cell cytotoxicity induced by activated macrophages. *Biochem. Biophys. Res. Comm.* **123**, 716–723.

Hider, R. C. (1984) Siderophore mediated absorption of iron. *Struct. Bonding* **58**, 25–87.

Higginson, J., Gerritsen, T. and Walker, A. R. P. (1953) Siderosis in the Bantu of South Africa. *Am. J. Path.* **29**, 779–815.

Higgs, J. M. and Wells, R. S. (1972) Chronic mucocutaneous candidiasis: associated abnormalities of iron metabolism. *Br. J. Dermatol.* **86** (Suppl.), 88–102.

Hoepelman, I. M., Bezemer, W. A., Vandenbroucke-Grauls, C. M. J. E., Marx, J. J. M. and Verhoef, J. (1990) Bacterial iron enhances oxygen radical-mediated killing of *Staphylococcus aureus* by phagocytes. *Infect. Immunity* **58**, 26–31.

Hoepelman, I. M., Jaarsma, E. Y., Verhoef, J. and Marx, J. J. M. (1988a) Polynuclear iron complexes impair the function of polymorphonuclear granulocytes. *Br. J. Haematol.* **68**, 385–389.

Hoepelman, I. M., Jaarsma, E. Y., Verhoef, J. and Marx, J. J. M. (1988b) Effect of iron on polymorphonuclear granulocyte phagocytic capacity: role of oxidation state and effect of ascorbic acid. *Br. J. Haematol.* **70**, 495–500.

Hoepelman, I. M., Bezmer, W. A., Van Doornmalen, E., Verhoef, J. and Marx, J. J. M. (1989) Lipid peroxidation of human granulocytes (PMN) and monocytes by iron complexes. *Br. J. Haematol.* **72**, 584–588.

Hoffbrand, A. V., Ganeshaguru, K., Hooton, J. W. L. and Tattersall, M. H. N. (1976) Effect of iron deficiency and desferrioxamine on DNA synthesis in human cells. *Br. J. Haematol.* **33**, 517–526.

Holland, J., Langford, P. R., Towner, K. J. and Williams, P. (1992) Evidence for in vivo expression of transferrin-binding proteins in *Haemophilus influenzae* type b. *Infect. Immunity* **60**, 2986–2991.

Horwitz, D. A., Bakke, A. C., Abo, W. and Nishiya, K. (1984) Monocyte and NK cell cytotoxic activity in human adherent cell preparations: discriminating affects of interferon and lactoferrin. *J. Immunol.* **132**, 2370–2374.

Huot, A. E., Gundel, R. M. and Hacker, M. P. (1990) Effect of erythrocytes on alveolar macrophage cytostatic activity induced by bleomycin lung damage in rats. *Cancer Res.* **50**, 2351–2355.

Jacobs, A. and Joynson, D. H. M. (1974) Lymphocyte function and iron-deficiency anaemia. *Lancet* **ii**, 844.

James, S. L. and Glaven, J. (1989) Macrophage cytotoxicity against schistosomula of *Schistosoma mansoni* involves arginine-dependent production of reactive nitrogen intermediates. *J. Immunol.* **143**, 4208–4212.

Jarvis, J. H. and Jacobs, A. (1974) Morphological abnormalities in lymphocyte mitochondria associated with iron-deficiency anaemia. *J. Clin. Pathol.* **27**, 973–979.

Jiménez, A., Sánchez, A., Vázquez, A. and Olmos, J. M. (1982) Alteraciones mitocondriales en los linfocitos de pacientes con anemia ferropénica. *Morfol. Norm. Patol.* **6B**, 279–287.

Johnson, C. S., Keckler, D. J., Topper, M. I., Braunschweiger, P. G. and Furmanski, P. (1989) *In vivo* hematopoietic effects of recombinant interleukin-1α in mice. Stimulation of granulocytic, monocytic, megakaryocytic, and early erythroid progenitors, and reversal of erythroid suppression with erythropoietin. *Blood* **73**, 678–683.

Joynson, D. H. M., Jacobs, A., Walker, D. M. and Dolby, A. E. (1972) Defect in cell-mediated immunity in patients with iron-deficiency anaemia. *Lancet* **ii**, 1058–1059.

Kaplan, J., Sarnaik, S., Gitlin, J. and Lusher, J. (1984) Diminished helper/suppressor lymphocyte ratios and natural killer activity in recipients of repeated blood transfusions. *Blood* **64**, 308–310.

Kemahli, A. S., Babacan, E. and Çavdar, A. O. (1988) Cell mediated immune responses on children with iron deficiency and combined iron and zinc deficiency. *Nutr. Res.* **8**, 129–136.

Kemp, J. D., Thorson, J. A., Stewart, B. C. and Naumann, P. W. (1992) Inhibition of hematopoietic tumor growth by combined treatment with deferoxamine and an IgG monoclonal antibody against the transferrin receptor: evidence for a threshold model of iron deprivation toxicity. *Cancer Res.* **52**, 4144–4148.

Kilstra, A. and Broersma, L. (1984) Lactoferrin stimulates the production of leucocyte migration inhibitory factor by human peripheral mononuclear phagocytes. *Clin. Exp. Immunol.* **55**, 459–464.

Klostergaard, J. (1987) Monokine-mediated release of intracellular iron in tumor target cells *in vitro*. *Lymphokine Res.* **6**, 19–28.

Kochanowski, B. A. and Sherman, A. R. (1985) Decreased antibody formation in iron-deficient rat pups – effect of iron repletion. *Am. J. Clin. Nutr.* **41**, 278–284.

Konijn, A. M. and Hershko, C. (1977) Ferritin synthesis in inflammation. I. Pathogenesis of impaired iron release. *Br. J. Haematol.* **37**, 7–16.

Konijn, A. M. and Hershko, C. (1989) The anaemia of inflammation and chronic disease. In: *Iron in Immunity, Cancer and Inflammation* (eds M. De Sousa and J. H. Brock), John Wiley, Chichester, pp. 111–143.

Konijn, A. M., Carmel, N., Levy, R. and Hershko, C. (1981) Ferritin synthesis in inflammation. II. Mechanism of increased ferritin synthesis. *Br. J. Haematol.* **49**, 361–370.

Konijn, A. M., Meyron-Holtz, E. G., Levy, R., Ben-Bassat, H. and Matzner, Y. (1990) Specific binding of placental acidic isoferritin to cells of the T-cell line HD-MDR. *FEBS Lett.* **263**, 229–232.

Konopka, K. and Neilands, J. B. (1984) Effect of serum albumin on siderophore-mediated utilization of transferrin iron. *Biochemistry* **23**, 2122–2127.

Krantman, H. J., Young, S. R., Ank, B. J., O'Donnell, C. M., Rachelefsky, G. S. and Stiehm, E. R. (1982) Immune function in pure iron deficiency. *Am. J. Dis. Child.* **136**, 840–844.

Kulapongs, P., Vithayasai, V., Suskind, R. M. and Olson, R. E. (1974) Cell-mediated immunity and phagocytosis and killing function in children with severe iron-deficiency anaemia. *Lancet* **ii**, 689–691.

Kulics, J. and Kijlstra, A. (1987) The effect of lactoferrin on the complement-mediated modulation of immune complex size. *Immunol. Lett.* **14**, 349–353.

Kumagai, N., Benedict, S. H., Mills, G. B. and Gelfand, E. W. (1988) Comparison of phorbol ester/calcium ionophore and phytohemagglutinin-induced signalling in human T lymphocytes. Demonstration of interleukin 2-independent transferrin receptor gene expression. *J. Immunol.* **140**, 37–43.

Kuvibidila, S. and Sarpong, D. (1990) Mitogenic response of lymph nodes and spleen lymphocytes from mice with moderate and severe iron deficiency anemia. *Nutr. Res.* **10**, 195–210.

Kuvibidila, S. and Wade, S. (1987) Macrophage function as studied by the clearance of ^{125}I-labelled polyvinylpyrollidone in iron-deficient and iron replete mice. *J. Nutr.* **117**, 170–176.

Kuvibidila, S. R., Baliga, B. S. and Suskind, R. M. (1981) Effects of iron deficiency anemia on delayed cutaneous hypersensitivity in mice. *Am. J. Clin. Nutr.* **34**, 2635–2640.

Kuvibidila, S. R., Baliga, B. S. and Suskind, R. M. (1983a) The effect of iron-deficiency anemia on cytolytic activity of mice spleen and peritoneal cells against allogenic tumor cells. *Am. J. Clin. Nutr.* **38**, 238–244.

Kuvibidila, S., Nauss, K. M., Bagila, B. S. and Suskind, R. M. (1983b) Impairment of blastogenic response of splenic lymphocytes from iron-deficient mice: in vivo repletion. *Am. J. Clin. Nutr.* **37**, 15–25.

Kuvibidila, S., Dardenne, M., Savino, W. and Lepault, F. (1990) Influence of iron-deficiency anemia on selected thymus functions in mice: thymulin biological activity, T-cell subsets, and thymocyte proliferation. *Am. J. Clin. Nutr.* **51**, 228–232.

Kuvibidila, S., Baliga, B. S. and Murthy, K. K. (1991) Impaired protein kinase C activation as one of the possible mechanisms of reduced lymphocyte proliferation in iron deficiency in mice. *Am. J. Clin. Nutr.* **54**, 944–950.

Lancaster, J. R. and Hibbs, J. B. (1990) EPT demonstration of iron–nitrosyl complex formation by cytotoxic activated macrophages. *Proc. Natl. Acad. Sci. USA* **87**, 1223–1227.

Lane, T. E., Wu-Hsieh, B. A. and Howard, D. H. (1991) Iron limitation and the gamma interferon-mediated antihistoplasma state of murine macrophages. *Infect. Immunity* **59**, 2274–2278.

Langman, L., Young, I. G., Frost, G., Rosenberg, H. and Gibson, F. (1972) Enterochelin system of iron transport in *Escherichia coli*: mutations affecting ferric-enterochelin esterase. *J. Bact.* **112**, 1142–1149.

Larrick, J. W. and Cresswell, P. (1979) Modulation of cell surface iron transferrin receptors by cellular density and state of activation. *J. Supramol. Struct.* **11**, 579–586.

Lee, B. C. (1991) Iron sources for *Haemophilus ducreyi*. *J. Med. Microbiol.* **34**, 317–322.

Lee, G. R. (1983) The anemia of chronic disease. *Semin. Hematol.* **20**, 61–80.

Lehker, M. W. and Alderete, J. F. (1992) Iron regulates growth of *Trichomonas vaginalis* and the expression of immunogenic trichomonad proteins. *Molec. Microbiol.* **6**, 123–132.

Letendre, E. D. and Holbein, B. E. (1983) Turnover in the transferrin iron pool during the hypoferremic phase of experimental *Neisseria meningitidis* infection in mice. *Infect. Immunity* **39**, 50–59.

Liew, F. Y. and Cox, F. E. G. (1991) Nonspecific defence mechanism: the role of nitric oxide. *Immunol. Today* **12**, A17–A21.

Lipinski, P., Jarzabek, Z., Broniek, S. and Zagulski, T. (1991) Protective effect of tissue ferritins in experimental *Escherichia coli* infection of mice *in vivo*. *Int. J. Exp. Pathol.* **72**, 623–630.

Lu, L., Broxmeyer, H. E., Meyers, P. A., Moore, M. A. S. and Thaler, H. T. (1983) Association of cell cycle expression of Ia-like antigenic determinants on normal human multipotential (CFU-GEMM) and erythroid (BFU-E) progenitor cells with regulation *in vitro* by acidic isoferritins. *Blood* **61**, 250–256.

Lukens, J. N. (1973) Control of erythropoiesis in rats with adjuvant-induced chronic inflammation. *Blood* **41**, 37–44.

Lum, J. B., Infante, A. J., Makker, D. M., Yang, F. and Bowman, B. H. (1986) Transferrin synthesis by inducer T-lymphocytes. *J. Clin. Invest.* **77**, 841–849.

Lundrigan, M. D. and Kadner, R. J. (1986) Nucleotide sequence of the gene for the ferrienterochelin receptor FepA in *Escherichia coli*. *J. Biol. Chem.* **261**, 10797–10801.

MacDougall, L. G. and Jacob, M. R. (1978) The immune response in iron-deficient children. Isohaemagglutinin titres and antibody response to immunization. *South Afr. Med.* **53**, 405–407.

MacDougall, L. G., Anderson, R., McNab, G. M. and Katz, J. (1975) The immune response in iron-deficient children: impaired cellular defense mechanisms with altered humoral components. *J. Pediatr.* **86**, 833–843.

Mackay, H. M. (1928) Anaemia in infancy; its prevalence and prevention. *Arch. Dis. Childh.* **3**, 117–147.

Mackler, B., Person, R., Ochs, H. and Finch, C. A. (1984) Iron deficiency in the rat: effects on neutrophil activation and metabolism. *Pediat. Res.* **18**, 549–551.

Magnusson, G., Flodh, H. and Malmfors, T. (1977) Oncological study in rats of Ferastral, and iron-poly-(sorbitol-gluconic acid) complex, after intramuscular administration. *Scand. J. Haematol. (Suppl.)* **32**, 87–98.

Mainou-Fowler, T. and Brock, J. H. (1985) Effect of iron deficiency on the response of mouse lymphocytes to concanavalin A: the importance of transferrin-bound iron. *Immunology* **54**, 325–332.

Marlon, A., Gentry, L. and Merigan, T. C. (1971) Septicemia and *Pasteurella pseudotuberculosis* and liver disease. *Arch. Int. Med.* **127**, 947–949.

Martino, M., Rossi, M. E., Resti, M., Vullo, C. and Vierucci, A. (1984) Changes in superoxide anion production in neutrophils from multitransfused β-thalassemia patients: correlation with ferritin levels and liver damage. *Acta Haematol.* **71**, 289–298.

Masawe, A. E. J., Muindi, J. M. and Swai, G. B. R. (1974) Infections in iron deficiency and other types of anaemias in the tropics. *Lancet* **ii**, 314–317.

Massad, G., Arceneaux, J. E. L. and Byers, B. R. (1991) Acquisition of iron from host sources by mesophilic *Aeromonas* species. *J. Gen. Microbiol.* **137**, 237–241.

Matzner, Y., Hershko, C., Polliack, A., Konijn, A. and Izak, G. (1979) Suppressive effect of ferritin on *in vitro* lymphocyte function. *Br. J. Haematol.* **42**, 345–353.

Matzner, Y., Konijn, A. M., Shlomai, Z. and Ben-Bassat, H. (1985) Differential effect of isolated placental isoferritins on *in vitro* T-lymphocyte function. *Br. J. Haematol.* **59**, 443–448.

Mauel, J., Ransijn, J. and Buchmuller-Rouillier, Y. (1991) Killing of *Leishmania* parasites in activated murine macrophages is based on an L-arginine-dependent process that produces nitrogen derivatives. *J. Leukocyte Biol.* **49**, 73–82.

McCormick, J. A., Markey, G. M. and Morris, T. C. M. (1991) Lactoferrin-inducible monocyte cytotoxicity for K562 cells and decay of natural killer lymphocyte cytotoxicity. *Clin. Exp. Immunol.* **83**, 154–156.

Means, R. T. and Krantz, S. B. (1992) Progress in understanding the pathogenesis of the anemia of chronic disease. *Blood* **80**, 1639–1647.

Means, R. T., Dessypris, E. N. and Krantz, S. B. (1990) Inhibition of human erythroid colony-forming units by tumor necrosis factor requires accessory cells. *J. Clin. Invest.* **86**, 538–541.

Melby, K., Slørdahl, S., Gutterberg, T. J. and Nordbø, S. A. (1982) Septicaemia due to *Yersinia enterocolitica* after oral overdoses of iron. *Brit. Med. J.* **285**, 467–468.

Mendelsohn, J. M., Trowbridge, I. S. and Castagnola, J. (1983) Inhibition of human lymphocyte proliferation by monoclonal antibody to transferrin receptor. *Blood* **62**, 821–826.

Miller, C. B., Jones, R. J., Piantadosi, S., Abeloff, M. D. and Spivak, J. L. (1990) Decreased erythropoietin response in patients with the anemia of cancer. *New Engl. J. Med.* **322**, 1689–1692.

Miller, L. L., Miller, S. C., Torti, S. V., Tsuji, Y. and Torti, F. M. (1991) Iron-dependent induction of ferritin H chain by tumor necrosis factor. *Proc. Nat. Acad. Sci. USA* **88**, 4946–4950.

Moore, L. L. and Humbert, J. R. (1984) Neutrophil bactericidal dysfunction towards oxidant radical-sensitive microorganisms during experimental iron deficiency. *Pediat. Res.* **18**, 684–689.

Moraes-de Souza, H., Kerbauym, J., Yamamoto, M., Da-Silva, M. P. and Dos-Santos, M. R. M. (1984) Depressed cell-mediated immunity in iron deficiency anemia due to chronic loss of blood. *Braz. J. Med. Biol. Res.* **17**, 143–150.

Moreau, M. C., Duval-Iflah, Y., Muller, M. C. *et al.* (1983) Effet de la lactoferrine bovine et des IgG bovines donnés per os sur l'implantation de *Escherichia coli* dans le tube digestif de souris gnotoxéniques et de nouveau nés humains. *Ann. Microbiol. (Inst. Pasteur)* **134B**, 429–441.

Moss, D., Powell, L. W., Arosio, P. and Halliday, J. W. (1992) Characterization of the ferritin receptors of human T-lymphoid (MOLT-4) cells. *J. Lab. Clin. Med.* **119**, 273–279.

Muirden, K. D. (1970) The anaemia of rheumatoid arthritis: the significance of iron deposits in the synovial membrane. *Austr. Ann. Med.* **2**, 97–104.

Munn, C. G., Markenson, A. L., Kapadia, A. and De Sousa, M. (1981) Impaired T cell mitogen responses in some patients with thalassemia intermedia. *Thymus* **3**, 119–128.

Murakawa, H., Bland, C. E., Willis, W. T. and Dallman, P. R. (1987) Iron deficiency and neutrophil function: different rates of the correction of the depressions in oxidative burst and myeloperoxidase activity after iron treatment. *Blood* **69**, 1464–1468.

Murray, M. J., Murray, A. B., Murray, N. J. and Murray, M. B. (1975) Refeeding malaria and hyperferraemia. *Lancet* i, 653–654.

Murray, M. J., Murray, A. B., Murray, M. B. and Murray, C. J. (1978) The adverse effect of iron repletion on the course of certain infections. *Brit. Med. J.* **2**, 1113–1115.

Nalder, B. N., Mahoney, A. W., Ramakrishnan, R. and Hendricks, D. G. (1972) Sensitivity of the immunological response to the nutritional status of rats. *J. Nutr.* **102**, 535–542.

Neckers, L. M. and Cossman, J. (1983) Transferrin receptor induction in mitogen-stimulated human T lymphocytes is required for DNA synthesis and is regulated by interleukin 2. *Proc. Natl. Acad. Sci. USA* **89**, 3494–3498.

Neckers, L. M., Yenokida, G. and James, S. P. (1984) The role of the transferrin receptor in human B-lymphocyte activation. *J. Immunol.* **133**, 2437–2441.

Neilands, J. B. (1982) Microbial envelope proteins related to iron. *Ann. Rev. Microbiol.* **36**, 285–309.

Nelson, R. L. (1992) Dietary iron and colorectal cancer risk. *Free Radical Biol. Med.* **12**, 161–168.

Nelson, R. L., Yoo, S. J., Tanure, J. C., Andrianopoulos, G. and Misumi, A. (1989) The effect of iron on experimental colorectal carcinogenesis. *Anticancer Res.* **9**, 1477–1482.

Niederau, C., Fischer, R., Sonnenberg, A., Stremmel, W., Trampish, H. J. and Strohmeyer, G. (1985) Survival and causes of death in cirrhotic and in non-cirrhotic patients with primary hemochromatosis. *N. Engl. J. Med.* **313**, 1256–1262.

Nonnecke, B. J. and Smith, K. L. (1984) Biochemical and antibacterial properties of bovine mammary secretions during mammary involution and at parturition. *J. Dairy Sci.* **67**, 2863–2872.

Nualart, P., Estévez, M. E., Ballart, I. J., de Miani, S., Peñalver, J. and Sen, L. (1987) Effect of alpha interferon on the altered T-B-cell immunoregulation in patients with thalassemia major. *Am. J. Hematol.* **24**, 151–159.

O'Brien, I. G. and Gibson, F. (1970) The structure of enterochelin and related 2,3-dihydroxy-N-benzoylserine conjugates from *Escherichia coli*. *Biochim. Biophys. Acta* **215**, 393–402.

Ogunnariwo, J. A. and Schryvers, A. B. (1990) Iron acquisition in *Pasteurella haemolytica*: expression and identification of a bovine-specific transferrin receptor. *Infect. Immunity* **58**, 2091–2097.

Oppenheimer, S. J. (1989) Iron and infection: the clinical evidence. *Acta Paediatr. Scand. Suppl.* **361**, 53–62.

Oria, R., Alvarez-Hernández, X., Licéaga, J. and Brock, J. H. (1988) Uptake and handling of iron from transferrin, lactoferrin and immune complexes by a macrophage cell line. *Biochem. J.* **252**, 221–225.

Otto, B. R., Verweij-van Vugt, A. M. J. J. and MacLaren, D. M. (1992) Transferrin and heme-compounds as iron sources for pathogenic bacteria. *Crit. Rev. Microbiol.* **18**, 217–233.

Pattananpanyasat, K. (1990) Expression of cell surface transferrin receptor following *in vitro* stimulation of peripheral blood lymphocytes in patients with β-thalassaemia and iron-deficiency anaemia. *Eur. J. Haematol.* **44**, 190–195.

Pattananpanyasat, K., Hoy, T. G. and Jacobs, A. (1987) The response of intracellular and surface ferritin after T-cell stimulation *in vitro*. *Clin. Sci.* **73**, 605–611.

Payne, S. M. (1989) Iron and virulence in *Shigella*. *Molec. Microbiol.* **3**, 1301–1306.

Pelosi-Testa, E., Samoggia, P., Giannella, G. *et al.* (1988) Mechanisms underlying T-lymphocyte activation: mitogen initiates and IL-2 amplifies the expression of transferrin receptors via intracellular iron level. *Immunology* **64**, 273–279.

Perry, R. D. and San Clemente, C. L. (1979) Siderophore synthesis in *Klebsiella pneumoniae* and *Shigella sonnei* during iron deficiency. *J. Bact.* **140**, 1129–1132.

Pincus, T., Olsen, N. J., Russell, I. J. *et al.* (1990) Multicenter study of recombinant human erythropoietin in correction of anemia of rheumatoid arthritis. *Amer. J. Med.* **89**, 161–168.

Pons, H. A., Soyano, A. and Romano, E. (1992) Interaction of iron polymers with blood mononuclear cells and its detection with the Prussian blue reaction. *Immunopharmacology* **23**, 29–35.

Powars, D. R. (1975) Natural history of sickle cell disease – the first ten years. *Semin. Hematol.* **12**, 267–285.

Prasad, J. S. (1979) Leukocyte function in iron-deficiency anemia. *Am. J. Clin. Nutr.* **32**, 550–552.

Prema, K., Ramalakshmi, B. A., Madhavapeddi, R. and Babu, S. (1982) Immune status of anaemic pregnant women. *Br. J. Obstet. Gynaecol.* **89**, 222–225.

Puschmann, M. and Ganzoni, A. M. (1977) Increased resistance of iron-deficient mice to *Salmonella* infection. *Infect. Immunity* **17**, 663–664.

Quastel, M. R. and Ross, J. F. (1966) The effect of acute inflammation on the utilization and distribution of transferrin-bound and erythrocyte iron. *Blood* **28**, 738–757.

Quinn, F. D. and Weinberg, E. D. (1988) Killing of *Legionella pneumophila* by human serum and iron-binding agents. *Curr. Microbiol.* **17**, 111–116.

Rabson, A. R., Hallett, A. F. and Koornhof, H. J. (1975) Generalised *Yersinia enterocolitica* infection. *J. Infect. Dis.* **131**, 447–451.

Reif, D. W. and Simmons, R. D. (1990) Nitric oxide mediates iron release from ferritin. *Arch. Biochem. Biophys.* **283**, 537–541.

Reissman, K. R. and Udupa, K. (1978) Effect of inflammation on erythroid precursors (BFU-E and CFU-E) in bone marrow and spleen of mice. *J. Lab. Clin. Med.* **92**, 22–29.

Richmond, H. G. (1959) Induction of sarcoma in the rat by iron-dextran complex. *Brit. Med. J.* **1**, 947–949.

Riss, T. L. and Sirbasku, D. A. (1987) Purification and identification of transferrin as a major pituitary-derived mitogen for MTW9/PL2 rat mammary tumor cells. *In Vitro Cell. Devel. Biol.* **28**, 841–849.

Roberts, A. K., Chierici, R., Sawatzki, G., Hill, M. J., Volpato, S. and Vigi, V. (1992) Supplementation of an adapted formula with bovine lactoferrin: 1. Effect on the infant faecal flora. *Acta Paediatr.* **81**, 119–124.

Rocha, E. R., de Uzeda, M. and Brock, J. H. (1991) Effect of ferric and ferrous iron chelators on growth of *Bacteroides fragilis* under anaerobic conditions. *FEMS Microbiol. Lett.* **84**, 45–50.

Rodríguez, M. H. and Jungery, M. (1986) A protein on *Plasmodium falciparum*-infected erythrocytes functions as a transferrin receptor. *Nature* **324**, 388–391.

Rogers, H. J., Bullen, J. J. and Cushnie, G. H. (1970) Iron compounds and resistance to infection: further experiments with *Clostridium welchii* type A *in vivo* and *in vitro*. *Immunology* **19**, 521–538.

Rogers, J., Lacroix, L., Durmowitz, G., Kasschau, K., Andriotakis, J. and Bridges, K. (1993) The role of cytokines in the regulation of ferritin expression. Abstract, 11th International Conference on Iron and Iron Proteins, Jerusalem, p. 37.

Rogers, J. T., Bridges, K. R., Durmowicz, G. P., Glass, J. Auron, P. E. and Munro, H. N. (1990) Translational control during the acute phase response. Ferritin synthesis in response to interleukin-1. *J. Biol. Chem.* **265**, 14572–14578.

Sakata, Y., Morimoto, A., Long, N. C. and Murakami, N. (1991) Fever and acute-phase response induced in rabbits by intravenous and intracerebroventricular injection of interleukin-6. *Cytokine* **3**, 199–203.

Sala, G., Worwood, M. and Jacobs, A. (1986) The effect of isoferritins on granulopoiesis. *Blood* **76**, 436–443.

Sánchez, L., Calvo, M. and Brock, J. H. (1992) Biological role of lactoferrin. *Arch. Dis. Childh.* **67**, 657–661.

Santos, P. C. and Falcão, R. P. (1990) Decreased lymphocyte subsets and K-cell activity in iron deficiency anemia. *Acta Hematol.* **84**, 118–121.

Sauvage, C. A., Mendelsohn, J. C., Lesley, J. F. and Trowbridge, I. S. (1987) Effect of monoclonal antibodies that block transferrin receptor function on the *in vivo* growth of a syngeneic murine leukemia. *Cancer Res.* **47**, 747–753.

Sawitsky, B., Kanter, R. and Sawitsky, A. (1976) Lymphocyte responses to phytomitogens in iron deficiency. *Am. J. Med. Sci.* **272**, 153–160.

Schade, A. L. and Caroline, L. (1946) An iron binding component in human blood plasma. *Science* **104**, 340–341.

Schade, S. G. and Fried, W. (1976) Suppressive effects of endotoxin on erythropoietin-responsive cells in mice. *Amer. J. Physiol.* **231**, 73–76.

Schell, D., Evers, R., Preis, D. *et al.* (1991) A transferrin-binding protein of *Trypanosoma brucei* is encoded by one of the genes in the variant surface glycoprotein gene expression site. *EMBO J.* **10**, 1061–1066.

Schryvers, A. B. (1989) Identification of the transferrin- and lactoferrin-binding proteins in *Haemophilus influenzae*. *J. Med. Microbiol.* **29**, 121–130.

Schryvers, A. B. and González, G. C. (1989) Comparison of the abilities of different sources of iron to enhance *Neisseria meningitidis* infection in mice. *Infect. Immunity* **57**, 2425–2492.

Schryvers, A. B. and Morris, L. J. (1988) Identification and characterization of the human lactoferrin-binding protein from *Neisseria meningitidis*. *Infect. Immunity* **56**, 1144–1149.

Sears, D. A. (1992) Anemia of chronic disease. *Med. Clin. N. Amer.* **76**, 567–579.

Selby, J. V. and Friedman, G. D. (1988) Epidemiologic evidence of an association between body iron stores and risk of cancer. *Int. J. Cancer* **41**, 677–682.

Seligman, P. A., Kovar, J. and Gelfand, E. W. (1992) Lymphocyte proliferation is controlled by both iron availability and regulation of iron uptake pathways. *Pathobiology* **60**, 19–26.

Shau, H., Shen, D. and Golub, S. H. (1986) The role of transferrin in natural killer cell and IL-2 induced cytotoxic cell function. *Cell. Immunol.* **97**, 121–130.

Shau, H., Kim, A. and Golub, S. H. (1992) Modulation of natural killer and lymphokine-activated killer cell cytotoxicity by lactoferrin. *J. Leukocyte Biol.* **51**, 343–349.

Sherman, A. R. and Lockwood, J. F. (1987) Impaired natural killer cell activity in iron-deficient rat pups. *J. Nutr.* **117**, 567–571.

Smith, C. H., Erlandson, M. E., Stern, G. and Hilgartner, M. W. (1964) Post splenectomy infection in Cooley's anemia. *Ann. NY Acad. Sci.* **119**, 748–758.

Smith, M. A., Knight, S. M., Maddison, P. J. and Smith, J. G. (1992) Anaemia of chronic disease in rheumatoid arthritis: effect of the blunted response to erythropoietin and of interleukin-1 production by marrow macrophages. *Ann. Rheum. Dis.* **51**, 753–757.

Snow, R. W., Bypass, P., Shenton, F. C. and Greenwood, B. M. (1991) The relationship between anthropometric measurements and measurements of iron status and susceptibility to malaria in Gambian children. *Trans. Royal Soc. Trop. Med. Hyg.* **85**, 584–589.

Soyano, A., Candellet, D. and Layrisse, M. (1982) Effect of iron-deficiency on the mitogen-induced proliferative response of rat lymphocytes. *Int. Arch. Allergy Appl. Immunol.* **69**, 353–357.

Soyano, A., Fernández, E. and Romano, E. (1985) Suppressive effect of iron on in vitro lymphocyte function: formation of iron polymers as a possible explanation. *Int. Arch. Allergy Appl. Immunol.* **76**, 376–378.

Spear, A. T. and Sherman, A. R. (1992) Iron deficiency alters DMBA-induced tumor burden and natural killer cell cytotoxicity in rats. *J. Nutr.* **122**, 46–55.

Srikantia, S. G., Prasad, J. S., Bhaskaram, C. and Krishnamachari, K. A. V. R. (1976) Anaemia and the immune response. *Lancet* **i**, 1307–1309.

Stevens, R. G., Kuvibidila, S., Kapps, M., Friedlaender, J. and Blumberg, B. S. (1983) Iron-binding proteins, hepatitis B virus, and mortality in the Solomon Islands. *Amer. J. Epidemiol.* **118**, 550–561.

Stevens, R. G., Beasley, R. P. and Blumberg, B. S. (1986) Iron-binding proteins and risk of cancer in Taiwan. *J. Natl. Cancer Inst.* **76**, 605–610.

Stevens, R. G., Jones, D. Y., Micozzi, M. S. and Taylor, P. R. (1988) Body iron stores and the risk of cancer. *New Engl. J. Med.* **319**, 1047–1052.

Stevens, R. G., Graubard, B. I. Neriishii, K. and Blumberg, B. S. (1993) Moderate elevation of iron stores and increased risk of cancer occurrence and death. *J. Natl. Cancer Inst.*, in press.

Stryckmans, P., Delforge, A., Amson, R. B. *et al.* (1984) Lactoferrin: no evidence for its role in regulation of CSA production by human lymphocytes and monocytes. *Blood Cells* **10**, 369–395.

Sturrock, A., Alexander, J., Lamb, J., Craven, C. M. and Kaplan, J. (1990) Characterization of a transferrin-independent uptake system for iron in HeLa cells. *J. Biol. Chem.* **265**, 3139–3145.

Sullivan, J. R., Till, G. O., Ward, P. A. and Newton, R. B. (1989) Nutritional iron restriction diminishes acute complement-dependent lung injury. *Nutr. Res.* **9**, 625–634.

Sussman, H. H. (1992) Iron in cancer. *Pathobiology* **60**, 2–9.

Taetle, R. and Honeysett, J. M. (1988) γ-Interferon modulates human monocyte/macrophage transferrin receptor expression. *Blood* **71**, 1590–1595.

Taetle, R., Rhyner, K., Catagnola, J., To, D. and Mendelsohn, J. (1985) Role of transferrin, Fe, and transferrin receptors in myeloid leukemia cell growth. *J. Clin. Invest.* **75**, 1061–1067.

Taetle, R., Honeysett, J. M. and Bergeron, R. (1989) Combination iron depletion therapy. *J. Nat. Cancer Inst.* **81**, 1229–1235.

Tanaka, T., Araki, E., Nitta, K. and Tateno, M. (1987) Recombinant human tumor necrosis factor depresses serum iron in mice. *J. Biol. Response Modifiers* **6**, 484–488.

Teixeira, S. and Kühn, L. C. (1991) Post-transcriptional regulation of the transferrin receptor and 4F2 antigen heavy chain mRNA during growth activation of spleen cells. *Eur. J. Biochem.* **202**, 819–826.

Thomas, T. K., Will, P. C., Srivastava, A. *et al.* (1991) Evaluation of an interleukin-1 receptor antagonist in the rat acetic acid-induced colitis model. *Agents and Actions* **34**, 187–190.

Thompson, H. J., Kennedy, K., Witt, M. and Juzefyk, J. (1991) Effect of dietary iron deficiency or excess on the induction of mammary carcinogenesis by 1-methyl-1-nitrosourea. *Carcinogenesis* **12**, 111–114.

Thorson, J. A., Smith, K. M., Gómez, F., Naumann, P. W. and Kemp, J. D. (1991) Role of iron in T cell activation: TH1 clones differ from TH2 clones in their sensitivity to inhibition of DNA synthesis caused by IGG Mabs against the transferrin receptor and the iron chelator desferrioxamine. *Cell. Immunol.* **134**, 126–137.

Trowbridge, I. S. (1989) Potential uses of anti-transferrin receptor monoclonal antibodies. In: *Iron in Immunity, Cancer and Inflammation* (eds M. De Sousa and J. H. Brock), John Wiley, Chichester, pp. 341–360.

Trowbridge, I. S. and Domingo, D. (1981) Anti-transferrin receptor monoclonal antibody and toxin-antibody conjugates affect growth of human tumour cells. *Nature* **294**, 171–173.

Tryon, V. V. and Baseman, J. (1987) The acquisition of human lactoferrin by *Mycoplasma pneumonia*. *Microb. Pathogenesis* **3**, 437–443.

Turgeon-O'Brien, H., Amiot, J., Lemieux, L. and Dillon, J.-C. (1985) Myeloperoxidase activity of polymorphonuclear leukocytes in iron deficiency anemia and the anemia of chronic disorders. *Acta Haematol.* **74**, 151–154.

Valenti, P., Visca, P., Antonini, G. and Orsi, N. (1986) Interaction between lactoferrin and ovatransferrin and *Candida* cells. *FEMS Microbiol. Lett.* **33**, 271–275.

Van Asbeck, B. S., Verbrugh, H. A., van Oost, B. A., Marx, J. J. M., Imhof, H. and Verhoef, J. (1982) *Listeria monocytogenes* meningitis and decreased phagocytosis associated with iron overload. *Br. Med. J.* **284**, 542–544.

Van Asbeck, B. S., Marx, J. J. M., Struyvenberg, J. and Verhoef, J. (1984) Functional defects in phagocytic cells from patients with iron overload. *J. Infect.* **8**, 232–240.

Van der Pouw-Kraan, T., van Kooten, C., van Oers, R. and Aarden, L. A. (1991) Human transferrin allows efficient IgE production by anti-CD3-stimulated human lymphocytes at low cell densities. *Eur. J. Immunol.* **21**, 385–390.

Vandewalle, B., Hornez, L., Revillion, F. and Lefebvre, J. (1991) Cyclic AMP stimulation of transferrin secretion by breast cancer cells grown on extracellular matrix or in two-compartment culture chambers. *Biochem. Biophys. Res. Comm.* **177**, 1041–1048.

Van Heerden, C., Oosthuizen, R., Van Wyk, H., Prinsloo, P. and Anderson, R. (1983) Evaluation of neutrophil and lymphocyte function in subjects with iron deficiency. *S. Afr. Med. J.* **24**, 111–113.

Van Miert, A. S. J. P. A. M., Van Duin, C. T. M. and Wensing, T. (1990) Fever and changes in plasma zinc and iron concentrations in the goat. The effects of interferon inducers and recombinant IFNα. *J. Comp. Path.* **103**, 289–300.

Van Snick, J. L., Masson, P. L. and Heremans, J. F. (1974) The involvement of lactoferrin in the hyposideremia of acute inflammation. *J. Exp. Med.* **140**, 1068–1084.

Vincendeau, P. and Daulouede, S. (1991) Macrophage cytostatic effect on *Trypanosoma musculi* involves an L-arginine-dependent mechanism. *J. Immunol.* **146**, 4338–4343.

Vodinelich, L., Sutherland, R., Schneider, C., Newman, R. and Greaves, M. (1983) Receptor for transferrin may be a 'target' structure for natural killer cells. *Proc. Natl. Acad. Sci. USA* **86**, 835–839.

Vostrejs, M., Moran, P. L. and Seligman, P. A. (1988) Transferrin synthesis by small cell lung cancer cells acts as an autocrine regulator of cellular proliferation. *J. Clin Invest.* **82**, 331–339.

Voyiatzaki, C. S. and Soteriadou, K. P. (1992) Identification and isolation of the *Leishmania* transferrin receptor. *J. Biol. Chem.* **267**, 9112–9117.

Wakabayashi, Y., Sugimoto, M., Ishiyama, T. and Hirose, S. (1988) Effect of iron on T-cell colony formation in patients with iron-deficiency anemia. *Acta Haematol. Jpn.* **51**, 691–697.

Walter, T., Arredondo, S., Arévalo, M. and Stekel, A. (1986) Effect of iron therapy on phagocytosis and bactericidal activity in neutrophils of iron deficient infants. *Am. J. Clin. Nutr.* **44**, 877–882.

Ward, C. G., Hammond, J. S. and Bullen, J. J. (1986) Effect of iron compounds on antibacterial function of human polymorphs and plasma. *Infect. Immunity* **51**, 723–730.

Warner, P. J., Williams, P. H., Bindereif, A. and Neilands, J. B. (1981) Col V plasmid-specified aerobactin synthesis by invasive strains of *Escherichia coli*. *Infect. Immunity* **33**, 540–545.

Waterlot, Y., Cantinieaux, B., Hariga-Muller, H. *et al.* (1985) Impaired phagocytic activity of neutrophils in patients receiving haemodialysis: the critical role of iron overload. *Br. Med. J.* **291**, 501–504.

Wei, Y., Miller, S. C., Tsuji, Y., Torti, S. V. and Torti, F. M. (1990) Interleukin-1 induces ferritin heavy chain in human muscle cells. *Biochem. Biophys. Res. Comm.* **169**, 289–296.

Weijmer, M. C., Neering, H. and Weltan, C. (1990) Preliminary report: furunculosis and hypoferraemia. *Lancet* **336**, 464–466.

Weinberg, E. D. (1984) Iron withholding: a defense against infection and neoplasia. *Physiol. Rev.* **64**, 65–102.

Weinberg, E. D. (1992a) Cellular acquisition of iron and the iron-withholding defense against microbial and neoplastic invasion. In: *Iron and Human Disease* (ed. R. B. Lauffer), CRC Press, Boca Raton, Florida, pp. 179–205.

Weinberg, E. D. (1992b) Roles of iron in neoplasia: promotion, prevention and therapy. *Biol. Trace Elements Res.* **34**, 123–140.

Weiss, G., Fuchs, D., Hausen, A. *et al.* (1992) Iron modulates interferon-gamma effects in the human myelomonocytic cell line THP-1. *Exp. Hematol.* **20**, 605–610.

Weiss, G., Goossen, B., Doppler, W. *et al.* (1993) Translational regulation via iron-responsive elements by the nitric oxide/NO synthase pathway. *EMBO J.* **12**, 3651–3657.

Weitman, S. D., Buchanan, G. R. and Kaman, B. A. (1991) Pulmonary toxicity of deferoxamine in children with advanced cancer. *J. Natl. Cancer Inst.* **83**, 1834–1835.

Westmacott, D., Hawkes, J. E., Hill, R. O., Clarke, L. E. and Bloxham, D. P. (1986) Comparison of the effects of recombinant murine and human interleukin-1 *in vitro* and *in vivo*. *Lymphokine Res.* **5**, S87–S91.

Wharton, M., Granger, D. L. and Durack, D. T. (1988) Mitochondrial iron loss from leukemia cells injured by macrophages. A possible mechanism for electron transport chain defects. *J. Immunol.* **141**, 1311–1317.

White, S., Taetle, R., Seligman, P., Rutherford, M. and Trowbridge, I. M. (1990) Combination of anti-transferrin receptor monoclonal antibodies inhibit human tumor cell growth *in vitro* and *in vivo*: evidence for synergistic antiproliferative effects. *Cancer Res.* **50**, 6295–6301.

Willett, W. C. and MacMahon, B. (1984) Diet and cancer – an overview. *New Engl. J. Med.* **310**, 633–638 [697–703].

Williams, P., Brown, M. R. W. and Lambert, P. A. (1984) Effect of iron deprivation on the production of siderophores and outer membrane proteins in *Klebsiella aerogenes*. *J. Gen. Microbiol.* **130**, 2357–2365.

Williams, P. H. (1979) Novel iron uptake system specified by Col V plasmids: an important component in the virulence of invasive strains of *Escherichia coli*. *Infect. Immunity* **26**, 925–932.

Yamashiro, K. M., Goldman, R. H. and Harris, D. (1971) *Pasteurella* pseudotuberculosis: acute sepsis with survival. *Arch. Int. Med.* **128**, 605–608.

Yancey, R. J., Breeding, S. A. L. and Lankford, C. E. (1979) Enterochelin (enterobactin): virulence factor for *Salmonella typhimurium*. *Infect. Immunity* **24**, 174–180.

Yetgin, S., Altay, C., Ciliv, G. and Laleli, Y. (1979) Myeloperoxidase activity and bactericidal function of PMN in iron deficiency. *Acta Haematol.* **61**, 10–14.

Yip, R. and Dallman, P. R. (1988) The roles of inflammation and iron deficiency as causes of anemia. *Amer. J. Clin. Nutr.* **48**, 1295–1300.

Yu, R. H., Gray-Owen, R. G., Ogunnariwo, J. and Schryvers, A. B. (1992) Interaction of ruminant transferrins with transferrin receptors in bovine isolates of *Pasteurella haemolytica* and *Haemophilus somnus*. *Infect. Immunity* **60**, 2992–2994.

Zimecki, M., Mazurier, J., Machnicki, M., Wieczorek, Z., Montreuil, J. and Spik, G. (1991) Immunostimulatory activity of lactotransferrin and maturation of CD4⁻ CD8⁻ murine thymocytes. *Immunol. Lett.* **30**, 119–124.

Zoumbos, N. C., Djeu, J. Y. and Young, N. S. (1984) Interferon is the suppressor of hematopoiesis generated by stimulated lymphocytes. *J. Immunol.* **133**, 769–774.

Zucali, J. R., Broxmeyer, H. E., Levy, D. and Morse, C. (1989) Lactoferrin decreased monocyte-induced fibroblast production of myeloid colony-stimulating activity by suppressing monocyte release of interleukin-1. *Blood* **74**, 1531–1536.

Zucker, S., Friedman, S. and Lysik, R. M. (1974) Bone marrow erythropoiesis in the anemia of infection, inflammation and malignancy. *J. Clin. Invest.* **53**, 1132–1138.

12. Iron Chelators

C. HERSHKO

Department of Medicine, Shaare Zedek Medical Center, and Department of Human Nutrition and
Metabolism, Hebrew University, Jerusalem, Israel, 91031, PO Box 3235

I. INTRODUCTION

Iron chelators are a unique class of drugs with a high and selective affinity to iron. Of the many natural and synthetic compounds available today, only desferrioxamine (DF), a siderophore produced by *Streptomyces pilosus*, has gained widespread clinical acceptance. The most obvious use of an iron chelator is promoting the excretion of excess and potentially toxic iron from the body. However, in view of the important physiological role of iron in electron transfer there is an increasing interest in recent years in the potential usefulness of iron chelators in conditions unrelated to iron overload, such as the prevention of free radical-induced injury or interference with cell proliferation.

This chapter will review the pharmacology of DF; consider the most likely compartments of iron available for interaction with iron chelators in the body; discuss the most promising new orally effective iron chelators presently considered for clinical use; and review the conditions unrelated to iron overload in which iron chelators may have a beneficial effect. The use of iron chelators in iron overload is discussed in Chapter 9.

2. THE PHARMACOLOGY OF DESFERRIOXAMINE

The iron chelating drug desferrioxamine B (DF) is a colourless crystalline substance produced by *Streptomyces pilosus*. It consists of a chain of three hydroxamic acids terminating in a free amino acid group (Fig. 12.1) which, in turn, enables it to form salts with organic and inorganic acids (Keberle, 1964). It combines with ferric (Fe^{3+}) iron at a 1:1 molar ratio and with a stability constant of 10^{31}. The affinity of DF to Fe^{2+} and other metal ions is much lower and ranges from 10^2 to 10^{14}. Studies published in the early 1960s (Wohler, 1963; Peters *et al.*, 1966; Meyer-Brunot and Keberle, 1967) have shown that ferrioxamine, the DF–iron complex, changes its configuration and becomes an extremely stable compound which is resistant to enzymatic degradation (Meyer-Brunot and Keberle, 1967). Ferrioxamine is distributed in the extracellular space and is unable to penetrate cells, as evidenced by a plateau in its serum concentrations following nephrectomy (Keberle, 1964). In the intact dog, 98% of labelled ferrioxamine is recovered in the urine within 3 days. In contrast to ferrioxamine, DF is capable of penetrating various tissues and is rapidly catabolized *in vivo*.

Studies in dogs employing tritium-labelled DF have shown that although 70% of labelled DF is excreted in the urine within 3 days, over half of this excretion is in

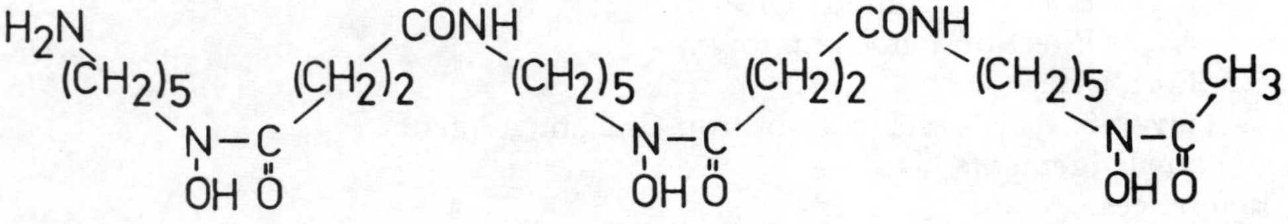

$$H_2N-(CH_2)_5-N(OH)-C(O)-(CH_2)_2-CONH-(CH_2)_5-N(OH)-C(O)-(CH_2)_2-CONH-(CH_2)_5-N(OH)-C(O)-CH_3$$

Fig. 12.1 Desferrioxamine B.

the form of DF metabolites (Keberle, 1964). DF is excreted by both glomerular filtration and tubular secretion, whereas ferrioxamine is partly reabsorbed following glomerular filtration (Peters et al., 1966). The combination of both of these tubular mechanisms tends to decrease the ability of injected DF to promote the urinary excretion of chelated iron. In contrast to ferrioxamine, the concentration in plasma of DF in nephrectomized dogs does not reach a plateau. Its disappearance curve is complex, reflecting a combination of metabolic breakdown, and penetration into various tissues. Bearing these limitations in mind, estimates such as the volume distribution of DF in 62% of the body, and a metabolic half-life of about 1 h (Peters et al., 1966) may be regarded as only rough approximations. Tissue concentrations of labelled DF in dogs following intravenous injection are highest in the bile and brain, intermediate in the spleen, kidney and plasma, and lowest in the heart, lungs and fatty tissues. Although the great efficiency of the liver in clearing DF from the circulation is clearly evidenced by the rapid concentration of labelled DF in the bile, DF is not retained in the liver to a significant extent. Most of the biliary and a great part of the urinary excretion of the tritiated compound is in the form of DF metabolites. Studies employing high-performance liquid chromatography (HPLC) and fast atom bombardment mass spectrometry in patients with hereditary haemochromatosis have shown that only 33% of iron is excreted in the form of ferrioxamine whereas 58% is bound to metabolite I produced by deamination of the terminal amino group and oxidation of the adjacent carbon atom to a carboxylic group (Lehmann and Heinrich, 1990). The metabolism of DF is largely confined to the N-terminal region of the molecule and is in many respects similar to the degradation of the amino acid lysine (Singh et al., 1990a). Studies employing HPLC have shown the existence of two major metabolites of DF in human plasma and up to five metabolites in the urine (Kruck et al., 1988; Singh et al., 1990a, 1992). By far the most active tissue in the enzymatic breakdown of DF is the plasma, followed by various parenchymatous organs (Meyer-Brunot and Keberle, 1967). Rat plasma is about four times more efficient in DF catabolism than plasma obtained from the dog, or man.

Although studies employing tritiated DF yielded valuable information in animals, the amounts of radioactivity required precluded the use of similar techniques in man. A useful substitute is the measurement of filtrable (chelated) plasma iron following DF administration. Using a saturating solution of iron in a manner similar to the measurement of latent iron binding capacity, both ferrioxamine and unbound DF can be measured simultaneously. Such studies have shown that following the intravenous bolus injection of DF, plasma levels of DF drop to half of the initial concentration within 5 to 10 minutes (Summers et al., 1979). After intramuscular injection of DF to healthy subjects, rapid and slow phases of DF clearance have been found with half-lives of 1.0 and 6.1 h respectively (Allain et al., 1987). Slow subcutaneous infusion of DF at a dose of 100 mg/kg/24 h results in a gradual build-up of plasma DF concentrations reaching a plateau in about 12 h. This is accompanied by a simultaneous increase in plasma ferrioxamine concentrations. There is a direct correlation between the total 48 h urinary excretion of iron and peak plasma concentrations of ferrioxamine during DF infusion. Similarly, a direct linear correlation was found between plasma ferrioxamine levels 2 hours after a bolus injection of DF, and the logarithm of 24 urinary excretion of chelated iron (Hershko and Rachmilewitz, 1979).

The gastrointestinal absorption of both DF and ferrioxamine is poor (Keberle, 1964). Oral administration of DF is effective in blocking the intestinal absorption of inorganic iron, but has only a marginal effect on urinary iron excretion. Although a slight, but consistent increase in urinary iron excretion has been shown following oral DF treatment at doses ranging from 3 to 9 g/d (Callender and Weatherall, 1980), the cost-effectiveness of such an approach is very low. Conversely, the intestinal absorption of food iron is inhibited by the parenteral administration of DF (Pippard et al., 1977).

In view of these observations, a number of factors should be considered in designing strategies for the optimal utilization of DF. Its rapid clearance from plasma, effective catabolism and active tubular secretion severely limit the effectiveness of single bolus injections given at large intervals. On the other hand, its apparent distribution in over 60% of the total body volume indicates ready access to intracellular compartments and availability in disease conditions in which interaction with chelatable intracellular iron might be of potential benefit.

3. THE NATURE OF CHELATABLE IRON

In normal subjects most of the body iron is unavailable for chelation and urinary excretion following DF treatment represents less than 0.03% of the total iron in the body. Iron in haemoglobin, representing over two-thirds of all iron, is unavailable for DF chelation in vivo or in vitro (Keberle, 1964). Likewise, transferrin-bound iron is a very poor source of iron for in vivo chelation by DF (Hershko et al., 1973). By exclusion then, the most likely source of chelatable iron is that stored in tissues in the form of ferritin or haemosiderin, or a labile iron compartment in dynamic equilibrium with the former.

3.1. Chelatable Labile Iron

A number of observations indicate that a labile iron pool in equilibrium with storage iron is a more likely direct source of chelatable iron than storage iron per se. In the rat model of hepatocellular storage iron labelled with exogenous ^{59}Fe-ferritin, optimal chelation occurs at 2–6 h prior to the incorporation of ^{59}Fe into endogenous ferritin (Pippard et al., 1982a). Likewise, hypertransfusion in thalassaemic patients results in diminished plasma iron turnover and a simultaneous suppression of DF-induced urinary iron excretion (Pippard et al., 1982b), whereas haemolysis, induced by phenylhydrazine, increases urinary DF-iron excretion (Cumming et al., 1967). In untreated megaloblastic anaemia urinary DF-iron is out of proportion to the magnitude of iron stores, but is rapidly decreased following resumption of normal erythropoiesis by specific treatment (Karabus and Fielding, 1967). A common feature of all of these examples is increased availability of iron for chelation by increased catabolism of ferritin- or haemoglobin-bound iron. These considerations lend support to the concept of a chelatable intermediate iron pool (Lynch et al., 1974) from which iron may either be released to the plasma to combine with transferrin, or diverted into ferritin stores. It is assumed that iron released from ferritin en route to plasma will first enter the same intermediate iron pool.

3.2. Cellular Origin of Chelatable Iron and Routes of Excretion

DF is able to interact with a number of cell types. Early studies with tritiated DF have shown significant uptake by liver, spleen, kidney and brain (Wohler, 1963; Keberle, 1964). More recent studies have shown that DF is able to interact *in vitro* with iron located in cultured liver cells (White and Jacobs, 1978; Octave *et al.*, 1983; Laub *et al.*, 1985), heart cells (Sciortino *et al.*, 1980; Link *et al.*, 1985) and monocytes (Esparza and Brock, 1981), although direct evidence for the cellular uptake of DF is available only in hepatocytes (Laub *et al.*, 1985). In iron overload, excess iron may be deposited in almost all tissues, but the bulk of iron is found in association with two cell types: reticuloendothelial (RE) cells found in the spleen, liver and bone marrow, and parenchymal tissues represented mainly by hepatocytes. In contrast to RE cells in which iron accumulation is relatively harmless, parenchymal siderosis may result in significant organ damage.

The source of iron, and the proportion of iron retained in ferritin stores or recycled into the circulation from the two cell types is quite different. RE cells are unable to assimilate transferrin iron and they derive iron from the catabolism of haemoglobin in non-viable erythrocytes (Hershko, 1977). Most of this catabolic iron is recycled within a few hours (Chapter 2). In contrast, hepatic parenchymal cells maintain a dynamic equilibrium with plasma transferrin, with iron uptake predominating when transferrin saturation is high, and release when serum iron and transferrin saturation are low (Cook *et al.*, 1970). Unlike RE cells, the turnover of parenchymal iron stores is extremely low. In general, iron overload associated with increased intestinal absorption, such as in hereditary haemochromatosis, results in predominant parenchymal siderosis, whereas in conditions wherein iron overload is caused by multiple blood transfusions the primary site of siderosis is the RE cells. Considerable redistribution of iron may take place subsequently.

It is possible to examine the selective interaction of an iron chelator with either parenchymal or RE iron stores by using radioiron-labelled probes targeted into one of these compartments (Hershko *et al.*, 1973). Several studies employing such selective storage iron labels in rats have shown that DF interacts preferentially with hepatocellular iron stores and that the contribution of RE cells to DF-induced iron excretion is limited (Pippard *et al.*, 1982a; Kim *et al.*, 1985). As hepatocytes are unable to incorporate circulating ferrioxamine (^{59}Fe-DF), the biliary excretion of ^{59}Fe-DF is clear evidence of intrahepatic chelation of biliary radioiron. In contrast, the interpretation of urinary radioiron excretion is more complicated. Such excretion is derived entirely from circulating ferrioxamine which in turn may originate from the chelation of iron in RE stores, or iron-in-transit to or from circulating transferrin (Pippard *et al.*, 1982a), which may be contributed by either RE or parenchymal cells. Considering the enormous volume of iron recycled by RE cells through haemolysis and ineffective erythropoiesis in thalassaemia and other iron-loading anaemias, the bulk of iron-in-transit for urinary iron excretion in such patients is most probably derived from RE cells.

A number of experimental and clinical observations support the assumption that the urinary excretion of chelated iron is derived mainly from RE cells. Studies in hypertransfused rats using continuous DF infusion to capture all chelatable iron have shown that, in contrast to hepatocellular radioiron excretion which is confined entirely to the bile, most of the radioiron excretion derived from the RE label is recovered in the urine (Hershko, 1975, 1978; Hershko et al., 1978b). Moreover, when DTPA, a water-soluble synthetic chelator which does not enter cells, is employed in the same experimental model, there is no enhancement at all of hepatocellular iron excretion, but the enhancement of urinary RE radioiron excretion is very similar to that observed previously with DF. According to the 'alternative pathways' hypothesis derived from these observations (Hershko and Weatherall, 1988), DF obtains iron for chelation by one of two alternative mechanisms; (a) in situ interaction with hepatocellular iron and subsequent biliary excretion, and; (b) chelation of iron derived from red cell catabolism in the RE system with subsequent urinary excretion. The observations described do not permit a firm conclusion as to whether RE-derived iron is chelated by DF within the RE cell or following its release into the plasma or upon the hepatocyte surface (Pippard et al., 1982a).

Clinical observations in patients with primary and secondary haemochromatosis lend strong support to the 'alternative pathways' hypothesis. In thalassaemic patients in whom the specific activity of storage iron in the spleen, representing RE stores, and the liver has been studied during splenectomy 10 to 12 days after ferrokinetic studies, the specific activity of splenic non-haem iron was identical with that of chelated urinary iron and both were 15 times higher than the specific activity of hepatic iron. These measurements indicate that chelated urinary iron is most probably derived from splenic and not from hepatic iron stores (Hershko and Rachmilewitz, 1979). In another study of thalassaemic patients (Pippard et al., 1982b), a reciprocal relation between urinary and faecal DF-induced iron excretion has been demonstrated. Hypertransfusion resulted in the suppression of plasma iron turnover, indicating decreased ineffective erythropoiesis and reduced RE breakdown of non-viable erythrocytes. This was associated with reduced urinary, and increased faecal excretion of chelated iron. The same study has also shown that increasing doses of DF administered to thalassaemic patients in whom the greatly increased plasma iron turnover is attributed to increased haemoglobin iron catabolism in RE cells, result in a predominant urinary iron excretion. In contrast, in hereditary haemochromatosis where plasma iron turnover is normal but hepatocellular iron stores are increased, the same treatment results in a predominant increase in faecal iron excretion. All of these studies indicate that urinary iron excretion is closely related to RE iron metabolism and is enhanced by increased RE haemoglobin catabolism. In contrast, faecal iron excretion depends mainly on hepatocellular iron concentrations and is actually increased when there is reduced plasma iron turnover.

3.3. Chemical Nature of Chelatable Iron

The chemical nature of the chelatable iron pool has been the subject of a number of studies. In cultured hepatocytes, radioiron supplied as ferric citrate is rapidly incorporated into cytosol ferritin. Such radioiron is readily available for chelation by DF (Octave et al., 1983). In subsequent studies employing tritiated DF-analogues, these chelators were shown to accumulate within plasma membrane related structures and in lysosomes (Laub et al., 1985). The authors proposed that autophagy of cytosolic ferritin may greatly facilitate the chelation of ferritin iron by DF due to the acidic pH and hydrolytic enzymes in lysosomes, and that this may represent the chelatable intracellular iron pool. Lysosomal/siderosomal iron was shown to be the most likely source of chelatable iron in iron-loaded heart cells in culture employing a combination of Mossbauer spectroscopy and electron microscopy in a recent study by Shiloh *et al.* (1992). Further support for the identification of lysosomal ferritin as the target of DF in hepatocytes may be derived from the observation that the phase of hepatocellular lysosomal degradation of injected ^{59}Fe-labelled exogenous ferritin coincides with the timing of maximal availability of ^{59}Fe for *in vivo* chelation by DF (Pippard *et al.*, 1982a; Unger and Hershko, 1974).

There is no available information on the chemical nature of chelatable RE iron although the ability of DF to mobilize iron directly from peritoneal macrophages has been clearly demonstrated *in vitro* (Esparza and Brock, 1981). It is possible that, similar to parenchymal cells, DF may enter secondary lysosomes in RE cells to interact directly with iron derived from haem catabolism. However, it is also possible that RE iron may be chelated following its release from these cells. The DTPA studies mentioned earlier (Hershko, 1975) have shown that RE iron may be chelated by a drug which is unable to enter these cells with an efficiency which is equal to that of DF both in experimental animals and in man (Hershko *et al.*, 1978b; Pippard *et al.*, 1986). The existence of a chelatable, low molecular weight plasma iron fraction (Hershko and Peto, 1987) has been documented in patients with severe iron overload by a number of investigators (Hershko *et al.*, 1978a; Batey *et al.*, 1978; Anuwatanakulchai *et al.*, 1984; Wang *et al.*, 1986; Wagstaff *et al.*, 1985; Gutteridge *et al.*, 1985; Singh *et al.*, 1990b). Such non-transferrin plasma iron (NTPI) is only found after complete saturation of circulating transferrin. NTPI was shown to promote the formation of free hydroxyl radicals and to accelerate the peroxidation of membrane lipids *in vitro* (Gutteridge *et al.*, 1985). The rate of low molecular weight iron uptake by cultured rat heart cells is over 300 times greater than that of transferrin iron (Link *et al.*, 1985). Such uptake was shown to result in increased myocardial lipid peroxidation and abnormal contractility, and these effects were reversed by *in vitro* treatment with DF. Recognition of NTPI as a potentially toxic component of plasma iron in haemochromatosis may be useful in designing better strategies for the effective administration of DF and other iron chelating drugs.

3.4. Site-directed Iron Chelation

The foregoing discussion indicates that pathophysiological determinants of the availability of chelatable iron at particular sites, and the pharmacology of the chelating agents used (particularly their tissue distribution), are both important in determining the efficiency and route(s) of iron excretion. Attempts have been made to enhance the amount of iron chelated by modifying the form in which such widely studied chelators as DF and DTPA are presented, thus altering the pattern of their subsequent tissue clearance. Incorporation of DF within red cell membrane 'ghosts' before intravenous injection led to prolongation and enhancement of iron excretion compared with subcutaneous DF infusions in patients with secondary iron overload (Green *et al.*, 1980). Studies with selective ^{59}Fe labels in rats suggested that this was attributable to clearance of the encapsulated DF by macrophages and consequent ready access by the drug to otherwise unavailable intracellular reticuloendothelial iron stores (Green *et al.*, 1981), rather than simply to prolongation of the duration of action of DF.

Liposomal delivery of parenterally administered chelators has also been suggested as a means to improve the excretion of metal ions in a variety of animal models (Rahman and Wright, 1975; Young et al., 1979), with the suggestion that the characteristics of the liposome might influence subsequent cellular uptake: in mice, large multilamellar liposomes and liposomes prepared without a glycolipid appeared to have a higher affinity for Kupffer cells than for hepatocytes, compared with unilamellar or glycolipid-containing liposomes (Lau et al., 1981, 1983). The synthesis of a water-insoluble amphiphilic chelator involving the covalent linkage of DTPA to a phospholipid, phosphatidylethanolamine (PE), allowed the chelator to be incorporated directly into liposomal membranes (Adams et al., 1991): in iron-loaded rats there was a 20-fold increase in the biliary excretion of iron using liposomal DTPA-PE compared with using either the water-soluble DTPA alone or liposomal DTPA without the amphiphilic phospholipid. Unfortunately, these approaches to improving the efficiency of iron chelation would still require parenteral administration of the chelators, and involve a complex drug preparation. Though of interest in exploring the nature of chelatable iron, they have thus not found a place in routine clinical practice, where regular use of subcutaneous infusions of DF is still the mainstay of effective iron chelation therapy in disorders associated with secondary iron overload.

4. DESFERRIOXAMINE TOXICITY

For many years DF was believed to be remarkably non-toxic and only occasional anaphylactic reactions (Miller et al., 1981), a few cataracts (Bloomfield et al., 1978) and mild local reactions at injection sites have been noted among hundreds of patients receiving long-term DF therapy. However, with the introduction of effective iron chelating therapy to an increasing number of patients with iron-loading anaemias (Chapter 9), the potential toxic effects of such treatment have been recognized.

Ocular toxicity, resembling tapeto-retinal dystrophy, was first described in two of four thalassaemic patients treated with high dose continuous i.v. DF by Davies et al. (1983). Additional cases of ocular toxicity associated with the use of DF have been reported in thalassaemic patients (Borgna-Pignatti et al., 1984; Olivieri et al., 1986), as well as in patients with rheumatoid arthritis (Polson et al., 1985; Blake et al., 1985) and patients on haemodialysis treated for aluminium toxicity (Simon et al., 1983; Rubinstein et al., 1985). Abnormal vision has been attributed to a mixed retinal cone and rod defect in some patients (Davies et al., 1983) and to atrophy of the optic nerve in others. Olivieri et al. (1986) studied 89 patients with transfusional iron overload treated by long-term s.c. DF at doses ranging from 34 to 150 mg/kg/d. Four of them developed visual loss attributed to optic neuropathy with delayed visual evoked potential in combination with loss of colour vision. In addition, five asymptomatic patients had changes in the pigment of the retinal epithelium. Symptoms were completely reversed within 4 weeks of discontinuing DF therapy.

Auditory neurotoxicity characterized by high-frequency sensorineural deficit was found in 22 of the 89 patients studied by Olivieri et al. (1986). In a major survey of 335 thalassaemic patients from Italy, significant sensorineural hearing loss of more than 50 dB was found in 6% of patients and mild defect in 21%. One year after reducing the dosage of DF significant improvement was observed among patients with mild hearing defect, but only minor improvement among severely affected patients (Gabutti, 1990). In contrast, of 52 patients reported by Cohen et al. (1990) receiving 26 to 136 mg DF/kg/d, only one has developed symptomatic loss of vision and hearing, and both problems improved when chelation therapy was stopped. Although it is generally recognized that the auditory neurotoxicity of DF is dose related and tends to occur in less iron-loaded patients (Porter et al., 1989), the gross differences in the incidence of these complications among the various treatment groups are at present unexplained.

Cerebral toxicity has only been described in patients treated for conditions unrelated to iron overload. Nausea and vomiting led to premature withdrawal of DF treatment in five of six adult patients treated for rheumatoid arthritis with 2.0 g/d DF s.c. given by portable pumps over 20 h (about 30 mg/kg/d). Transient confusion was reported in one haemodialysis patient treated for aluminium toxicity (Rubinstein et al., 1985), and coma lasting for 48 to 72 h developed in two patients with rheumatoid arthritis receiving 3 g DF/d in combination with prochlorperazine (Blake et al., 1985).

The neuro-ophthalmic complications of DF treatment are dose-related, but strongly modified by an inverse correlation with the magnitude of iron stores. Thus, in the rheumatoid arthritis patients reported by Polson et al. (1985), subjects with low iron stores developed symptoms of DF toxicity earlier than those with normal or increased stores. Similarly, in the series reported by Olivieri et al. (1986), patients with impaired visual or auditory function had lower serum ferritin, received higher doses of DF, and were of a younger age. Thus, DF toxicity appears to be a function of the amounts of iron-free drug available to interact with alternative iron or other trace metal compartments in excess of the chelatable storage iron pool.

Impaired growth velocity was first described in 1985 when it was recognized in about 50% of prepubertal Italian patients receiving DF. This problem was particularly common among subjects with low ferritin levels receiving the highest doses of DF. Following the reduction of DF dosage to 50 mg/kg/d impairment in growth velocity has no longer been observed (Gabutti, 1990). Abnormal bone growth has been observed in two of five children who were started on DF before the age of 3 years (Brill et al., 1991). The radiographic changes included flattening of the thoracic and lumbar vertebral bodies, circumferential metaphyseal osseous defects, sharp zones of provisional calcification and widened growth plates. Healing was noted in one patient after decreasing the dose of DF. No radiological abnormalities have been encountered in 22 other patients from the same group in whom treatment was started after 3 years of age.

A pulmonary syndrome of moderate to life-threatening severity characterized by tachypnoea, hypoxaemia and diffuse interstitial pulmonary infiltrates, has been reported in four of eight patients within 5 to 9 days of starting continuous intravenous DF therapy (Freedman et al., 1990). Lung biopsies showed diffuse alveolar damage, interstitial fibrosis and inflammation. Demonstration of IgE-fixation to mast cells suggested a hypersensitivity reaction. Continuous intravenous DF therapy has been used by many other groups without similar complications, and the difference in the incidence of such reactions between the various treatment groups is at present unexplained.

The mechanism of DF toxicity is at present unknown. Interaction with copper or zinc is unlikely, since the relative affinity of DF to these trace elements is low, and no evidence of altered plasma levels of these trace metals has been found following DF treatment (Simon *et al.*, 1983; Borgna-Pignatti *et al.*, 1984). A more likely explanation is direct interaction of DF with metabolically active iron compartments which may be critical for normal visual or neurological function. Although access of DF is normally limited by the blood–brain and blood–retinal barrier, this barrier is decreased by diabetic angiopathy, and drugs such as prochlorperazine and urethane, all of which are known to potentiate DF-toxicity (Arden *et al.*, 1984). Direct access of DF to the CNS has been elegantly demonstrated by the measurement of bleomycin-reactive (low molecular weight) iron in the cerebrospinal fluid of patients with DF + prochlorperazine associated coma (Blake *et al.*, 1985). These authors have suggested that DF-induced brain iron depletion may result in abnormal serotonin uptake by synaptic vesicles or inactivation of tryptophan hydroxylase. Obviously, more studies are required to elucidate the mechanism of DF-induced neuro-ophthalmic complications. Inhibition of ribonucleotide reductase (Hoffbrand *et al.*, 1976; Lederman *et al.*, 1984) resulting in interference with cell proliferation may be responsible at least in part for the interference with growth velocity and skeletal abnormalities observed in small children. The methyl sulfonate carrier of DF is remarkably toxic *in vitro*, and it is possible that some of the clinical toxicities observed following DF treatment are not directly related to DF. Steady-state pharmacokinetics of DF compared in thalassaemic children developing severe neurotoxicity with asymptomatic thalassaemic children have shown identical clearance rates of DF implying that DF induced neurotoxicity is dose-dependent and cannot be explained by drug accumulation caused by slower clearance rates (Bentur *et al.*, 1990). Another study of DF toxicity in Alzheimer's disease has suggested that DF metabolites, and not DF *per se* may be responsible for some of the toxic effects observed (Kruck *et al.*, 1990).

On a practical level, these observations underline the need for increased awareness of toxic complications of DF therapy, in particular in patients at increased risk such as subjects with limited iron stores, patients receiving unusually high dosage, small children, and patients with impaired blood–brain or blood–retinal barrier. Pre-treatment evaluation and periodic monitoring for adverse neurological effects during long-term DF therapy is strongly recommended, with prompt discontinuation or modification of treatment at the earliest evidence of toxicity.

Rarely, DF treatment may be complicated by opportunistic infections. *Yersinia enterocolitica*, an organism of low virulence in humans and with no siderophores of its own (Robins-Browne and Prpic, 1985), has receptors for siderophores and, if supplied with DF-bound iron, may produce serious clinical infection (Gallant *et al.*, 1986). *Mucormycosis* associated with the use of DF in haemodialysis patients has been described in several cases, although the mechanism of this complication is at present unclear (Calescibetta *et al.*, 1986; Goodill and Abuelo, 1987).

5. DEVELOPMENT OF NEW ORAL IRON CHELATORS

There is an obvious need for the development of alternative, orally effective iron chelating drugs which would be more convenient for use than DF and therefore available to a larger number of patients who at present are unable to comply with the need for long-term subcutaneous infusion by portable pumps (Chapter 9).

Several hundred candidate compounds have been screened over the last decade, using *in vitro* and *in vivo* animal models or a combination of both. These studies have led to the identification of several interesting compounds of possible clinical usefulness (Hershko and Weatherall, 1988). For the sake of convenience and simplicity, the present discussion will be limited to the most outstanding of these compounds, all of which are effective by oral administration. These are the polyanionic amines, the aryl hydrazones and the 3-hydroxypyrid-4-ones.

5.1. Polyanionic Amines

The search for useful orally effective iron chelating compounds has led to the rediscovery of two very powerful polyanionic amines synthesized over 20 years ago by the group led by Martell (Frost *et al.*, 1958; L'Eplattenier, 1967; Pitt *et al.*, 1979; Grady and Hershko, 1990): N,N'-ethylenebis (2-hydroxyphenylglycine) (EHPG), and N,N'-bis (2-hydroxybenzoyl) ethylenediamine-N,N'-diacetic acid (HBED) (Fig. 12.2). They both form hexadentate ligands with ferric iron by their secondary or tertiary nitrogens and their hydroxyl and carboxyl groups. The affinity constant for iron of EHPG is 33.9 and that of HBED is 39.6 (Martell, 1981). Their affinity for other metals is relatively low. Conversion of the carboxylic groups of HBED to methyl esters (Pitt,

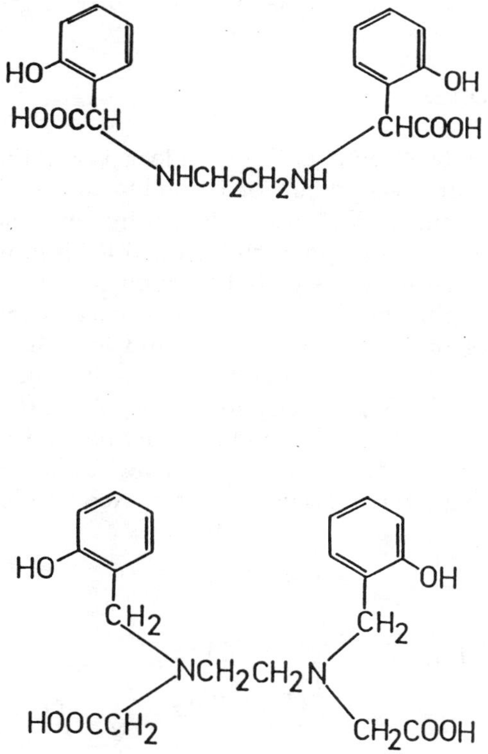

Fig. 12.2 N,N'-ethylenebis-(2-hydroxyphenylglycine) (EHPG) (above), and N,N'-bis-(2-hydroxybenzoyl) ethylenediamine-N,N'-diacetic acid (HBED) (below).

1981) results in a marked improvement in its intestinal absorption and a further increase in iron excretion.

Studies in hypertransfused rats injected with ^{59}Fe-ferritin to label hepatocellular iron stores have shown an accurate inverse relation between biliary iron excretion and residual hepatic radioactivity (Hershko *et al.*, 1984). Faecal radioiron excretion (percentage of injected dose) following a single i.m. injection of dimethyl-HBED 200 mg/kg was 80%, with a simultaneous decrease in hepatic radioactivity from 88% to 8%. Dose-response relations indicated that at the dose range of 25 to 50 mg/kg HBED and dimethyl HBED were 12 to 15 times more effective than DF. Finally, chemical measurements have shown that a single dose of dimethyl-HBED 200 mg/kg i.m. decreased hepatic non-haem iron stores from 2247 ± 185 µg/liver to 632 ± 59, and ferritin iron stores from 1082 ± 62 to 280 ± 90 µg. Animal studies involving prolonged EHPG administration disclosed significant toxicity manifested in weight loss, anaemia, hepatic and pulmonary damage (Rosenkrantz *et al.*, 1986). In contrast, HBED and dimethyl-HBED are remarkably non-toxic and their LD_{50} is in excess of 800 mg/kg as against 100 for EHPG (Grady and Hershko, 1990). Clearly, dimethyl-HBED is one of the most promising oral iron chelators identified so far, and if its low toxicity in rodents is confirmed by long-term toxicity studies in higher animal species, it may represent a significant advance in the development of drugs for the management of clinical iron overload. HBED has been licensed quite recently in the USA for clinical trial in a small number of thalassaemic paitents (Grady, personal communication), and results of this trial are awaited with great interest.

5.2. Aryl Hydrazones

The prototype of this family of compounds is pyridoxal isonicotinoyl hydrazone (PIH) (Fig. 12.3) introduced after recognition of its ability to mobilize iron from ^{59}Fe-labelled reticulocytes (Ponka *et al.*, 1970, 1979). In hypertransfused rats (Hershko *et al.*, 1981) PIH is able to remove parenchymal and RE iron with equal efficiency and practically all chelated iron is excreted through the bile. Its *in vivo* chelating efficiency is equal to or slightly better than DF and its oral and parenteral effectiveness is similar. No evidence of toxicity has been found at doses up to 500 mg/kg/d. However, results of long-term oral treatment with PIH in rats have been disappointing (Williams *et al.*, 1982). At the end of 10 weeks of treatment, no decrease in hepatic iron stores or in whole body radioactivity beyond that found in control animals could be demonstrated. Studies in patents with iron overload treated with PIH at a dose of 30 mg/kg/d have shown a net iron excretion of 0.12 ± 0.07 mg/kg/d

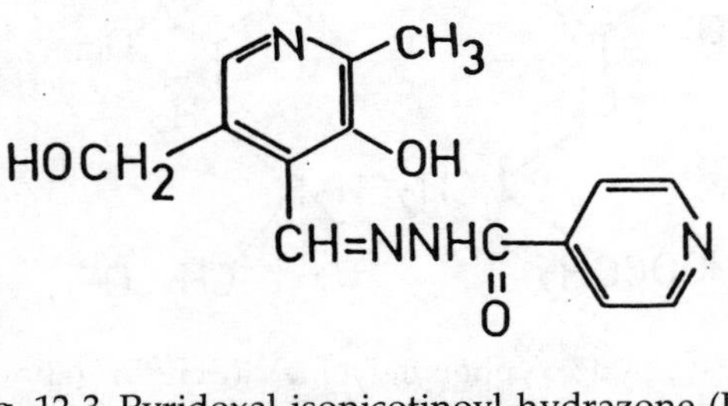

Fig. 12.3 Pyridoxal isonicotinoyl hydrazone (PIH).

and it was estimated that this degree of iron excretion may be sufficient for achieving a negative iron balance in non-transfusion-dependent patients with iron-loading anaemias (Brittenham, 1990).

Other Schiff base compounds are readily formed by pyridoxal, and a large number of such derivatives have been investigated (Ponka et al., 1979; Hershko et al., 1981; Johnson et al., 1982; Williams et al., 1982). In studies of over 40 such new derivatives in recent years (Hershko et al., 1981, 1988; Avramovici-Grisaru et al., 1983), most were found to be inferior to PIH both in their ability to promote iron excretion and in their oral effectiveness. However, more recently some powerful new derivatives have been identified. The most effective of these, pyridoxalpyrimidinyl-ethoxy-carbonyl methbromide (PPH15), is able to remove 79% of hepatocellular radioiron stores following a single parenteral dose of 200 mg/kg, and its oral effectiveness exceeds that of parenteral DF. Results of preliminary toxicity studies in rats have been encouraging, but studies in Cebus monkeys disclosed significant toxicity which may preclude the use of this drug for clinical purposes.

5.3. 3-Hydroxypyrid-4-ones

This new class of iron chelators has been designed by Hider and Kontoghiorghes to permit optimal intestinal absorption (Hider et al., 1990; Kontoghiorghes, 1990). These bidentate chelators bind to iron in a 3:1 ratio with a stability constant of 10^{37}, about six orders of magnitude higher than DF. Increasing the size of the alkyl function substitution on the ring N atom enhances lipophilicity without altering affinity to iron (Table 12.1). Low lipophilicity is associated with decreased chelating efficiency, whereas high lipophilicity is associated with increased toxicity (Porter et al., 1990). The chelating properties of the 3-hydroxypyrid-4-ones (CP compounds) have been studied both in vitro in hepatocyte cultures, and in vitro in several species of animals including mice, rats and rabbits.

A variety of 3-hydroxypyrid-4-ones have been studied in cultured, iron-loaded heart cells to explore their ability to remove iron directly from the heart (Hershko et al., 1991a). At a concentration of 1.0 mM, all CP compounds were more effective in removing radioiron from iron-loaded myocardial cells than DF. Conversely, at 0.1 mM DF was considerably more effective than all CP compounds tested. LDH release into the culture medium, used as an indicator of cellular damage, was

Table 12.1 Chemical structure and partition coefficient of 3-hydroxypyrid-4-ones

Chelator	R_1	R_2	Partition coefficient	
			Free ligand	Iron complex
CP 20	CH_3	CH_3	0.21	<0.002
CP 40	CH_3	CH_2CH_2OH	<0.002	<0.002
CP 51	CH_3	$CH_2CH_2OCH_3$	0.3	0.005
CP 94	C_2H_5	C_2H_5	0.85	0.07
CP 96	C_2H_5	$CH_2CH_2OCH_3$	0.83	0.05

negligible. The most effective chelators in these *in vitro* studies at 1.0 mM were CP 51, CP 94 and CP 96 (Table 12.1).

In vivo studies in rats treated by DF or CP compounds by 8-hourly s.c. injections at a dose of 300 mg/kg/d for 13 consecutive days (Hershko *et al.*, 1990) showed a clear distinction between CP 20 and 40, which were unable to decrease liver iron stores, and CP 51, 94 and 96, which have been effective in depleting hepatic iron. However, increased *in vivo* chelating efficiency was associated with increased toxicity manifested in weight loss which, in the case of CP 51, was quite remarkable. Of the compounds tested, CP 94 represented the optimal combination of increased efficiency and minimal toxicity. The ability of CP 20 and CP 94, the two most important CP compounds, to interact with hepatocellular and reticuloendothelial (RE) iron stores was studied in hypertransfused rats labelled with ^{59}Fe-ferritin and ^{59}Fe-DRBC (heat-damaged erythrocytes) respectively (Zevin *et al.*, 1992). Both chelators promoted the biliary excretion of hepatocellular iron and the urinary as well as biliary excretion of RE iron. The *in vivo* effect of CP 20 was comparable with that of DF, whereas CP 94 was considerably more effective. Contrary to previous observations in cell cultures, there was no *in vivo* evidence for a diminishing chelating efficiency at the lowest doses employed.

A number of clinical studies are presently under way to determine the safety and efficiency of oral treatment by CP 20 (L1) in patients with transfusional iron overload (Kontoghiorghes *et al.*, 1990; Olivieri *et al.*, 1990; Tondury *et al.*, 1990; Bartlett *et al.*, 1990). Results of these trials and those to be conducted in the future with some of the most promising CP compounds will provide decisive information regarding the suitability of these compounds for clinical use. Of concern are observations in rats indicating involution of the thymus and spleen and interference with lymphocyte function following L1 treatment at 300 mg/kg/d (Grady *et al.*, 1991). Arthropathy requiring discontinuation of treatment has been reported in 12 of 52 thalassaemic patients on long-term L1 therapy at 50 to 100 mg/kg/d. One of these patients died of a severe SLE-like reaction (Agarwal *et al.*, 1991). Severe agranulocytosis has been encountered in several groups receiving L1 therapy (Hoffbrand *et al.*, 1991; Korkina *et al.*, 1991). On the other hand, no serious side-effects of L1 have been found among several other groups of patients on long-term L1 treatment (Olivieri *et al.*, 1990; Tondury *et al.*, 1990).

5.4. Characteristics of an Ideal Iron Chelator

A number of considerations should be borne in mind in the selection of an optimal compound for future use in iron chelating therapy. Such a compound should have improved *in vivo* chelating activity, but this is not an absolute need since a new drug with an oral effectiveness comparable to parenteral DF would be quite acceptable. High intestinal absorption is mandatory, but care should be taken that *in situ* chelation of luminal iron within the gut may not enhance iron absorption instead of promoting its excretion. A preferential interaction with liver and heart cell iron deposits would be desirable since iron accumulated within such cells is more harmful than in RE cells. This in turn is a function of the partition coefficient (lipid vs. water solubility) which in some compounds such as the 3-hydroxypyrid-4-ones may be modified at will by altering the side-chain of the molecule. An ideal compound should also have a prolonged effect to ensure the continued presence of the chelator in the circulation which in turn would protect tissues from the accumulation of non-transferrin iron in plasma. This objective could be easier to achieve with an oral medication, possibly in slow-release form, than with parenteral drugs which are rapidly cleared from the blood. Finally, an improved iron chelator should have low toxicity and should be inexpensive to make it available for a maximal number of patients.

Although we do not yet have a drug available for large-scale clinical use to replace DF, significant progress has been made in recent years. The hope that some of the compounds discussed above may prove suitable for long-term clinical use is based on encouraging preliminary results. With increasing interest on the part of the pharmaceutical industry on one hand, and public awareness of the need for developing improved iron chelating medications, it is reasonable to expect that such drugs may indeed be introduced for clinical use in the near future.

6. IRON CHELATION IN CONDITIONS UNRELATED TO IRON OVERLOAD

The rationale for using DF and other iron chelators in conditions unrelated to iron overload is based on (a) the central role of iron in oxygen toxicity and the ability of iron chelators to prevent hydroxyl radical formation by inhibiting the iron-driven Haber-Weiss reaction; (b) the ability of iron chelators to inhibit cell growth by reversible inactivation of ribonucleotide reductase, a rate controlling enzyme in DNA synthesis, and; (c) the beneficial effect of iron depletion on uroporphyrinogen decarboxylase in porphyria cutanea tarda.

6.1. Interference with Hydroxyl Radical Formation

Interest in the therapeutic potential of DF in biological processes not directly related to iron overload has been stimulated by the important work of Halliwell and Gutteridge on the role of iron and iron chelation in oxygen toxicity (Editorial, 1985; Halliwell and Gutteridge, 1984, 1986; Halliwell, 1989). Activation of the respiratory burst in granulocytes and macrophages is associated with a sharp increase in the production of superoxide (O_2^-) and peroxide (O_2^{2-}). At physiological pH, peroxide is rapidly protonated to hydrogen peroxide (H_2O_2). The superoxide radical and H_2O_2 are poorly reactive in aqueous solution, but the hydroxyl radical ($^{\cdot}OH$) is a highly reactive, toxic species. Unlike O_2^-, H_2O_2 readily crosses biological membranes, and may function as a propagator of oxygen-related damage. Free hydroxyl radicals ($^{\cdot}OH$) are produced from O_2^- and H_2O_2 through the Haber-Weiss reaction which is catalysed by iron:

$$(1)\ Fe^{3+} + O_2^- \rightarrow Fe^{2+} + O_2$$

$$(2)\ Fe^{2+} + H_2O_2 \rightarrow Fe^{3+} + {}^{\cdot}OH + OH^-$$

The hydroxyl radical is extremely reactive, and combines with other molecules at its site of formation. Hydroxyl radicals, and possibly other oxygen-derived species may cause considerable damage by the degradation of DNA, proteins and hyaluronic acid, and by membrane lipid peroxidation (Halliwell and Gutteridge, 1984; Johnson *et al.*, 1981). Because of the central role of iron in ˙OH formation, DF has been introduced into free radical research as a specific *in vitro* and *in vivo* probe for iron-dependent radical reactions (Gutteridge *et al.*, 1979). DF has a very high, and specific affinity to Fe^{3+}. It is very efficient in preventing its reduction to Fe^{2+} and the participation of iron in the Haber-Weiss reaction. In view of the extensive experience gained in the management of transfusional iron overload, DF is believed to be reasonably safe for *in vivo* use.

6.1.1. Tissue Injury with Neutrophil Activation

Tissue injury associated with the activation of complement and neutrophils is closely related to ˙OH production, and can be inhibited by DF. The systemic activation of complement by cobra venom factor in rats is followed by leukoagglutination in pulmonary capillaries, endothelial cell destruction, intra-alveolar haemorrhage, and fibrin deposition (Ward *et al.*, 1983). Such lung injury can be prevented by pre-treatment with DF or lactoferrin, both of which bind iron and prevent the conversion of O_2^- and H_2O_2 produced by granulocyte activation into free hydroxyl radicals. Conversely, infusion of ionic iron greatly potentiates lung injury. In another study by the same authors, immune complex-induced vasculitis was also shown to be attenuated by DF, lactoferrin or catalase, and potentiated by the administration of ionic iron (Fligiel *et al.*, 1984). Phorbol myristate acetate (PMA) stimulates neutrophils to produce superoxide and other harmful oxygen derivatives. This in turn results in marked damage to endothelial cells manifested in increased vascular permeability and resistance in blood-perfused dog lungs. Pretreatment with DF results in significant protection from PMA-induced endothelial damage in this experimental model of free radical-induced vascular injury (Allison *et al.*, 1988).

In the adult respiratory distress syndrome (ARDS) toxic oxygen metabolites produced by stimulated neutrophils may be responsible for alveolar injury (Cochrane *et al.*, 1983). Expiratory hydrogen peroxide levels in ARDS patients are five times higher than in other patients receiving mechanical ventilation, and are directly related to plasma lysozyme levels indicating neutrophil turnover. They are also directly related to the fluctuations in clinical status of individual ARDS patients (Baldwin *et al.*, 1986). These data lend further support to the assumption that toxic oxygen metabolites produced by activated neutrophils may have a role in the pathogenesis of ARDS. At present, no information is available on the possible protective effect of DF or other agents preventing the participation of iron in the Haber-Weiss reaction in human ARDS.

6.1.2. Postischaemic Reperfusion Injury

Postischaemic reperfusion injury is another condition where DF may be useful in preventing further damage to cells. It has been proposed that injury initiated during ischaemia may be aggravated by re-exposure to normal oxygen concentrations, causing further damage to vital cellular membranes by lipid peroxidation (White et al., 1985).

(a) Brain. The brain is one of the most sensitive organs to lipid peroxidation, because of its high polyunsaturated fatty acid content. Earlier studies in dogs have shown that following resuscitation from cardiac arrest, both brain MDA and low molecular weight iron concentrations are increased (Nayini et al., 1985). Both of these were prevented by post-resuscitation DF therapy. These findings were interpreted as evidence of a cause and effect relation between the release of low molecular iron from the brain and increased lipid peroxidation during the post-resuscitation period. While it is reasonable to assume that iron chelation prevented lipid peroxidation, there is no evidence in these studies to indicate that lipid peroxidation has been responsible for brain damage, or that its prevention by DF resulted in the protection of the brain from anatomic or functional injury associated with either ischaemia or reperfusion. Indeed, in another study in dogs, no improvement in neurological outcome following DF treatment could be shown after 11 minutes of complete cerebral ischaemia (Fleischer et al., 1987). In other studies, the effect of post-resuscitation DF treatment on survival was investigated in rats. Two days following cardiac arrest and successful resuscitation, 75% of treated animals were alive as compared with 25% of controls (Babbs, 1985; Badylak and Babbs, 1986). Unfortunately, in addition to DF, these animals were also treated by lidoflazine to block calcium uptake and by CO_2 to improve cerebral perfusion. Thus, the role of DF in improving survival in these studies cannot be evaluated. Nevertheless, these studies have shown that it is conceivable that the production of toxic oxygen metabolites may contribute to the severity of damage initiated by ischaemia. In order to substantiate this claim, direct evidence was needed to demonstrate that preventing the formation of harmful oxygen derivatives by iron chelation may lead to improved cellular survival or function.

Table 12.2 summarizes the results of subsequent studies in which the value of DF in reducing damage to the brain has been evaluated. Unfortunately, in most of these studies more than one treatment has been given simultaneously. Thus, if a favourable effect has been observed, it is hard to tell whether this may be attributed

Table 12.2 Prevention of brain damage by desferrioxamine

Model	Treatment	Timing	Effect	Author (year)
Dogs 15 min cardiac arrest	DF + lidoflazine	Post	Decreased number of micro-haemorrhages. No improvement in anoxic neuronal injury	Kumar et al. (1988)
Cats cortical freezing	DF	Pre or Post	Decreased brain oedema and less disruption of blood–brain barrier in pre- but not post-treated animals	Ikeda et al. (1989)
Dogs 7 min cardiac arrest	DF + superoxide dismutase	Post	Improved post-arrest EEG recovery. No improvement in brainstem auditory evoked potentials	Cerchiari et al. (1987, 1990)
Gerbils carotid occlusion	DF + low iron diet	Pre	Decreased severity of neurological deficit. Decreased brain oedema	Patt et al. (1990)

to superoxide dismutase, the calcium antagonist lidoflazine, iron depletion by dietary restriction, or DF. None of the studies resulted in a dramatic reduction of damage compared with the changes observed in the control groups. In spite of these limitations, some favourable effects have been observed in all studies, and this was more pronounced in studies where DF treatment had been started prior to the induction of primary brain insult by anoxia or freezing.

(b) *Heart*. The heart is the second organ receiving much attention regarding the potential usefulness of iron chelators in preventing or limiting post-anoxic tissue damage. Several studies have shown that DF treatment is capable of limiting myocardial stunning and increasing the rate of recovery following reversible myocardial ischaemia in experimental animals. In dogs, DF treatment introduced prior to coronary occlusion improved the recovery of contractile function, reduced tissue oedema and increased endocardial ATP content following reperfusion (Bolli *et al.*, 1987; Farber *et al.*, 1988). DF treatment was also effective in some models when started after ischaemia and shortly before reperfusion, as evidenced by an improved recovery

Table 12.3 Prevention of postischaemic myocardial damage by desferrioxamine

Model	Treatment	Timing	Effect	Author (year)
Rabbits 30 min global ischaemia	DF	Post or Pre	Increased ATP, phosphocreatine and developed pressure with both pre- and post-ischaemic DF	Williams *et al.* (1988)
Dogs 15 min LAD occlusion	DF	Pre and through-out	Improved postperfusion contractile function	Bolli *et al.* (1987)
Dogs 20 min LAD occlusion	DF	Post and during cardio-plegia	Elimination of regional stunning after ischaemia	Illes *et al.* (1989)
Dogs 90 min LAD occlusion	DF	Pre and Post	Decreased infarct size	Lesnefsky (1990)
Dogs 2 h coronary occlusion 4 h reperfusion	DF	Pre or Post	Decreased infarct size in pretreated group but no effect with post-ischaemic DF treatment	Reddy *et al.* (1989)
Rats 30 min ischaemia 2 h cardioplegia	DF or per-oxidase	Pre	Improved post-ischaemic aortic flow, higher ATP content	Bernard *et al.* (1988)
Rats 5 h cold storage 1 h hypothermic ischaemia	DF	Through-out study	Improved postperfusion ventricular pressure, compliance and coronary flow	Menasche *et al.* (1990b)
Man cardiopulmonary bypass	DF	Pre	Decreased production of superoxide radicals by phorbol-myristate stimulated granulocytes	Menasche *et al.* (1988)
Man cardiopulmonary bypass	DF	Pre and through-out	Inhibition of LDL peroxidation measured by thiobarbituric acid reactive substances	Menasche *et al.* (1990a)
Man cardiopulmonary bypass	DF	Through-out	Inhibition of peroxidative damage and preservation of mitochondrial morphology	Ferreira *et al.* (1990)

of developed pressure, intracellular pH and phosphocreatine content in isolated rabbit hearts (Ambrosio *et al.*, 1987). Finally, DF was also able to improve pressure development, ventricular dP/dt, left ventricular compliance and coronary blood flow upon reperfusion of rat hearts subjected to prolonged cardioplegic arrest (Menasche *et al.*, 1987). Table 12.3 summarizes the results of several recent studies where DF was used to limit reperfusion injury. In general, the beneficial effects of DF were more pronounced when treatment was started prior to reperfusion and preferably prior to ischaemia as well. Although most of these observations were made in experimental animal models, the three studies in man where preliminary information is available on lipid peroxidation, superoxide production by granulocytes and on mitochondrial morphology, are encouraging (Menasche *et al.*, 1988, 1990a; Ferreira *et al.*, 1990).

All of these observations imply that iron may play a significant role in the pathogenesis of myocardial stunning, and that DF treatment may result in a significant attenuation of myocardial dysfunction in the above conditions. The practical implications of these observations for the management of analogous clinical situations remain to be explored. Because of the importance of introducing the chelator prior to reperfusion damage, the most promising situations in clinical medicine where DF may be useful are elective surgical procedures in which DF treatment may be started before and throughout cardioplegia and hypothermic anoxia.

(c) *Intestine.* Apart from the brain and heart, DF has also been found to be effective in attenuating damage to the intestine, as manifested in the suppression of granulocytic infiltration of the small intestinal mucosa following ischaemia/reperfusion in cats (Zimmerman *et al.*, 1990).

6.1.3. *Organ Transplantation*

Free radicals may interfere with the successful transplantation of organs at two distinct stages: (a) in impairing the viability of stored organs assigned for transplantation, and (b) by mediating their immune rejection.

(a) *Organ storage.* Normothermic ischaemia in rabbit kidneys results in increased lipid-soluble Schiff bases and diene conjugates indicating increased lipid peroxidation. This, in turn, is well correlated with subsequent derangement in function and morphology (Green *et al.*, 1986a,b). Single passage arterial flushing of cold, ischaemic rabbit kidneys with saline and 60 mM DF results in a significant decrease in lipid peroxidation (Green *et al.*, 1986b). DF treatment attenuates lung reperfusion injury following cold ischaemia of auto-transplanted lungs in dogs, and results in improved alveolar–arterial oxygen gradients (Bonser *et al.*, 1990; Pickford *et al.*, 1990). Similarly, as indicated earlier (Menasche *et al.*, 1990b) DF treatment of isolated rat hearts maintained under conditions that closely mimic heart transplantation results in improved postperfusion ventricular pressure and better compliance and coronary flow. All of these observations indicate that DF may be useful in organ transplantation by improving the viability and accelerating the recovery of organs subjected to hypothermic anoxia because of the requirements of temporary storage pending revascularization.

(b) *Graft rejection.* The beneficial effects of DF on transplant survival and on graft-versus-host diseases are more complex, and its mechanism of action is at present a topic of speculation. The inflammatory response associated with organ rejection involves activation of the respiratory burst and the subsequent formation of toxic hydroxyl radicals may be directly responsible for organ rejection. This hypothesis was tested by Bradley *et al.* (1986) in a mouse model of pancreatic islet cell allografts. DF was administered by a subcutaneously implanted osmotic pump delivering 4 mg drug per day for 28 d. Chronic islet allograft rejection occurred in 18 of 29 control mice as against only three of 23 DF treated animals after 100 days. This striking effect of DF on graft survival could not be attributed to immunosuppression since (a) DF had no effect *in vivo* on the activation of a specific response by cytotoxic T-lymphocytes (CTL) to P815 tumour cells; (b) DF had no effect on the ability of activated T-cells to lyse target cells, and; (c) it had no effect on the release of lymphokine IL-3 by activated T-cells. These findings are compatible with the assumption that chronic islet cell allograft rejection as well as damage to beta cells in insulin-dependent diabetes are the consequence of direct damage by hydroxyl radicals produced by inflammatory cells accumulating at the site of the inflammatory reaction (Okamoto, 1985). In another study by the same group of investigators, the fate of allogeneic islet cell transplants was studied in a strain of non-obese rats with a high incidence of spontaneous type I diabetes (Nomikos *et al.*, 1986). In addition to DF, nicotinamide, a week free-radical scavenger and inhibitor of poly(ADP-ribose) synthetase, has also been tested. Combined treatment with DF and nicotinamide was more effective in preventing islet cell destruction than either treatment alone. Similarly, in a more recent study by Mendola *et al.* (1989) combined DF and nicotinamide treatment was effective in preventing the rejection of cultured islet cell transplants. On the other hand, DF alone was more effective in preventing streptozotocin-induced insulitis and diabetes than either nicotinamide or a combination of nicotinamide and DF. While some of the apparent discrepancies between the results of the above studies are not easy to reconcile, all of these data underline the potential usefulness of DF in prolonging the survival of transplanted islet allografts, and possibly in the prevention of the spontaneous development of insulitis.

Finally, DF treatment in patients with poorly controlled type II diabetes was reported to result in a dramatic clinical improvement in subjects with increased serum ferritin levels (Cutler, 1989). This improvement was manifested in improved fasting glucose, triglyceride and HbA_{1c} levels, and independence from continued hypoglycaemic therapy in eight of nine subjects. These beneficial effects of DF are surprising, as the dose of DF employed (10 mg/kg i.v. ×2 weekly) was much less than that used in the treatment of iron overload, and since on the basis of animal studies type I diabetes and not type II would be a more likely disease to respond to DF therapy. Nevertheless, these intriguing data deserve further investigations.

In a preliminary report in children receiving allogeneic bone marrow trans-plantation (BMT) prompt resolution of graft-versus-host disease (GvHD) has been described following DF administration, in association with inhibition of interleukin-2 receptor expression in lymphocytes (Weinberg *et al.*, 1986). However, DF also interferes with cell proliferation (*vide infra*), and in a group of 15 thalassaemic patients receiving DF pre- and post-BMT to prevent GvHD, delay in bone marrow engraftment appeared to be a problem (Lucarelli *et al.*, 1989). Thus, interference with bone marrow engraftment may preclude the future use of DF in GvHD.

Although more direct evidence is obviously needed to document the role of free radicals in the pathogenesis of graft rejection, the impressive improvement in the survival of transplanted islet allografts shown in the above studies underlines the need for examining the possible beneficial effects of DF on graft survival and possibly on graft-versus-host disease in other animal models of allotransplantation (Weinberg, 1990).

6.1.4. Drug Toxicity

(a) *Bleomycin*. This antibiotic is useful in the management of some malignant tumours. Its antitumour effect requires the formation of an O_2-Fe^{2+}-bleomycin complex which results in DNA cleavage together with the release of O_2^- and $\cdot OH$ radicals which, in turn, may attack other cellular components. Unfortunately, progressive lung fibrosis is an important dose-related side-effect of bleomycin, limiting its clinical usefulness. In view of the critical role of iron in the pathogenesis of bleomycin toxicity and the effectiveness of DF in preventing lung damage in other experimental models associated with free radical toxicity (Ward et al., 1983), it was anticipated that DF may be effective in limiting bleomycin-induced lung toxicity. Indeed, studies in hamsters pretreated with DF showed a significant reduction in lung collagen accumulation, lipid peroxidation, inhibition of DNA synthesis, as well as morphological evidence of less lung fibrosis following bleomycin administration (Chandler and Fulwer, 1985; Chandler et al., 1988). However, other studies in rats employing similar experimental protocols failed to demonstrate any beneficial effects of DF on bleomycin-induced lung toxicity (Cross et al., 1985; Ward et al., 1988). Species differences have been proposed as a possible explanation for these seemingly conflicting results. Another possible explanation for the failure of DF to prevent lung toxicity in rats is inability of DF to penetrate the relevant effector cells to interact with intracellular low molecular iron compartments participating in complex formation with bleomycin.

(b) *Paraquat*. A similar dilemma exists in relation to the role of DF in paraquat toxicity. Paraquat is a widely used herbicide causing rapidly progressive respiratory failure after accidental ingestion. *In vivo*, paraquat is reduced into a cation radical which, upon reoxidation yields superoxide anions. The final product of this chain of events is $\cdot OH$ formation through the metal-driven Haber-Weiss reaction. Studies in mice and in vitamin D deficient rats have shown that DF treatment reduces the mortality and prolongs the survival of paraquat-treated animals whereas iron administration aggravates paraquat toxicity (Kohen and Chevion, 1985; Van Asbeck et al., 1989). *In vitro* studies with alveolar type II cells have shown that the protective effect of DF ($500\,\mu M$) in paraquat toxicity involves inhibition of paraquat-induced iron-catalysed free radical generation, as well as a decrease in the cellular uptake of paraquat (Van der Wal et al., 1990). However, other studies in rats failed to demonstrate a protective effect of DF (Osheroff et al., 1985). In the latter studies bolus injections of DF have been employed, delivered once or twice daily. It is possible that the failure to elicit a protective effect of DF is explained by the mode of drug administration, and that a continuous supply of DF is mandatory in conditions where the objective of treatment is effective inhibition of iron-driven free hydroxyl radical formation.

(c) *Anthracyclines*. The anthracycline antineoplastic drugs are highly effective agents with a curative potential in the treatment of leukaemias, lymphomas, and a number of other malignancies. One of the important factors limiting their use is the risk of severe toxicity to the heart. Any measure preventing the cardiotoxicity of anthracyclines would increase their curative effect by permitting dose escalation without an increased risk of cardiac mortality (Young *et al.*, 1981). Anthracyclines promote the formation of free radicals which are believed to play a central role in their cardiotoxicity, but there is no evidence that free radical formation is essential to their tumour-cell killing effect (Powis, 1989).

It is possible to dissociate the antineoplastic effect of anthracyclines from their cardiotoxic effect and to interfere with one without affecting the other. Tocopherol treatment in mice receiving adriamycin prevents both lipid peroxidation and cardiac toxicity without diminishing the response to therapy of P388 ascites tumour (Myers *et al.*, 1977). Similarly, methylene blue treatment aimed at modifying intracellular redox balance and preventing the *in vivo* reduction of doxorubicin, results in a marked decrease in drug toxicity without interfering with the antineoplastic effect against L1210 ascites tumour cells in mice (Hrushesky *et al.*, 1985).

Iron plays an important role in the formation of oxygen radicals by anthracyclines. Daunorubicin or doxorubicin are reduced to a semiquinone free radical which, in turn, reduces molecular oxygen to the superoxide ion. Superoxide and peroxide are converted into the highly toxic hydroxyl radical by the iron-driven Haber-Weiss reaction (Powis, 1989). Recent studies in cultured heart cells have shown that iron loading prior to doxorubicin treatment causes a two- to three-fold increase in doxorubicin toxicity manifested in LDH release, a sharp decrease in spontaneous heart cell beating, and the emergence of irregular and ineffective heart cell beats (Hershko *et al.*, 1992). DF treatment of iron-loaded cells prior to doxorubicin therapy resulted in decreased doxorubicin toxicity as manifested in all of the above abnormalities.

These observations provide strong support for the claim that iron loading may aggravate and iron chelating treatment may limit the cardiotoxicity of anthracycline drugs. In view of the low toxicity of DF and the extensive clinical experience accumulated within the last two decades, such treatment may easily be applicable for clinical use provided animal studies are found to be encouraging. DF itself is an inhibitor of cell proliferation via inactivation of ribonucleotide reductase (Hoffbrand *et al.*, 1976; Lederman *et al.*, 1984). Thus, it is reasonable to assume that concurrent DF therapy may prevent the toxicity and enhance the tumouricidal effect of anthracyclines simultaneously.

6.2. Effect on Cell Proliferation

The proliferation of mammalian cells is inhibited by severe iron deficiency. Decreased thymidine incorporation was first described in 1970 in iron deficient human bone marrow cells (Hershko *et al.*, 1970), and subsequently in iron deficient lymphocytes stimulated by PPD or *Candida* antigen (Joynson *et al.*, 1972). A similar inhibition of DNA synthesis may be achieved by *in vitro* DF treatment of human lymphocytes (Hoffbrand *et al.*, 1976; Lederman *et al.*, 1984). Reversible S-phase inhibition of lymphocyte proliferation can be achieved by overnight incubation with DF at 20 to

$50\,\mu$M concentrations. This inhibition is equally effective in stimulated normal human T- and B-lymphocytes or in lymphoblastoid cell lines. The mechanism of this inhibition by DF is interaction with ribonucleotide reductase, a rate-controlling enzyme in DNA synthesis. This enzyme contains a tyrosine free-radical structure which is essential for its activity, and which requires the presence of iron and oxygen (Reichard and Ehrenberg, 1983). The binding of chelatable iron by DF results in the inactivation of ribonucleotide reductase, similar to the effect of hydroxyurea, a known inhibitor of this enzyme.

6.2.1. Effect on Tumour Growth

In a preliminary report, DF was shown to achieve temporary control of drug-resistant acute leukaemia (Estrow et al., 1987). Table 12.4 summarizes a number of subsequent studies on the effect of iron chelators on normal and tumour cell growth. Although various experimental models have been used, and the dose of chelators employed ranged from 1 to $120\,\mu$M, a number of generalizations can be made.

(a) Despite claims to the contrary (Hann et al., 1990), the cytostatic effect of iron chelators is not selective for tumour cells as normal human and murine haematopoietic progenitor cells in culture are inhibited by DF at concentrations employed for treating tumour cells in vitro (Nocka and Pelus, 1988). The latter observation is in line with the clinical experience of delayed bone marrow engraftment in thalassaemic patients receiving DF for prophylaxis against graft-versus-host disease (Lucarelli et al., 1989).

Table 12.4 Suppression of tumour cell growth by desferrioxamine

Model	Treatment	Effect	Author (year)
Neuroblastoma cell lines	DF $60\,\mu$M	90% cell death within 5 d	Blatt and Stitely (1987)
Human neuro-blastoma cells	DF $50\,\mu$M	Maximal killing at 72 h exposure	Becton and Bryles (1988)
Neuroblastoma cell line	DF $60\,\mu$M	Block of cell cycle progression at the early DNA synthesis phase after 24 h	Blatt et al. (1988)
Neuroblastoma patients	DF 150 mg/kg/d i.v. for 5 d	Clinical response in seven of nine patients	Donfrancesco et al. (1990)
Human and murine haematopoietic progenitor cells	DF 1–$60\,\mu$M i.v. for 5 d	Dose-dependent S-phase inhibition of GM and erythroid colonies	Nocka and Pelus (1988)
Cell cultures: HL60 leukaemia KB carcinoma	Parabactin 3–$10\,\mu$M + Gallium + anti-Tf receptor	Arrest of cell growth in G1 phase or G1/S interface	Taetle et al. (1989)
Friend cell culture	Liposome-entrapped DF	Inhibition of cell proliferation without interfering with erythroid differentiation	Nastruzzi et al. (1989)
Hepatoma cell lines and diploid cells	DF 2.5–$120\,\mu$M	DF $>15\,\mu$M caused 30–50% tumour cell death. Minimal effect on normal cells	Hann et al. (1990)
Murine lymphoid tumour cultures	DF 5–$25\,\mu$g/ml + anti-Tf receptor	Synergistic inhibition of in vitro tumour growth	Kemp et al. (1990)

(b) In line with earlier studies, all subsequent work indicates a dose-dependent S-phase inhibition as the mechanism of DF action on cell growth. This inhibition is reversible after short-term incubation with the chelator, but exposure for several days results in cell death.

(c) The inhibitory effect of DF is iron-specific. It is reversible by the addition of iron to the *in vitro* system without removing DF. It is enhanced by other selective measures employed simultaneously to deprive iron from tumour cells such as anti-transferrin-receptor antibodies or gallium. In most studies, the effective inhibitory molar concentration of the chelator was about 20 to 50 μM or above. Although this may be a very crude estimate, similar inhibitory concentrations have been encountered in the parasite studies (*vide infra*), and this figure may represent the magnitude of the intracellular chelatable pool.

(d) Tumour cell inhibition by iron chelators is not restricted to experimental systems. The early observations of Estrow *et al.* (1987) in drug-resistant acute leukaemia, and the recent observations of Donfrancesco *et al.* (1990) in neuroblastoma patients indicate that DF is able to inhibit tumour growth in cancer patients as well. Whether or not this antiproliferative effect of DF may be of practical usefulness in the management of malignant disease remains to be seen.

6.2.2. *Effect on Parasite Growth*

Interest in the therapeutic potential of iron chelating agents in the control of infection originated in the belief that iron depletion may suppress the proliferation of pathogens. If pathogens are dependent on iron for their unimpeded growth, it might be possible to interfere specifically with their proliferation by the use of selective iron-binding agents. Several recent studies have shown that this may be feasible (Table 12.5). *In vitro* and *in vivo* studies with *Leishmania donovani* (Segovia *et al.*, 1989), *Trypanosoma cruzi* (Lalonde and Holbein, 1984), *Pneumocystis carinii* (Clarkson *et al.*, 1990), *Legionella pneumophila* (Byrd and Horwitz, 1989), *Plasmodium falciparum*, *P. vinckei* and *P. berghei* in mice, rats and monkeys (Raventos-Suarez *et al.*, 1982; Fritsch *et al.*, 1985; Hershko and Peto, 1988; Pollack *et al.*, 1987) have shown that it is possible to inhibit the proliferation of these microorganisms by the iron chelating agent desferrioxamine (DF). *In vivo* studies with *P. berghei* in rats have shown that parasite inhibition is independent of host iron status (Hershko and Peto, 1988), and that the therapeutic effect of DF is explained by its direct interaction with a chelatable labile iron pool within the infected erythrocyte. It is assumed that parasite inhibition is caused by inactivation of ribonucleotide reductase, an iron-dependent rate-limiting enzyme in DNA synthesis (Hoffbrand *et al.*, 1976). Since the ability of DF to penetrate the red cell membrane is limited, other iron chelating compounds with a higher lipid solubility have been studied and several of these have shown improved antimalarial activity (Hershko *et al.*, 1991a). Preliminary studies in patients with asymptomatic *P. falciparum* parasitaemia (Gordeuk *et al.*, 1992a), and in children with cerebral malaria conducted in Zambia (Gordeuk *et al.*, 1992b) have shown that DF given by continuous infusion at 100 mg/kg/d for 72 hours results in the disappearance of parasites from the circulation, and a significant shortening of the duration of altered consciousness.

Table 12.5 Inhibition of parasite growth by iron chelators

Model	Treatment	Effect	Author (year)
Trypanosoma cruzi in macrophages	DF 20–40 μM	Dose-dependent inhibition of amastigotes	Loo *et al.* (1984)
Trypanosoma cruzi in mice	DF 10 mg/d ×2 + iron deficient diet	Mortality decreased from 23% to 0	Lalonde and Holbein (1984)
Leishmania donovani amastigotes in macrophages	DF 90 μM	Up to 60% of amastigotes killed No effect on promastigotes	Segovia *et al.* (1989)
Legionella pneumophila in monocytes	DF 15 μM	Complete inhibition of intracellular multiplication	Byrd and Horwitz (1989)
Pneumocytosis carinii pneumonia in rats	DF 0.25–1.0 g/kg/d i.p.	Dose-dependent decrease in cyst counts in infected lungs	Clarkson *et al.* (1990)
Plasmodium falciparum cultures	DF 20–100 μM	Dose-dependent inhibition of parasite growth	Raventos-Suarez *et al.* (1982)
Plasmodium falciparum in aotus monkeys	DF continuous infusion by osmotic pump	Suppression of clinical infection	Pollack *et al.* (1987)
Plasmodium vinckei in mice	DF 1 g/kg/d q8h i.p.	Suppression of clinical infection	Fritsch *et al.* (1985)
Plasmodium berghei in rats	DF 1 g/kg/d q8h i.p.	Suppression of clinical infection	Hershko *et al.* (1988)
Plasmodium falciparum in man	DF 100 mg/kg/d continuous s.c. 72 h	Enhanced parasite clearance in asymptomatic subjects	Gordeuk *et al.* (1992a)
Plasmodium falciparum cultures	DF or DF–dextran	Ability to enter the parasitic compartment is essential for antimalarial effect	Scott *et al.* (1990)
Plasmodium falciparum cultures	desferrithiocin 25–30 μM	Dose-dependent inhibition of parasite growth	Fritsch *et al.* (1987)
Plasmodium berghei in rats *Plasmodium falciparum* in culture	HBED 50–200 mg/kg/d q8h i.p. *in vivo* 5–20 μM *in vitro*	Dose-dependent inhibition of parasite growth. Importance of stability constant	Yinnon *et al.* (1989)
Plasmodium berghei in rats *Plasmodium falciparum* in culture	Hydroxypyrid-4-ones 200 mg/kg/d q8h i.p. *in vivo* 5–40 μM *in vitro*	Dose-dependent inhibition of parasite growth. Importance of partition coefficient	Hershko *et al.* (1991b)

Studies on the intracellular biology of L. *pneumophila* in human monocytes have shown that activated monocytes are able to limit the availability of iron for invading organisms by downregulating the number of transferrin receptors on the cellular surface (Byrd and Horwitz, 1989). In addition, the sharp increase in apoferritin synthesis induced by inflammation may result in a shift of labile intracellular iron to the relatively unavailable compartment of ferritin iron stores (Konijn and Hershko, 1977). Thus, the alterations in iron homeostasis associated with inflammation may limit the availability of intracellular iron for invading organisms by reducing transferrin iron uptake as well as by diverting the labile iron pool into relatively unavailable storage compartments (Chapter 11). DF may represent a compound which simulates this intracellular protective mechanism. Comparison of all available *in vitro* studies on the antimicrobial effect of DF and other chelators reveals a striking similarity in the inhibitory concentration of these drugs. Without exception, the inhibitory concentration is about 20 μM, and a maximal effect is achieved between 40 to 100 μM. These figures may represent the approximate magnitude of the intracellular chelatable iron pool.

These intriguing new observations on the antimicrobial effects of DF and other iron chelators lend new meaning to the term nutritional immunity and open new channels for exploring the possibility of controlling infection by means of selective intracellular iron deprivation. Experimental models for studying the effect of iron chelators on other intracellular pathogens such as *Toxoplasma gondii*, *Chlamydia psittaci*, or *Mycobacterium tuberculosis* should be established. Packaging the chelator in liposomes or red cell ghosts, or manipulating their lipid solubility to improve their delivery to appropriate target organs such as the macrophage system may greatly improve their efficiency. In view of its short half-life and poor oral effectiveness it is unlikely that DF *per se* will be suitable for clinical use as a practical antimicrobial agent. However, with the introduction of simple, orally effective new chelators, it is reasonable to expect that future research may lead to the identification of iron chelators with considerable usefulness in the control of infectious disease.

6.3. Porphyria

Porphyria cutanea tarda is an inherited disease characterized by a deficiency of uroporphyrinogen decarboxylase (UD), the enzyme responsible for the conversion of uroporphyrinogen into coproporphyrinogen (Chapter 9). Hepatic siderosis, often associated with porphyria, plays an important role in inhibiting UD activity (Kushner *et al.*, 1979) and, conversely, storage iron depletion by phlebotomy results in a striking improvement in the clinical and biochemical expressions of the disease (Ramsay *et al.*, 1975). Although phlebotomy is accepted as the treatment of choice in porphyria cutanea tarda, this form of therapy may not be easily applicable in patients with additional underlying problems such as refractory anaemia or advanced liver disease.

Rocchi *et al.* (1986) have shown that in such patients DF treatment may be a reasonable alternative. The time to complete recovery was 14 months in patients treated by phlebotomy compared with 11 months in patients receiving 1.5 g DF by slow s.c. infusion daily five times weekly. Improvement in liver function and other biochemical parameters of disease activity occurred at the same rate. However, manifestations of cutaneous photosensitivity such as skin pigmentation, bullae and fragility, regressed within 2 to 3 months of DF treatment, much earlier than with phlebotomy. This may be attributed to direct interference by DF with free radical formation involved in the cutaneous manifestations of this variant of porphyria. DF therapy is much more expensive and tedious than phlebotomy and the latter should remain the preferred therapeutic modality in porphyria cutanea tarda. The study of Rocchi *et al.* and the recent reports on haemodialysis-related porphyria (Praga *et al.*, 1987; Stockenhuber *et al.*, 1990) demonstrate, however, that in the occasional patient in whom phlebotomy is contraindicated, DF is an equally effective form of treatment.

6.4. Overview of Novel Uses of Iron Chelating Agents

Conditions in which DF has been proposed as a useful pharmacological agent interfering with iron-dependent reactions may be classified according to the strength of evidence supporting the clinical usefulness of DF. The highest level of evidence exists in situations where the clinical efficacy of DF has been clearly demonstrated in human disease. Only porphyria cutanea tarda would appear to fulfil this requirement at present. The second level of evidence is in conditions where experimental *in vivo* models have shown clear-cut functional and anatomical evidence of improvement. Immune-complex-induced vasculitis, islet cell allograft survival and inhibition of malaria are convincing examples of this category, although confirmation by other investigators and extension to other experimental models would be highly desirable. In the third category of diseases, evidence of a beneficial effect of DF is at present insufficient either because of conflicting reports of efficiency, or because of poor experimental design.

Familiarity with the specific pharmacological features of metal chelators is a prerequisite for their successful therapeutic application. Interaction with a rapidly exchanging intracellular low molecular weight chelatable iron pool requires a steady supply of a drug capable of penetrating the relevant effector cells. The effectiveness of continuous DF infusion in preventing paraquat toxicity as against the failure of bolus injections illustrates this problem. Similarly, the failure of DF to interact with synovial bleomycin-reactive iron in a treatment schedule involving once-weekly injections is hardly surprising. These problems also underline the need for developing new orally effective iron chelators which, by virtue of their slower absorption, would be more suitable for providing a continuous supply of circulating drug.

Modification of disease by preventing the formation of free radicals, the powerful final effectors of tissue damage resulting from the respiratory burst of granulocytes and macrophages participating in the inflammatory response, or by S-phase inhibition of cell proliferation through selective iron depletion, is an exciting new concept in pharmacological intervention. Although much experimental work is still required, this novel approach may have wide ranging implications in the management of autoimmune disease, adult respiratory distress syndrome, organ transplantation and the control of protozoal infection.

ACKNOWLEDGEMENTS

Supported by grant HL 34062-06 of the National Heart, Lung and Blood Institute, and grant G-33-042.2/87 of the German-Israeli Foundation for Scientific Research and Development.

REFERENCES

Adams, P. C., Lin, E., Barber, K. R. and Grant, C. W. M. (1991) Enhanced biliary iron excretion with amphiphilic diethylenetriamine-pentaacetic acid. *Hepatology* **14**, 1230–1234.

Agarwal, M. B., Gupte, S., Vishwanathan, C. *et al.* (1991) L1 (1,2-dimethyl-3-hydroxypyrid-4-one) arthropathy in iron overloaded thalassaemia major may not be immune mediated. 3rd International Conference on Oral Iron Chelators in the Treatment of Thalassaemia and Other Diseases. Acropolis, Nice 4–5th November 1991, Abstract 16.

Allain, P., Mauras, Y., Chaleil, D. *et al.* (1987) Pharmacokinetics and renal elimination of desferrioxamine and ferrioxamine in healthy subjects and patients with haemochromatosis. *Brit. J. Clin. Pharmac.* **24**, 207–212.

Allison, R. C., Hernandez, E. M., Prasad, V. R., Grisham, M. G. and Taylor, A. E. (1988) Protective effects of O_2 radical scavengers and adenosine in PMA-induced lung injury. *J. Appl. Physiol.* **64**, 2175–2182.

Ambrosio, G., Zweier, J. L., Jacobus, W. E., Weisfeldt, M. L. and Flaherty, J. T. (1987) Improvement of postischemic myocardial function and metabolism induced by administration of deferoxamine at the time of reflow: the role of iron in the pathogenesis of reperfusion injury. *Circulation* **76**, 906–915.

Anuwatanakulchai, M., Pootrakul, P., Thuvasethakul, P. and Wasi, P. (1984) Non-transferrin plasma iron in β-thalassaemia/HbE and haemoglobin H diseases. *Scand. J. Haematol.* **32**, 153–158.

Arden, G. B., Wonke, B., Kennedy, C. and Huehns, E. R. (1984) Ocular changes in patients undergoing longitudinal desferrioxamine treatment. *Br. J. Ophthalmol.* **68**, 873–877.

Avramovici-Grisaru, S., Sarel, S., Link, G. and Hershko, C. (1983) Synthesis of pyridoxal isonicotinoyl hydrazones and the *in vivo* iron-removal properties of some pyridoxal derivatives. *J. Med. Chem.* **26**, 298–302.

Babbs, C. F. (1985) Role of iron ions in the genesis of reperfusion injury following successful cardiopulmonary resuscitation: preliminary data and a biochemical hypothesis. *Ann. Emerg. Med.* **14**, 777–783.

Badylak, S. F. and Babbs, C. F. (1986) The effect of carbon dioxide, lidoflazine and deferoxamine upon long term survival following cardiorespiratory arrest in rats. *Resuscitation* **13**, 165–173.

Baldwin, S. R., Grum, C. M., Boxer, L. A., Simon, R. H., Ketai, H. and Devall, L. J. (1986) Oxidant activity in expired breath of patients with adult respiratory distress syndrome. *Lancet* i, 11–14.

Bartlett, A. N., Hoffbrand, A. V. and Kontoghiorghes, G. J. (1990) Long-term trial with the oral iron chelator 1,2-dimethyl-3-hydroxypyrid-4-one (L_1). II. Clinical observations. *Br. J. Haematol.* **76**, 301–304.

Batey, R. G., Lai Chung Fong, P. and Sherlock, S. (1978) The nature of serum iron in primary haemochromatosis. *Clin. Sci.* **55**, 24–25.

Becton, D. L. and Bryles, P. (1988) Deferoxamine inhibition of human neuroblastoma viability and proliferation. *Cancer Res.* **48**, 7189–7194.

Bentur, Y., Koren, G., Tesoro, A., Carley, H., Olivieri, N. and Freedman, M. H. (1990) Comparison of deferoxamine pharmacokinetics between asymptomatic thalassemic children and those exhibiting severe toxicity. *Clin. Pharmacol. Ther.* **47**, 478–482.

Bernard, M., Menasche, P., Pietri, S., Grousset, C., Piwnica, A. and Cozzone, P. J. (1988) Cardioplegic arrest superimposed on evolving myocardial ischemia. Improved recovery after inhibition of hydroxyl radical generation by peroxidase and deferoxamine. *Circulation* **78** (Suppl. III), 164–172.

Blake, D. R., Winyard, P., Lunec, J. *et al.* (1985) Central and ocular toxicity induced by desferrioxamine. *Quart. J. Med.* **56**, 345–355.

Blatt, J. and Stitely, S. (1987) Antineuroblastoma activity of desferroxamine in human cell lines. *Cancer Res.* **47**, 1749–1750.

Blatt, J., Taylor, S. R. and Stitely, S. (1988) Mechanism of antineuroblastoma activity of deferoxamine in vitro. *J. Lab. Clin. Med.* **112**, 433–436.

Bloomfield, S. E., Markenson, A. L., Miller, D. R. and Peterson, C. M. (1978) Lens opacities in thalassemia. *J. Ped. Ophth. Strab.* **15**, 154–156.

Bolli, R., Patel, B. S., Zhu, W. X. *et al.* (1987) The iron chelator desferrioxamine attenuates postischemic ventricular dysfunction. *Am. J. Physiol.* **253**, H1372–H1380.

Bonser, R. S., Fragomeni, L. S., Edwards, B. J. *et al.* (1990) Allopurinol and deferroxamine improve canine lung preservation. *Transplant. Proc.* **22**, 557–558.

Borgna-Pignatti, C., De Stefano, P. and Broglia, A. M. (1984) Visual loss in a patient on high-dose subcutaneous desferrioxamine. *Lancet* i, 681.

Bradley, B., Prowse, S. J., Bauling, P. and Lafferty, K. J. (1986) Desferrioxamine treatment prevents chronic islet allograft damage. *Diabetes* **35**, 550–555.

Brill, P. W., Winchester, P., Giardina, P. J. and Cunningham-Rundles, S. (1991) Deferoxamine-induced bone dysplasia in patients with thalassemia major. *Amer. J. Roentgenol.* **156**, 561–565.

Brittenham, G. M. (1990) Pyridoxal isonicotinoyl hydrazone: Effective iron chelation after oral administration. In: *Sixth Cooley's Anemia Symposium* (ed. A. Bank), *Ann. New York Acad. Sci.* **612**, 315–326.

Byrd, T. F. and Horwitz, M. A. (1989) Interferon gamma-activated human monocytes downregulate transferrin receptors and inhibit the intracellular multiplication of *Legionella pneumophila* by limiting the availability of iron. *J. Clin. Invest.* **83**, 1457–1465.

Calescibetta, C. C., Eribaum, A. I. and Coburn, J. W. (1986) Fatal disseminated phycomycosis (mucormycosis) in patients on deferoxamine for aluminium toxicity. *Amer. J. Kidney Dis.* **8**, A20 (abstract).

Callender, S. T. and Weatherall, D. J. (1980) Iron chelation with oral desferrioxamine. *Lancet* **ii**, 689.

Cerchiari, E. L., Hoel, T. M., Safar, P. and Sclabassi, R. J. (1987) Protective effects of combined superoxide dismutase and deferoxamine on recovery of cerebral blood flow and function after cardiac arrest in dogs. *Stroke* **18**, 869–878.

Cerchiari, E. L., Sclabassi, R. J., Safar, P. and Hoel, T. M. (1990) Effects of combined superoxide dismutase and deferoxamine on recovery of brainstem auditory evoked potentials and EEG after asphyxial cardiac arrest in dogs. *Resusc.* **19**, 25–40.

Chandler, D. B. and Fulwer, J. D. (1985) The effect of deferoxamine on bleomycin-induced lung fibrosis in the hamster. *Amer. Rev. Respir. Dis.* **131**, 596–598.

Chandler, D. B., Butler, T. W., Briggs, D. D., Grizzle, W. E., Barton, J. C. and Fulmer, J. D. (1988) Modulation of the development of bleomycin-induced fibrosis by deferoxamine. *Toxic. Appl. Pharm.* **92**, 358–367.

Clarkson, A. B., Saric, S. and Grady, R. W. (1990) Deferoxamine and eflornitine (DF-α-difluoromethylornithine) in a rat model of *Pneumocystis carinii* pneumonia. *Antimicrob. Agent. Chemother.* **34**, 1833–1835.

Cochrane, C. G., Spragg, R. and Revak, S. D. (1983) Pathogenesis of the adult respiratory distress syndrome: evidence of oxidant activity in bronchoalveolar lavage fluid. *J. Clin. Invest.* **71**, 754–761.

Cohen, A., Martin, M., Mizanin, J., Konkle, D. F. and Schwartz, E. (1990) Vision and hearing during deferoxamine therapy. *J. Pediatr.* **117**, 326–330.

Cook, J. D., Marsaglia, G. and Eschbach, J. W. (1970) Ferrokinetics: A biologic model for plasma iron exchange in man. *J. Clin. Invest.* **49**, 197–205.

Cross, C. E., Warren, D., Gerriets, J. E., Wilson, D. W., Halliwell, B. and Last, J. A. (1985) Deferoxamine injection does not affect bleomycin-induced lung fibrosis in rats. *J. Lab. Clin. Med.* **106**, 433–438.

Cumming, R. L. C., Goldberg, A., Morrow, J. and Smith, J. A. (1967) Effect of phenylhydrazine-induced haemolysis on the urinary excretion of iron after desferrioxamine. *Lancet* **i**, 71–74.

Cutler, P. (1989) Deferoxamine therapy in high-ferritin diabetes. *Diabetes* **38**, 1207–1210.

Davies, S. C., Hungerford, J. L., Arden, J. B., Marcus, R. E., Miller, M. H. and Huehns, E. R. (1983) Ocular toxicity of high-dose intravenous desferrioxamine. *Lancet* **ii**, 181–184.

Donfrancesco, A., Deb, G., Dominici, C., Pileggi, D., Castello, M. A. and Helson, L. (1990) Effects of single course of deferoxamine in neuroblastoma patients. *Cancer Res.* **50**, 4929–4930.

Editorial (1985) Metal chelation therapy, oxygen radicals, and human disease. *Lancet* **i**, 143–145.

Esparza, I. and Brock, J. H. (1981) Release of iron by resident macrophages following ingestion and degradation of transferrin–antitransferrin immune complexes. *Br. J. Haematol.* **49**, 603–614.

Estrow, Z., Tawa, A., Wang, X. H. *et al.* (1987) In vitro and in vivo effects of deferoxamine in neonatal acute leukemia. *Blood* **69**, 757–761.

Farber, N. E., Vercellotti, G. M., Jacob, H. S., Pieper, G. M. and Gross, G. J. (1988) Evidence for a role of iron-catalyzed oxidants in functional and metabolic stunning in the canine heart. *Circulation Res.* **63**, 351–360.

Ferreira, R., Burgos, M., Milei, J. *et al.* (1990) Effect of supplementing cardioplegic solution with deferoxamine on reperfused human myocardium. *J. Thorac. Cardiovasc. Surg.* **100**, 708–714.

Fleischer, J. E., Lanier, W. L., Milde, J. H. and Michenfelder, J. D. (1987) Failure of deferoxamine, an iron chelator, to improve neurologic outcome following complete cerebral ischemia in dogs. *Stroke* **18**, 124–127.

Fligiel, S. E. G., Ward, P. A., Johnson, K. J. and Till, G. O. (1984) Evidence for a role of hydroxyl radical in immune-complex-induced vasculitis. *Amer. J. Pathol.* **115**, 375–382,

Freedman, M. H., Grisaru, D., Olivieri, N., MacLusky, I. and Thorner, P. S. (1990) Pulmonary syndrome in patients with thalassemia major receiving intravenous deferoxamine infusions. *Am. J. Dis. Child.* **144**, 565–569.

Fritsch, G., Treumer, J., Spira, D. T. and Jung, A. (1985) *Plasmodium vinckei*: suppression of mouse infections with desferrioxamine B. *Exp. Parasitol.* **60**, 171–174.

Fritsch, G., Sawatzki, G., Treumer, J., Jung, A. and Spira, D. T. (1987) Plasmodium falciparum: Inhibition in vitro with lactoferrin, desferrithiocin, and desferriocrocin. *Exp. Parasitol.* **63**, 1–9.

Frost, A. E., Freedman, H. H., Westerback, S. J. and Martell, A. E. (1958) Chelating tendencies of N,N'-Ethylenebis [2-(o-hydroxyphenyl)]-glycine. *J. Amer. Chem. Soc.* **80**, 530–536.

Gabutti, V. (1990) Current therapy for thalassemia in Italy. In: *Sixth Cooley's Anemia Symposium* (ed. A. Bank), *Ann. New York Acad. Sci.* **612**, 268–274.

Gallant, T., Freedman, M. H., Vellend, H. and Francombe, W. H. (1986) *Yersinia* sepsis in patients with iron overload treated with deferoxamine. *New Engl. J. Med.* **314**, 1643.

Goodill, J. J. and Abuelo, J. G. (1987) Mucormycosis – a new risk of deferoxamine therapy in dialysis patients with aluminum or iron overload? *New Engl. J. Med.* **317**, 54.

Gordeuk, V. R., Thuma, P. E., Brittenham, G. M. *et al.* (1992a) Iron chelation with deferoxamine B in adults with asymptomatic *Plasmodium falciparum* parasitemia. *Blood* **79**, 308–312.

Gordeuk, V., Thuma, P., Brittenham, G. *et al.* (1992b) Effect of iron chelation therapy on recovery from deep coma in children with cerebral malaria. *New Engl. J. Med.* **327**, 1473–1477.

Grady, R. W. and Hershko, C. (1990) HBED: A potential iron chelator. In: *Sixth Cooley's Anemia Symposium* (ed. A. Bank), *Ann. New York Acad. Sci.* **612**, 361–368.

Grady, R. W., Srinivasan, R., Lemert, R. and Hilgartner, M. W. (1991) DMHP (L1) and DEHP (CP4): Evidence of toxicity in rats. 3rd International Conference on Oral Iron Chelators in the Treatment of Thalassaemia and Other Diseases. Acropolis, Nice 4–5th November 1991, Abstract 11.

Green, J. C., Healing, G., Simpkin, S., Lunec, J. and Fuller, B. J. (1986a) Increased susceptibility to lipid peroxidation in rabbit kidneys: a consequence of warm ischaemia and subsequent reperfusion. *J. Comp. Biochem. Physiol.* **83**, 603–606.

Green, C. J., Healing, G., Simpkin, S., Fuller, B. J. and Lunec, J. (1986b) Reduced susceptibility to lipid peroxidation in cold ischemic rabbit kidneys after addition of desferrioxamine, mannitol and uric acid to the flush solution. *Cryobiology* **23**, 358–365.

Green, R., Lamon, J. and Curran, D. (1980) Clinical trial of desferrioxamine entrapped in red cell ghosts. *Lancet* **ii**, 327–330.

Green, R., Miller, J. and Crosby, W. (1981) Enhancement of iron chelation by desferrioxamine entrapped in red blood cell ghosts. *Blood* **57**, 866–872.

Gutteridge, J. M. C., Richmond, R. and Halliwell, B. (1979) Inhibition of the iron-catalysed formation of hydroxyl radicals from superoxide and of lipid peroxidation by desferrioxamine. *Biochem. J.* **184**, 469–472.

Gutteridge, J. M. C., Rowley, D. A., Griffiths, E. and Halliwell, B. (1985) Low-molecular-weight iron complexes and oxygen radical reactions in idiopathic haemochromatosis. *Clin. Sci.* **68**, 463–467.

Halliwell, B. and Gutteridge, J. M. C. (1984) Oxygen toxicity, oxygen radicals, transition metals and disease. *Biochem. J.* **219**, 1–14.

Halliwell, B. and Gutteridge, J. M. C. (1986) Oxygen, free radicals and iron in relation to biology and medicine: some problems and concepts. *Arch. Biochem. Biophys.* **246**, 540–544.

Halliwell, B. (1989) Protection against tissue damage in vivo by desferrioxamine: what is its mechanism of action? *Free Radic. Biol. Med.* **7**, 645–651.

Hann, H. W. L., Stahlhut, M. W. and Hann, C. L. (1990) Effect of iron and desferoxamine on cell growth and in vitro ferritin synthesis in human hepatoma cell lines. *Hepatology* **11**, 566–569.

Hershko, C. (1975) A study of the chelating agent diethylenetriamine pentaacetic acid using selective radioiron probes of reticuloendothelial and parenchymal iron stores. *J. Lab. Clin. Med* **85**, 913–921.

Hershko, C. (1977) Storage iron regulation. *Progr. Hematol.* **10**, 105–148.

Hershko, C. (1978) Determinants of fecal and urinary iron excretion in desferrioxamine treated rats. *Blood* **51**, 415–424.

Hershko, C. and Peto, T. E. A. (1987) Non-transferrin iron. *Br. J. Haematol.* **66**, 149–152.

Hershko, C. and Peto, T. E. A. (1988) Deferoxamine inhibition of malaria is independent of host iron status. *J. Exper. Med.* **168**, 375–387.

Hershko, C. and Rachmilewitz, E. A. (1979) Mechanism of desferrioxamine-induced iron excretion in thalassaemia. *Br. J. Haematol.* **42**, 125–132.

Hershko, C. and Weatherall, D. J. (1988) Iron chelating therapy. *CRC Crit. Rev. Clin. Lab. Sci.* **26**, 303–345.

Hershko, C., Karsai, A., Eylon, L. and Izak, G. (1970) The effect of chronic iron deficiency on some biochemical functions of the human hemopoietic tissue. *Blood* **36**, 321–329.

Hershko, C., Cook, J. D. and Finch, C. A. (1973) Storage iron kinetics III. Study of desferrioxamine action by selective radioiron labels of RE and parenchymal cells. *J. Lab. Clin. Med.* **81**, 876–886.

Hershko, C., Graham, G., Bates, G. W. and Rachmilewitz, E. A. (1978a) Non-specific serum iron in thalassaemia: an abnormal serum iron fraction of potential toxicity. *Br. J. Haematol.* **40**, 255–263.

Hershko, C., Grady, R. W. and Cerami, A. (1978b) Mechanism of iron chelation in the hypertransfused rat: definition of the two alternative pathways of iron mobilization. *J. Lab. Clin. Med.* **92**, 144–151.

Hershko, C., Avramovici-Grisaru, S., Link, G., Gelfand, L. and Sarel, S. (1981) Mechanism of in vivo iron chelation by pyridoxal isonicotinoyl hydrazone and other imino derivatives of pyridoxal. *J. Lab. Clin. Med.* **98**, 99–107.

Hershko, C., Grady, R. W. and Link, G. (1984) Phenolic ethylenediamine derivatives: a study of orally effective iron chelators. *J. Lab. Clin. Med.* **103**, 337–346.

Hershko, C., Link, G., Pinson, A. *et al.* (1988) Iron toxicity and chelating therapy. In: *Trace Elements in Man and Animals 6* (L. S. Hurley, C. L. Keen, B. Lonnerdal and R. B. Rucker), Plenum Press, New York, pp. 67–71.

Hershko, C., Link, G., Pinson, A. *et al.* (1990) New orally effective iron chelators: animal studies. In: *Sixth Cooley's Anemia Symposium* (ed. A. Bank), *Ann. New York Acad. Sci.* **612**, 3351–3360.

Hershko, C., Link, G., Pinson, A., Peter, H. H., Dobbin, P. and Hider, R. C. (1991a) Iron mobilization from myocardial cells by 3-hydroxypyridin-4-one chelators: Studies in rat heart cells in culture. *Blood* **77**, 2049–2053.

Hershko, C., Theanacho, E. N., Spira, D. T., Peter, H. H., Dobbin, P. and Hider, R. C. (1991b) The effect of N-alkyl modification on the antimalarial activity of 3-hydroxypyrid-4-one oral iron chelators. *Blood* **77**, 637–643.

Hershko, C., Link, G. and Pinson, A. (1992) Preventing anthracycline toxicity: Cardioprotective effect of iron chelating therapy in cultured rat heart cells. 3rd NIH Symposium on Development of Iron Chelators for Clinical Use, 20–22 May, Gainesville, Florida. (Abstract).

Hider, R. C., Singh, S., Porter, J. B. and Huehns, E. R. (1990) The development of hydroxypyridin-4-ones as orally active iron chelators. In: *Sixth Cooley's Anemia Symposium* (ed. A. Bank), *Ann. New York Acad. Sci.* **612**, 327–338.

Hoffbrand, A. V., Ganeshaguru, K., Hooton, J. W. L. and Tattersall, M. H. N. (1976) Effect of iron deficiency and desferrioxamine on DNA synthesis in human cells. *Br. J. Haematol.* **33**, 517–526.

Hoffbrand, A. V., Al-Refaie, F. A., Bartlett, A., Wonke, B. and Kontoghiorghes, G. J. (1991) Updated protocol and monitoring of efficacy and toxicity in clinical trials with the oral iron chelator 1,2-dimethyl-3-hydroxypyrid-4-one (L1). 3rd International Conference on Oral Iron Chelators in the Treatment of Thalassaemia and Other Diseases. Acropolis, Nice 4–5 November 1991, Abstract 24.

Hrushesky, W. J. M., Olshefski, R., Wood, P. *et al.* (1985) Modifying intracellular redox balance: an approach to improving therapeutic index. *Lancet* **i**, 565–567.

Ikeda, Y., Ikeda, K. and Long, D. M. (1989) Protective effect of the iron chelator deferoxamine on cold-induced brain edema. *J. Neurosurg.* **71**, 233–238.

Illes, R. W., Silverman, N. A., Krukenkamp, I. B., del Nido, P. J. and Levitsky, S. (1989) Amelioration of postischemic stunning by deferoxamine-blood cardioplegia. *Circulation* **80** (Suppl. III) 30–35.

Johnson, D. K., Pippard, M. J., Murphy, T. B. and Rose, N. J. (1982) An in vivo evaluation of iron chelating drugs derived from pyridoxal and its analogs. *J. Pharm. Exp. Ther.* **221**, 399–403.

Johnson, K. J., Fantone, J. C., Kaplan, J. and Ward, P. A. (1981) In vivo damage of rat lungs by oxygen metabolites. *J. Clin. Invest.* **67**, 983–993.

Joynson, D. H. M., Jacobs, A., Murray-Walker, D. and Dolby, A. E. (1972) Defect of cell-mediated immunity in patients with iron-deficiency anaemia. *Lancet* **ii**, 1058–1059.

Karabus, C. D. and Fielding, J. (1967) Desferrioxamine chelatable iron in haemolytic, megaloblastic and sideroblastic anaemias. *Br. J. Haematol.* **13**, 924–933.

Keberle, H. (1964) The biochemistry of desferrioxamine and its relation to iron metabolism. *Ann. NY Acad. Sci.* **119**, 758–768.

Kemp, J. D., Smith, K. M., Kanner, L. J., Gomez, F., Thorson, J. A. and Naumann, P. W. (1990) Synergistic inhibition of lymphoid tumor growth in vitro by combined treatment with the iron chelator deferoxamine and an immunoglobulin G monoclonal antibody against the transferrin receptor. *Blood* **76**, 991–995.

Kim, B. K., Huebers, H., Pippard, M. J. and Finch, C. A. (1985) Storage iron exchange in the rat as affected by desferrioxamine. *J. Lab. Clin. Med.* **105**, 440–448.

Kohen, R. and Chevion, M. (1985) Paraquat toxicity is enhanced by iron and reduced by desferrioxamine in laboratory mice. *Biochem. Pharm.* **34**, 1841–1843.

Konijn, A. M. and Hershko, C. (1977) Ferritin synthesis in inflammation: I. Pathogenesis of impaired iron release. *Brit. J. Haematol.* **37**, 7–16.

Kontoghiorghes, G. J. (1990) Design, properties, and effective use of the oral chelator L1 and other α-ketohydroxypyiridines in the treatment of transfusional iron overload in thalassemia. In: *Sixth Cooley's Anemia Symposium* (ed. A. Bank), *Ann. New York Acad. Sci.* **612**, 339–350.

Kontoghiorghes, G. J., Bartlett, A. N., Hoffbrand, A. V. et al. (1990) Long-term trial with the oral iron chelator 1,2-dimethyl-3-hydroxypyrid-4-one (L_1). Iron chelation and metabolic studies. *Br. J. Haematol.* **76**, 295–300.

Korkina, L. G., Maschan, A. A. Samochatova, E. V. and Kontoghiorghes, G. J. (1991) Treatment of Diamond-Blackfan child patients with chelating drug L1. 3rd International Conference on Oral Iron Chelators in the Treatment of Thalassaemia and Other Diseases. Acropolis, Nice 4–5 November 1991, Abstract 18.

Kruck, T. P. A., Teichert-Kuliszewska, K., Fisher, E. et al. (1988) HPLC analysis of desferrioxamine: Pharmacokinetic and metabolic studies. *J. Chromatogr.* **433**, 207–216.

Kruck, T. P. A., Fisher, E. A. and McLachan, D. R. (1990) Suppression of deferoxamine mesylate treatment-induced side effects by coadministration of isoniazid in a patient with Alzheimer's disease subject to aluminum removal by nonspecific chelation. *Clin. Pharmacol. Ther.* **48**, 439–446.

Kumar, K., White, B. C., Krause, G. S. et al. (1988) A quantitative morphological assessment of the effect of lidoflazine and deferoxamine therapy on global brain ischemia. *Neurol. Res.* **10**, 136–140.

Kushner, J. P., Steinmuller, D. P. and Lee, G. R. (1979) The role of iron in the pathogenesis of porphyria cutanea tarda. II. Inhibition of uroporphyrinogen decarboxylase. *J. Clin. Invest.* **56**, 661–667.

Lalonde, R. G. and Holbein, B. E. (1984) Role of iron in *Trypanosoma cruzi* infection in mice. *J. Clin. Invest.* **73**, 470–476.

Lau, E. H., Cerny, E. A. and Rahman, Y. E. (1981) Liposome-encapsulated desferrioxamine in experimental iron overload. *Br. J. Haematol.* **47**, 505–518.

Lau, E. H., Cerny, E. A., Wright, B. J. and Rahman, Y. E. (1983) Improvement of iron removal from the reticuloendothelial system by liposome encapsulation of N,N'-bis(2-hydroxybenzyl)-ethylenediamine-N,N'-diacetic acid (HBED). Comparison with desferrioxamine. *J. Lab. Clin. Med.* **101**, 806–816.

Laub, R., Schneider, Y. J., Octave, J. N., Trouet, A. and Crichton, R. R. (1985) Cellular pharmacology of desferrioxamine B and derivatives in cultured rat hepatocytes in relation to iron mobilization. *Biochem. Pharm.* **34**, 1175–1183.

Lederman, H. M., Cohen, A., Lee, J. W. W., Freedman, M. H. and Gelfand, E. W. (1984) Deferoxamine: a reversible S-phase inhibitor of human lymphocyte proliferation. *Blood* **64**, 748–753.

Lehmann, W. D. and Heinrich, H. C. (1990) Ferrioxamine and its hexadentate iron-chelating metabolites in human post-desferal urine studied by high-performance liquid chromatography and fast atom bombardment mass spectrometry. *Anal. Biochem.* **184**, 219–227.

L'Eplattenier, F., Murase, I. and Martell, A. E. (1967) New multidentate ligands. VI. Chelating tendencies of N,N'-Di(2-hydroxybenzoyl) ethylenediamine-N,N'-diacetic acid. *J. Amer. Chem. Soc.* **89**, 837–843.

Lesnefsky, E. J., Repine, J. E. and Horwitz, L. D. (1990) Deferoxamine pretreatment reduces canine infarct size and oxidative injury. *J. Pharm. Exper. Therap.* **253**, 1103–1109.

Link, G., Pinson, A. and Hershko, C. (1985) Heart cells in culture: a model of myocardial iron overload and chelation. *J. Lab. Clin. Med.* **106**, 147–153.

Loo, V. G. and Lalonde, R. G. (1984) Role of iron in intracellular growth of *Trypanosoma cruzi*. *Infect. Immun.* **45**, 726–730.

Lucarelli, G., Galimberti, M., Polchi, P. *et al.* (1989) Bone marrow transplantation in thalassemia. The experience of Pesaro. In: *Advances and Controversies in Thalassemia Therapy: Bone Marrow Transplantation and Other Approaches* (eds C. D. Buckner, R. P. Gale and G. Lucarelli), Alan R. Liss Inc. New York, pp. 163–171.

Lynch, S. R. Lipschitz, D. A., Bothwell, T. H. and Charlton, R. W. (1974) Iron and the reticuloendothelial system. In: *Iron in Biochemistry and Medicine* (eds A. Jacobs and M. Worwood), Academic Press, London, pp. 563–587.

Martell, A. E. (1981) The design and synthesis of chelating agents. In: *Development of Iron Chelators for Clinical Use* (eds A. E. Martell, W. F. Anderson and D. G. Badman), Elsevier North-Holland, New York, pp. 67–104.

Menasche, P., Grousset, C., Gaudel, Y., Mouas, C. and Piwnica, A. (1987) Prevention of hydroxyl radical formation: A critical concept for improving cardioplegia. *Circulation* **76** (Suppl. V), V180–V185.

Menasche, P., Pasquier, C., Bellucci, S., Lorente, P., Jaillon, P. and Piwnica, A. (1988) Deferoxamine reduces neutrophil-mediated free radical production during cardiopulmonary bypass in man. *J. Thorac. Cardiovasc. Surv.* **96**, 582–589.

Menasche, P., Antebi, H., Alcindor, L. G. *et al.* (1990a) Iron chelation by deferoxamine inhibits lipid peroxidation during cardiopulmonary bypass in humans. *Circulation* **82** (Suppl. IV), 390–396.

Menasche, P., Grousset, C., Mouas, C. and Piwnica, A. (1990b) A promising approach for improving the recovery of heart transplants. Prevention of free radical injury through iron chelation by deferoxamine. *J. Thorac. Cardiovasc. Surg.* **100**, 13–21.

Mendola, J., Wright, J. R. and Lacy, P. E. (1989) Oxygen free-radical scavengers and immune destruction of murine islets in allograft rejection and multiple low-dose streptozocin-induced insulitis. *Diabetes* **38**, 379–385.

Meyer-Brunot, H. G. and Keberle, H. (1967) The metabolism of desferrioxamine B. *Biochem. Pharm.* **16**, 527–537.

Miller, K. B., Rosenwasser, L. J., Bessette, J. M., Beer, D. J. and Rocklin, R. E. (1981) Rapid desensitization for desferrioxamine anaphylactic reaction. *Lancet* **i**, 1059.

Myers, C. E., McGuire, W. P., Liss, R. H. *et al.* (1977) Adriamycin: the role of lipid peroxidation in cardiac toxicity and tumor response. *Science* **197**, 165–167.

Nastruzzi, C., Walde, P., Menegatti, E. and Gambari, R. (1989) Differential effects of liposome-entrapped desferrioxamine on proliferation and erythroid differentiation of murine erythroleukemic Friend cells. *Biochim. Biophys. Acta* **1013**, 36–41.

Nayini, N. R., White, B. C., Aust, S. D. *et al.* (1985) Post resuscitation iron delocalization and malondialdehyde production in the brain following prolonged cardiac arrest. *J. Free Radic. Biol. Med.* **1**, 111–116.

Nocka, K. H. and Pelus, L. M. (1988) Cell cycle specific effects of deferoxamine on human and murine hematopoietic progenitor cells. *Cancer Res.* **48**, 3571–3575.

Nomikos, I. N., Prowse, S. J., Carotenuto, P. and Lafferty, J. (1986) Combined treatment with nicotinamide and desferrioxamine prevents islet allograft destruction in NOD mice. *Diabetes* **35**, 1302–1304.

Octave, J. N., Schneider, Y. J., Crichton, R. R. and Trouet, A. (1983) Iron mobilization from cultured hepatocytes: effect of desferrioxamine B. *Biochem. Pharm.* **32**, 3413–3418.

Okamoto, H. (1985) Molecular basis of experimental diabetes: degeneration, oncogenesis and regeneration of pancreatic b-cells of islets of Langerhans. *Bioessays* **2**, 15–21.

Olivieri, N. F., Buncic, J. R., Chew, E. *et al.* (1986) Visual and auditory neurotoxicity in patients receiving subcutaneous deferoxamine infusions. *N. Engl. J. Med.* **314**, 869–873.

Olivieri, N. F., Koren, G., Hermann, C. *et al.* (1990) Comparison of oral iron chelator L1 and desferrioxamine in iron-loaded patients. *Lancet* **336**, 1275–1279.

Osheroff, M. R., Schaich, K. M., Drew, R. T. and Borg, D. C. (1985) Failure of desferrioxamine to modify the toxicity of paraquat in rats. *J. Free Radic. Biol. Med.* **1**, 71–82.

Patt, A., Horesh, I. R., Berger, E. M., Harken, A. H. and Repine, J. E. (1990) Iron depletion or chelation reduces ischemia/reperfusion-induced edema in gerbil brains. *J. Pediat. Surg.* **25**, 224–228.

Peters, G., Keberle, H., Schmid, K. and Brunner, H. (1966) Distribution and renal excretion of desferrioxamine and ferrioxamine in the dog and in the rat. *Biochem. Pharm.* **15**, 93–109.

Pickford, M. A., Green, C. J., Sarathchandra, P. and Fryer, P. R. (1990) Ultrastructural changes in rat lungs after 48h cold storage with and without reperfusion. *Int. J. Exp. Pathol.* **71**, 513–528.

Pippard, M. J., Warner, G. T., Callender, S. T. and Weatherall, D. J. (1977) Iron absorption in iron-loading anaemias: effect of subcutaneous desferrioxamine infusions. *Lancet* **ii**, 737–739.

Pippard, M. J., Johnson, D. K. and Finch, C. A. (1982a) Hepatocyte iron kinetics in the rat explored with an iron chelator. *Br. J. Haematol.* **52**, 221–224.

Pippard, M. J., Callender, S. T. and Finch, C. A. (1982b) Ferrioxamine excretion in iron-loaded man. *Blood* **60**, 288–294.

Pippard, M. J., Jackson, M. J., Hoffman, K., Petrou, M. and Modell, C. B. (1986) Iron chelation using subcutaneous infusions of diethylene triamine penta-acetic acid (DTPA). *Scand. J. Haematol.* **36**, 466–472.

Pitt, C. G. (1981) Structure and activity relationships of iron chelating drugs. In: *Development of Iron Chelators for Clinical Use* (eds A. E. Martell, W. F. Anderson and D. G. Badman), Elsevier North-Holland, New York, pp. 105–131.

Pitt, C. G., Gupta, G., Estes, W. E. *et al.* (1979) The selection and evaluation of new chelating agents for the treatment of iron overload. *J. Pharm. Exper. Therap.* **208**, 12–18.

Pollack, S., Rossan, R. N., Davidson, D. E. and Escajadillo, A. (1987) Desferrioxamine suppresses *Plasmodium falciparum* in aotus monkeys. *Proc. Soc. Exp. Biol. Med.* **184**, 162–165.

Polson, R. J., Jawed, A., Bomford, A., Berry, H. and Williams, R. (1985) Treatment of rheumatoid arthritis with desferrioxamine: relation between stores of iron before treatment and side effects. *Br. Med. J.* **291**, 448.

Ponka, P., Borova, J., Neuwirt, J. and Fuchs, O. (1970) Mobilization of iron from reticulocytes. *FEBS Letters* **97**, 317–321.

Ponka, P., Borova, J., Neuwirt, J., Fuchs, O. and Necas, E. (1979) A study of intracellular iron metabolism using pyridoxal isonicotinoyl hydrazone and other synthetic chelating agents. *Biochim. Biophys. Acta* **586**, 278–297.

Porter, J. B., Jaswon, M. S., Huehns, E. R., East, C. A. and Hazell, J. W. P. (1989) Desferrioxamine ototoxicity: evaluation of risk factors in thalassaemic patients and guidelines for safe dosage. *Br. J. Haematol.* **73**, 403–409.

Porter, J. B., Morgan, J., Hoyes, K. P., Burke, L. C., Huehns, E. R. and Hider, R. C. (1990) Relative oral efficacy and acute toxicity of hydroxypyridin-4-one iron chelators in mice. *Blood* **76**, 2389–2396.

Powis, G. (1989) Free radical formation by antitumor quinones. *Free Radical Biol. & Med.* **6**, 63–101.

Praga, M., de Salamanca, R. E., Andres, A. *et al.* (1987) Treatment of hemodialysis-related porphyria cutanea tarda with deferoxamine. *N. Engl. J. Med.* **316**, 547–548.

Ramsay, C. A., Magnus, I. A., Turnbull, A. and Baker, H. (1974) The treatment of porphyria cutanea tarda by venesection. *Q. J. Med.* **43**, 1–24.

Rahman, Y. E. and Wright, B. J. (1975) Liposomes containing chelating agents: cellular penetration and possible mechanisms of metal removal. *J. Cell Biol.* **65**, 112–122.

Raventos-Suarez, C., Pollack, S. and Nagel, R. L. (1982) *Plasmodium falciparum*: inhibition of in vitro growth by desferrioxamine. *Am. J. Trop. Med. Hyg.* **31**, 919–922.

Reddy, B. R., Kloner, R. A. and Przyklenk, K. (1989) Early treatment with deferoxamine limits myocardial ischemic/reperfusion injury. *Free Radic. Biol. Med.* **7**, 45–52.

Reichard, P. and Ehrenberg, A. (1983) Ribonucleotide reductase – A radical enzyme. *Science* **221**, 514–519.

Rocchi, E., Gilbertini, P., Cassanelli, M. *et al.* (1986) Iron removal therapy in porphyria cutanea tarda: phlebotomy versus slow subcutaneous desferrioxamine infusion. *Br. J. Dermatol.* **114**, 621–629.

Robins-Browne, R. M. and Prpic, J. K. (1985) Effects of iron and desferrioxamine on infections with *Yersinia enterocolitica*. *Infect. Immun.* **47**, 774–779.

Rosenkrantz, H., Metterville, J. J. and Fleischman, R. W. (1986) Preliminary toxicity findings in dogs and rodents given the iron chelator ethylenediamine-N,N' bis (2-hydroxyphenylacetic acid) (EDHPA). *Fundam. Appl. Toxicol.* **6**, 292–298.

Rubinstein, M., Dupont, P., Doppee, J. P., Dehon, C., Ducobu, J. and Hainaut, J. (1985) Ocular toxicity of desferrioxamine. *Lancet* **i**, 817–818.

Sciortino, C. V., Byers, B. R. and Cox, P. (1980) Evaluation of iron-chelating agents in cultured heart muscle cells. Identification of a potential drug for chelation therapy. *J. Lab. Clin. Med.* **96**, 1081–1085.

Scott, M. D., Ranz, A., Kuypers, F. A., Lubin, B. H. and Meshnick, S. R. (1990) Parasite uptake of desferrioxamine: a prerequisite for antimalarial activity. *Br. J. Haematol.* **75**, 598–602.

Segovia, M., Navarro, A. and Artero, J. M. (1989) The effect of liposome-entrapped desferrioxamine on *Leishmania donovani* in vitro. *Ann. Trop. Med. Parasit.* **83**, 357–360.

Shiloh, H., Iancu, T. C., Bauminger, E. R., Link, G., Pinson, A. and Hershko, C. (1992) Deferoxamine-induced iron mobilization and redistribution of myocardial iron in cultured rat heart cells: Studies of the chelatable iron pool by electron microscopy and Mossbauer spectroscopy. *J. Lab. Clin. Med.* **119**, 428–436.

Simon, P., Ang, K. S., Meyvier, A., Allain, P. and Mauras, Y. (1983) Desferrioxamine ocular toxicity, and trace metals. *Lancet* **ii**, 512–513.

Singh, S., Hider, R. C. and Porter, J. B. (1990a) Separation and identification of desferrioxamine and its iron chelating metabolites by high-performance liquid chromatography and fast atom bombardment mass spectrometry: choice of complexing agent and application to biological fluids. *Anal. Biochem.* **187**, 212–219.

Singh, S., Hider, R. C., and Porter, J. B. (1990b) A direct method for quantification of non-transferrin-bound iron. *Anal. Biochem.* **186**, 320–323.

Singh, S., Mohammed, N, Ackerman, R., Porter, J. B. and Hider, R. C. (1992) Quantification of desferrioxamine and its iron chelating metabolites by high-performance liquid chromatography and simultaneous ultraviolet-visible/radioactive detection. *Anal. Biochem.* **203**, 116–120.

Stockenhuber, F., Kurz, R., Grimm, G., Moser, G. and Balcke, P. (1990) Successful treatment of hemodialysis-related porphyria cutanea tarda with deferoxamine. *Nephron.* **55**, 321–324.

Summers, M. R., Jacobs, A., Tudway, D., Perera, P. and Ricketts, C. (1979) Studies in desferrioxamine and ferrioxamine metabolism in normal and iron-loaded subjects. *Br. J. Haematol.* **42**, 547–555.

Taetle, R., Honeysett, J. M. and Bergeron, R. (1989) Combination iron depletion therapy. *J. Natl. Cancer Inst.* **81**, 1229–1235.

Tondury, P., Kontoghiorghes, G. J., Ridolfi-Luthy, A. *et al.* (1990) L1 (1,2-dimethyl-3-hydroxypyrid-4-one) for oral iron chelation in patients with beta-thalassaemia major. *Br. J. Haematol.* **76**, 550–553.

Unger, A. and Hershko, C. (1974) Hepatocellular uptake of ferritin in the rat. *Br. J. Haematol.* **28**, 169–176.

Van der Wal, N. A. A., Van Oirschot, J. F. L. M., Van Dijk, A., Verhoef, J. and Van Asbeck, B. S. (1990) Mechanism of protection of alveolar type II cells against paraquat-induced cytotoxicity by deferoxamine. *Biochem. Pharm.* **39**, 1665–1671.

Van Asbeck, B. S., Hillen, F. C., Boonen, H. C. M. *et al.* (1989) Continuous intravenous infusion of deferoxamine reduces mortality by paraquat in vitamin-E deficient rats. *Am. Rev. Respir. Dis.* **139**, 769–773.

Wagstaff, M., Peters, S. W., Jones, B. M. and Jacobs, A. (1985) Free iron and iron toxicity in iron overload. *Br. J. Haematol.* **61**, 566–567.

Wang, W. C., Ahmed, N. and Hanna, M. (1986) Non-transferrin-bound iron in long-term transfusion in children with congenital anemias. *J. Pediatr.* **108**, 552–557.

Ward, P. A., Till, G. O., Kunkel, R. and Beauchamps, C. (1983) Evidence for role of hydroxyl radical in complement and neutrophil-dependent tissue injury. *J. Clin. Invest.* **72**, 789–801.

Ward, H. E., Hicks, M., Nicholson, A. and Berend, N. (1988) Deferoxamine infusion does not inhibit bleomycin-induced lung damage in the rat. *Am. Rev. Respir. Dis.* **137**, 1356–1359.

Weinberg, K. (1990) Novel uses of deferoxamine. *Am. J. Pediatr. Hematol. Oncol.* **12**, 9–13.

Weinberg, K., Champagne, J., Lenarsky, C. *et al.* (1986) Desferrioxamine (DFO) inhibition of interleukin 2 receptor (IL2R) expression: potential therapy of graft versus host disease (GVHD). *Blood* **68** (Suppl. 1), 286a.

White, B. C., Krause, G. S., Aust, S. D. and Eyster, G. E. (1985) Postischemic tissue injury by iron-mediated free radical-lipid peroxidation. *Ann. Emerg. Med.* **14**, 804–809.

White, G. P. and Jacobs, A. (1978) Iron uptake by Chang cells from transferrin, nitriloacetate and citrate complexes. The effects of iron-loading and chelation with desferrioxamine. *Biochim. Biophys. Acta* **543**, 217–225.

Williams, A. Hoy, T., Pugh, A. and Jacobs, A. (1982) Pyridoxal complexes as potential chelating agents for oral therapy in transfusional iron overload. *J. Pharm. Pharmacol.* **34**, 730–732.

Williams, R. E., Zweier, J. L. and Flaherty, J. T. (1988) Reduction of free radical injury at reperfusion by intraischemic treatment with deferoxamine. *J. Amer. Coll. Cardiol.* **11**, 48A (Abstract).

Wohler, F. (1963) The treatment of haemochromatosis with desferrioxamine. *Acta Haemat.* **30**, 65–87.

Yinnon, A. M., Theanacho, E. N., Grady, R. W., Spira, D. Y. and Hershko, C. (1989) Antimalarial effect of HBED and other phenolic and catecholic iron chelators. *Blood* **74**, 2166–2171.

Young, R. C., Ozols, R. F. and Myers, C. E. (1981) The anthracycline neoplastic drugs. *N. Engl. J. Med.* **305**, 139–153.

Zevin, S., Link, G., Grady, R. W., Hider, R. C. and Hershko, C. (1992) Origin and fate of iron mobilized by the 3-hydroxypyridin-4-one oral chelators: Studies in hypertransfused rats by selective radioiron probes of RE and hepatocellular iron stores. *Blood* **79**, 248–253.

Zimmerman, B. J., Grisham, M. B. and Granger, D. N. (1990) Role of oxidants in ischemia/reperfusion-induced granulocyte infiltration. *Am. J. Physiol.* **258**, G185–190.

13. Changes in Iron Metabolism with Age

R. YIP

Division of Nutrition and Prevention (CDC), Centers for Disease Control, Atlanta, Georgia 30333, USA

I. INTRODUCTION

Iron metabolism can best be summarized as the maintenance of iron-related physiological functions through the balance of intake, transport, stores and loss of iron. There are a number of factors that affect the iron balance, and the role of these factors vary at different stages of the life cycle. For example, dietary iron, an external factor which can affect iron balance, is a major limiting factor in infancy because of low iron content in most infant diets, including breast milk. The increased iron requirement related to rapid blood volume expansion and maternal and fetal growth is an example of an internal factor that affects iron balance during pregnancy. The purpose of this chapter is to review the various factors and conditions that affect iron metabolism at different parts of the life cycle. To do so, several aspects need to be considered beyond the major factors which affect iron balance: (1) normal developmental changes of major laboratory parameters commonly used to assess iron status; (2) the iron status and vulnerability to iron deficiency at different ages; and (3) factors that can interfere with the utilization of iron other than the balance between intake and loss.

2. MAJOR PARAMETERS OF IRON BALANCE

Iron requirement and intake is governed by the need to maintain iron balance relative to loss and growth. In addition to iron intake and loss, iron stores in the body play a major role in maintaining the supply of iron for metabolic need. There are various methods to assess the different aspects of iron metabolism. For this discussion, emphasis will be placed on two major parameters of iron metabolism: the functional component of iron related to oxygen transport, haemoglobin in red cells; and the storage component assessed by serum ferritin assay. A large part of the information used in this chapter is based on haematological and iron biochemistry results of the US National Health and Nutritional Examination Surveys (NHANES). The first survey (NHANES I) was conducted from 1970 to 1975, and the second survey was conducted from 1976 to 1980. Both surveys utilized a national probability sample of healthy children and adults (Dallman et al., 1984).

2.1. Factors that Affect Iron Uptake

There are several components that govern iron uptake by the body. The quantity and quality of iron in the diet, and the compounds in food that can either promote or inhibit iron absorption can all be regarded as external factors affecting iron availability and uptake. The internal factor that affects iron uptake is the efficiency of iron absorption, and to a great extent this is related to the iron status or the haematological status of an individual.

2.1.1. Dietary Factors

Even though dietary factors are not in themselves physiological parameters, at different stages of development their interaction with iron requirements affects iron status. Because iron requirements are greater during periods of rapid tissue growth such as infancy, early childhood, adolescence and pregnancy, relatively greater intake is needed to meet these requirements (Dallman et al., 1980). The most difficult period to meet this greater iron requirement is in infancy. Because of the limited diversity of diet in infancy, the majority of infant diets are marginal in iron content. For this reason, late infancy and early childhood is a period of high risk for iron deficiency (Dallman et al., 1980).

Beyond infancy, the constraints of dietary iron quantity and quality are still a major problem in most developing parts of the world. Dietary haem iron is better absorbed than non-haem iron, and there are many dietary factors that either promote or inhibit non-haem iron absorption (Chapter 6). Any dietary deficiencies affect women more than men because of the obligatory blood loss during the menstrual cycle that renders iron requirements higher for women during the child-bearing years (Bothwell and Charlton, 1981).

2.1.2. Absorption Factors

The efficiency of iron absorption from the intestinal lumen is regulated by the iron status: greater absorption efficiency is related to greater severity of iron deficiency or anaemia. Because at different parts of the life cycle (such as during late infancy and pregnancy) the vulnerability to iron deficiency is greater, efficiency of iron absorption also tends to be greater at those times. However, there is no evidence to suggest that in a non-iron depleted state there is an age or sex difference in iron absorption.

2.2. Factors that Affect Iron Utilization and Loss

There are two major pathways in the output part of the iron balance equation: utilization by tissue, and loss from the body. The demands of these two outputs vary at different ages.

2.2.1. Tissue Utilization

By far the greatest component of tissue iron need is for the haemoglobin of red blood cells. Aside from specific circumstances which result in greater red cell mass and more iron being needed for higher haemoglobin levels (such as residing at higher altitude and cigarette smoking), the greatest demand for tissue iron is during rapid growth periods – infancy, early childhood, adolescence and pregnancy – related to expanding blood volume. During these periods of increasing tissue mass, the increased iron requirement results in a greater risk of iron deficiency.

2.2.2. *Blood Loss*

Under normal conditions, a small amount of iron is lost daily from stool, urine and skin. Within this normal loss related to metabolic turnover, the minute blood loss from the gastrointestinal (GI) tract constitutes the greatest proportion. During infancy, some infants can experience exaggerated occult GI blood loss as a result of exposure to cow's milk proteins and this can further increase the risk of iron deficiency (Fomon *et al.*, 1981). Another type of exaggerated normal GI blood loss is related to a high level of strenuous physical activity (Stewart *et al.*, 1984).

For women of child-bearing age, the normal menstrual blood loss represents a major source of iron loss in addition to the daily loss through GI tract, urine and skin. The range of menstrual blood loss is rather wide, and those women with greater blood loss certainly are at greater risk of negative iron balance (Bothwell and Charlton, 1981). Pregnancy is a period of high iron requirement to meet the iron needs of maternal and fetal tissue growth. The estimated basal iron loss for women is 0.8 mg per day, and to meet the iron loss related to menstrual blood loss the average requirement increases to 2.2 mg per day (Hallberg *et al.*, 1966). During pregnancy, the cessation of menstruation actually reduces iron loss to the basal level, but the overall iron requirement is increased to 5 mg/day during the second and third trimester because of blood volume expansion and growth of maternal and fetal tissue (Bothwell and Charlton, 1981). Even though a substantial amount of iron is transferred to the fetus, a net positive iron balance may remain after completion of the pregnancy if the iron intake has been sufficient. However, because it is difficult to achieve sufficient intake, especially in developing parts of the world where diet quality is limited, most women end up with a negative iron balance after pregnancy.

3. NORMAL DEVELOPMENTAL VARIATION OF LABORATORY PARAMETERS RELATED TO IRON METABOLISM

There are a number of well established haematological and biochemical tests that can be used to assess the iron status for an individual and on a population basis (Chapter 14). However, there are significant developmental variations of some of these laboratory tests, independent of the iron status, that need to be taken into account when characterizing iron status throughout the life cycle (Yip *et al.*, 1984).

The commonly used iron related tests can be grouped into three types: (1) haematological or red blood cell related tests – haemoglobin (Hb), haematocrit (Hct), red cell indices including mean corpuscular volume (MCV) and red cell distribution width (RDW), and erythrocyte protoporphyrin (EP); (2) iron transport related tests – serum iron, transferrin or total iron binding capacity (TIBC), transferrin saturation (SAT) and transferrin receptors; and (3) iron store related – serum ferritin. It appears that most of the red cell related tests, and transferrin saturation, undergo normal developmental changes, making age- and sex-specific criteria a requirement for the proper interpretation of test results. Serum ferritin also changes significantly across age groups, but the variation is dependent on the iron status of the particular population under study. For this reason, it is more difficult to define a true physiological range of serum ferritin for normal individuals.

3.1. Variation of Red Blood Cell Parameters

A number of studies have used similar strategies in determining the normal range of haematological parameters by excluding individuals with abnormal biochemical tests of iron metabolism (Yip et al., 1984; LSRO, 1985). For example, to define the normal range of haemoglobin, a sample can be utilized after excluding all individuals with other abnormal iron related tests such as low transferrin saturation and low serum ferritin. In general, the normal haematological range established using such an exclusionary approach was similar in different studies. This suggests that, when iron status is normal, most populations have similar haematological values. The only exception is that blacks in general have a 0.5 g/dl lower haemoglobin level than whites, and this is not related to iron status (Perry et al., 1992).

3.1.1. Haematological Variation during Infancy

Red cell parameters undergo the greatest changes during infancy, especially during the neonatal period. The most comprehensive study of normal developmental changes was carried out by Sarrinen and Siimes (1977) using a sample of healthy Finnish infants after exclusion of those with questionable iron status (transferrin saturation below 16% or serum ferritin values below 10 µg/l). Table 13.1 details values for the mean and mean − 2 SD of haemoglobin, haematocrit and red cell indices, and Fig. 13.1 details the changes of haemoglobin distribution from 1 to 12 months of age. It is quite evident that marked changes take place among these haematological parameters during the first year of life, especially during the first six months. A more recent study of low-income black and Hispanic children in New York City found similar patterns of developmental changes of haemoglobin level from 6 to 12 months of age for infants with lower haemoglobin values but no evidence of iron deficiency (Irigoyen et al., 1991). It is evident from these studies that the age-related changes

Table 13.1 Normal haematological values for infants up to 12 months of age based on the study of Sarrinen and Siimes (1977) of a sample of healthy Finnish infants after excluding those with low transferrin saturation and serum ferritin concentrations

Age (mo)	0.5	1	2	4	6	9	12
Hb (g/dl)Mean	16.6	13.9	11.2	12.2	12.6	12.7	12.7
−2 SD	13.4	10.7	9.4	10.3	11.1	11.4	11.3
Hct (%) Mean	53	44	35	38	36	36	37
−2 SD	41	33	28	32	31	32	33
RBC count ($\times 10^{12}$/l) Mean	4.9	4.3	3.7	4.3	4.7	4.7	4.7
−2 SD	3.9	3.3	3.1	3.5	3.9	4.0	4.1
MCV (fl) Mean	105	101	95	87	76	78	78
−2 SD	88	91	84	76	68	70	71
MCH (pg) Mean	33.6	32.5	30.4	28.6	26.8	27.3	26.8
−2 SD	30	29	27	25	24	25	24
MCHC (g/l) Mean	31.4	31.8	31.8	32.7	35.0	34.9	34.3
−2 SD	28.1	28.1	28.3	28.8	32.7	32.4	32.1

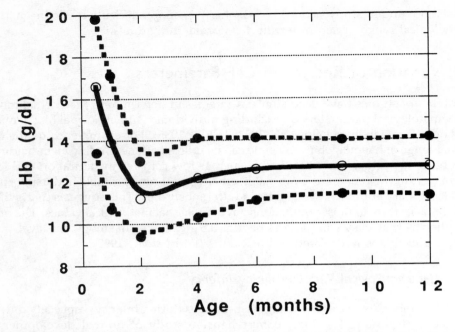

Fig. 13.1 Normal haemoglobin ranges (mean ±2 SD) during infancy. Redrawn from Saarinen and Siimes (1977).

in haemoglobin value during infancy are large enough to warrant separate criteria to define anaemia.

3.1.2. *Haematological Variation during Childhood and Adolescence*

Two studies have defined the normal ranges in haematological parameters for children and adolescents using an approach similar to that used for infants by excluding individuals with evidence of abnormal iron related tests. One report by Dallman and Siimes (1979), using several study samples from California and Finland, developed the percentile curves for Hb and MCV from 1 to 15 years of age. The other study by Yip *et al.* (1984) used a representative sample of the US children from the second National Health and Nutrition Examination Survey, 1976–1980 (NHANES II). The later study defined the normal range of haematological values for adults as well as for parameters other than Hb and MCV, such as Hct, MCH and RBC counts. The Hb and MCV values for both studies are quite similar. Table 13.2 details the values for the mean and mean − 2 SD of haematological values based on the NHANES II sample, and Fig. 13.2 illustrates the mean haemoglobin values from childhood to adulthood. It is evident that normal haemoglobin values undergo changes throughout childhood.

3.1.3. *Haematological Variation in Adulthood*

Starting in early adolescence, boys begin to have a greater haemoglobin level than girls. The difference stabilizes at late adolescence and persists throughout adulthood

Table 13.2 Normal age-related changes of haematological values for children and adults based on the US NHANES II survey after excluding those with abnormal tests related to iron (Yip et al., 1984)

Age (year) M=Male; F=Female	1–1.9	2–4.9	5–7.9	8–11.9	F12–14	F15–18	F18–44	M12–14	M15–17	M18–44
Hb (g/dl) Mean	12.3	13.9	12.5	12.8	13.4	13.5	13.5	14.0	14.8	15.3
−2 SD	10.7	10.7	10.9	11.0	11.5	11.7	11.7	12.0	12.3	13.2
Hct (%) Mean	35.9	36.3	37.2	38.4	39.0	39.54	40.0	40.5	43.0	44.5
−2 SD	32.0	32.0	33.0	34.0	34.0	34.0	34.0	35.0	37.0	39.0
RBC count (×10^{12}/l)										
Mean	4.34	4.34	4.41	4.51	4.47	4.48	4.42	4.71	4.92	4.99
−2 SD	3.8	3.7	3.31	3.8	3.9	3.9	3.8	4.1	4.2	4.3
MCV (fl) Mean	79	81	82	84	86	88	90	85	87	89
−2 SD	67	73	74	76	77	78	81	77	79	80
MCH (pg) Mean	27.4	28.1	28.6	28.7	29.4	30.0	30.6	29.1	29.9	30.5
−2 SD	22	25	25	26	26	26	26	26	27	27
MCHC (g/l) Mean	34.4	34.5	34.5	34.5	34.1	33.9	33.9	34.4	34.4	34.5

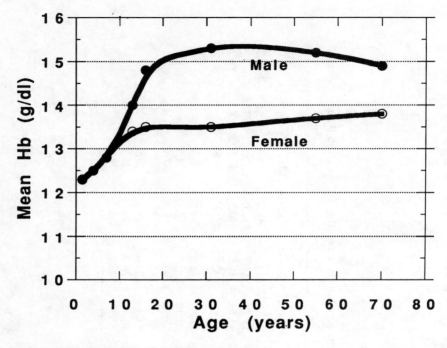

Fig. 13.2 Mean haemoglobin values of the US children and adults based on the sample of NHANES II after excluding subjects with abnormal iron related tests. Redrawn from Yip *et al.* (1984).

(Fig. 13.2). For this reason, sex-specific haemoglobin criteria are needed to define anaemia after 10 years of age. The mean haemoglobin value appears to decline slightly in older age groups in the NHANES II sample even after exclusion of those individuals with abnormal iron related tests (Fig. 13.2) (Yip *et al.*, 1984). One theory to explain such a decline in relation to ageing is a normal reduction of erythropoietic capacity with age or the 'physiological anaemia of ageing' (Freedman and Marcus, 1980). However, based on a study of the effect of inflammation, as represented by elevated erythrocyte sedimentation rate (ESR), on iron and haemoglobin status, it appears that pathological factors can interfere with iron metabolism and may explain at least part of the decline of haemoglobin level among the elderly (Yip and Dallman, 1988). Chronic disease and inflammatory conditions, even when mild, can affect the haemoglobin and red cell production at all ages, including younger children (Reeves *et al.*, 1984).

3.1.4. Haematological Variation during Pregnancy

Haematological parameters undergo significant changes throughout a normal pregnancy. Figure 13.3 details the values for the mean and mean – 2 SD of haemoglobin concentrations throughout pregnancy based on the composite results from four studies where all pregnant women were adequately supplemented with iron (Sjosted *et al.*, 1977; CDC, 1989; Puolakka *et al.*, 1980; Taylor *et al.*, 1982). The decline of haemoglobin, starting early in pregnancy and reaching a low point in the second

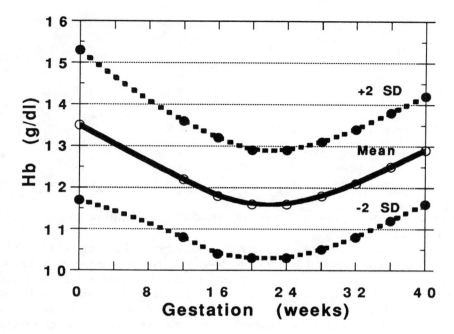

Fig. 13.3 Normal haemoglobin ranges during pregnancy based on women with adequate iron supplementation from four different studies (see text).

trimester, can be regarded as a haemodilution phenomenon: an expansion of plasma volume exceeds the accompanying increase in red cell mass (McFee, 1973). There is an increased iron requirement related to the expanding maternal red cell mass and growth of maternal, placental and fetal tissue, the major increase in iron needs being in the second and third trimesters (Chapter 7). A rise of haemoglobin concentration toward the end of the pregnancy occurs in those receiving iron supplements, at a time when expansion in plasma volume has slowed down. A failure of haemoglobin to rise during the third trimester is indicative of negative maternal iron balance (Svanberg et al., 1976) as the iron requirements of the fetus are met. Postpartum, haematological values resume the non-pregnant state within 2 to 3 months. Currently, there are no well-defined normal haematological ranges for the postpartum period.

3.1.5. *Factors that Affect Haemoglobin Levels Independent of Developmental Stage*

There are a few non-pathological conditions that can affect haemoglobin levels independent of developmental changes. These factors cause a significant shift in the distribution of haemoglobin values in a population, and this can affect the interpretation of anaemia or iron status. The most important of these factors are altitude, cigarette smoking and race, and will be briefly discussed here.

   (a) *Altitude*. Long-term exposure to mild to moderate hypoxia results in a higher haemoglobin level to compensate for the reduced oxygen supply. The relationship of haemoglobin level and altitude is a curvilinear one (Hurtado et al., 1945). Table 13.3 details this relationship (CDC, 1989). The increase in haemoglobin concentration

Table 13.3 Normal increase of haemoglobin and haematocrit values
related to long-term altitude exposure (adapted from CDC, 1989)

	Hb (g/dl)	Hct (%)
<900 m	0	0
900–1199 m	+0.2	+0.5
1200–1499 m	+0.3	+1.0
1500–1799 m	+0.5	+1.5
1800–1999 m	+0.7	+2.0
2000–2199 m	+1.0	+3.0
2200–2399 m	+1.3	+4.0
2400–2599 m	+1.6	+5.0
2600–2800 m	+2.0	+6.0

related to altitude requires an exposure period of one month or longer to reach a
steady state.

(b) *Cigarette smoking*. Smokers consistently have higher haemoglobin levels than
non-smokers. The higher haemoglobin level is a compensatory response for a
reduced oxygen carrying capacity: carbon monoxide renders a portion of the
haemoglobin non-functional by forming carboxyhaemoglobin (Smith and Landaw,
1978; Nordenberg *et al.*, 1990). Table 13.4 details the relationship between
haemoglobin changes and the quantity of cigarettes smoked based on a national
sample studied in the United States (CDC, 1989).

(c) *Race*. A number of studies consistently found black children and adults to have
lower haemoglobin levels than comparable white groups. The observed difference is
approximately 0.5 to 0.8 g/dl and it is independent of iron nutrition status (Perry *et al.*,
1992). Even though it is not clear whether this race difference represents a physiological variation or is the result of a higher frequency of mild hereditary haemoglobin
or red cell production defects among blacks, the magnitude of the difference warrants
attention in the interpretation of tests for iron status in screening for iron deficiency.

3.2. Variation of Iron Stores

Iron stores represent a substantial part of the total body iron that serves as a reservoir
of extra iron beyond that needed for iron metabolism. Monitoring the status of iron
stores is helpful in assessing conditions that affect iron metabolism. During the early
phase of a negative iron balance, gradual depletion of iron stores presents no
significant physiological consequence in itself. However, causes which lead to
persistent negative iron balance such as abnormal blood loss can be of clinical
significance. Similarly, an increase in iron stores may signal iron overload, or a

Table 13.4 Smoking adjustment for haemoglobin and haematocrit
values (adapted from CDC, 1989)

	Hb (g/dl)	Hct (%)
Non-smoker	0	0
Smoker (all)	+0.3	+1.0
1/2–1 pack/day	+0.3	+1.0
1–2 packs/day	+0.5	+1.5
2+ packs/day	+0.7	+2.0

disturbance of iron metabolism where there is a block to the normal iron supply for the production of haemoglobin. Under normal conditions (without significant illness or poor iron intake), the body's iron stores vary tremendously with age, and differ between men and women (Cook *et al.*, 1974). However, unlike haemoglobin or red cell parameters, which are maintained within a narrow and normally distributed range (defined as the optimal distribution for healthy individuals with adequate iron status), there is a wide variation of iron stores, with no set physiological upper limit. For this reason, the developmental variation of iron stores, as reflected by the statistical distribution of serum ferritin values, is specific for the population under study and does not imply an optimal functional range, in contrast to the haemoglobin distribution. It is quite possible that among different populations of comparable age and sex, the statistical distribution of serum ferritin may vary because of variation in iron intake. Even though the upper end of the serum ferritin distribution may vary widely across age and between sex, there is a relatively narrow range of values at the lower end of the serum ferritin distribution that represents depleted iron stores. In fact, the range is so narrow that use of a common cut-off value can be justified for different ages and sexes. In general, when serum ferritin falls below 20 µg/l, the probability of abnormal results in other iron tests starts to increase (Yip *et al.*, 1983). When serum ferritin falls below 10–12 µg/l, it can be regarded as diagnostic for absent iron stores (Lipschitz *et al.*, 1974). There are few if any conditions that can cause falsely low serum ferritin values, and a low serum ferritin value is thus specific for iron depletion. However, the reverse is not true; a serum ferritin value above the range of iron depletion does not exclude iron deficiency. This is because serum ferritin is an acute phase reactant and tends to become elevated during infection or inflammation (Lipschitz *et al.*, 1974; see also Chapter 11).

3.2.1. Iron Stores during Infancy

Infants are born with an endowment of iron stores which is in proportion to birth weight (Widdowson and Spray, 1951). Because of this strong relationship between body iron endowment and birth weight, preterm infants become depleted of stored iron significantly earlier than term infants and hence are at greater risk of iron deficiency. Figure 13.4 details the changes of serum ferritin during the first year of life based on a study of healthy Finnish infants (Saarinen and Siimes, 1978). The relatively high level of body iron stores in the neonatal period reflects the iron endowment from the intrauterine period. The further rise in storage iron during the first few days of life is the result of rapid degradation of haemoglobin when the high red cell mass required for intrauterine oxygen transport is no longer needed for the extrauterine respiratory function. The iron from the degraded red cells further adds to the high iron stores at birth. However, these iron stores are usually depleted by 6 months of age as a result of tissue iron needs during this rapid growth period when the infant doubles in body weight by 3 to 4 months of age. The rapid decline of body iron stores can be viewed as a dilution effect – the existing iron in stores becomes distributed to a greater mass of tissue, including red cells, as iron absorbed from the gastrointestinal tract cannot keep pace with the requirement of rapid growth.

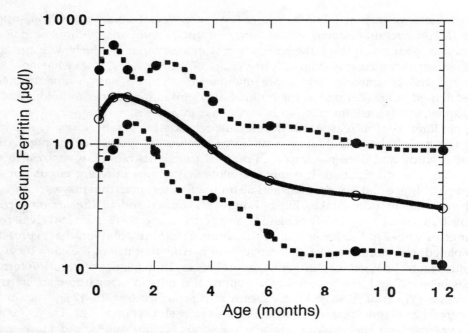

Fig. 13.4 Serum ferritin ranges (geometric mean ±2 SD) during infancy. Redrawn from Saarinen and Siimes (1978).

By 6 months of age, most infants have only marginal iron stores even when iron intake is regarded as adequate. It is not until 2–3 years of age when the growth rate has slowed down considerably that iron stores start to build up again. Even before the availability of the serum ferritin assay, the changing pattern of body iron stores for infants and younger children was well studied by Smith *et al.* (1955) who measured the liver iron content of autopsy specimens. They found iron content to be at its lowest between 12 and 24 months of age, corresponding to the age of the highest incidence of iron deficiency. This study demonstrated that iron stores do not become depleted until 6–12 months of age, and there is little risk of iron deficiency before 6 months of age. For this reason, screening for iron deficiency anaemia in a term infant under 6 months of age is not indicated. Because of the marginal iron stores by 6 months of age, it is from this age onwards that the risk of iron deficiency may warrant screening and iron supplementation for iron deficiency anaemia (see below).

3.2.2. Iron Stores during Childhood and Adolescence

Figure 13.5 shows the distribution of values for serum ferritin in a group of children less than 1 and up to 12 years of age for a group of children studied in Minneapolis, Minnesota (Deinard *et al.*, 1983). It is evident that serum ferritin distribution gradually shifted upwards with increasing age. The serum ferritin distribution of children between the ages of 1 and 2 years showed the greatest variation and the lowest value for the mean – 2 SD. Figure 13.6 (male) and Fig. 13.7 (female) detail the serum ferritin distributions from 3 years to adulthood based on the US sample of NHANES II

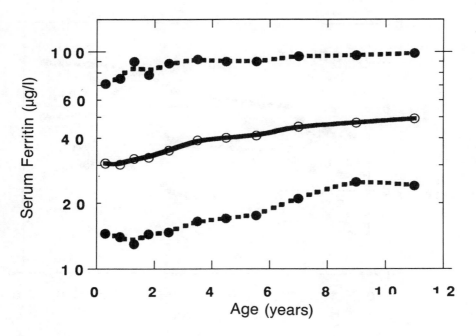

Fig. 13.5 Serum ferritin ranges (geometric mean ± 2 SD) during childhood. Redrawn from Deinard *et al.* (1983).

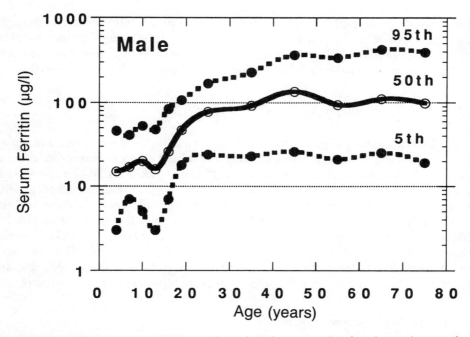

Fig. 13.6 Serum ferritin ranges (5th, 50th and 95th percentile) for the male sample of NHANES II after exclusion of subjects with low transferrin saturation and/or elevated erythrocyte protoporphyrin values.

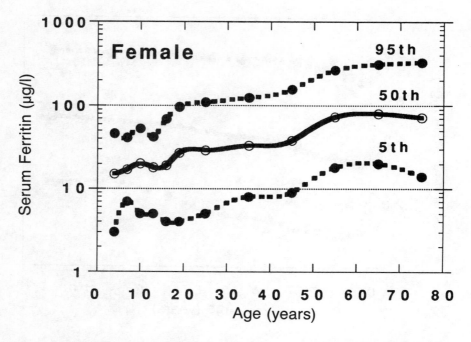

Fig. 13.7 Serum ferritin ranges (5th, 50th and 95th percentile) for the female sample of NHANES II after exclusion of subjects with low transferrin saturation and/or elevated erythrocyte protoporphyrin values.

after excluding individuals with abnormalities in other iron parameters (low transferrin saturation, low haemoglobin and high erythrocyte protoporphyrin). Until about 13–14 years of age, boys and girls have comparable serum ferritin values. After this age, males consistently have higher serum ferritin values than females.

3.2.3. Iron Stores during Adulthood

Figure 13.8 compares the geometric mean serum ferritin values of males and females in the US NHANES II sample after excluding individuals with low transferrin saturation and/or elevated erythrocyte protoporphyrin values. There are distinct sex-specific patterns of iron stores with increasing age: males have a progressive increase in serum ferritin until the fifth decade of life, whereas from adolescence females maintain a stable value which only increases after the fourth decade of life. The levelling off observed among elderly males from this US sample may be explained by the cross-sectional nature of the study, where different age groups represented different cohorts with different iron nutritional backgrounds. The changing pattern observed for women is probably the result of greater iron accumulation after cessation of menstruation.

3.2.4. Iron Stores during Pregnancy

The usual high iron requirement related to expanding red cell mass and tissue growth during pregnancy places an increased demand on iron stores. Even in women with

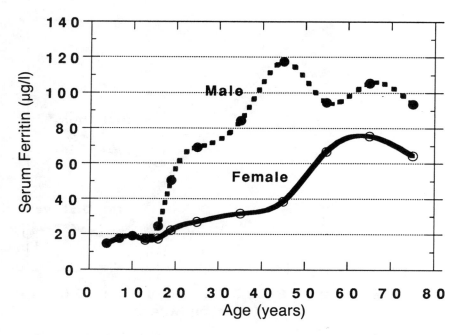

Fig. 13.8 Comparison of the geometric mean serum ferritin values in men and women. Data from NHANES II after exclusion of subjects with other abnormal iron test results.

a positive iron balance, most of the stored iron would be mobilized to meet this high requirement. Figure 13.9 illustrates the serum ferritin value throughout pregnancy for a group with adequate iron supplementation (Fenton et al., 1977). As with haemoglobin (Fig. 13.3) serum ferritin declined progressively throughout the first two-thirds of pregnancy and gradually rose toward the end of pregnancy (Fenton et al., 1977; Romslo et al., 1983). However, for those women who were not supplemented during pregnancy, the serum ferritin declined steadily throughout the entire pregnancy and, by the third trimester, the mean serum ferritin was in the range characteristic of iron depletion.

3.3. Age-related Variation of Transferrin Saturation and Erythrocyte Protoporphyrin

As with haemoglobin, two other commonly used laboratory iron parameters, transferrin saturation and erythrocyte protoporphyrin, vary significantly with age and appear to be independent of iron status (Koerper and Dallman, 1977; Deinard et al., 1983; Yip and Dallman, 1984; Yip et al., 1984). Unlike serum ferritin, which does not have a set upper limit, both of these tests appear to maintain a relatively narrow physiological range of values among healthy individuals with normal iron status. Figure 13.10 details the changes of transferrin saturation based on the US sample from the NHANES II study after excluding those individuals with abnormal haematological and elevated erythrocyte protoporphyrin values (Yip et al., 1984). During pregnancy, the transferrin saturation undergoes changes which parallel

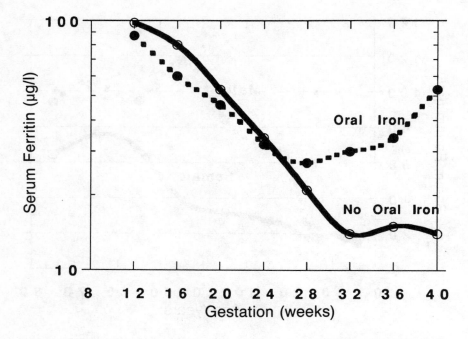

Fig. 13.9 Comparison of changes of mean serum ferritin values during pregnancy in women with and without oral iron supplementation. Redrawn from Fenton *et al.* (1977).

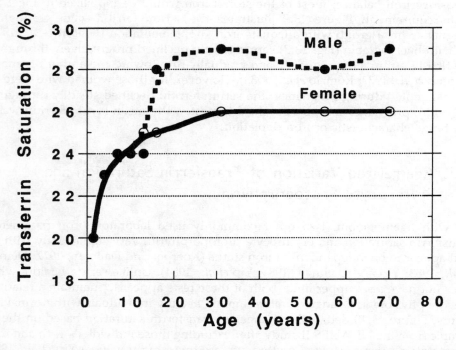

Fig. 13.10 Age- and sex-specific mean values for transferrin saturation in NHANES II. Redrawn from Yip *et al.* (1984).

those of serum ferritin: if iron intake is adequate, transferrin saturation continues to decline until the end of the second trimester and then starts to rise; if iron intake is inadequate, it continues to decline throughout the third trimester (Romslo *et al.*, 1983).

Elevated erythrocyte protoporphyrin indicates insufficient iron supply for haem synthesis (Yip *et al.*, 1983). However, there are other conditions that interfere with haem synthesis that are not related to iron deficiency, the most prominent example being exposure to lead. Apart from occupational lead exposure among certain industrial workers, the greatest risk of lead exposure occurs in young children, and this may give rise to protoporphyrin levels higher than those which would otherwise be expected in relation to their iron status (Yip and Dallman, 1984). Figure 13.11 details the developmental changes of erythrocyte protoporphyrin based on the US NHANES II sample (Yip *et al.*, 1984), excluding individuals with abnormal iron metabolism. Erythrocyte protoporphyrin remains relatively stable throughout pregnancy with iron supplementation, but shows a tendency to increase with advancing gestation if iron intake is insufficient (Schifman *et al.*, 1987).

4. AGE- AND SEX-SPECIFIC SUSCEPTIBILITY TO IRON DEFICIENCY

Even though there are a variety of iron related tests with well-defined reference ranges, the fact that each test reflects a different aspect of iron metabolism means that

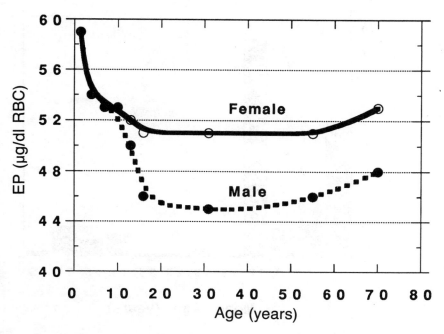

Fig. 13.11 Age- and sex-specific mean values for erythrocyte protoporphyrin in NHANES II. Redrawn from Yip *et al.* (1984).

444   R. YIP

there is no single test that can define iron status or diagnose iron deficiency with a high degree of certainty. One strategy to bypass the limitation of a single test in defining iron status is to utilize multiple iron related tests in parallel (see also Chapter 7). Those individuals with abnormalities in multiple tests have a greater likelihood of iron deficiency. Currently, there are two well accepted multiple-test models to define the likelihood of iron deficiency. Both models define a case as iron deficient or of 'impaired iron status' based on two or more abnormal tests out of three tests utilized (LSRO, 1985). One model is referred to as the MCV model, which uses MCV, transferrin saturation and erythrocyte protoporphyrin as the multiple tests, and the other as the ferritin model, which uses serum ferritin, transferrin saturation and erythrocyte protoporphyrin (LSRO, 1985). For epidemiological studies, if two of the three tests are in the abnormal range for defining iron deficiency, then a case would be regarded as iron deficient or of 'impaired iron status'. In some cases the term 'impaired iron status' is preferred because the combination of abnormal tests such as low transferrin saturation and elevated protoporphyrin can be the result of metabolic disturbance related to inflammation rather than nutritional iron deficiency. Figures 13.12 and 13.13 summarize the prevalence of iron deficiency in males and females, respectively, from the US NHANES II study. This study used a modified ferritin model where serum ferritin is required to be one of

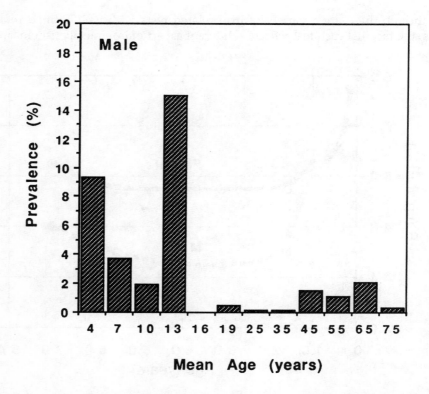

Fig. 13.12 Prevalence of iron deficiency in US males in relation to age, based on a modified serum ferritin model to define iron deficiency (NHANES II).

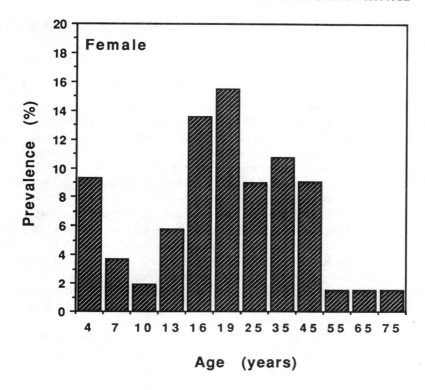

Fig. 13.13 Prevalence of iron deficiency in US females in relation to age, based on a modified serum ferritin model to define iron deficiency (NHANES II).

the abnormal tests in defining a case of iron deficiency. Because low serum ferritin is specific for iron deficiency, this modified approach can justify the definition of iron deficiency without resorting to use of the term impaired iron status. The criteria for each test within the model is based on the sex- and age-specific cut-off values (LSRO, 1985). It is evident that the ages of susceptibility to iron deficiency are during early childhood and for women during child-bearing years.

The greater susceptibility to iron deficiency in late infancy and early childhood is the net result of inadequate intake relative to the high iron requirements of rapid growth, and the gradual depletion of iron stores during infancy. Recent studies of Chilean infants demonstrated that the most important determinant of iron status in late infancy is the adequacy of the iron content of infant feeds (Pizarro *et al.*, 1991). Depending on the type of infant feeding, the need subsequently to screen for iron deficiency can differ. Use of cow's milk or formula without iron fortification presents the greatest risk for iron deficiency, but breast-feeding infants not receiving iron supplements should also be screened (Dallman and Yip, 1989). Infants fed with iron fortified formula have little or no risk for iron deficiency, and routine screening is therefore unnecessary. The use of screening tests in groups at high risk of iron deficiency is discussed further in Chapter 7.

5. INFLAMMATION-RELATED DISTURBANCES OF IRON METABOLISM

It is well known that a significant inflammatory process can cause interference of iron delivery for haem synthesis resulting in reduced haemoglobin level, elevated erythrocyte protoporphyrin, elevated serum ferritin level and reduced transferrin saturation (Chapter 11). This complex of metabolic changes related to the inflammatory process has been characterized as the 'anaemia of chronic disorders' (Cartwright, 1966). This process may cause particular confusion at two periods of life – during infancy and early childhood, and among the elderly – when it is often mistaken for nutritional iron deficiency anaemia.

In the case of infants and children, the inflammatory process is most commonly related to mild childhood infections. A study by Reeves *et al.* (1984) of 1-year-old infants illustrates that recent upper respiratory infections and otitis media are associated with elevated erythrocyte sedimentation rates and changes of iron metabolism characteristic of the anaemia of chronic disorders, even though these are relatively mild acute infections. Since younger children often suffer from common infections, many children may have mild anaemia as a result of illness-related changes in iron metabolism that can be misclassified as nutritional iron deficiency anaemia (Yip *et al.*, 1987). Among hospitalized children with severe infections and chronic inflammatory processes, it is well documented that many have a significant anaemia that fits the classic description of the anaemia of chronic disorders (Abshire and Reeves, 1983).

Among the elderly, the role of chronic disorders appears to play a major role in the observed decline of the mean haemoglobin level and the increased prevalence of anaemia with advancing age. In an earlier US survey (NHANES I) where erythrocyte sedimentation rates (ESR) were also measured, it was evident that elevated ESR, an indicator of inflammation, was closely associated with anaemia, and that among the elderly there was an increased proportion of individuals with an elevated ESR (Yip and Dallman, 1988). In that survey, the overall mean haemoglobin for men aged 60 to 69 years was 15.26 ± 1.36 g/dl, significantly lower than the mean haemoglobin of 15.73 ± 1.01 g/dl for the 20 to 29 year old group. However, if individuals with elevated ESR (> 20 mm/h) and low transferrin saturation ($< 16\%$) were excluded, the mean haemoglobin increased to 15.56 ± 1.19 g/dl for the 60 to 69 year old group, but remained unchanged for the 20 to 29 year old group because few of them had elevated ESR or low transferrin saturation. This evidence from the NHANES I study strongly suggests that changes in the parameters of iron metabolism such as haemoglobin level or transferrin saturation observed among elderly individuals are to a large extent related to chronic disease or to an inflammatory process, rather than normal developmental changes in iron metabolism. This proposition is further strengthened by the follow-up of the cohort of the NHANES I study after 17 years: those with low haemoglobin or low transferrin saturation levels had significantly higher mortality than those with normal haemoglobin and transferrin saturation (Yip, unpublished observation). Existing evidence suggests that the concept of 'normal ageing' of haematopoiesis may not be a correct explanation for the lower haemoglobin levels observed in the elderly population (Freedman and Marcus, 1980).

6. SUMMARY

From the discussion in this chapter, it is evident there are marked variations in measures of iron metabolism throughout the life cycle. Some of the variations can be attributed solely to developmental or physiological differences, and it is important to take them into account in the evaluation of iron status. Others are more directly related to changes in iron status, with differences in iron requirements at different periods of the life cycle, including increased susceptibility to iron deficiency during the high demand periods of infancy and pregnancy. Lastly, apart from the balance of iron intake and output, there are pathological factors, such as infections in childhood and chronic disorders among elderly, which can affect iron metabolism and potentially lead to misinterpretation of iron status. Awareness of these factors that can influence iron metabolism is essential in the evaluation and interpretation of measures of iron status.

REFERENCES

Abshire, T. C. and Reeves, J. D. (1983) Anemia of acute inflammation in children. *J. Pediatr.* **103**, 868–871.

Bothwell, T. H. and Charlton, R. W. (1981) Iron deficiency in women. A report of the International Nutritional Anaemia Consultative Group (INACG). The Nutrition Foundation, Washington, DC.

Cartwright, G. E. (1966) The anemia of chronic disorders. *Semin. Hematol.* **3**, 351–375.

CDC criteria for anemia in children and childbearing age women (1989) *MMWR* **38**, 400–404.

Cook, J. D., Lipschitz, D. A., Miles, L. E. and Finch, C. A. (1974) Serum ferritin as a measure of iron stores in normal subjects. *Am. J. Clin. Nutr.* **27**, 681–687.

Dallman, P. R. and Siimes, M. A. (1979) Percentile curves for hemoglobin and red cell volume in infancy and childhood. *J. Pediatr.* **94**, 26–31.

Dallman, P. R. and Yip, R. (1989) Changing characteristics of childhood anemia. *J. Pediatr.* **114**, 161–164.

Dallman, P. R., Siimes, M. A. and Stekel, A. (1980) Iron deficiency in infancy and childhood. *Am. J. Clin. Nutr.* **33**, 86–118.

Dallman, P. R., Yip, R. and Johnson, C. (1984) Prevalence and causes of anemia in the United States. *Am. J. Clin. Nutr.* **39**, 437–445.

Fenton, V., Cavill, I. and Fisher, J. (1977) Iron stores in pregnancy. *Br. J. Haematol.* **37**, 145–149.

Fomon, S. J., Ziegler, E. E., Nelson, S. E. and Edwards, B. (1981) Cow milk feeding in infancy: Gastrointestinal blood loss and iron nutritional status. *J. Pediatr.* **98**, 540–545.

Freedman, M. L. and Marcus, D. L. (1980) Anemia and the elderly: is it physiology or pathology? *Am. J. Med. Sci.* **280**, 81–85.

Hallberg, L., Hogdahl, A. M., Nilsson, L. and Rybo, G. (1966) Menstrual blood loss – a population study: variation at different ages and attempts to define normality. *Acta Obstet. Gynaec. Scand.* **45**, 320–351.

Hurtado, A., Merino, C. and Delgado, E. (1945) Influence of anoxemia on the hematopoietic activity. *Arch. Int. Med.* **75**, 284–323.

Irigoyen, M., Davidson, L. L., Damaris, C. and Seaman, C. (1991) Randomized, placebo-controlled trial of iron supplementation in infants with low hemoglobin levels fed iron fortified formula. *Pediatrics* **88**, 320–326.

Koerper, M. A. and Dallman, P. R. (1977) Serum iron concentration and transferrin saturation in the diagnosis of iron deficiency in children. *J. Pediatr.* **91**, 870–874.

LSRO (Life Science Research Office) Expert Scientific Working Group (1985) Summary of a report on assessment of the iron nutritional status of the United States population. *Am. J. Clin. Nutr.* **42**, 1318–1330.

Lipschitz, D. A., Cook, J. D. and Finch, C. A. (1974) A clinical evaluation of serum ferritin as an index of iron stores. *N. Engl. J. Med.* **290**, 1213–1216.

McFee, J. G. (1973) Anemia in pregnancy – a reappraisal. *Obstet. Gynecol. Surv.* **28**, 769–793.

Nordenberg, D. F., Yip, R. and Binkin, N. J. (1990) The effect of cigarette smoking on haemoglobin levels and the diagnosis of anemia. *JAMA* **264**, 1556–1559.

Perry, G. S., Byers, T., Yip, R. and Margen, S. (1992) Iron nutrition does not account for the hemoglobin differences between blacks and whites. *J. Nutr.* **122**, 1417–1424.

Pizarro, F., Yip, R., Dallman, P. R., Olivares, M., Hertrampf, E. and Walter T. (1991) Iron status with different infant feeding regimens: relevance to screening and prevention of iron deficiency. *J. Pediatr.* **118**, 687–692.

Puolakka, J., Janne, O., Pakarinen, A., Jarvinen, A. and Vihko, R. (1980) Serum ferritin as a measure of iron stores during and after normal pregnancy with and without iron supplements. *Acta Obstet. Gynecol. Scand. Suppl.* **95**, 43–51.

Reeves, J. D., Yip, R., Kiley, V. A. and Dallman, P. R. (1984) Iron deficiency in infants: The influence of mild antecedent infection. *J. Pediatr.* **105**, 874–879.

Romslo, I., Haram, K., Sagen, N. and Augensen, K. (1983) Iron requirement in normal pregnancy as assessed by serum ferritin, serum transferrin saturation and erythrocyte protoporphyrin determinations. *Br. J. Obstet. Gynaecol.* **90**, 101–107.

Saarinen, U. M. and Siimes, M. A. (1978a) Developmental changes in red blood cell counts and indices of infants after exclusion of iron deficiency by laboratory criteria and continued iron supplementation. *J. Pediatr.* **92**, 412–416.

Saarinen, U. M. and Siimes, M. A. (1978b) Serum ferritin in assessment of iron nutrition in healthy infants. *Acta Pediatr. Scand.* **67**, 745–751.

Schifman, R. B., Thomasson, J. E. and Evers, J. M. (1987) Red blood cell zinc protoporphyrin testing for iron-deficiency anemia in pregnancy. *Am. J. Obstet. Gynecol.* **157**, 304–307.

Sjosted, J. E., Manner, P., Nummi, S. and Ekenved, G. (1977) Oral iron prophylaxis during pregnancy – a comparative study on different dosage regimens. *Acta Obstet. Gynecol. Scand. Suppl.* **60**, 3–9.

Smith, J. R. and Landaw, S. R. (1978) Smokers' polycythemia. *N. Engl. J. Med.* **298**, 6–10.

Smith, N. J., Rosello, S., Say, M. B. and Yeya, K. (1955) Iron storage in the first five years of life. *Pediatrics* **16**, 166–173.

Stewart, J. G., Ahlquist, D. A., McGill, D. B., Ilstrup, D. M., Schwartz, S. and Owen, R. A. (1984) Gastrointestinal blood loss and anemia in runners. *Ann. Int. Med.* **100**, 843–845.

Svanberg, B., Arvidsson, B., Norrby, A., Rybo, G. and Solvell, L. (1976) Absorption of supplemental iron during pregnancy. A longitudinal study with repeated bone marrow studies and absorption measurements. *Acta Obstet. Gynecol. Scand. Suppl.* **48**, 87–108.

Taylor, D. J., Mallen, C., McDougall, N. and Lind, T. (1982) Effect of iron supplementation on serum ferritin levels during and after pregnancy. *Br. J. Obstet. Gynaecol.* **89**, 1011–1017.

Widdowson, E. M. and Spray, C. M. (1951) Chemical development in utero. *Arch. Dis. Child.* **26**, 205–214.

Yip, R. and Dallman, P. R. (1984) Developmental changes in erythrocyte protoporphyrin: the roles of iron deficiency and lead toxicity. *J. Pediatr.* **104**, 710–713.

Yip, R. and Dallman, P. R. (1988) The role of inflammation and iron deficiency as causes of anemia. *Am. J. Clin. Nutr.* **48**, 1295–1300.

Yip, R., Deinard, A. S. and Schwartz, S. (1983) Age-related changes in serum ferritin and erythrocyte protoporphyrin in normal (non-anemic) children. *Am. J. Clin. Nutr.* **38**, 71–76.

Yip, R., Johnson, C. and Dallman, P. R. (1984) Age-related changes in laboratory values used in the diagnosis of anemia and iron deficiency. *Am. J. Clin. Nutr.* **39**, 427–438.

Yip, R., Walsh, K. M., Goldfarb, M. G. and Binkin, N. J. (1987) Declining prevalence of anemia in childhood in a middle-class setting: a pediatric success story. *Pediatrics* **80**, 330–334.

14. Laboratory Determination of Iron Status

M. WORWOOD

Department of Haematology, University of Wales College of Medicine, Heath Park, Cardiff CF4 4XN, UK

I. INTRODUCTION: WHAT IS IRON STATUS?

The body of a normal, well-fed man contains about 4 g iron, most of which is found in haemoglobin (Chapter 2, Fig. 2.1). Among other functional iron compounds, muscle myoglobin accounts for about 10% of body iron, but the many other iron-containing enzymes (Wrigglesworth and Baum, 1980), such as the cytochromes and iron–sulfur proteins which take part in redox reactions throughout the tissues, account for only a small percentage of total iron. Transport iron, bound to transferrin in plasma and extravascular fluids, is also a very small fraction, and the remaining iron is the so-called storage iron, which represents the balance between uptake and loss. Men may have up to 2 g storage iron, although about 1 g is usual, but women of child-bearing age may have little or none.

Normal iron status may therefore be defined as the presence of sufficient haemoglobin in the circulation for normal physical activities and a small reserve of 'storage iron' to cope with 'normal' losses of iron due to menstruation and childbirth. The ability to cope with the more acute loss of blood (iron) which may result from injury is also an advantage. The limits of normality are difficult to define but the extremes of iron deficiency anaemia and iron overload are well understood.

Apart from too little or too much iron in the body there is also the possibility of a maldistribution of iron. An example is the anaemia often associated with inflammation or infection (Chapter 11) where there is partial failure of iron release from the phagocytic cells in liver, spleen and bone marrow, to circulating transferrin. This results in anaemia and accumulation of iron as ferritin and haemosiderin in phagocytic cells. Thus determination of iron status requires an estimate of the total amount of haemoglobin iron (usually by measuring the haemoglobin concentration in the blood) and the level of storage iron (Fig. 14.1). Though transport iron is quantitatively unimportant, measures of iron supply to the tissues may sometimes yield additional diagnostic information, particularly in assessing the likelihood of excessive iron uptake. Assays on blood samples are commonly used to assess all three compartments of body iron (functional, storage and transport). Occasionally, further investigations into iron loss (Chapter 7), iron absorption (Chapter 6) and flow rates within the body (Chapter 2) are also required. Reference values for measures of iron status are shown in Table 14.1.

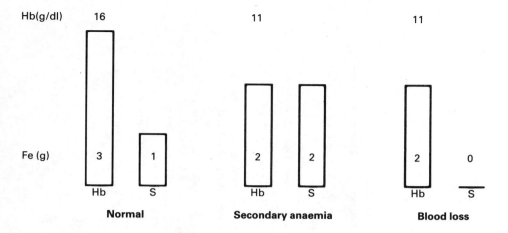

Fig. 14.1 Body iron: relationship between total haemoglobin iron (Hb) and storage iron (S) normally, in the anaemia of chronic disease, and in iron deficiency anaemia.

2. ASSESSMENT OF BODY IRON COMPARTMENTS

2.1. Haemoglobin and Red Cell Indices

The measurement of haemoglobin concentration is straightforward and well standardized (Dacie and Lewis, 1991). The method depends on the conversion of haemoglobin to cyanmethaemoglobin and determination of the absorbance at 540 nm. An international standard is widely available for calibration, and the measurement is included in the analysis provided by electronic blood cell counters in most haematology laboratories.

The investigation of anaemia must begin with a full blood count, since information about the different blood cell numbers and red cell size and haemoglobinization will give important diagnostic clues as to the aetiology of the anaemia. For example, the microcytic hypochromic red cells associated with impaired haemoglobin synthesis (e.g. with an inadequate iron supply) may be distinguished from the macrocytes associated with impaired nuclear maturation (e.g. due to B$_{12}$ or folate deficiency). The full blood count will also reveal clues to other causes of anaemia which require haematological investigation such as hypoproliferative disorders, a haemolytic process or the presence of thalassaemia or haemoglobinopathy. Modern automated cell counters provide a rapid and sophisticated way to detect the changes in red cells which accompany a reduced supply of iron to the bone marrow.

There are two basic principles of cell counting in common use: the optical method where the passage of a blood cell in a narrow channel interrupts a light or laser beam, and the electrical impedance method where the passage of a blood cell through a narrow aperture causes a change in current between electrodes (Williams, 1990). These machines provide measurement of red cell volume and haemoglobin content (although in different ways) and by counting large numbers of cells provide much greater accuracy than the manual techniques which they have largely replaced.

Table 14.1 Assessment of body iron status

Measurement	Representative reference range (adults)	Diagnostic Use
Functional iron		
Haemoglobin concentration – Males	13–18 g/dl	Assess severity of IDA; response to a therapeutic trial of iron confirms IDA. Not applicable to assessment of iron overload
– Females	12–16 g/dl	
Red cell indices – MCV	80–94 fl	
– MCH	27–32 pg	
Tissue iron supply		
Serum iron	10–30 μmol/l	Raised saturation of TIBC used to assess risk of tissue iron loading (e.g. in haemochromatosis or iron-loading anaemias)
Saturation of TIBC	16–60%	Decreased saturation of TIBC, reduced red cell ferritin, increased zinc protoporphyrin, and increased serum transferrin receptors indicate impaired iron supply to the erythroid marrow. Particular value in identifying early iron deficiency and, in conjunction with a measure of iron stores, distinguishing this from ACD
Red cell zinc protoporphyrin	<80 μmol/mol Hb (<70 μg/dl red cells)	
Red cell ferritin (basic)	3–40 ag/cell	
Serum transferrin receptor	2.8–8.5 mg/l	
Iron stores		
Quantitative phlebotomy	<2 g iron	All measures are positively correlated with iron stores except TIBC which is negatively correlated
Tissue biopsy iron – liver (chemical assay)	3–33 μmol/g dry weight	Quantitative phlebotomy, liver iron concentration, chelatable iron and MRI are of value only in iron overload
– bone marrow (Prussian Blue stain)	–	Bone marrow iron may be graded as absent, normal or increased, and is most commonly used to differentiate ACD from IDA. In IDA a raised TIBC is also characteristic
Serum ferritin	15–300 μg/l	Serum ferritin is of value throughout the range of iron stores
Urine chelatable iron (after 0.5 g I.M. desferrioxamine)	<2 mg/24 h	
Non-invasive methods (MRI, etc.)	–	
Serum TIBC/transferrin	47–70 μmol/l	

IDA, Iron deficiency anaemia; ACD, anaemia of chronic disorders; TIBC, total iron-binding capacity

The changes in red cell parameters associated with iron deficiency anaemia are well known – a low mean cell volume (MCV), mean cell haemoglobin (MCH) and a high red cell distribution width (RDW). These changes indicate a reduced supply of iron to the erythroblasts in the bone marrow but do not necessarily indicate an absence of storage iron. There is now considerable interest in detecting the very earliest changes which accompany the development of iron deficiency anaemia and this appears to be hypochromasia – the presence of red cells with a reduced haemoglobin content. Erythropoietin therapy is widely used to treat anaemia in patients with renal failure who are undergoing dialysis. In such patients the rapid regeneration of haemoglobin means that a functional iron deficiency may develop even though storage iron levels (as assessed by serum ferritin concentration) would be considered to be adequate. Macdougall *et al.* (1992) suggest that determination of the percentage of hypochromic red cells provides a simple and rapid way of detecting functional iron deficiency and preventing this by giving oral or parenteral iron.

Modern blood counters can thus indicate that the cause of anaemia is a reduced supply of iron to the bone marrow. Further tests are usually necessary to distinguish between simple iron deficiency (absence of storage iron) and a deficiency secondary to another disease process.

2.2. Methods for Estimating Iron Stores

The methods which have been used to estimate the level of iron stores are summarized in Table 14.1.

2.2.1. Quantitative Phlebotomy

The most accurate method for measuring iron stores is by quantitative phlebotomy (Haskins *et al.*, 1952; Weinfeld, 1970). This gives a measure of the amount of iron available for haemoglobin synthesis. Blood is removed at a rate of 500 ml/week so that most of the iron used for synthesis of replacement haemoglobin (250 mg Fe/week) is obtained from the stores rather than by absorption. After a number of venesections the subject is unable to maintain his or her normal haemoglobin level, and at this point it is assumed that the available iron stores have been used up. The total amount of iron removed is then calculated. Iron lost in reducing the haemoglobin level from the initial to the final value is calculated and a further correction is applied for the amount of iron absorbed during the study (Torrance and Bothwell, 1980). This pragmatic way of assessing iron stores has been applied to validate the concept that serum ferritin concentrations in normal subjects reflect the level of available storage iron (Walters *et al.*, 1973). It is also applied to the determination of the initial level of storage iron during treatment of haemochromatosis by phlebotomy (Chapter 8). However it has no practical applications otherwise. Furthermore 'available iron' may not always equate to the total amount of ferritin and haemosiderin iron in tissues. Torrance *et al.* (1968) have suggested that storage iron in muscle is not as readily available for mobilization as that at other sites. The amounts of storage iron detected by chemical estimation of iron concentration, quantitative phlebotomy and isotopic dilution analysis vary somewhat and the reasons for this have been discussed by Torrance and Bothwell (1980).

2.2.2. *Estimation of Tissue Iron Concentrations*

The liver and bone marrow are important and accessible storage sites and the amount of iron present can be estimated either visually, using the Prussian Blue reaction on tissue sections, or chemically. There is generally a good relationship between iron concentrations in liver and bone marrow (Gale *et al.*, 1963). Methods for chemical and histological assessment of tissue iron concentration have been described in detail by Torrance and Bothwell (1980). Most tissues contain significant amounts of functional haem iron compounds as well as storage non-haem iron, and methods which assess total liver iron (e.g. Barry and Sherlock, 1971) will therefore give an overestimate of iron stores, particularly when these are low. However, chemical determination of liver iron concentration is most widely applied to the demonstration of iron overload, where either total or non-haem iron determinations give a satisfactory assessment. Mean liver, non-haem iron concentrations lie between 80 and 300 μg (1.4–5.4 μmol)/g wet weight in most countries (Charlton *et al.*, 1970). The dry liver iron concentration is approximately four times that of wet liver (Frey *et al.*, 1968), and a reference range for total liver iron, based on 40 adult autopsy samples, is 3–33 μmol/g dry weight (Bassett *et al.*, 1986). The important distinction between the relatively minor elevations of liver non-haem iron sometimes found in patients with cirrhosis of the liver, and iron overload associated with inherited haemochromatosis, is discussed in Chapter 8. Estimation of iron concentration in bone marrow is, in contrast, usually by the histochemical method, and is often applied to the detection of iron deficiency. In particular, assessing marrow iron histologically distinguishes between 'true' iron deficiency and other chronic disorders in which there is accumulation of iron within reticuloendothelial cells (Chapter 11). However it should be noted that this is not a reliable way of diagnosing inherited haemochromatosis as the level of bone marrow iron is often within the normal range even when liver parenchymal iron concentrations are high.

Normal red cell precursors which contain some Prussian Blue staining granules in their cytoplasm are called sideroblasts and the number of sideroblasts is diminished in iron deficiency. Accurate sideroblast counts are tedious and are therefore rarely carried out. The absence of sideroblasts is diagnostic of an impairment of iron delivery to the developing red cells, and may be associated with a lack of storage iron but may also be found in a variety of acute and chronic inflammatory conditions. Ring sideroblasts are nucleated red cells with iron-loaded mitochondria. These are found in inherited or acquired sideroblastic anaemias and their detection is important in the haematological investigation of these conditions (Chapter 9).

2.2.3. *Chelatable Iron*

Some indication of storage iron levels is given after the intramuscular injection of an iron chelator such as desferrioxamine (Chapter 12) and determination of the amount of iron excreted in the urine. There has been considerable debate about the origin of the chelated iron – either parenchymal or from reticuloendothelial cells. Torrance and Bothwell (1980) concluded that desferrioxamine can chelate both parenchymal and reticuloendothelial iron, with the major source being the hepatocyte in inherited haemochromatosis and the reticuloendothelial cell in conditions associated with ineffective erythropoiesis.

Chelator-induced iron excretion is not useful for the detection of iron deficiency but may provide a useful way of confirming the diagnosis of iron overload (Chapters 8 and 9).

2.2.4. Serum Ferritin

(a) *Methodology*. It was only after the development of a sensitive immunoradiometric assay (IRMA) that ferritin was detected in normal serum or plasma (Addison *et al.*, 1972). The original assay was simple in concept but tedious and very dependent on reagent quality, and did not attract much attention until the introduction of the '2-site IRMA' (Miles *et al.*, 1974). Reliable assays, both RIA (labelled ferritin) and IRMA (labelled antibody), have been described in detail (Worwood, 1980). More recently radioactive labels have been supplanted by enzyme-linked immunoassays (ELISA) with colorimetric and fluorescent substrates, or by antibodies with chemi-luminescent labels. The solid phase may be a tube, bead, microtitre plate or (magnetic) particle. Numerous variations have been described and serum ferritin is included in the latest batch and random access automated analysers for immunoassay. A simple, enzyme-linked assay with standard reagents has been described and may have application as a reference method (Worwood *et al.*, 1991b) in evaluating automated methods.

Overall assay times have now been reduced to a few hours, and labour and reagent costs are clearly of primary importance. However, there are technical considerations which need to be evaluated when introducing any new procedure.

(i) Limit of detection

Two-site immunoradiometric assays are intrinsically more sensitive than radio-immunoassays. For example, concentrations of ferritin in buffer solution as low as $0.01 \, \mu g/l$ may be detected. Serum effects (see below) require dilution of samples, however, and for practical purposes, the lower limit of detection is of the order of $1 \, \mu g/l$. For some radioimmunoassays limits of detection may approach $10 \, \mu g/l$ and this may cause difficulties in using the assay for detection of iron deficiency. This point should be examined carefully. The detection limits for enzyme-linked assays are now usually adequate.

(ii) The 'high dose hook'

This is a problem peculiar to labelled antibody assays, particularly two-site immunoradiometric assays. As the amount of ferritin added increases, the radio-activity bound to the solid phase increases to a maximum and then declines with increasing ferritin concentrations. Two causes have been suggested (Rodbard *et al.*, 1978): (a) heterogeneity of the solid phase antiserum; and (b) incomplete washing after the first reaction (binding of ferritin to the solid phase). Exhaustive washing may move the 'hook' to higher ferritin concentrations (Casey *et al.*, 1979) but does not usually eliminate it. Our experience is that selection of high affinity antibodies for the first reaction is not effective and the hook effect is also seen with a monoclonal antibody (Perera and Worwood, 1984a). A related phenomenon is seen with labelled antibody assays in which ferritin is incubated with the solid phase antibody and labelled antibody simultaneously. At high concentrations of ferritin the solution phase reaction is so rapid that little ferritin binds to the solid phase and a 'hook' is seen (Perera and Worwood, 1984b). If a 'hook effect' is present then the only safe procedure is to assay each sample at two dilutions in order to be certain that the upward part of the calibration curve has been selected. In view of the wide range of serum ferritin concentrations which may be encountered in hospital patients (0–40 000 μg/l) this is, in any case, a good practice.

(iii) Serum effects

These may be found with any method but particularly with labelled antibody assays. It is usually found that the serum proteins inhibit the binding of ferritin to the solid phase when compared with the binding in buffer solutions alone. Serum effects may be avoided by diluting the standards in a buffer containing a suitable serum and by diluting serum samples as much as possible (Miles et al., 1974). For example, for the two-site immunoradiometric assay with rabbit antiferritin serum, the sample may be diluted 20 times with buffer while the standards are prepared in 5% normal rabbit serum in buffer. Further dilutions of the sera are carried out with this solution. Occasionally human sera may be found which appear to contain antibodies to the species used to make the antiferritin antibodies. Dilution of standards and samples with serum of the same species should prevent interference with the assay of ferritin.

(iv) Reproducibility

Most assays are satisfactory, but this must always be established for any method introduced into the laboratory. Particular problems may be encountered with enzyme-linked assays which have microtitre plates as the solid phase. Edge effects and assay drift need to be eliminated.

(v) Dilution of serum samples

It should be established that both standard and serum samples dilute in parallel over at least a ten-fold range.

(vi) Accuracy

The use of a reference ferritin preparation to calibrate the assay is recommended. The second WHO reference for the assay of serum ferritin is reagent 80/578 (ICSH, 1984). This may be obtained from the National Institute of Biological Standards and Control, PO Box 1193, Potters Bar, Herts EN6 3QH, UK. There is a small handling charge.

(b) *Relationship with iron status (Worwood, 1982)*. Serum ferritin concentrations are normally within the range 15–300 μg/l, are lower in children than adults, and from puberty to middle age mean concentrations are higher in men than in women (Chapter 13). In older men and women, mean concentrations are similar. Good correlations have been found between serum ferritin concentrations and storage iron mobilized by phlebotomy, stainable iron in the bone marrow, and the concentration of both non-haem iron and ferritin in the bone marrow. This suggests a close relationship between the total amount of storage iron and serum ferritin concentration in normal individuals. Serum ferritin concentrations are relatively stable in healthy persons (but see later). In patients with iron deficiency anaemia, serum ferritin concentrations are less than 15 μg/l, and a reduction in the level of reticuloendothelial stores is the only common cause of a low serum ferritin concentration. This is the key to the use of the serum ferritin assay in clinical practice.

In infection, inflammation and chronic disease in which iron is transferred from haemoglobin to the reticuloendothelial stores, the increased level of storage iron is reflected in the serum ferritin concentration (compare this with the fall in serum iron discussed below). The serum ferritin concentration can be used in these circumstances to assess the adequacy of the iron stores. Unfortunately, interpretation of serum ferritin concentrations in patients with chronic disease is not quite as straightforward as this and the use of the assay in clinical practice is discussed later.

Iron overload causes high concentrations of serum ferritin, but so may liver disease and some forms of cancer. High concentrations of serum ferritin can only be ascribed to iron overload after careful consideration of the clinical situation; a normal serum ferritin concentration, however, provides good evidence against iron overload. Serum ferritin concentrations are always high in patients with advanced idiopathic haemochromatosis, but the serum ferritin assay alone should not be used for screening for the disorder (Chapter 8).

(c) *Biochemistry and physiology of plasma ferritin.* (See also Chapter 4) Immunologically plasma ferritin resembles liver or spleen ferritin. Only low concentrations of ferritin are usually measurable with antibodies to heart or HeLa cell ferritin (Hann et al., 1988; Worwood, 1990). Plasma ferritin from patients with iron overload (Worwood et al., 1976; Cragg et al., 1981) has a low iron content (0.02–0.07 µg Fe/µg protein) compared with 0.2 µg Fe/µg protein in the liver and spleen of such patients. By immunoprecipitation, Pootrakul et al. (1988) found a mean value of 0.06 µg Fe/µg protein in normal subjects. On isoelectric focusing both native and purified serum ferritin display a wide range of isoferritins encompassing the isoelectric points found in both liver and heart (McKeering et al., 1976; Worwood et al., 1976), yet on anion exchange chromatography it behaves as a relatively basic isoferritin (Worwood et al., 1976). This seems to be due to glycosylation rather than variation in the ratio of H- to L-subunits as about 60% of ferritin from normal serum binds to the lectin concanavalin A, whereas tissue ferritins show little binding (Worwood et al., 1979). On incubation with neuraminidase the acidic isoferritins of serum are converted to the more basic isoferritins, whereas tissue isoferritins are unaffected (Cragg et al., 1980). It has been shown that ferritin from plasma of patients with iron overload has an additional subunit (which has been called the G-subunit), which stains for carbohydrate and has an apparent molecular weight of 23 000 (Cragg et al., 1981; Santambrogio et al., 1987).

The origin of plasma ferritin is not known. The presence of glycosylation suggests secretion of ferritin, possibly from phagocytic cells degrading haemoglobin. This possibility is supported by the very high ferritin levels in patients demonstrating erythrophagocytosis (Esumi et al., 1988) and studies in rats which indicate that macrophages release ferritin after erythrophagocytosis (Kleber et al., 1978; Kondo et al., 1988; Rama et al., 1988; Sibille et al., 1988). However, there is no evidence for such release in cultured human macrophages (Custer et al., 1982). In liver disease another mechanism is clearly important: that of direct release of cellular ferritin through damaged cell membranes. In patients with ferritinaemia due to necrosis of the liver very little of the plasma ferritin binds to concanavalin A (Worwood et al., 1979). Various isoferritins may also be cleared from the circulation at different rates. On injection of ^{131}I-labelled spleen ferritin into two normal subjects it was found that clearance was very rapid ($T_{1/2}$ approximately 9 min), with uptake and degradation of ferritin by the liver (Cragg et al., 1983). Rapid clearance of liver ferritin has also been found in dogs (Pollock et al., 1978). ^{131}I-labelled plasma ferritin was removed only slowly from the plasma and radioactivity had only decreased by 50% after 30 h (Worwood et al., 1982). Rapid clearance of tissue isoferritins may be initiated by interaction with ferritin-binding proteins in the plasma (Covell et al., 1984; Bellotti *et al.*, 1987; Santambrogio and Massover, 1989). It is not known how such findings relate to the demonstration of ferritin receptors on liver parenchymal cells (Halliday *et al.*, 1979; Adams *et al.*, 1988) which, at least in the rat, have a higher affinity for liver ferritin than serum ferritin. Many isoferritins are released into the plasma but the only ones which accumulate are L_{24} molecules and glycosylated molecules which are also rich in L-subunits and contain little iron (Fig. 14.2). It should be noted that clearance studies with labelled, purified ferritins described above have not confirmed estimates of plasma ferritin turnover derived from measurements of plasma ferritin during exchange transfusions (Siimes *et al.*, 1975). In these studies plasma ferritin half-lives ranging from 3–95 min have been estimated. However, it is possible that in the neonatal period there are differences in both properties of ferritin in the plasma and clearance mechanisms. Similar studies in two adults with lysinuric protein intolerance gave computed ferritin half-lives of 65 and 95 mins (Rajantie *et al.*, 1981) and it was suggested that the high plasma ferritins in these patients (with low iron stores) may be due to an impaired clearance from the plasma.

2.2.5. *Detection of Iron Overload – Non-invasive Techniques*

Despite the range of biochemical assays available for the investigations of levels of storage iron major practical problems remain. Although determination of transferrin saturation and serum ferritin will identify almost all cases of inherited haemo-chromatosis with hepatic iron overload there will be many 'false positives'. A high

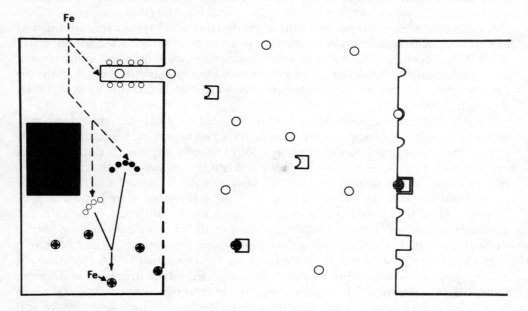

Fig. 14.2 Cytosolic ferritin (◉) is released directly (bottom left-hand cell) from damaged cell membranes into plasma or secreted (top) after synthesis on membrane-bound polysomes and glycosylation (○). In the circulation non-glycosylated ferritin may interact with ferritin-binding proteins followed by removal of the complex from the circulation. Many cells also carry ferritin receptors (see text). Injection of spleen ferritin into the circulation in man is followed by rapid uptake by the liver (Worwood, 1990). Reproduced with permission from Longman Group.

proportion are eliminated by a repeat test but in the remainder confirmation of iron overload can only be achieved by liver biopsy and iron determination, or by venesection. What is required is a sensitive, non-invasive technique which can quantitate liver iron concentration within and above the normal range.

There is the same requirement for monitoring the treatment of transfusional iron overload by chelation. Although a falling serum ferritin concentration indicates effective treatment it may be due to a reduction in tissue iron concentration, an improvement in liver function, or both.

Three scanning methods have been adapted for determining tissue iron content. Their application to the diagnosis and screening of patients with iron overload is discussed in Chapters 8 and 9.

  (i) Dual-energy computed tomography relates X-ray attenuation to liver iron levels but so far does not have sufficient sensitivity for quantitation of liver iron within the clinically important range (Howard et al., 1983; Stark, 1991).

 (ii) The magnetic susceptibility of liver iron can be measured accurately by means of superconducting quantum interference (SQUID). This allows quantitation of iron levels in the normal to mildly elevated range (Brittenham et al., 1982) but only two such instruments (one in USA and one in Germany) are currently available for investigation of patients.

(iii) Magnetic resonance imaging (MRI) is now in widespread use in hospitals. Interest in detection of iron overload has followed from the early demonstration that iron overload caused a reduction in signal intensity of the liver. Later it was shown that there was selective enhancement of transverse relaxation (T2) but none of longitudinal relaxation. The enhancement of the T2 relaxation rate (1/T2) gave a linear relationship with tissue iron levels from 250–3000 μg/g (Stark, 1991). Although MR imaging can distinguish between the predominantly parenchymal iron overload of inherited haemochromatosis and the reticuloendothelial distribution of secondary iron overload it still lacks the sensitivity to detect early iron overload and follow treatment (Kaltwasser et al., 1990; Gomori et al., 1991).

2.3. Measures of Iron Supply to the Tissues

The various measures used to assess the transport iron fraction and the adequacy of iron delivery to the tissues are shown in Table 14.1.

2.3.1. Serum Iron, Total Iron-binding Capacity and Percentage Saturation

(a) *Methodology*. The assay of serum iron and the saturation of transferrin with iron have been intensively investigated since the 1950s (ICSH, 1972). The International Committee for Standardization in Hematology (Expert Panel on Iron) has recommended a reference method which is simple and reliable (ICSH, 1978b, 1990). This requires the simultaneous precipitation of serum proteins and the release of iron from transferrin (in the presence of a reducing agent) in the ferrous state. This is followed by centrifugation to remove denatured protein and detection of the iron in the supernatant by adding a chromogen (originally bathophenanthroline but now ferrozine). The method avoids non-specific absorbance caused by interference with serum proteins and there is relatively little interference by copper. However when EDTA anti-coagulated blood is used to prepare plasma at least 15 min should be allowed for colour formation (INACG, 1985). Methods which do not require centrifugation have obvious advantages in terms of automation, and techniques in which iron is released from transferrin without precipitating serum proteins are also widely applied (for example, Persijn et al., 1971). Conditions must be carefully controlled to allow rapid and complete release of iron from transferrin while maintaining the released iron in soluble form and without denaturing protein. It is also necessary to run a 'blank' sample (without chromogen) in order to allow for absorbance due to the serum proteins. Procedures for measuring serum iron are available for most clinical chemistry autoanalysers but it is advisable to validate the method selected by comparison with the reference method (ICSH, 1990). Serum iron concentrations may also be measured by atomic absorption spectroscopy but this has the disadvantage of measuring any form of iron present, including haem or ferritin.

(b) *Relationship with iron status*. Measurement of the serum iron concentration alone provides little useful clinical information because of the considerable variation from hour to hour and day to day in normal individuals (see later). Transferrin iron is only 0.1% of the total body iron, and the transferrin iron pool turns over 10 to 20 times each day. Changes in supply and demand due to infection, inflammation, or surgery therefore cause rapid changes in serum iron concentration. The serum iron concentration is normally within the range of 10 to 30 μmol/l. Concentrations below the normal range are found in patients with iron deficiency anaemia, and those above the normal range are found in patients with iron overload (Bothwell et al., 1979). However many hospital patients have a low serum iron concentration which is a response to inflammation, infection, surgery or chronic disease. Low serum iron concentrations do not therefore necessarily indicate an absence of storage iron. High concentrations are found in liver disease, conditions associated with marrow hypoplasia, ineffective erythropoiesis and iron overload.

(c) *Total iron-binding capacity/transferrin*. More information may be obtained by measuring both the serum iron concentration and the total iron-binding capacity (TIBC), from which the percentage of transferrin saturation with iron may be calculated. The TIBC is a measurement of transferrin concentration and may be estimated by saturating the transferrin iron-binding capacity with excess iron and removing the excess unbound iron with solid magnesium carbonate, charcoal or an ion exchange resin. This is followed by determination of the iron content of the saturated serum. The unsaturated iron-binding capacity (UIBC) may be determined by methods which detect iron remaining, and able to bind to chromogen, after adding a standard excess iron to the serum and incubating for sufficient time to saturate the binding sites (Persijn et al., 1971). The problems inherent in these direct assays have been summarized by Bothwell et al. (1979). An alternative technique involves the addition of radioactive iron in order to saturate the binding sites followed by measurement of the radioactivity present in the supernatant after treatment with $MgCO_3$ and centrifugation (Fielding, 1980). As for the serum iron determination, protocols for clinical chemistry analysers often include a method for UIBC. Such methods should be validated with standard techniques (ICSH, 1978a, 1990). An alternative approach is to measure transferrin directly by an immunological assay. Nephelometric methods are the most rapid and easily automated and there is generally a good correlation between the chemical and immunological TIBC (Huebers *et al.*, 1987). However, Bandi *et al.* (1985) reported great variability among a number of immunochemical assays for transferrin.

TIBC (or transferrin) concentrations are inversely related to iron stores (Chapter 1): a raised TIBC (greater than 70 μmol/l or 390 μg/dl) is characteristic of a deficiency of storage iron, while normal or reduced values may be seen in iron overload or in association with the anaemia of chronic diseases.

(d) *Transferrin saturation*. A transferrin saturation of 16% or less is usually considered to indicate an inadequate iron supply for erythropoiesis (Bainton and Finch, 1964). The closer correlation of iron supply with transferrin saturation than with serum iron concentration probably reflects the importance of the higher proportion of iron present as diferric transferrin as transferrin saturation increases, since this has a greater affinity for transferrin receptors on the cell surface than monoferric transferrin (Chapters 2 and 3). A low transferrin saturation is a feature of iron deficiency, but is also sometimes found in inflammation, infection, etc., as mentioned above. The measurement of TIBC or transferrin may sometimes lead to an apparent saturation of greater than 100% if there is non-transferrin iron present in the serum. Such non-transferrin iron may be ferritin if there is significant liver damage which releases ferritin into the blood. Some of the ferritin iron may be assayed in the determination of serum iron (Pootrakul *et al.*, 1988). Other low molecular weight forms of iron may also be present in iron-overload patients (Grootveld *et al.*, 1989; Singh *et al.*, 1989). It is possible that such iron is potentially damaging to tissues and its measurement may provide a useful index of potential toxicity in iron overload (Hershko and Peto, 1987).

These measurements of serum iron, which for many years formed the basis of much clinical investigation of iron metabolism, are now seen to provide an inadequate index of storage iron and for this purpose they have been to a large extent replaced by the assay of serum ferritin. In screening for idiopathic haemochromatosis, however, it is essential to measure both the serum iron concentration and the TIBC (or transferrin concentration) and to calculate the percentage of saturation (Chapter 8).

2.3.2. *Erythrocyte Protoporphyrin*

This assay has been performed for many years as a screening test for lead poisoning. More recently, there has been considerable interest in its use in evaluating the iron supply to the bone marrow. The protoporphyrin concentration of red blood cells increases in iron deficiency. A widely used technique directly measures the fluorescence of zinc protoporphyrin (μmol/mol haem) in an instrument called a haematofluorometer (Labbe and Rettmer, 1989). The small sample size (about 20 μl of venous or skin-puncture blood), simplicity, rapidity and reproducibility within a laboratory are advantages. However, the necessity to transfer drops of blood to glass slides and dispose of the slides safely means that the procedure is too time-consuming and potentially dangerous to be suitable for laboratories processing large numbers of samples. Presumably automation would overcome these problems. Furthermore, the test has an interesting retrospective application. Because it takes some weeks for a significant proportion of the circulating red blood cells to be replaced with new cells, it is possible to make a diagnosis of iron deficiency anaemia some time after iron therapy has commenced. Chronic diseases that reduce serum iron concentration, but do not reduce iron stores, also increase protoporphyrin levels (Hastka *et al.*, 1993).

The measurement of erythrocyte protoporphyrin levels as an indicator of iron deficiency has particular advantages in paediatric haematology and in large-scale surveys in which the small sample size and simplicity of the test are important. The normal range in adults is $<80\,\mu$mol/mol haem. In the general clinical laboratory, however, it provides less information about iron storage levels in anaemic patients than the serum ferritin assay and no help in the diagnosis of iron overload.

2.3.3. Red Cell Ferritin

The ferritin in the circulating erythrocyte is but a tiny residue of that present in its nucleated precursors in the bone marrow. Normal erythroblasts contain ferritin which is immunologically more similar to heart than liver ferritin (i.e. ferritin rich in H-subunits) and mean concentrations are about 10 fg ferritin protein/cell (Hodgetts *et al.*, 1986). Concentrations decline in late erythroblasts, decline further in reticulocytes and only about 10 ag/cell (10^{-18} g/cell) remains in the erythrocyte (measured with antibodies to L-ferritin), again with somewhat higher levels detected with antibodies to H-type ferritin (Cazzola *et al.*, 1983; Peters *et al.*, 1983). Red cell ferritin concentrations have been measured in many disorders of iron metabolism, usually with antibodies to L-ferritin. In general red cell ferritin levels reflect the iron supply to the erythroid marrow and tend to vary inversely with red cell protoporphyrin levels (Cazzola *et al.*, 1983). Thus in patients with rheumatoid arthritis and anaemia low values of red cell ferritin are found in those with microcytosis and low serum iron concentrations regardless of the serum ferritin levels (Davidson *et al.*, 1984). Red cell ferritin levels do not therefore necessarily indicate levels of storage iron. It has however been noted that red cell ferritin levels may be useful in the differential diagnosis of hereditary haemochromatosis from alcoholic liver disease (van der Weyden *et al.*, 1983) and possibly in distinguishing heterozygotes for haemochromatosis from normal subjects (Cazzola *et al.*, 1983). Van der Weyden *et al.* (1983) found that the mean red cell ferritin content in patients with untreated inherited haemochromatosis was about 70 times the normal mean and fell during phlebotomy. However, in some patients levels were still elevated after phlebotomy even when serum ferritin concentrations were within the normal range. This was shown to reflect liver parenchymal cell iron concentrations which were still elevated. Van der Weyden *et al.* (1983) showed that the ratio of red cell ferritin (ag/cell) to serum ferritin (μg/l) was about 0.5 in hereditary haemochromatosis but only 0.03 in patients with alcoholic cirrhosis thus clearly separating the two conditions. There may also be advantages over the assay of serum ferritin in determining iron stores in patients with liver damage as red cell ferritin levels should not be greatly influenced by the release of ferritin from damaged liver cells. It should be noted that high levels of red cell ferritin are also found in thalassaemia (Piperno *et al.*, 1984; van der Weyden *et al.*, 1989), megaloblastic anaemia (Yamada *et al.*, 1983; van der Weyden and Fong, 1984) and myelodysplastic syndromes (Peters *et al.*, 1983) presumably indicating a disturbance of erythroid iron metabolism in these conditions.

Despite these specific, diagnostic advantages (Cazzola and Ascari, 1986) the assay of red cell ferritin has seen little routine application. This is because it is necessary to have fresh blood in order to prepare red cells free of white cells (which have much higher ferritin levels).

2.3.4. Serum Transferrin Receptor

Immunoreactive transferrin receptors are detectable in the circulation by immunoassay and, in the absence of iron deficiency, appear to reflect the level of bone marrow erythropoiesis (Cazzola and Beguin, 1992). This is potentially of considerable value as it provides an alternative to the very cumbersome ferrokinetic studies which were previously necessary (Chapter 2), and a guide to the pathophysiological classification of anaemia for clinical purposes. The serum transferrin receptor level also provides a sensitive indicator of an early impairment of iron delivery to the erythron in subjects with absent iron stores but who have not yet developed iron deficiency anaemia (Skikne et al., 1990). As well as being quantitatively related to the degree of tissue iron deficiency, the serum transferrin receptor distinguishes any anaemia due to iron deficiency from that associated with chronic disease (Chapter 7) (Cook et al., 1993). The levels determined depend on the assay and a mean normal concentration of 250 μg/l has been reported by Kohgo et al. (1987) but a mean level of 5600 μg/l by Flowers et al. (1989). These differences reflect the application of different monoclonal antibodies. The combination of serum transferrin receptor and ferritin may provide a quantitative measure of body iron over a broad range from tissue iron deficiency to iron overload (Cook et al., 1993).

3. VARIABILITY OF ASSAYS

3.1. Methodological and Biological Variability

The blood assays vary greatly in both methodological and biological stability. Haemoglobin concentrations are stable and the simple and well-standardized method of determination (Dacie and Lewis, 1991) ensures relatively low day-to-day variation in individuals (Table 14.2). Automated cell counters analyse at least 10 000 cells and thus reduce errors. The more complicated procedures involved in immunoassays mean higher methodological variation for ferritin assays (CV around 5%) and this, coupled with some physiological variation, gives an overall coefficient of variation for serum ferritin for an individual over a period of weeks of the order of 15%. There is however little evidence of any significant diurnal variation in serum ferritin concentration (Dawkins et al., 1979). The serum iron determination has a contrast between reasonably low methodological variation and extreme physiological variability, giving an overall 'within subject' CV of approximately 30% when venous samples are taken at the same time of day. A diurnal rhythm has been reported with higher values in the morning than in late afternoon when the concentration may fall to 50% of the morning value (Bothwell et al., 1979). The circadian fluctuation is due largely to variation in the release of iron from the reticuloendothelial system to the plasma. Results from a number of more recent studies of overall variability are given in Table 14.2 but it should be noted that the type of blood sample, length of study period and statistical analysis vary from study to study. The somewhat

Table 14.2 Overall variability of assays for iron status: within-subject, day-to-day CV (%) for healthy subjects

Reference	Haemoglobin	Serum ferritin	Serum iron	TIBC	EP
Dawkins et al. (1979)	—	15 (MF)	—	—	—
Gallagher et al. (1989)	1.6(F)	15F	—	—	—
Statland and Winkel (1977)	—	—	29(F)	—	—
Statland et al. (1976)	—	—	27(M)	—	—
Statland et al. (1977)	3(MF)	—	29(MF)	—	—
Pilon et al. (1981)	—	15(MF)	29(MF)	—	—
Romslo and Talstad* (1988)	—	13(MF)	33(MF)	11(MF)	12(MF)
Borel et al. (1991)	4(MF)	14(M)	27(M)	—	—
		26(F)	28(M)	—	—

*Hospital patients
F, female; M, male.

higher variability for Hb and ferritin reported by Borel et al. (1991) may be due to their use of capillary blood and plasma. Pootrakul et al. (1983) have demonstrated that mean plasma ferritin concentration is slightly higher in capillary specimens than venous specimens and that within and between sample variation was approximately three times greater. Variability was less in capillary serum but still greater than venous serum.

These results have clear implications for the use of these assays in population studies (Dallman, 1984; Looker et al., 1990; Wiggers et al., 1991) or in the assessment of patients (Borel et al., 1991). For accurate diagnosis either a multiparameter analysis is required or the assay of several samples. However, in hospital practice decisions are usually based on the analysis of a single blood sample without formal consideration of the effects of either methodological or biological variation and this limits interpretation to a semiquantitative approach at best.

3.2. Developmental Changes

The use of all the blood assays in clinical practice requires an understanding of the changes which take place during development. Figure 14.3 summarizes these in terms of percentage change from mean or median adult male values, and Chapter 13 gives a full account of changes in iron metabolism with age.

4. APPLICATION OF BLOOD ASSAYS FOR DETERMINATION OF IRON STATUS

Two important applications need to be considered. The first is in population surveys and the second in the evaluation of individual patients in hospital or general practitioner clinic. Details of the use of blood assays in the detection of iron deficiency and iron overload are discussed in Chapters 7 and 8 respectively.

% change

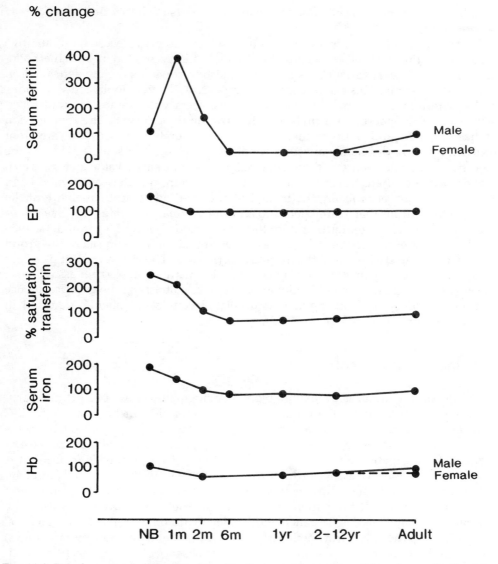

Fig. 14.3 Developmental changes in blood indicators of iron status. Mean (or median) values for normal subjects are expressed as a percentage of adult male mean (median). Median values have been taken for ferritin, per cent saturation and serum iron: means for EP and Hb. This figure is intended to give an impression of changes and shows the great variation in ferritin and transferrin saturation which reflect corresponding changes in the level of storage iron. Erythrocyte protoporphyrin (EP) levels are remarkably constant in non-anaemic subjects. Detailed information is given in Chapter 13.

4.1. Population Surveys

In considering a population survey, factors other than variation in iron stores which might influence the analytes should be considered. In older people there may be a higher incidence of chronic disease or in some parts of the world infection may be prevalent.

The serum ferritin assay is the only method which can provide a semiquantitative indication of the levels of storage iron but its application is limited by both methodological and biological variation. A common question concerns the incidence of iron deficiency anaemia. This can be assessed simply from haemoglobin concentrations or by determining the number of anaemic subjects with values for transferrin saturation, ZPP or serum ferritin below the lower limit of normal. The combination of haemoglobin and another measurement considerably reduces the apparent incidence of iron deficiency anaemia (Cook et al., 1986). The same applies to the detection of iron deficiency without anaemia, the use of a single value giving a much higher incidence than the combination of serum ferritin, transferrin saturation and ZPP. One reason is probably the biological and methodological variability of the assays which means that a number of subjects with normal iron status will give values below the normal range. Furthermore the cut-off value selected for iron deficiency needs to be carefully assessed for the assay used and for age and sex of the group of subjects being studied, and this is rarely carried out. The measurement of serum transferrin receptor concentration, in combination with serum ferritin assay, looks extremely promising as an epidemiological tool for establishing the true prevalence of iron deficiency and distinguishing unrelated causes of anaemia detected in population surveys (Cook et al., 1993).

4.2. Individual Patients

In combination with measurement of blood haemoglobin, assays of ZPP and transferrin saturation can indicate iron deficient erythropoiesis. Furthermore high TIBC provides good evidence that there is no storage iron. However, most hospital patients have anaemia which is secondary to infection, inflammation, malignant disease or surgery. If information about the amount of storage iron present is required it is in general necessary to assay serum ferritin or to assess tissue iron levels directly.

The serum ferritin concentration must always be assessed in terms of the total iron content of the body. If the patient is not anaemic then concentrations within the normal range (say 15–300 μg/l for men) indicate levels of storage iron within the normal range. If the patient has iron deficiency anaemia (anaemia caused by blood loss) then a ferritin concentration of $<15\,\mu$g/l indicates an absence of storage iron (Worwood, 1982). If the patient has an anaemia secondary to another disease then the iron released from haemoglobin should be present in the tissues as ferritin and haemosiderin unless there has been blood loss (Cavill et al., 1986). For a normal man (body mass 65 kg) a reduction in blood haemoglobin concentration of 1 g/dl is equivalent to the diversion of about 160 mg iron into stores. Using the very approximate relationship that 8 mg storage iron is equivalent to a serum ferritin concentration of 1 μg/l (Walters et al., 1973) then there should be an approximate increase in serum ferritin concentration of 20 μg/l. Thus a patient with an initially normal haemoglobin concentration of 15 g/dl and a serum ferritin concentration of 200 μg/l may subsequently present with a reduced haemoglobin concentration of 10 g/dl. If no iron has been lost the expected serum ferritin concentration would be 300 μg/l. Unfortunately the laboratory rarely has information about a patient's iron status in good health.

There is good evidence, in patients with the anaemia of chronic disease, that the most important factor controlling serum ferritin concentration is the level of storage iron. However, serum ferritin levels are higher than those found in patients with similar levels of storage iron but without infection and inflammation. Early studies were reviewed by Worwood (1979). There is experimental evidence from studies of rat liver that the rapid drop in serum iron concentration which follows the induction of inflammation may be due to an increase in apoferritin synthesis which inhibits the release of iron in the plasma (Konijn and Hershko, 1977). The possible role of cytokines as mediators of the process is discussed in Chapter 11.

Many clinical studies have demonstrated that patients with the anaemia of chronic disease and no stainable iron in the bone marrow may have serum ferritin concentrations considerably in excess of $15 \mu g/l$ and there has been much debate (Witte, 1991) about the application of the serum ferritin assay in this situation: for example, is the assay of any practical use, and if so, what 'cut-off' points for distinguishing between adequate and inadequate iron stores are appropriate? (See also Table 11.4, Chapter 11). It would seem logical to combine the assay of serum ferritin with a measure of disease severity such as the plasma viscosity, ESR or C-reactive protein, in order to exclude or confirm the absence of storage iron. Witte *et al.* (1986) have described such an approach and claim to be able to confirm iron deficiency (absence of storage iron in the bone marrow) or to exclude iron deficiency in almost all patients with secondary anaemia. However, these conclusions have been challenged (Coenen *et al.*, 1991).

In chronic disease a simpler approach may be adopted: a low serum ferritin concentration indicates absent iron stores, values within the normal range indicate either low or normal levels or storage iron and high values may indicate either normal or high levels. In terms of the adequacy of iron stores for replenishing haemoglobin, the degree of anaemia must also be considered. Thus a patient with haemoglobin concentration 10 g/dl may benefit from iron therapy if the serum ferritin concentration is below $100 \mu g/l$.

The other major influence confounding the use of the serum ferritin assay to determine iron stores is liver disease. The liver contains much of the storage iron in the body and any process damaging liver cells will release ferritin. It is also possible that liver damage may interfere with clearance of ferritin from the circulation (see earlier). In the early days of the serum ferritin assay it was suggested that the ratio of serum ferritin to aspartate aminotransferase activity might provide a good index of liver iron concentration (Prieto *et al.*, 1975). Another possibility is that determination of glycosylated serum ferritin concentration might relate directly to storage iron concentrations while non-glycosylated levels would relate to the degree of liver damage (Worwood *et al.*, 1979; Cazzola *et al.*, 1982). However, neither the ferritin aspartate aminotransferase ratio (Batey *et al.*, 1978; Valberg *et al.*, 1978) nor the measurement of glycosylated ferritin levels (Worwood *et al.*, 1980; Chapman *et al.*, 1982a) have proved to be any better than the simple assay of serum ferritin in providing a good index of liver iron concentration. In patients with liver damage a low value always indicates absent iron stores, normal values indicate absent or normal levels but rule out iron overload, whereas high values of serum ferritin in patients with liver damage may indicate either normal or high iron stores and further investigation may be necessary to distinguish between the two.

4.3. Specific Applications

In the previous section the general application of the ferritin assay for the determination of iron storage level has been described. There are however a number of
common diagnostic applications where a more specific application of the various
indicators of iron metabolism is justified.

4.3.1. Iron Deficiency in Infancy and Childhood

The serum ferritin concentration is a less useful guide to iron deficiency than in adults
partly because of the low concentrations generally found in children over 6 months of
age (Chapter 12). ZPP provides a useful indicator of iron deficient erythropoiesis (Yip
et al., 1983) although high values may indicate lead poisoning rather than iron deficiency.
The small sample volume for ZPP determination is also an advantage in paediatric
practice. Hershko et al. (1981) studied children in villages from the Golan Heights
(Israel) and concluded that erythrocyte protoporphyrin was a more reliable index of
iron deficiency than serum ferritin and serum iron. They suggested that a significant
incidence of chronic disease affected both ferritin and iron values. However, Zanella
et al. (1989) did not find that EP was a better predictor of iron deficiency than ferritin.

4.3.2. Thalassaemia

Screening for carriers of thalassaemias, or other haemoglobinopathies giving rise
to reduced haemoglobinization of red cells, requires differentiation from iron
deficiency anaemia, but there may also be co-existing thalassaemia and iron deficiency
(particularly in pregnancy). Many attempts have been made to devise 'discriminant
functions' based on haemoglobin concentration and red cell indices in order to
provide a simple, rapid method of distinguishing between iron deficiency anaemia
and thalassaemia (England and Frazer, 1973). More recently the red cell distribution
width (RDW) has been proposed as a useful discriminator (Bessman et al., 1983).
Further developments have been described (Bessman et al., 1989; England, 1989;
Green and King, 1989; Houwen, 1989; Makris, 1989; Paterakis et al., 1989; Shine,
1989). However, although providing a valuable screening method, these approaches
are not sufficiently reliable to be used without supplementary testing (Osborne et
al., 1989). A screening procedure which includes measurement of haemoglobin
concentration and MCV or MCH (depending on the type of blood counter in use)
can be followed by measurements of HbF and HbA_2 to allow the detection of β-
thalassaemia trait. Confirmation of a diagnosis of alpha-thalassaemia requires either
measurement of the globin-chain synthesis ratio or genotyping (Old and Higgs, 1983).
Abnormal haemoglobins are detected by electrophoresis (Dacie and Lewis, 1991).
A serum ferritin determination is also made and in the absence of any indication
of a globin defect the combination of a low MCV and low ferritin suggests simple
iron deficiency anaemia. However, it does not exclude alpha-thalassaemia trait, since
iron deficiency with a low ferritin concentration, may also be found in thalassaemia
trait. This is more likely in patients with alpha-thalassaemia (White et al., 1986) than
in β-thalassaemia trait (Hershko et al., 1979). This may be related to the greater
degree of ineffective erythropoiesis in β-thalassaemia trait which may be associated
with enhanced iron absorption (White et al., 1986).

4.3.3. Iron Stores in Renal Failure

One of the first benefits resulting from the introduction of the serum ferritin assay was the demonstration that many patients with renal failure undergoing dialysis had high levels of serum ferritin which were indicative of raised levels of storage iron in the bone marrow. The increased levels of storage iron were often caused by giving intravenous iron (iron-dextran, for example) to compensate for the blood losses which occur during the dialysis. Serum ferritin has been shown to be a valuable indicator of iron stores (Hussein et al., 1975; Mirahmadi et al., 1977; Aljama et al., 1978; Hofman et al., 1978; Milman et al., 1983). Concentrations should normally be maintained in the range 100–400 µg/l to ensure that the patient neither develops iron deficiency anaemia nor iron overload. However, following the changes in the serum ferritin level is not valuable if there are additional complications such as active hepatitis or infectious disease (Muller et al., 1981). There has also been much interest in the association between the gene for haemochromatosis and iron overload in haemodialysis patients. In practice this means the demonstration of association between HLA A3, B7, or B14 and high levels of serum ferritin (Bregman et al., 1980). Simon (1985) has reviewed these studies and concluded that the combination of an inadequate genetic analysis (A3 is the only consistent marker of the haemochromatosis allele and B7 and B14 cannot be used independently) and inadequate demonstration of high levels of storage iron (selection of ferritin levels >1000 µg/l without regard to blood or therapeutic iron administration or presence of inflammation or liver damage) means that an association of haemochromatosis and iron overload in dialysis patients has not been proved. Nevertheless, in European populations, around 10% of the population may carry the haemochromatosis gene and identification of carriers may prevent overload caused by unnecessary iron administration.

4.3.4. Diagnosis and Treatment of Haemochromatosis (HC)

In screening for HC it is essential to determine the transferrin saturation, which provides the most sensitive way of detecting the early stages of iron accumulation (Chapter 8). The serum ferritin concentration gives an indication of the degree of whole body iron loading. Liver damage is rarely seen at concentrations of <700 µg/l but is increasingly likely as the ferritin concentration rises (Bassett et al., 1984).

Treatment by venesection can be effectively monitored by measuring serum ferritin, although in patients with liver damage there may be some initial fluctuation. After excess iron has been removed it is better to attempt to keep the transferrin saturation less than 60% by occasional venesection rather than waiting until the serum ferritin concentration becomes abnormal. At this stage there will probably be significant, parenchymal cell iron overload.

4.3.5. Monitoring Treatment of Secondary Iron Overload

A falling serum ferritin concentration is a valuable indicator of successful chelation therapy (Aldouri et al., 1987; Maurer et al., 1988; Pippard, 1989). Concentrations should eventually be reduced to about 1000 µg/l and maintained at this level. It is not usually possible to distinguish between the contribution of reducing levels of storage iron and improving liver function to the drop in serum ferritin level. In patients who are ascorbic acid replete, there is a close correlation between serum ferritin concentrations and the amount of blood transfused, but this is not so for patients deficient in ascorbic acid (Chapman *et al.*, 1982b).

4.3.6. *Diagnosis of Iron Deficiency after Starting Iron Treatment*

Replacement of hypochromic red cells by normochromic cells during oral iron therapy takes some weeks and it is therefore possible to make a retrospective diagnosis by measuring ZPP even after the patient has commenced a course of treatment. Oral iron therapy at conventional dose (60 mg Fe, three times daily) has little immediate effect on serum ferritin levels which rise slowly as the haemoglobin concentration increases. However, with double doses there is a rapid rise of serum ferritin to within the normal range (within a few days) which probably does not represent the increase in storage iron (Wheby, 1980). Intravenous iron causes a rapid rise to concentrations which may be above the normal range and ferritin concentrations then gradually drop back to the normal range.

4.3.7. *Screening Blood Donors for Iron Deficiency*

Regular blood donation reduces storage iron levels and this has been demonstrated in a number of surveys of blood donors (see review by Skikne *et al.*, 1984 and Milman *et al.*, 1991). Another, well-known difficulty is that the conventional screening test for anaemia (the 'copper sulfate' test, see Mollison *et al.*, 1988) is somewhat inaccurate and donors may be deferred unnecessarily. It has been suggested that secondary screening using ZPP would provide an immediate confirmation of iron deficiency (Raftos *et al.*, 1983; Schifman and Rivers, 1986). Despite the availability of the serum ferritin assay during the last 20 years there has been little attention to the fundamental relationship between storage iron levels and the ability to give blood. In populations of European origin the high prevalence of HC gives an added value for screening all donors by measuring serum ferritin. Screening blood donors by routinely assaying serum ferritin may make it possible to predict the development of iron deficiency anaemia, identify donors with high iron stores who may give blood more frequently than usually permitted, and also identify donors with homozygous HC who are beginning to develop iron overload (Worwood *et al.*, 1991; Worwood and Darke, 1993).

It remains to be seen whether or not serum ferritin levels are sufficiently stable, and assays sufficiently reproducible, for such a widespread application.

REFERENCES

Adams, P.C., Powell, L. W. and Halliday, J. W. (1988) Isolation of a human hepatic ferritin receptor. *Hepatology* **8**, 719–721.

Addison, G. M., Beamish, M. R., Hales, C. N., Hodgkins, M., Jacobs, A. and Llewellin, P. (1972) An immunoradiometric assay for ferritin in the serum of normal subjects and patients with iron deficiency and iron overload. *J. Clin. Pathol.* **25**, 326–329.

Aldouri, M. A., Wonke, B., Hoffbrand, A. V. *et al.* (1987) Iron state and hepatic disease in patients with thalassaemia major, treated with long term subcutaneous desferrioxamine. *J. Clin. Pathol.* **40**, 1353–1359.

Aljama, P., Ward, M. K., Pierides, A. M. *et al.* (1978) Serum ferritin concentration: a reliable guide to iron overload in uremic and hemodialyzed patients. *Clin. Nephrol.* **10**, 101–104.

Bainton, D. F. and Finch, C. A. (1964) The diagnosis of iron deficiency anaemia. *Am. J. Med.* **37**, 62–70.

Bandi, Z. L., Schoen, I. and Bee, D. E. (1985) Immunochemical methods for measurement of transferrin in serum: Effects of analytical errors and inappropriate reference intervals on diagnostic utility. *Clin. Chem.* **31**, 1601–1605.

Barry, M. and Sherlock, S. (1971) Measurement of liver-iron concentration in liver-biopsy specimens. *Lancet* **i**, 100–103.

Bassett, M. L., Halliday, J. W., Ferris, R. A. and Powell, L. W. (1984) Diagnosis of hemochromatosis in young subjects: predictive accuracy of biochemical screening tests. *Gastroenterology* **87**, 628–633.

Bassett, M. L., Halliday, J. W. and Powell, L. W. (1986) Value of hepatic iron measurements in early hemochromatosis and determination of the critical iron level associated with fibrosis. *Hepatology* **6**, 24–29.

Batey, R. G., Hussein, S., Sherlock, S. and Hoffbrand, A. V. (1978) The role of serum ferritin in the management of idiopathic haemochromatosis. *Scand. J. Gastroenterol.* **13**, 953–957.

Bellotti, V., Arosio, P., Cazzola, M. *et al.* (1987) Characteristics of a ferritin-binding protein present in human serum. *Br. J. Haematol.* **65**, 489–493.

Bessman, J. D., Gilmer, P. R. and Gardner, F. H. (1983) Improved classification of anaemias by MCV and RDW. *Am. J. Clin. Pathol.* **80**, 322–326.

Bessman, J. D., McClure, S. and Bates, T. (1989) Distinction of microcytic disorders: comparison of expert, numerical discriminant and microcomputer analysis. *Blood* **85**, 533–540.

Borel, M. J., Smith, S. M., Derr, J. and Beard, J. L. (1991) Day-to-day variation in iron-status indices in healthy men and women. *Am. J. Clin. Nutrition* **54**, 729–735.

Bothwell, T. H., Charlton, R. W., Cook, J. D. and Finch, C. A. (1979) *Iron Metabolism in Man.* Oxford: Blackwell Scientific Publications.

Bregman, H., Winchester, J. F., Knepshield, J. H., Gelfand, M. C., Manz, J. H. and Schreiner, G. E. (1980) Iron-overload-associated myopathy in patients on maintenance haemodialysis: a histocompatibility-linked disorder. *Lancet* **ii**, 882–885.

Brittenham, G. M., Farrell, D. E., Harris, J. W. *et al.* (1982) Magnetic-susceptibility measurement of human iron stores. *N. Engl. J. Med.* **307**, 1671–1675.

Casey, G. J., Rudzki, Z. and Kimber, R. J. (1979) Reduction of the 'high dose hook effect' in the serum ferritin assay. *Br. J. Haematol.* **43**, 675–677.

Cavill, I., Jacobs, A. and Worwood, M. (1986) Diagnostic methods for iron status. *Ann. Clin. Biochem.* **23**, 168–171.

Cazzola, M. and Ascari, E. (1986) Annotation. Red cell ferritin as a diagnostic tool. *Br. J. Haematol.* **62**, 209–213.

Cazzola, M. and Beguin, Y. (1992) Annotation. New tools for clinical evaluation of erythron function in man. *Br. J. Haematol.* **80**, 278–284.

Cazzola, M., Bergamaschi, G., Dezza, L., Barosi, G. and Ascari, E. (1982) The origin of serum ferritin in acquired transfusional iron overload in adults. Studies with concanavalin A-sepharose absorption. *Haematologica* **67**, 818–824.

Cazzola, M., Dezza, L., Bergamaschi, G. *et al.* (1983) Biologic and clinical significance of red cell ferritin. *Blood* **62**, 1078–1087.

Chapman, R. W. G., Gorman, A., Laulight, M., Hussain, M. A. M., Sherlock, S. and Hoffbrand, A. V. (1982a) Binding of serum ferritin to concanavalin A in patients with iron overload and with chronic liver disease. *J. Clin. Pathol.* **35**, 481–486.

Chapman, R. W. G., Hussain, M. A. M., Gorman, A. *et al.* (1982b) Effect of ascorbic acid deficiency on serum ferritin concentration in patients with B-thalassaemia major and iron overload. *J. Clin. Pathol.* **35**, 487–491.

Charlton, R. W., Hawkins, D. M., Mavor, W. O. and Bothwell, T. H. (1970) Hepatic iron storage concentrations in different population groups. *Am. J. Clin. Nutrition* **23**, 358–371.

Coenen, J. L. L. M., van Dieijen-Visser, M. P., van Pelt, J. *et al.* (1991) Measurements of serum ferritin used to predict concentrations of iron in bone marrow in anemia of chronic disease. *Clin. Chem.* **37**, 560–563.

Cook, J. D., Skikne, B. S. and Baynes, R. D. (1993) Serum transferrin receptor. *Ann. Rev. Med.* **43**, 63–74.

Cook, J. D., Skikne, B. S., Lynch, S. R. and Reusser, M. E. (1986) Estimates of iron sufficiency in the US population. *Blood* **68**, 726–731.

Covell, A. M., Jacobs, A. and Worwood, M. (1984) Interaction of ferritin with serum: implications for ferritin turnover. *Clinica Chimica Acta* **139**, 75–84.

Cragg, S. J., Wagstaff, M. and Worwood, M. (1980) Sialic acid and the microheterogeneity of human serum ferritin. *Clin. Sci.* **58**, 259–262.

Cragg, S. J., Wagstaff, M. and Worwood, M. (1981) Detection of a glycosylated subunit in human serum ferritin. *Biochem. J.* **199**, 565–571.

Cragg, S. J., Covell, A. M., Burch, A., Owen, G. M., Jacobs, A. and Worwood, M. (1983) Turnover of ^{131}I-human spleen ferritin in plasma. *Br. J. Haematol.* **55**, 83–92.

Custer, G., Balcerzak, S. and Rinehart, J. (1982) Human macrophage hemoglobin-iron metabolism in vitro. *Am. J. Hematol.* **13**, 23–36.

Dacie, Sir J. V. and Lewis, S. M. (1991) *Practical Haematology*, Churchill Livingstone, Edinburgh.

Dallman, P. R. (1984) Diagnosis of anemia and iron deficiency: analytic and biological variations of laboratory tests. *Am. J. Clin. Nutrition* **39**, 937–941.

Davidson, A., van Der Weyden, M. B., Fong, H., Breidahl, M. J. and Ryan, P. F. J. (1984) Red cell ferritin content: a re-evaluation of indices for iron deficiency in the anaemia of rheumatoid arthritis. *Br. Med. J.* **289**, 648–650.

Dawkins, S. J., Cavill, I., Ricketts, C. and Worwood, M. (1979) Variability of serum ferritin concentration in normal subjects. *Clin. Lab. Haematol.* **1**, 41–46.

England, J. M. (1989) Discriminant function. *Blood Cells* **15**, 463–474.

England, J. M. and Fraser, P. (1973) Differentiation of iron deficiency from thalassaemia trait by routine blood count. *Lancet* **i**, 449.

Esumi, N., Ikushima, S., Hibi, S., Todo, S. and Imashuku, S. (1988) High serum ferritin level as a marker of malignant histiocytosis and virus-associated hemophagocytic syndrome. *Cancer* **61**, 2071–2076.

Fielding, J. (1980) *Serum Iron and Iron Binding Capacity in Iron, Methods in Hematology Volume 1* (ed. J. D. Cook), Churchill Livingstone, New York, pp. 15–43.

Flowers, C. H., Skikne, B. S., Covell, A. M. and Cook, J. D. (1989) The clinical measurement of serum transferrin receptor. *J. Lab. Clin. Med.* **114**, 368.

Frey, W. G., Gardner, M. H. and Pillsbury, J. A. (1968) Quantitative measurements of liver iron by needle biopsy. *J. Lab. Clin. Med.* **72**, 52–57.

Gale, E., Torrance, J. and Bothwell, T. (1963) The quantitative estimation of total iron stores in human bone marrow. *J. Clin. Invest.* **42**, 1076–1082.

Gallagher, S. A., Johnson, L. K. and Milne, D. H. (1989) Short-term and long-term variability of indices related to nutritional status I: Ca, Cu, Fe, Mg, and Zn. *Clin. Chem.* **35**, 369–373.

Gomori, J. M., Horev, G., Tamary, H. *et al.* (1991) Hepatic iron overload: quantitative MR imaging. *Radiology* **179**, 367–369.

Green, R. and King, R. (1989) A new red cell discriminant incorporating volume dispersion for differentiating iron deficiency anaemia from thalassemia minor. *Blood Cells* **15**, 481–488.

Grootveld, M., Bell, J. D., Halliwell, B., Aruoma, O. I., Bomford, A. and Sadler, P. J. (1989) Non-transferrin-bound iron in plasma or serum from patients with idiopathic hemochromatosis. *J. Biol. Chem.* **264**, 4417–4422.

Halliday, J. W., Mack, U. and Powell, L. W. (1979) The kinetics of serum and tissue ferritins: relation to carbohydrate content. *Br. J. Haematol.* **42**, 535–546.

Hann, H-W. L., Stahlhut, M. W. and Evans, A. E. (1988) Basic and acidic isoferritins in the sera of patients with neuroblastoma. *Cancer* **62**, 1179–1182.

Haskins, D., Stevens, A. R., Jr, Finch, S. C. and Finch, C. A. (1952) Iron metabolism: iron stores in man as measured by phlebotomy. *J. Clin. Invest.* **31**, 543–547.

Hastka, J., Lasserre, J. J., Schwartzbeck, A., Strauch, M. and Hehlmann, R. (1993) Zinc protoporphyrin in anemia of chronic disorders. *Blood* **81**, 1200–1204.

Hershko, C. and Peto, T. E. A. (1987) Annotation: Non-transferrin plasma iron. *Br. J. Haematol.* **66**, 149–151.

Hershko, C., Konijn, A. M. and Loria, A. (1979) Serum ferritin and mean corpuscular volume measurement in the diagnosis of β-thalassaemia minor and iron deficiency. *Acta Haematologica* **62**, 236–239.

Hershko, C., Bar-Or, D., Gaziel, Y. *et al.* (1981) Diagnosis of iron deficiency anemia in a rural population of children. Relative usefulness of serum ferritin, red cell protoporphyrin, red cell indices, and transferrin saturation determinations. *Am. J. Clin. Nutrition* **34**, 1600–1610.

Hodgetts, J., Peters, S. W., Hoy, T. G. and Jacobs, A. (1986) The ferritin content of normoblasts and megaloblasts from human bone marrow. *Clin. Sci.* **70**, 47–51.

Hofman, V., Descoeudres, C., Montandon, A., Galeazzi, R. L. and Straub, P. W. (1978) Serum ferritin bei Neireninsuffizienz Hamodialyse and nach Nierentransplantation. *Schweizerische Medizinische Wochenschrift* **108**, 1835–1838.

Houwen, B. (1989) The use of inference strategies in the differential diagnosis of microcytic anaemia. *Blood Cells* **15**, 509–532.

Howard, J. M., Ghent, C. N., Carey, L. S., Flanagan, P. R. and Valberg, L. S. (1983) Diagnostic efficacy of hepatic computed tomography in the detection of body iron overload. *Gastroenterology* **84**, 209–215.

Huebers, H. A., Eng, M. J., Josephson, B. M. *et al.* (1987) Plasma iron and transferrin iron-binding capacity evaluated by colorimetric and immunoprecipitation methods. *Clin. Chem.* **33**, 273–277.

Hussein, S., Prieto, J., O'Shea, M., Hoffbrand, A. V., Baillod, R. A. and Moorhead, J. F. (1975) Serum ferritin assay and iron status in chronic renal failure and haemodialysis. *Br. Med. J.* **1**, 546–548.

International Committee for Standardization in Haematology (1972) Studies on the standardization of serum iron and iron-binding capacity assays. In: *Modern Concepts in Hematology* (eds G. Izak and S. M. Lewis), New York, Academic Press, pp. 69–162.

International Committee for Standardization in Haematology (1978a) The measurement of total and unsaturated iron-binding capacity in serum. *Br. J. Haematol.* **38**, 281.

International Committee for Standardization in Haematology (1978b) Recommendations for measurement of serum iron in human blood. *Br. J. Haematol.* **38**, 291.

International Committee for Standardization in Haematology (1984) Preparation, characterization and storage of human ferritin for use as a standard for the assay of serum ferritin. *Clin. Lab. Haematol.* **6**, 177–191.

International Committee for Standardization in Haematology (1990) Revised recommendations for the measurements of the serum iron in human blood. *Br. J. Haematol.* **75**, 615–616.

INACG (1985) Measurements of Iron Status: A report of the International Nutritional Anemia Consultative Group (INACG). The Nutritional Foundation, Inc. Washington DC.

Kaltwasser, J. P., Gottschalk, R., Schalk, K. P. and Hartl, W. (1990) Non-invasive quantitation of liver iron-overload by magnetic resonance imaging. *Br. J. Haematol.* **74**, 360–363.

Kleber, E. E., Lynch, S. R., Skikne, B., Torrance, J. D., Bothwell, T. H. and Charlton, R. W. (1978) Erythrocyte catabolism in the inflammatory peritoneal moncyte. *Br. J. Haematol.* **39**, 41–54.

Kohgo, Y., Niitsu, Y., Kondo, H. *et al.* (1987) Serum transferrin receptor as a new index of erythropoiesis. *Blood* **70**, 1955–1958.

Kondo, H., Saito, K., Grasso, J. P. and Aisen, P. (1988) Iron metabolism in the erythro-phagocytosing Kupffer cell. *Hepatology* **8**, 32–38.

Konijn, A. M. and Hershko, C. (1977) Ferritin synthesis in inflammation 1. Pathogenesis of impaired iron release. *Br. J. Haematol.* **37**, 7–16.

Labbe, R. F. and Rettmer, R. L. (1989) Zinc protoporphyrin: a product of iron-deficient erythropoiesis. *Seminars Hematol.* **26**, 40–46.

Looker, A. C., Sempos, C. T., Liu, K., Johnson, C. L. and Gunter, W. E. (1990) Within-person variance in biochemical indicators of iron status: effects on prevalence estimates. *Am. J. Clin. Nutrition* **52**, 541–547.

Macdougall, I. C., Cavill, I., Hulme, B. *et al.* (1992) Detection of functional iron deficiency during erythropoietin treatment: a new approach. *Br. Med. J.* **304**, 225–226.

Makris, P. E. (1989) Utilization of a new index to distinguish heterozygous thalassemic syndromes: comparison of its specificity to five other discriminants. *Blood Cells* **15**, 497–508.

Maurer, H. S., Lloyd-Still, J. D., Ingrisano, C., Gonzalez-Crussi, F. and Honig, G. R. (1988) A prospective evaluation of iron chelation therapy in children with severe β-thalassemia. *Am. J. Dis. Children* **142**, 287–292.

McKeering, L. V., Halliday, J. W., Caffin, J. A., Mack, U. and Powell, L. W. (1976) Immunological detection of isoferritins in normal human serum and tissue. *Clinica Chimica Acta* **67**, 189–197.

Miles, L. E. M., Lipschitz, D. A., Bieber, C. P. and Cook, J. D. (1974) Measurement of serum ferritin by a 2-site immunoradiometric assay. *Anal. Biochem.* **61**, 209–224.

Milman, N. and Kirchhoff, M. (1991) Influence of blood donation on iron stores assessed by serum ferritin and haemoglobin in a population survey of 1433 Danish males. *Eur. J. Haematol.* **47**, 134–139.

Milman, N., Bangsboll, S., Pedersen, N. S. and Visfeldt, J. (1983) Serum ferritin in non-dialysis patients with chronic renal failure: relation to bone marrow iron stores. *Scand. J. Haematol.* **30**, 337–344.

Mirahmadi, K. S., Paul, W. L., Winer, R. L. *et al.* (1977) Determinant of iron requirement in hemodialysis patients. *J. Am. Med. Assoc.* **238**, 601–603.

Mollison, P. L., Engelfriet, C. P. and Contreras, M. (1988) *Blood Transfusion in Clinical Medicine*, Blackwell Scientific Publications, Oxford.

Muller, H. A. G., Schneider, H., Hovelborn, U. and Streicher, E. (1981) Ferritin: A reliable indicator of iron supplementation in patients on chronic hemodialysis/hemofiltration treatment? *Artificial Organs* **5**, 168–174.

Old, J. M. and Higgs, D. R. (1983) Gene analysis. In: *Methods in Hematology* (ed. D. J. Weatherall), Churchill Livingstone, Edinburgh pp. 74–102.

Osborne, P. T., Burkett, L. L., Ryan, G. M., Jr and Lane, M. (1989) An evaluation of red blood cell heterogeneity (increased red blood cell distribution width) in iron deficiency of pregnancy. *Am. J. Obstet. Gynecol.* **160**, 336–339.

Paterakis, G. G., Teizoglou, G. and Vasilioy, E. (1989) The performance characteristic of an expert system for the 'on-line' assessment of thalassemia trait and iron deficiency. *Blood Cells* **15**, 541–562.

Perera, P. and Worwood, M. (1984a) Antigen binding in the two-site immunoradiometric assay for serum ferritin: the nature of the hook effect. *Ann. Clin. Biochem.* **21**, 393–397.

Perera, P. and Worwood, M. (1984b) A single-step immunoradiometric assay for the measurement of serum ferritin. *Ann. Clin. Biochem.* **21**, 389–392.

Persijn, J.-P., van der Slik, W. and Riethorst, A. (1971) Determination of serum iron and latent iron-binding capacity (LIBC). *Clinica Chimica Acta* **35**, 91–98.

Peters, S. W., Jacobs, A. and Fitzsimons, E. (1983) Erythrocyte ferritin in normal subjects and patients with abnormal iron metabolism. *Br. J. Haematol.* **53**, 211–216.

Pilon, V. A., Howantitz, P. J., Howanitz, J. H. and Domres, N. (1981) Day-to-day variation in serum ferritin concentration in healthy subjects. *Clin. Chem.* **27**, 78–82.

Piperno, A., Taddei, M. T., Sampietro, M., Fargion, S., Arosio, P. and Fiorelli, G. (1984) Erythrocyte ferritin in thalassemia syndromes. *Acta Haematologica* **71**, 251–256.

Pippard, M. J. (1989) Desferrioxamine-induced iron excretion in humans. *Baillière's Clin. Haematol.* **2**, 323–343.

Pollock, A. S., Lipschitz, D. A. and Cook, J. D. (1978) The kinetics of serum ferritin. *Proc. Soc. Experimental Biology and Medicine* **157**, 481–485.

Pootrakul, P., Skikne, B. S. and Cook, J. D. (1983) The use of capillary blood for measurements of circulating ferritin. *Am. J. Clin. Nutrition* **37**, 307–310.

Pootrakul, P., Josephson, B., Huebers, H. A. and Finch, C. A. (1988) Quantitation of ferritin iron in plasma, an explanation for non-transferrin iron. *Blood* **71**, 1120–1123.

Prieto, J., Barry, M. and Sherlock, S. (1975) Serum ferritin in patients with iron overload and with acute and chronic liver diseases. *Gastroenterology* **68**, 525–533.

Raftos, J., Schuller, M. and Lovric, V. A. (1983) Iron stores assessed in blood donors by hematofluorometry. *Transfusion* **23**, 226–228.

Rajantie, J., Rapola, J. and Siimes, M. A. (1981) Ferritinemia with subnormal iron stores in lysinuric protein intolerance. *Metabolism* **30**, 3–5.

Rama, R., Sanchez, J. and Octave, J.-N. (1988) Iron mobilization from cultured rat bone marrow macrophages. *Biochimica et Biophysica Acta* **968**, 51–58.

Rodbard, D., Feldman, Y., Jaffe, M. L. and Miles, L. E. M. (1978) Kinetics of two-site immunoradiometric ('sandwich') assays – II. Studies on the nature of the 'high-dose hook' effects. *Immunochemistry* **15**, 77–82.

Romslo, I. and Talstad, I. (1988) Day-to-day variations in serum iron, serum iron binding capacity, serum ferritin and erythrocyte protoporphyrin concentrations in anaemic subjects. *Eur. J. Haematol.* **40**, 79–82.

Santambrogio, P. and Massover, W. H. (1989) Rabbit serum α-2-macroglobin binds to liver ferritin: association causes a heterogeneity of ferritin molecules. *Br. J. Haematol.* **71**, 281–290.

Santambrogio, P., Cozzi, A., Levi, S. and Arosio, P. (1987) Human serum ferritin G-peptide is recognized by anti-L ferritin subunit antibodies and concanavalin A. *Br. J. Haematol.* **65**, 235–237.

Schifman, R. B. and Rivers, S. L. (1987) Red blood cell zinc protoporphyrin to evaluate anemia risk in deferred blood donors. *Am. J. Clin. Pathol.* **87**, 511–514.

Shine, I. (1989) Non random distribution of genotypes among red cell indices. *Blood Cells* **15**, 475–480.

Sibille, J.-C., Kondo, H. and Aisen, P. (1988) Interactions between isolated hepatocytes and Kupffer cells in iron metabolism: a possible role for ferritin as an iron carrier protein. *Hepatology* **8**, 296–301.

Siimes, M. A., Koerper, M. A., Licko, V. and Dallman, P. R. (1975) Ferritin turnover in plasma: an opportunistic use of blood removed during exchange transfusion. *Ped. Res.* **9**, 127–129.

Simon, M. (1985) Annotation. Secondary iron overload and the haemochromatosis allele. *Br. J. Haematol.* **60**, 1–5.

Singh, S., Hider, R. C. and Porter, J. B. (1989) Quantification on non-transferrin-bound iron in thalassaemic plasma. *Analytical Biochemistry* **17**, 697–698.

Skikne, B., Lynch, S., Borek, D. and Cook, J. (1984) Iron and blood donation. *Clin. Haematol.* **13**, 271–287.

Skikne, B. S., Flowers, C. H. and Cook, J. D. (1990) Serum transferrin receptor: a quantitative measure of tissue iron deficiency. *Blood* **75**, 1870–1876.

Stark, D. D. (1991) Hepatic iron overload: paramagnetic pathology. *Radiology* **179**, 333–335.

Statland, B. E. and Winkel, P. (1977) Relationship of day-to-day variation of serum iron concentrations to iron-binding capacity in healthy young women. *Am. J. Clin. Pathol.* **67**, 84–90.

Statland, B. E., Winkel, P. and Bokieland, H. (1976) Variation of serum iron concentration in healthy young men: within day and day-to-day changes. *Clin. Biochem.* **9**, 26–29.

Statland, B. E., Winkel, P., Harris, S. C., Burdsall, M. J. and Saunders, A. M. (1977) Evaluation of biologic sources of variation of leucocyte counts and other hematologic quantities using very precise automated analyzers. *Am. J. Clin. Pathol.* **69**, 48–54.

Torrance, J. D. and Bothwell, T. H. (1980) Tissue iron stores. In: *Iron. Methods in Hematology, Vol. I.* (ed. J. D. Cook), Churchill Livingstone, New York, pp. 90–115.

Torrance, T. D., Charlton, R. W., Schmaman, A., Lynch, S. R. and Bothwell, T. H. (1968) Storage iron in 'muscle'. *J. Clin. Pathol.* **21**, 495–500.

Valberg, L. S., Ghent, C. N., Lloyd, D. A., Frei, J. V. and Chamberlain, M. J. (1978) Diagnostic efficacy of tests for the detection of iron overload in chronic liver disease. *Can. Med. Assoc. J.* **119**, 229–236.

Van der Weyden, M. B. and Fong, H. (1984) Red cell basic ferritin content of patients with megaloblastic anaemia due to vitamin B_{12} folate deficiency. *Scand. J. Haematol.* **33**, 373.

Van der Weyden, M. B., Fong, H., Salem, H. H., Batey, R. C. and Dudley, F. J. (1983) Erythrocyte ferritin content in idiopathic haemochromatosis and alcoholic liver disease with iron overload. *Br. Med. J.* **286**, 752.

Van der Weyden, M. B., Fong, H., Hallam, L. J. and Harrison, C. (1989) Red cell ferritin and iron overload in heterozygous β-thalassemia. *Am. J. Hematol.* **30**, 201–205.

Walters, G. O., Miller, F. M. and Worwood, M. (1973) Serum ferritin concentration and iron stores in normal subjects. *J. Clin. Pathol.* **26**, 770–772.

Weinfeld, A. (1970) Iron stores. In: *Iron Deficiency: Pathogenesis, Clinical Aspects and Therapy* (eds L. Hallberg, H. G. Harweth and A. Vannotti), Academic Press, London and New York, pp. 329–372.

Wheby, M. S. (1980) Effect of iron therapy on serum ferritin levels in iron-deficiency anemia. *Blood* **56**, 138–140.

White, J. M., Richards, R., Jelenski, G., Byrne, M. and Ali, M. (1986) Iron state in alpha and β-thalassaemia trait. *J. Clin. Pathol.* **39**, 256–259.

Wiggers, P., Dalhoj, J., Hyltoft Peterson, P., Blaabjerg, O. and Horder, M. (1991) Screening for haemochromatosis: influence of analytical imprecision diagnostic limit and prevalence on test validity. *Scand. J. Clin. Lab. Invest.* **51**, 143–148.

Williams, W. J. (1990) Clinical evaluation of the patient. In: *Hematology* (4th edn) (eds W. J. Williams, A. J. Erslev and M. A. Lichtman), McGraw-Hill, New York, pp. 9–23.

Witte, D. L. (1991) Can serum ferritin be effectively interpreted in the presence of the acute-phase response? *Clin. Chem.* **37**, 484–485.

Witte, D. L., Kraemer, D. F., Johnson, G. F., Dick, F. R. and Hamilton, H. (1986) Prediction of bone marrow iron findings from tests performed on peripheral blood. *Am. J. Clin. Pathol.* **85**, 202–206.

Wrigglesworth, J. M. and Baum, H. (1980) The biochemical function of iron. In: *Iron in Biochemistry and Medicine II* (eds A. Jacobs and M. Worwood), Academic Press, London and New York, pp. 29–86.

Worwood, M. (1979) Serum ferritin. In: *Critical Reviews in Clinical Laboratory Sciences* (eds J. Batsakis and J. Savory), CRC Press, Boca Raton, Florida.

Worwood, M. (1980) Serum ferritin. In: *Methods in Hematology, Vol 1* (ed. J. D. Cook), Churchill-Livingstone, New York, pp. 59–89.

Worwood, M. (1982) Ferritin in human tissues and serum. *Clin. Haematol.* **11**, 275–307.

Worwood, M. (1990) Ferritin. *Blood Reviews* **4**, 259–269.

Worwood, M. and Darke, C. (1993) Serum ferritin, blood donation, iron stores and haemochromatosis. *Transfusion Med.* **3**, 21–28.

Worwood, M., Dawkins, S., Wagstaff, M. and Jacobs, A. (1976) The purification and properties of ferritin from human serum. *Biochem. J.* **157**, 97–103

Worwood, M., Cragg, S. J., Wagstaff, M. and Jacobs, A. (1979) Binding of human serum ferritin to concanavalin A. *Clin. Sci.* **56**, 83–87.

Worwood, M., Cragg, S. J., Jacobs, A., McLaren, C., Rickets, C. and Economidou, J. (1980) Binding of serum ferritin to concanavalin A: patients with homozygous β-thalassaemia and transfusional iron overload. *Br. J. Haematol.* **46**, 409–416.

Worwood, M., Cragg, S. J., Williams, A. M., Wagstaff, M. and Jacobs, A. (1982) The clearance of ^{131}I-human plasma ferritin in man. *Blood* **60**, 827–833.

Worwood, M., Darke, C. and Trenchard, P. (1991a) Hereditary haemochromatosis and blood donation. *Br. Med. J.* **302**, 59.

Worwood, M., Thorpe, S. J., Heath, A., Flowers, C. H. and Cook, J. D. (1991b) Stable lyophilised reagents for the serum ferritin assay. *Clin. Lab. Haematol.* **13**, 297–305.

Yamada, H., Hirano, A., Maeda, H. and Saito, H. (1983) Human red cell ferritin. Its physicochemical and clinicopathological characterization. In: *Structure and Function of Iron Storage and Transport Proteins* (eds I. Urushizaki, P. Aisen, I. Listowsky and J. W. Drysdale), Elsevier Science Publishers, Amsterdam, pp. 202–207.

Yip, R., Schwartz, S. and Deinard, A. S. (1983) Screening for iron deficiency with the erythrocyte protoporphyrin test. *Pediatrics* **72**, 214–219.

Zanella, A., Gridelli, L., Berzuini, A. *et al.* (1989) Sensitivity and predictive value of serum ferritin and free erythrocyte protoporphyrin for iron deficiency. *J. Lab. Clin. Med.* **113**, 73–78.

Index